Contributors

FRED L. ALLMAN, JR., M.D.

Director, Sports Medicine Clinic, Atlanta, and
Orthopaedic Consultant, Georgia Tech and the
Atlanta Public Schools, Atlanta, Georgia

Rehabilitation Following Athletic Injuries

GAEL R. FRANK, M.D.

Bothwell Memorial Hospital, Sedalia, Missouri,
Fitzgibbon Memorial Hospital, Marshall, Missouri,
and Courtesy Staff, Research Hospital,
Kansas City, Missouri

Injuries of the Hand

BOB J. RUTLEDGE, M.D.

Clinical Professor of Neurosurgery
Oklahoma Health Sciences Center and
Teaching Hospitals and Chief of Staff
St. Anthony Hospital, Oklahoma City, Oklahoma

Injuries to the Cranium and
Central Nervous System During Athletics

C.P. WILKINSON, M.D.

Clinical Professor of Ophthalmology,
Oklahoma Health Sciences Center
and Teaching Hospitals, Oklahoma City, Oklahoma

Injury in the Vicinity of the Eye

TREATMENT OF INJURIES TO ATHLETES

Fourth Edition

DON H. O'DONOGHUE, M.D.

Professor Emeritus of Orthopaedic Surgery
Oklahoma Health Sciences Center and
Teaching Hospitals
Oklahoma City, Oklahoma

W. B. SAUNDERS COMPANY   1984
Philadelphia / London / Toronto / Mexico City / Rio de Janeiro / Sydney / Tokyo

W. B. Saunders Company: West Washington Square
Philadelphia, PA   19105

1 St. Anne's Road
Eastbourne, East Sussex BN21 3UN, England

1 Goldthorne Avenue
Toronto, Ontario M8Z 5T9, Canada

Apartado 26370—Cedro 512
Mexico 4, D.F., Mexico

Rua Coronel Cabrita, 8
Sao Cristovao Caixa Postal 21176
Rio de Janeiro, Brazil

9 Waltham Street
Artarmon, N.S.W. 2064, Australia

Ichibancho, Central Bldg., 22-1 Ichibancho
Chiyoda-Ku, Tokyo 102, Japan

Library of Congress Cataloging in Publication Data

O'Donoghue, Don H.

Treatment of injuries to athletes.

Includes index.

1. Sports—Accidents and injuries.   I. Title. [DNLM: 1. Athletic injuries—Therapy. QT 260 026t]

RD97.036 1984   617′.1027   83–4501

ISBN 0-7216-6928-X

Listed here is the latest translated edition of this book together
with the language of the translation and the publisher.

Italian (*3rd Edition*)—Piccin Editore, Padova, Italy

Treatment of Injuries to Athletes   ISBN   0-7216-6928-X

Last digit is the print number: 9   8   7   6   5   4   3   2   1

This book is dedicated to the delightful and devoted members of my personal staff, whose unstinting efforts made the preparation of this fourth edition not only possible but pleasurable.

PREFACE
TO THE
FOURTH EDITION

The question may rightfully be what is innovative about the fourth edition? The original edition and succeeding ones have been very basic, with emphasis on the basic principles of care. However, each succeeding edition has better defined the actual care of the athlete, just as I hope this fourth edition will.

Actually, there have been many developments in medicine and in the health care of the athlete, with a change in emphasis, particularly among the public and school personnel, who have become much more conscious of prevention than ever before. Also amazing advances have been made in sports medicine teaching. I do not know of a major medical center that does not now have a division, or section, relating to sports medicine. In the previous editions I denied myself the privilege of discussing reconstruction in any detail, since sophisticated care of the athlete was not as readily available as it is now. In this edition I have added information on reconstruction that I have found useful through the years, particularly in regard to the knee but also in regard to the shoulder. When, because of space limitations, I could not provide certain information, I have suggested references that give more detail.

My personal status has changed somewhat: after more than 50 years I have discontinued doing any orthopaedic surgery. I do have a diagnostic and referral clinic and am tremendously interested in rehabilitation. In fact, I am the medical director of a new rehabilitative facility at the University of Oklahoma Medical Center in Oklahoma City. I am so fascinated by this work that I do not really feel too bad about abandoning the surgery. My confrères do an exemplary job when I refer a patient to them for one of my "pet" operations. My interest in sports medicine has not changed one whit, since much of sports medicine is, indeed, rehabilitation.

DON H. O'DONOGHUE, M.D.

PREFACE
TO THE
THIRD EDITION

In considering the purpose of a preface for this third edition, many thoughts come to mind. The first one is to acknowledge my profound admiration for my confrères involved in the development of the specialty of sports medicine. Within the last relatively few years, sports medicine, which had been considered a hobby for the frustrated athlete who had not quite gotten over his pregraduation days, has blossomed to include some of the most sophisticated procedures and certainly has supported some of the most important precepts of the physician.

With each new edition I ponder the problem of a bibliography. A bibliography is extremely important in noting the sources of information, more detailed information than is permissible in a single volume. On the other hand, the specialty has developed so rapidly with so much talent that I find myself at a complete loss to know what to recommend and what to omit. Perhaps I do not solve anything by omitting all of it, but as I look through some of the modern articles and notice references to 200 or more sources, I wonder how much this really contributes to the practical knowledge of the physician who is going to treat the injured or ill athlete. Hence, for this reason and also, I suppose, for an inherent compulsion not to credit the wrong person with the right thing, I have omitted the bibliography. I refer the reader to the Bibliography of Sports Medicine, prepared under the auspices of the Committee on Sports Medicine of the American Academy of Orthopaedic Surgeons, which does list a great many authoritative articles on the subject. This volume is available from the American Academy of Orthopaedic Surgeons, 444 North Michigan Avenue, Chicago, Illinois, 60611, and is well worth the minimum charge.

Originality I do not claim. As I have said before, everything I know I learned at my mother's knee or some other joint. Seriously, however, I do bow long and deep to the many capable, earnest, enthusiastic, altruistic, dedicated, young and old, orthopaedists, and others, who have involved themselves in the care of the athlete. As I have not personally credited my many friends for their contributions, so I do not myself expect any credit for the material published in this book. Originality of a certain procedure is not my interest; rather, it is its application and sustained effectiveness in the care of the athlete that is important.

I still greatly appreciate the American athlete. The exigencies of my personal situation have made it possible, and desirable, for me to travel with the University of Oklahoma football team on their weekends away from home. No more delightful group of people could be assembled. If there ever was a day of the football bum, this day has long since passed. We see the cream of American manhood involved in a highly competitive situation, with innumerable examples of total unselfishness and dedication to the greatest good for the greatest number. Their ready acceptance of the fact that the doctor is on their side and is dedicated to doing what is best for them is, indeed, reassuring. My association with the University of Oklahoma Department of Intercollegiate Athletics continues to be a highly salutary one, a unit to which I owe a debt of gratitude for their complete cooperation in our study of and advancement of the care of the American athlete.

Again, a word of appreciation to all of my long-suffering staff who have personally helped me in the revision of this book. My secretaries, my radiology technician, my surgical nurse and my long-time secretary-manager, without whom I could not function, have especially been involved in the work we have been carrying on. Their organizational ability, their memory, their careful preservation of specific cases and their patience have rendered this research much easier.

Then, finally, to the many orthopaedic surgeons who have unstintedly shared their feelings, beliefs, problems and cases with me, particularly to the Sports Medicine Committee of the American Academy of Orthopaedic Surgeons and to the newly formed but very viable American Orthopaedic Society for Sports Medicine, I express my gratitude. Without these people this work would not have been possible.

DON H. O'DONOGHUE, M.D.

PREFACE
TO THE
SECOND EDITION

I see no reason to alter any of the original Preface. The eight years since it was published have seen further advances in the vital field of sports medicine. There has been a tremendous increase in interest in this area, with attention to many aspects other than injury. I have made no attempt here to expand into the fields of physiology, biochemistry, metabolism, neurology, biomechanics and psychiatry. There remain many verdant areas for expansion, research and application in these and many other disciplines.

The University of Oklahoma, through its Medical Center, its Physical Education Department, its advanced Student Health Program and, most particularly, its Department of Intercollegiate Athletics, has continued to lead the way in seeking to guard the welfare not only of the students of the University but of young athletes throughout our area.

I must extend a final word of appreciation to my secretaries, my radiology technologist, my nurse, and many others who helped make the preparation of this edition not only possible but enjoyable. A deep bow to my many anonymous associates in sports medicine, not only locally but throughout the United States and the world, who have shared unstintedly their ideas and their techniques. I am particularly grateful to the members of the Sports Medicine Committee of the American Academy of Orthopaedic Surgeons for their cooperation and support.

DON H. O'DONOGHUE, M.D.

PREFACE
TO THE
FIRST EDITION

I have given a great deal of thought to the advisability of including a bibliography in this volume. The material in this book is in large part basic. No claim is made for originality of concept or of procedures. Indeed, it is so fundamental that proper acknowledgment is well nigh impossible. I give full credit to my confrères, both present and past, for all I know about the subject. I had at first considered that I might credit those procedures which are generally understood to have been advanced by a specific man. Further consideration made it seem unjustifiable to credit some things but to leave the greater number unacknowledged. So a very grateful bow is offered to those members of the medical profession who take the pains to reduce their thinking to print and so make it available for all who want to, and can, read. By the same token, the thoughts in this book are freely available to anyone and no credit need be given me. My reward will be in your perusal of this book.

I also owe a debt of gratitude to the American athlete. That which in the beginning was an interesting sideline in a life devoted largely to pediatric orthopaedics, has burgeoned to become perhaps my major interest. The young athlete with his tremendous enthusiasm and his desire to recover is a stimulation to anyone who has the privilege of caring for him. He makes a splendid antidote to the rapidly increasing group of "freeloaders" who would rather be supported by their brothers than return to work.

Finally, I must express my sincere appreciation to the Athletic Department of the University of Oklahoma, which has to my personal knowledge never permitted selfish considerations to interfere in any way with the proper medical management of its athletes. It has presented a shining example which has spread throughout our state and has been particularly valuable in our successful efforts to improve the overall care of the young athlete in our public schools. The combined efforts of school administrators, teachers, coaches, trainers and physicians are resulting in a steady improvement in this vital area which will be rewarded manyfold by notable improvement in the physical condition of our people.

DON H. O'DONOGHUE, M.D.

The BILL OF RIGHTS for the SCHOOL and COLLEGE ATHLETE

Participation in athletics is a privilege involving both responsibilities and rights. The athlete has the responsibility to play fair, to give his best, to keep in training, to conduct himself with credit to his sport and his school. In turn he has the right to optimal protection against injury as this may be assured through good technical instruction, proper regulation and conditions of play, and adequate health supervision. Included are:

Good Coaching:

The importance of good coaching in protecting the health and safety of athletes cannot be minimized. Careful conditioning and technical instruction leading to skillful performance are significant factors in lowering the incidence and decreasing the severity of injuries. Also, good coaching includes the discouragement of tactics, outside either the rules or the spirit of the rules, which may increase the hazard and thus the incidence of injuries.

Good Officiating:

The rules and regulations governing athletic competition are made to protect players as well as to promote enjoyment of the game. To serve these ends effectively the rules of the game must be thoroughly understood by players as well as coaches and be properly interpreted and enforced by impartial and technically qualified officials.

Good Equipment and Facilities:

There can be no question about the protection afforded by proper equipment and right facilities. Good equipment is now available and is being improved continually; the problem lies in the false economy of using cheap, worn out, outmoded, or ill-fitting gear. Provision of proper areas for play and their careful maintenance are equally important.

Good Health Supervision . . . Including:

FIRST . . . a thorough preseason history and medical examination. Many of the sports tragedies which occur each year are due to unrecognized health problems. Medical contraindications to participation in contact sports must be respected.

SECOND . . . a physician present at all contests and readily available during practice sessions. It is unfair to leave to a trainer or coach decisions as to whether an athlete should return to play or be removed from the game following injury. In serious injuries the availability of a physician may make the difference in preventing disability or even death.

THIRD . . . medical control of the health aspects of athletics. In medical matters, the physician's authority should be absolute and unquestioned. Today's coaches and athletic trainers are happy to leave medical decisions to the medical profession. They also assist in interpreting this principle to students and the public.

American Medical Association
Committee on the Medical Aspects of Sports

9801—141F: 369-2M-D243 OP-37

CONTENTS

3
THE TREATMENT OF INJURIES IN SPECIFIC AREAS

5
INJURIES TO THE CRANIUM AND CENTRAL NERVOUS SYSTEM
by Bob J. Rutledge

6
INJURIES OF THE FACE.. 105

7
INJURIES OF THE SHOULDER GIRDLE.. 118

Introduction ⎯⎯⎯⎯ *1*

INTRODUCTION TO THE FOURTH EDITION

In approaching the subject of the Introduction to the Fourth Edition, I thought it seemed proper to review the Introduction to the First Edition. I urge readers of this edition to give themselves the time to read the Introduction to the First Edition, bearing in mind that it is over 20 years old. In spite of the passage of these years and in spite of the tremendous developments that have taken place in the field of sports medicine, I find that the principles expressed in that introduction are as valid today as they were in 1962. This is not to say there have been no improvements. Many of the suggestions in the first edition have, indeed, been followed. Much more has been done in the lower age groups to match competitors by strength and size rather than wholly by age. So too at the college level, the strong gridiron power's knocking off two or three teams with far fewer resources is pretty much a thing of the past. The practice of setting up a team as a patsy for the satisfaction of beating it 60 to 0 no longer seems either proper or valuable. For example, the University of Oklahoma in 1982 started with West Virginia, Kentucky and Southern California. There is not too much heard anymore about the seven blocks of granite who are proud of playing both offense and defense and 60 minutes of the football game.

Then, too, the first introduction discussed the attitude considering the physician as more or less a last resort in helping the players. This situation has certainly changed since 1962. It is now well understood and universally accepted that the physician is an important element in the successful management of the sports program. In the first introduction I state that diagnosis is the single most important thing in the handling of the athlete. There has been no change in my opinion.

The Sports Medicine Committee of the American Academy of Orthopaedic Surgeons progressed into the organization of the American Orthopaedic Society for Sports Medicine (AOSSM) in 1971, and the AOSSM has had tremendous acceptance among physicians throughout the United States. Its educational meetings are overattended on every occasion. Such new societies as the International Society for the Knee will spread the gospel further afield and, it is hoped, will bring the knowledge of other parts of the world closer to our own door. As noted in the Preface, sports medicine divisions at the major medical centers are now fairly universal.

Again, I have made no effort to list my sources, since they are so voluminous that to do so would be meaningless. Throughout the years since the publication of the first edition, a large part of my time has been spent not only in the care of the athlete but also in the development of new concepts of care. Care, of course, includes prevention. I never attend a session on sports medicine without coming home with some improvement in my basic knowledge, and I fully expect to relate this new information here without specific recognition of any individual involved. As I have said before, it is virtually impossible to find the true origin of any new idea, which in my mind negates the value of the eponym.

Another notable advancement in the field of sports has been the tremendously increased involvement of females. There have always been female athletes, and I have always provided them with the same care that I have given male athletes, with possible exceptions due to differences in physical make-up. Now there is, indeed, a considerable effort to try to equalize the involvement of the two sexes in sports. Semantically, there is the same difficulty in writing a text. No one has come up yet with any single word that implies both sexes. In some foreign languages, such as Latin, each noun is either male, female or neuter. In English, however, gender is usually contingent on the sex of the subject. When I say athlete or player, I make no sexual distinc tion. If in some contexts I use the word "man," meaning a genetic result of evolution, no distinction of sex is intended. To artificially add throughout the text "and boy" when "girl" is mentioned or "and female" when "male" is mentioned would border on the ridiculous. I see, treat and care for a great many female athletes. They are a gorgeous people. They are a great pleasure to work with, and they have a great desire to get well. They are in no way downgraded or negated in any of the material presented in this volume.

INTRODUCTION TO THE THIRD EDITION *(1976)*

Time marches on and with it marches the care of the athlete. Further advances in organized efforts have occurred in the past five years. The American Orthopaedic Society for Sports Medicine has been organized to encourage dissemination of knowledge among the orthopaedists. The AOSSM is particularly designed to provide a forum for orthopaedists who are interested in improvement of health care to the American athlete. The drive of this important new society has been to alert the orthopaedist, primarily but not exclusively, to the proper means by which improved care can be provided the athlete. Several foundations that are dedicated to the health of the athlete are operating for the common good. The activities of the Sports Medicine Committee of the American Academy of Orthopaedic Surgeons, which was formed in 1962, have greatly expanded from the original one postgraduate course per year, until in 1975, eight courses were presented in diverse parts of the country.

Sports Medicine is coming of age, but I see no signs of senescence. On the contrary, a great number of eager young orthopaedists are pushing the older group and are receiving proper recognition for their efforts for the good of the athlete. Much in this third edition evolves from past volumes, since basic principles do not change. An effort has been made to provide more clarity, to establish principles and to make room for new concepts as they develop. We are trying hard to eliminate old eponyms and to prevent the establishment of new ones, since semantics is a very important factor in education.

Since the previous editions of this book have been published, there have been marked changes in the athletic picture, particularly related to female contestants. Importance has always been attached to the female contestants through the many years in which records were kept. There has always been, however, a slight reserve about whether or not the distaff side of the show should be granted equal time with the spear side. There must be many areas in which the competition can be equal. Certainly up to the age of puberty, girls may be further developed than boys, but from then on, males begin to get more physical characteristics and females more romantic ones. In this work we have made no effort to discriminate between male and female. Since the book is basically on athletic injuries, there is little here that applies to the male that doesn't apply equally as well to the female. Since there is, to my knowledge, no short word to imply "he" or "she", my "he" and "his" will refer to both sexes to the disparagement of neither. I love them all.

Since rehabilitation has become of maximum importance in the treatment of the athlete, whether he be young or old, we have included a chapter devoted to rehabilitation. Fred Allman, the author of this chapter, has devoted a major part of his professional life to the advancement of this aspect of treatment of musculoskeletal conditions, and I extend a most grateful thanks to him for his help in adding this aspect. Dr. Allman has also been kind enough to add shorter sections on rehabilitation in regard to specific injuries, particularly some of the more common ones. Once again, Dr. Gael Frank has cooperated very much in the preparation of the material on the hand, and I appreciate his efforts in this direction. The section on craniocerebral injuries has been carefully reviewed with the idea of some more definitive recommendations. This has been done by Dr. Bob Rutledge, an eminent neurosurgeon at the University of Oklahoma School of Medicine, with my sincere appreciation. For the first time we have included some authoritative material on treatment of injuries to the eye. Although this is an infrequent injury, it is one that causes great dismay on the part of the team physician who is hard put to decide just what level of care it requires. Ophthalmologist Dr. Pat Wilkinson, who has a long background in athletics, has contributed to this effort and has our heartfelt thanks for giving authenticity to an area in which my personal opinions are far less than authoritative.

INTRODUCTION TO THE SECOND EDITION *(1970)*

I had intended to completely rewrite the introduction to this second edition. However,

I find the comments made in the Introduction to the First Edition as valid today as they were when written a number of years ago. The principles remain the same.

In the intervening years there has been a vast expansion of athletic participation and, I am happy to say, an even more comprehensive program to improve the young athlete. Most of the points referred to in the Introduction to the First Edition have developed amazingly well. The educational programs have vastly expanded, as will be noted. Many excellent books and articles have been published. There has been a notable expansion of the breadth of participation. Most responsible athletic programs today make a real effort to provide participation for every young person who desires it. Responsible medical organizations have awakened to realize not only the tremendous increase in the importance of trauma in relation to economic loss, morbidity and mortality but also that sports medicine has attained great stature. The same precepts which serve to make sports medicine unique have contributed to the development of methods of prevention, diagnosis and treatment which can be and have been applied to nonathletic situations.

There has also been a sweeping evolution in the medical care of the young athlete. Led by the American Medical Association Committee on the Medical Aspects of Sports, many organizations throughout the United States have organized very active committees dedicated to the health of American youth. This AMA committee has invited the participation of other organizations with interest in sports medicine. Under this committee's aegis a coordination committee has been formed with representation from similar committees of other associations, medical and nonmedical, concerned with the problem. Annual meetings of this group committee have been held since 1964. The total number of associations represented in this group is rapidly approaching 50. A subcommittee on standard sports nomenclature from the AMA committee has published a thesaurus of definitions in an attempt to clarify the language and so improve communications. I shall follow this terminology in so far as it is possible in this book.

Led by the Sports Medicine Committee of the American Academy of Orthopaedic Surgeons, which was activated in 1962, the orthopaedic aspects of this development have greatly expanded. The Committee promotes instructional courses, presents exhibits and encourages scientific study of musculo-skeletal conditions relative to sports. The American Academy of Orthopaedic Surgeons Committee has encouraged and promoted programs for coaches, trainers, team physicians and orthopaedists all about the country. More recently the Committee has presented an increasing number of postgraduate seminars developed for orthopaedic surgeons. This interest is not confined to orthopaedic surgeons, however. It has been taken up by internists, pediatricians, physiatrists, physiologists, neurologists and indeed the whole gamut of the medically oriented professions. Sophisticated courses are given for specialists, more practical ones for generalists, and still others directed to trainers and physical therapists. In fact, at this time the coverage of the field seems complete. In spite of all this, each new program develops new ideas which may bring about some breakthrough in treatment, conditioning or prevention.

My present effort is to try to bring this volume up to date and in line with the progress made in this and other fields. Methods change, but general principles are remarkably constant.

Finally, a few words of appreciation for the many colleagues who have contributed to this volume. They shall remain largely anonymous, but without this constant contact I should have little to offer. Most of the actual cases are my own, since I find that I write better and with more confidence about cases with which I am wholly familiar. I shall never fail to appreciate the many contacts that I have had with members of my profession, both in the United States and abroad, by personal association, by direct correspondence and by study of their excellent reports. I cannot close this introduction without acknowledging a great debt of gratitude to my dedicated and long-suffering personal staff who serve as my memory for cases and who patiently put up with my constant desire for improvement by substituting new material at the last minute. Without their efforts this book would have been impossible.

INTRODUCTION TO THE FIRST EDITION *(1962)*

A book devoted entirely to injuries to a special group must have justification. Why injuries to athletes alone? Why not just injuries in general? Certainly the athlete is a human being, subject to the same frailties as the rest of the race, and one might reasonably expect him to be treated in the same manner. Could not the physician refer for guidance to one or more of the multitude of books that have been written on the subject of injury?

The very fact that you are reading this book to some extent justifies it. Obviously you recognize the athletic injury as a special situation—an area in which we as physicians can render a unique service. I believe that a few paragraphs explaining our approach to this stimulating subject will give added meaning to the later sections on specific injuries.

There is, indeed, real significance in the fact that a separate volume on the subject of injuries to athletes is considered warranted. Ten years ago this would not have been likely. Lately, however, there has been a tremendous upsurge of interest in this subject, not only among orthopaedists but among physicians in general, and indeed among the laity. An increasing number of postgraduate seminars and medical sessions have been concerned with it. At a postgraduate course on athletic injuries sponsored by the University of Colorado at Denver less than four years ago at which from 30 to 40 registrants were expected, an amazing total of almost 300 very interested and enthusiastic physicians, orthopaedists, coaches and trainers appeared. In the following years the attendance was markedly increased. The injuries discussed at this and other meetings have been largely those of college athletes, but there is presently a ground swell in various parts of the country to develop these educational sessions to include secondary school and even grade school athletics.

Organized athletics has been extended to involve a major segment of our youth. In many areas not only the junior high schools but the grade schools participate in competitive sports. Whether or not this is good, it must be recognized as a fait accompli which cannot be ignored. There is no present trend toward less athletics. On the contrary, the trend is toward a more inclusive program. Indeed, one of the major criticisms leveled at athletic programs has been their tendency to include the few to the neglect of the many. It should be recalled that in this country the various types of organized athletics, many of them competitive, must serve almost the whole function of physical conditioning, whereas in other countries there are various health clubs, hiking clubs, ski societies, etc. Organizations of the latter type have not been popular in the United States. Our citizens are a keenly competitive group and exercise for exercise's sake; the calisthenic drill or the regimentation into marching clubs, has not appealed to them, one reason being the fact that in other countries these various groups have been used as spring-

boards for political activity. Our youth have an almost paranoid dislike of anything smacking of regimentation. The effort, therefore, must be not to decry athletics and demand less participation but, on the contrary, to demand greater participation and then see to it that the whole background of organized athletics is improved.

There can be no denying that competitive athletics has a great appeal to the mass of our people. However, the public is more inclined to look at the score, to observe the outstanding player and to foster the competitive contest than to direct its attention toward those facets of the program which are best calculated to return the major good to the greatest number. Comparatively little attention outside the confines of sport itself has been paid to conditioning or to prevention of injury. An occasional blare of publicity follows a major injury to a stellar athlete or the untimely death of a budding prep school player. Occasionally this triggers a lay magazine article on the importance of equipment and the value of physical conditioning as important factors in the prevention of injury. The greater emphasis, however, is placed on the injury itself. The sports pages eagerly play up injury to the star. Wryly enough, the reporter moans that the star has been disabled by his operation rather than by his injury.

In the final analysis, however, the lay public and, I fear, the majority of our medical profession have little knowledge of the actual processes of training and the actual mechanics of athletic injury.

Competitive Athletics: Benefits and Risks

Why is it important for young men to participate in athletics? Certainly it does carry an element of risk. Perhaps the solution to the problem of athletic injuries lies in the prayer of the timorous mother that her boy not compete. Abandonment of sports would certainly be the quickest way to prevent injury to the contestant.

In common with many others, I believe there are tangible benefits to be derived from athletic competition that greatly outweigh the element of risk. Certainly some of them are obvious. No one seriously doubts that the athlete does develop a stronger, healthier body. Most of the myths of catastrophic sequelae from strenuous athletic activity have been dispelled. The "athlete's heart" is a bogeyman which has finally been exorcised. The ex-athlete who "turns to fat" has at least postponed his impending adiposity throughout his years of training. The trained athlete is superior to his more sedentary fellow in drive and stamina and better fitted for both work and play.

I think most of us would agree that competitive athletics does have a salutary effect upon the character of the participant. This is particularly true if the program is managed so that the major emphasis is placed on the development of the ability in the athlete to value his own and respect his opponent's capabilities rather than to win at any cost. The player learns the importance of team participation, that he must sacrifice immediate gain to the final end, that desire is one of the key factors in success. The fact that the word "sportsmanship" seems trite has in no way changed its reality as a trait of character. Team effort as opposed to individual glory, ability to take a job and to follow it through, the necessity for taking it as well as dishing it out, are all basic lessons learned by the successful athlete.

There are certainly material benefits for the athlete in our present educational system that have much importance. Many a young man goes to school because of his athletic ability. Much has been said about scholarships, especially by those who know the least about them. Suffice it to say that the athletic scholarship does permit many a lad to finish his education who otherwise would have dropped out of school long before. Who are we to say that the athletic scholarship is not as worthwhile as the scholarship for merit in other fields? In most of the better schools of the country the scholarship athlete has to maintain a scholastic average higher than the average of his school. A good estimate of the quality of the scholarship program in a given institution can be made from the proportion of the scholarship boys who go ahead to graduation.

So much for the benefit of athletics to the students in school. But after graduation, what? It has been said that the athlete out of school is as a fish out of water. Not so! Many athletes develop their careers in some form of physical education or a related field. The conditioning of our youth depends upon the organized type of athletic training which he gets in the elementary and secondary schools and in such organizations as the YMCA and the Boy Scouts. Without the trained athlete to provide capable leadership, these programs would be in sorry straits, indeed. We need these people.

Indeed, we will find that much of the physical education of our youth is in the hands of former athletes. On a more personal plane, many an athlete makes contacts during his school years with men who are seeking his very type of qualifications to fill the leading jobs in industry. In many years of knowing athletes, I have seen most of them display the same fine enthusiasm and attain the same success in life that they did in school. Certainly there are real advantages to an athletic program from many standpoints.

Why then is there such bitter opposition to organized competitive athletics as such? Not because of any interference with scholastic pursuits, not because of any moral implications, not because the aftereffects of training impair the physique in later life, but because of one principal thing, namely, physical injuries. Do athletes get physical injuries? The answer is "Yes, they do." Here is a very real objection to the athletic program—in fact, almost the only real objection. Our youngsters do get injured—on occasion even seriously or fatally injured. It must be the duty of the medical profession to accept this challenge and do everything in its power to minimize those things which interfere with the goals of the athletic program.

The Role of the Physician

What can we as physicians do to prevent injury, to minimize temporary disability and to prevent permanent disability? Much indeed has been accomplished in the past few years toward these ends. A few years ago the trainer in the average scholastic institution was a fugitive from the supply room, having graduated into the "wrapping and taping" club largely by osmosis. He had no real knowledge of injuries, and his main concern actually was to "keep 'em rollin'." We all remember the famous men who attained a great deal of notoriety by reason of their ability to keep the athlete in the game. Too many times this goal of immediate playing was a more vital one than the final goal of complete recovery of the patient. During this era the physician was a necessary evil. The player felt that once he reached the doctor his days as an athlete were over. In too many instances this feeling was justified for two very pertinent reasons. First, since the doctor was the last resort, he did not see the player until long after treatment should ideally have been instituted. Second, and I think of almost equal importance, was the sad reality that it was not of any immediate concern to the doctor whether or not the patient was an athlete or was able to remain one after treatment was completed. All too often the first recommendation the doctor made was "Well, give up football," or "You must not play any more baseball." This simply tended to confirm the conviction of the player, the coach and the public that athletes and physicians were incompatible. Also, in the past there has been a tendency on the part of the coaching staff to demand that the player continue in spite of injury or be labeled "yellow." The trainer was urged to "tape her up" and "run him back in" —often to the detriment of the player, the team and the game. In our major institutions this is no longer true.

A more enlightened approach has demonstrated that everyone is better served by having the injured player promptly and ably treated, thereby obtaining recovery before he does himself irreparable damage. The successful coach seeks to protect the player and seeks to prevent damage to either body or mind. In the well-run athletic program of today, the coach, trainer, team physician and specialist *all* combine in one effective unit designed to keep the player well equipped and in ideal condition. In fact, more emphasis is placed, and actually more time is spent, on preparing a player to participate and on preventing his injury than is spent on treatment. The player, coach, trainer and physician are no longer working at cross purposes in most institutions. Athletic injuries are much less frequent and they are less severe than in the past. The period of disability is shorter. The degree of recovery is more complete. Many factors have combined to produce this vast improvement in the one area in which it must be conceded that athletics may have a bad effect.

So we find that once again the physician must become not only the doer but the teacher. The physician with an especial interest in athletes must prepare himself to handle their injuries, and he must in turn pass this information on to other physicians. It must be recognized that there is one overriding difference in the management of injuries to athletes. That is, the patient must completely recover from his injury or he is no longer an athlete. True enough, this axiom *should* apply to any injury the physician sees, but nowhere else is it dramatized quite so constantly as in the care of the athlete.

Diagnostic Judgment

The outstanding consideration in the treatment of athletic injury is early detection not only of the nature of the injury but of its degree. The optimum time to examine an athlete for injury is as soon as possible after he is hurt. There must be no compromise with this statement. It may be impossible to examine the patient or to make a complete diagnosis at once, but if it can be done precious time has been saved. Frequently the initial examination is by the coach, the trainer or the physician on the field. Whoever this is, he must make as careful an evaluation of the injured player's condition as he is capable of doing and must pass this information on to each succeeding link in the chain of therapy. The doctor must conscientiously and objectively examine the player. Does the injury seem serious enough that the boy should not return to the game, or should he be strapped up and allowed to play? To err is human, but the margin of error can be drastically reduced by comprehensive consideration of the patient's injury. There is no place here for wishful thinking. The player is eager to continue and should not be deprived unnecessarily of this privilege. On the other hand, if continued competition adds to the hazard of injury, he should not be permitted to compete. It is, of course, always better to err on the side of conservatism.

After the injury sidelines the player, what then? The prevalent habit of packing the injured part in ice and delaying examination until a convenient time the next day, or even later, is to be deplored. Your examination as a physician should be done at the earliest possible moment, even at considerable inconvenience to yourself, the coach or the player. It should be obvious that the part should be undressed, all taping or strapping removed, and a meticulous examination carried out. Frequently the diagnosis, which will be easy in the early stage, becomes exceedingly difficult as pain increases apprehension, and swelling, edema and hemorrhage interfere with an accurate evaluation of the injury. If consultation with a specialist is needed, seek it promptly so that the specialist, too, may be able to take advantage of the optimum time for treatment. The specialist should have enough integrity to be able to cooperate with the referring physician and to "take the monkey off his back," as it were, in regard to the severity of the injury. This is particularly true of the decision on whether or not the player should be allowed to compete, either at once or later.

Concepts of Treatment

Once treatment is decided upon, the physician should proceed to carry it out with confidence. If the treatment is within the capabilities of the team physician, he should be permitted to conduct it. If the specialist's attention is required, the specialist himself should not hesitate to say so. The physician should be encouraged to seek the specialist's advice early, and this will be done only when there is good rapport between the player, the referring physician and the specialist.

The following concepts ("Five A's") of treatment have proved to be of great value: (1) accept athletics; (2) avoid expediency; (3) adopt the best method; (4) act promptly; (5) achieve perfection.

1. *Accept athletics.* The physician—not the player, not the coach, not the parents, but the physician—must recognize the value of competitive athletics. He must believe that it is vital to this particular patient to be restored to competitive athletics. If the physician fails in this, the patient-doctor relationship suffers and rapport is lost. The doctor who deprecates the player's ambition should not be treating him.

2. *Avoid expediency.* Outside influence must not be permitted to outweigh sound medical judgment. Many pressing factors will tend to influence the doctor's decision. All concerned are extremely unwilling to believe that the player is really hurt. The boy's desire to compete, his fear of failing his teammates, the parents' desire to see their son excel, the coach's hope that the player is not really hurt—all must be ignored if the proper conclusion is to be reached. Procrastination, vacillation and so-called "conservative" attitudes must not prevail. Temporary convenience must be sacrificed for the ultimate goal.

3. *Adopt the best method of treatment.* Medical evaluation of the nature and extent of injury must be the controlling factor in the choice of treatment. A temporizing attitude will not accomplish the best results. If you really believe that one method is distinctly better than another, you should recommend it and then carry it out. This must be an entirely objective decision. How often do we hear the statement "Well, perhaps it would be better to operate on this knee, but I'll put it in a cast" or "We really should have put the boy on crutches, but. . . . "

4. *Act promptly.* A definitive decision as to the proper method of treatment must be made at the earliest possible moment and then that method must be carried out. We have been able to show conclusively that delay very often spells the difference between success and failure of treatment.

5. *Achieve perfection.* Make complete recovery your goal. While this may not be possible in any given case, it must always be the goal. The athlete is basically in good condition and can well tolerate any reasonable measure if it serves to increase his chances for a complete recovery.

Will such a program be accepted? Yes, but not without some educational effort on the part of the physician. He must be able to show conclusively that the program is better not only for the physician but for the school, the coach and especially for the player. This will require time. He must be interested and capable. As his program develops, those most concerned will recognize the benefits. They will observe that the sprained ankle responds to treatment, that a short, complete layoff is followed by normal ability as opposed to an ineffectual season. The coach will note that prompt treatment restores the player more rapidly and permits more actual playing in the long run and so is better for the team. The player will not fear the physician who has a sympathetic and understanding attitude. He notes that his buddy gets well. He also expects to get well and will accept the physician's recommendation for treatment. He may fear some specific part of the treatment, such as the insertion of a needle into a joint, but never to the extent of failing to return or refusing the treatment, provided he believes that the doctor is sincerely trying to restore him to his normal ability.

These are not idle dreams of Utopia. The type of program described is practical and has been established in a number of institutions. It must be our aim to make it the rule, not the exception. Nor is a full scale, university-type training program necessary. The program does require an able, conscientious coach and a physician who will interest himself in the peculiar problems of the athlete.

PREVENTION
OF INJURIES

Prevention of Injuries 2

The prevention of injuries should be the major goal of anyone responsible for the physical and mental conditioning of athletes. If we grant that the athletic program is important from the standpoint of the improvement of the physical and mental condition of our young people, we must adopt every possible means to see that it has no detrimental effect. There may be differences of opinion concerning the benefits of athletics, but one cannot deny that almost the only deleterious effect is physical injury. We spend much time devising ways and means to relieve the effects of injury. If we spent even a small percentage of this time in striving to prevent the injury from occurring, a major portion of our problem could be solved.

Prevention of injuries has many facets. In a university-type training program, more attention will be given to prevention of injuries by one means or another than to their treatment. In the secondary school programs, someone must be made responsible for the physical welfare of the players. There has been a steady improvement in this facet of the problem for many years. The trainer has become a skilled professional person. Unfortunately, most secondary schools have not employed full-time trainers. The role of the physician here must be that of advisor to whatever amateur trainer is available. It is neither fair nor advisable to put the whole responsibility of physical conditioning upon the busy coach, however capable he may be. The coach must of necessity concentrate his attention on the practice session or on the game. His training duties must be incidental to this. The team physician should be the one who is especially interested in this problem. He must be willing to accept the responsibility for it even at some inconvenience to himself. It may seem very tedious to supervise the details of strapping, wrapping, equipment, weight control and all of the other areas of training, but the team physician is not worthy of the name if he is not willing to do

it. This is particularly important in the preseason training period. Prevention of injury is as much the sphere of the doctor as is prevention of disease. The overall aim of the athletic program is to improve the participant. If the participant leaves the program in poorer condition than when he started, it has failed regardless of how many games have been won.

THE INDIVIDUAL PLAYER

Physical Condition (General Health)

Before the prospective player is permitted to enter an athletic program, he should have an intelligent and complete physical examination. It is not necessary to take a multitude of laboratory tests. The general physical examination should, however, provide leads to needed supplemental measures. For example, if there seems to be a defect in vision, a detailed examination of the eye should be recommended. If a cardiac murmur is discovered, it should be investigated. It is not enough simply to examine a player and record the findings. The physician should be willing to give an opinion as to the boy's physical ability to participate in the sport concerned. If he does not feel himself capable of doing this, he should recommend special examinations. It is not proper to request a boy to drop the program simply because the physician does not know whether or not he has a physical defect which would contraindicate his participation. It is almost as bad to err by overconservatism as it is to overlook serious hazards. Does this functional heart murmur really constitute a hazard? Can this boy's adiposity be controlled? Are this young man's bones to be judged overbrittle because he has had several fractures? To each individual the answers are extremely vital. They must be vital to the examining physician as well.

Once it has been decided that the candidate may compete in athletics, every effort must be made to *improve* his physical condition. He should be given advice as to his diet and told to avoid faddish eating, to avoid overeating and to eat regularly. He should be advised not to snack between meals at the expense of his regular meals. Many young people are subject to constipation. This can usually be completely controlled by regulation of the diet, which is far better than the habitual use of laxatives. An effort should be made to determine the proper weight for the individual player. His diet then is regulated so that he may reach this weight, using a high caloric regimen if he is undernourished or a low caloric, high protein diet if he is adipose. On every squad there will be several players who are in dire need of regulation in dietary matters.

The player should be instructed in good living habits. He should get plenty of rest and sleep. The two are not necessarily synonymous. If he has irregular study and sleeping hours, an effort should be made to find a schedule more in keeping with his general surroundings. There is no point in forcing him to go to bed early and to get up early if the habit of his family is to go to bed late and to get up late. There is nothing magical in certain specific hours of sleep. The benefit is in the number of hours and the degree of relaxation. The well-regulated program should permit the player to have 30 to 40 minutes of relative relaxation between practice or competition and eating. It goes without saying that he should be instructed not to eat just before strenuous practice periods. Great emphasis is put on regulating eating before an actual game, but too often the practice session is not so well regulated. The player's blood may be concentrated in his muscles by extreme physical exercise when it should be busy aiding in the digestion of his food.

The player should be instructed to avoid all drugs except on the specific prescription of a physician. This includes intoxicants and nicotine. Stimulants not only are useless but may cause irreparable overexertion. Various fads should be discouraged.

Conditioning

The physical conditioning of a player should be a coninuous thing. If the player can be kept in good condition throughout the year, one of the major goals of the athletic program will have been accomplished—namely, the im-

provement of the general condition of the youth of America. Nonetheless, there are certain sports that require concentration of conditioning far beyond the others. Ideally, the conditioning should be fitted to the sport. In our University of Oklahoma program, for example, the football player is urged to keep in condition the year round. It is fully understood that he probably will not keep in game condition for the full 12 months, but it is fatuous to believe that he can be put in game condition in two or three weeks. Hence, each individual player is instructed when he leaves school on exactly what he should do that summer. The following summer conditioning program for high school athletes was recommended by Mr. Ken Rawlinson, former head trainer of the University of Oklahoma, and is quoted directly from his book.*

A Recommended Summer High School Conditioning Program

It is my belief that a high school athlete needs even more incentive to carry on a summer conditioning program than a college athlete. There follows a summer or off-season conditioning plan that can be inaugurated in any high school.

I. Squad meeting—end of school—tell boys why of everything.
  1. Start in June—peak in August.
  2. Calisthenic program.
  3. Weight training program.
  4. Isometric program.
  5. 6:30 mile.
  6. Wind sprints.
  7. Run circles, figure 8's.
  8. Stadium steps.
  9. Rope skipping.
  10. Rehabilitative exercises.
  11. Temperate living.
    A. Sleep—"the great restorer"—a minimum of nine hours. Two hours before midnight is better than four after.
    B. No intoxicants. The A.M.A. has stated that "alcohol is a detriment to the human organism. Its use in therapeutics, as a tonic, food, or stimulant has no scientific value. It attacks the central nervous system. It is not a food; it is a poison."
    C. No smoking. Nowhere is there any medical evidence that states that it improves an athlete's ability. It actually slows him up. Nicotine is a poison. If one smokes a pack of cigarettes a day for a week, he inhales 400 mg. of nicotine, which in

---

*Rawlinson, K.: Modern Athletic Training. Englewood Cliffs, New Jersey, Prentice-Hall Inc., 1961, page 25.

a single injection would kill him instantly.
D. No drugs. The United States Olympic Committee has recently ruled that any competitor who uses drugs, stimulants, or other substances known as "dope" for any purpose will be disqualified.
E. Good diet.
12. Possibly assign weight for first practice.
13. Date and place of physical exam.
14. Pre-season physical test.
6:30 mile
Push-ups—30
Sit-ups—50
Pull-ups—10
II. Personal letters or calls in summer—incentive, challenge.
1. Season's objectives (offense, defense, etc.)
2. Conditioning hints.
3. Rehabilitative exercises.
4. Physical exam—reminder.
5. Pre-season physical condition test.

"What Makes a Champion" by Bud Wilkinson

1. Condition.
2. Will to win.
3. Physically tougher than opponent.
4. Execution of fundamentals.
5. Fewer errors.

A Recommended Summer College or University Conditioning Program

Short sprints develop speed. Distance running develops endurance. Running in circles, figure 8's (around goal posts), strengthens ankles, knees, hips and back.
JUNE:
Daily exercises (see below).
Run 2 to 3 days a week—distance running, 440's—jog 1, walk 1, etc. Minimum 2 miles
JULY:
Daily exercises (see below).
Run 3 to 4 days a week—distance running plus a few sprints, 880's—jog 1, walk 1, etc. Minimum 2 miles. Sprints: 10–20–30 yards. Three of each at ½ speed.
AUGUST:
Take your salt tablets daily. If possible work out at 4:00 p.m. daily—climatic conditions are thus about equal to our practice sessions. Work 5 to 7 days a week with emphasis on:
A. Daily exercise program.
B. Sprints (10–20–30 yards—start with 5 of each at ¾ speed and work up to 10 at full speed).
C. Be able to run a mile. Objective: backs, 6:00; lineman, 6:30.

D. Football drills (wave, quarter eagles, pass cuts, etc.).
E. You should be within 3 pounds of your assigned playing weight by August 1.

Daily Exercises

Follow the daily exercise program during June, July and August (increase tempo in August). For a variation on many of the daily exercises you may use the INTENSITY SYSTEM—maximum effort over a limited time (example: number of push-ups you can do in 20 seconds—decrease time interval as you progress).
EVERYDAY:
1. Rope jumping (objective: 15 minutes).
2. Step bench. Using an 18 to 21 in. bench or chair, do at least 45 steps each leg once a day.
3. Wrestler's bridge. Position: Weight supported on feet and head—rotate in circles to right and left.
4. Weight training—at least three times a week.

Daily Exercise Guide

Do five exercises per day for six days a week during the months of June and July. Increase the tempo in August. These exercises are set up specifically to reach every area of the body and can be done daily in the athlete's room or back yard. He should start exercises by jumping rope.

MONDAY:
Side Bender. Position: Stand with feet apart, hands clasped overhead, arms straight. Bend sideward to the right, bending right knee and slowly going as far as possible. Repeat to left. Repeat ten times each side.
Knee Stretcher. Position: Stand with feet apart, knees slightly flexed and hands on outside of knees. Press knees together with hands, knees offering resistance. Repeat outward 20 times.
Shoulder Hang. Position: Grasp an overhead crossbar, ladder, tree limb, etc., and hang, elbows straight. Hang one minute, relax, and repeat ten times. Especially good for boys with acromioclavicular, muscular or nerve shoulder trouble. (If shoulder will permit, walk hand-over-hand across overhead ladder.)
Hurdle Spread. Position: Sit in hurdle position with right leg forward. Bend trunk forward and touch right foot with both hands. Repeat 40 times, then extend left leg and repeat 40 times.

TUESDAY:
Groin Stretch. Position: Stand with feet apart, hands on groin. Bend body obliquely to right and left (forward and backward). Stretch it out.
Bicycle Ride. Position: Support body on shoulders with elbows on ground and hands on hips supporting the body. Move feet and legs in motion necessary for riding a bicycle as rapidly as possible for count of 40. Repeat four to five times.

Stomach Drill. Position: Flat on back with hands under hips, with legs straight together and toes pointed. Raise feet slowly with a slow count of ten until the legs are perpendicular to the ground, lower them slowly halfway and stop; here spread the legs and bring them together eight times, then lower legs to within six inches from the ground and repeat the spread eight times. Raise legs slowly to the perpendicular position and lower them to the ground very slowly. Repeat eight times.

WEDNESDAY:

Wood Chopper. Position: Stand with feet apart, trunk turned right, hands together and over right shoulder. In a chopping movement bring arms down vigorously between the legs. Uncoil over left shoulder and repeat. Repeat 20 times each side.

Quarter Eagles. Position: Feet width of shoulders, parallel, and heels on ground. Bend at knees so thighs are parallel to ground. Maintaining the above base, jump ¼ turns to right and left.

THURSDAY:

Trunk Twister. Position: Stand with feet apart, hands clasped behind head and elbows back. Bend and bounce downward and simultaneously rotate trunk far to left. Recover and repeat to right. Repeat 15 times to each side.

All Fours. Position: Face down. Weight on hands and feet, and walk forward, backward, sideward, etc.

Sit Up and Paw Dirt. Position: Flat on back with arms extended overhead. Sit up, thrust arms forward and touch toes, knees straight. Return to starting position. Swing legs overhead until feet touch ground behind neck. Dig the dirt with running motion of legs, for 15 counts. Return to original position and repeat.

FRIDAY:

Mountain Climber. Position: Squatting with hands on ground, right leg drawn up to chest and left leg extended to rear with knee straight. With a fast cadence extend right foot backward and bring left leg to chest. Repeat 25 times.

Leg-Back Stretch. Position: Flat on back with arms bracing shoulders against the turn. With knee stiff, raise one leg to perpendicular position and swing it across body until foot touches hand on opposite side, shoulders flat throughout. Repeat 20 times with right, left and both legs (good for low back injuries).

Toe and Heel Dance. Position: One-half squat position with trunk erect. Remaining in this position, jump with the right heel extended in front and the left toe extended behind. Jump again, reversing the order of the feet. Repeat rapidly 40 times. From same position jump with the right heel to the side and left foot in place. Repeat to left.

SATURDAY:

Leg Stretch. Position: Stand erect with hands at sides. Bend forward without bending knees, and touch toes. Repeat 20 to 30 times. Repeat same with legs crossed.

High Step-Dive. Position: Stationary high step run-dive forward, weight on hands and let chest strike ground lightly, then abdomen, thighs and feet. Jump to feet and repeat 15 times.

SUNDAY: Optional.

The major portion of this conditioning must be carried out by the athlete himself. He cannot be expected to do it without proper direction and instruction. Each boy is given a set of exercises which he is to use three or four times a week until the first part of August and then daily until the beginning of the fall practice. He is encouraged to supplement these exercises by jogging, running for endurance, wind sprints and other types of exercise. He is encouraged to maintain, at least to some degree, his training program by getting rest, sleep, and proper food and by avoiding dissipation throughout the summer. Furthermore, each boy is assigned the weight at which he is expected to be when he reports for the first day of practice in the fall. The player is told that he should report in such condition that he could play a game on the first day of practice.

Obviously, such a program cannot be fitted entirely to the secondary school. However, the essence of the program is there. If the boy is to participate in football, he should start conditioning himself early in the summer. It will not suffice simply to tell him to keep himself in shape. He must be given a specific program to follow. Most of the eager young athletes will be glad to carry out such a program if they know what is really expected of them. There is probably less trouble with physical conditioning for football than for any other sport, since it is recognized as a rugged sport. It is equally important for the player to be conditioned for such games as basketball, baseball and particularly for track. Many a track career has been nipped in the bud because the participant has not been "brought along" by gradually increasing effort. A single major effort by the broad jumper or the sprinter may be responsible for losing the whole season of competition, since he may develop tenosynovitis of the tendo Achilles or a strain of the hamstring muscle or a *stress* fracture of the foot or fibula (see Fig. 49, page 70.) A runner should not be permitted to run the mile under competitive conditions until he has paced himself many times through this same distance at a gradually accelerating rate. The baseball player who needs to get his arms as well as his legs in top shape may require a wholly different set of exercises, although the goal remains the same. He must not be permitted to exert the maximum strength of any muscle until it has been suitably conditioned for this effort. This is well known as it applies to the pitcher, but it may be equally disastrous for the outfielder or third baseman to start his practice with maximum throws to the plate or across to first. These factors are particularly pertinent in secondary school players, who have a maximum of desire and a minimum of regulatory common sense. They require supervision and this is one of the major advantages of organized athletics. In a regulated program the player can have supervision and so be developed gradually until his full potential is reached.

It should be noted that the physician has a real responsibility to eliminate any exercise that he feels to be bad for the athlete, no matter how traditional or popular it may be. Any orthopaedist handling injuries knows all too well the danger of the popular "deep knee bends" and "duck waddle." In these exercises, as the heel is forcibly jammed against the buttock, there is a real danger of a posterior tear of the medial or lateral meniscus. They have no advantage over three-quarter knee bends. Obviously, all doctors will not agree on which exercises are particularly bad and which are good. The doctor must first inform himself and then have the strength of his convictions when offering his advice to the athletic administration.

The conditioning program at the University of Oklahoma naturally has been expanded and refined throughout the years. The latest edition of Ken Rawlinson's book, Modern Athletic Training,* co-authored by Dan Pickett, Ken's very able successor as head trainer at the University of Oklahoma, covers the sophisticated conditioning program currently being used for the college athlete at the University of Oklahoma. The initial program developed by the late Ken Rawlinson is still quite valid today, particularly at the high school level. The following examples of conditioning exercises for certain sports are quoted from the original version of his book.†

Conditioning Athletes' Bodies

For top performance, body conditioning is absolutely necessary. A conditioned boy is less susceptible to injuries. Conditioning affects:

---

*Rawlinson, K.: Modern Athletic Training. 200 Castlewood St., North Palm Beach, Florida, The Athletic Institute, 1980.

†Rawlinson, K.: Modern Athletic Training. Englewood Cliffs, New Jersey, Prentice-Hall, Inc., Chapter III, 1961.

1. Ability to play.
2. Mental attitude.
3. Determination.
4. Teamwork.
5. Spirit.

Many fail to make the team because they do not have the desire. They will not pay the price to get themselves into shape both physically and mentally. Mental conditioning is a phase often overlooked, but it is very vital. Many athletes do not think it is important, but it goes hand-in-hand with physical conditioning. If an athlete is going to be great, he must have both.

Conditioning at Oklahoma

The conditioning program for the fall season at the University of Oklahoma begins at the close of spring football practice (approximately the middle of May). This portion of the conditioning program must be carried on by the athlete himself. He cannot be expected to do this without proper direction and instruction. It is our firm conviction that if athletes have the desire to be great, they must be, and are, willing to pay the price to help accomplish their goal.

Basic Principles of Running

An important phase of conditioning is running. Every athlete should learn how to run correctly. Anyone can be taught to run a little faster, if he has the desire. Following are a few suggestions:

1. Relax. The body must be supple to attain best performance.
2. Run on the balls of the feet.
3. Point the toes straight ahead. You lose at least one-half inch on each step if toes are not straight ahead.
4. Run in a straight line. It is the shortest distance between two points.
5. Develop your proper stride. The average stride is the height of your body. Lengthen your stride as much as possible but do not overstride. It is worse than an understride.
6. Running angle is important; body leaning, head up, ankles, hips, shoulders and head in a straight line. Do not bend too far backward. You should be in the proper running angle and with the proper stride 12 to 15 yards from the starting point.
7. Arm action is very important; opposite arm and leg move in unison. Keep arm relaxed and shoot uppercuts to height of shoulder and not beyond center of body. Bring arm back so hand does not go beyond crest of hip, a relaxed piston-like movement.

* * *

Short sprints develop speed.
Distance running develops endurance.
Running in circles and figure 8's strengthens ankles, knees, hips and back.

* * *

The yearly conditioning program at the University of Oklahoma follows. (Take into consideration that we work on rehabilitation the year round.)

JUNE:

Run two or three times a week, distance plus exercises.

JULY-AUGUST:

Five weeks before the start of fall football practice we send each boy a weekly post card of activities that we request be performed daily. The cards are to be properly marked and returned to our office at the close of each week. A sample of the daily activities are:

Mile jog.

15 minutes of calisthenics and stretching exercises.

10 to 30 yard quick starts.

Mile at a good pace.

By the first day of fall football practice each athlete should be in condition to play a regulation game if it were necessary. If he watches his weight and works hard and faithfully, he will have no trouble reporting back in tip-top condition. The athlete should post the daily exercises in his bedroom.

If Post-Season Game:

December—practice.

January—nothing.

February-March—an organized off-season conditioning program (HPER 103) which meets three times a week for a period of 50 minutes of all-out activity. The class consists of strength, quickness, mat, running, and agility drills. Weights are assigned for spring practice.

If No Post Season Game:

December—nothing.

January—run, exercises, handball, weights, etc.

February-March—same as above.

April-May—spring practice: Tuesday, Wednesday, Thursday and Saturday for five weeks. Assign weights for fall practice.

Weight Lifting as Part of the Program

Weight lifting, like any other activity, is an ideal form of exercising if not carried to an extreme. Weight lifting alone is not recommended. It should be a part of an over-all program.

In regard to agility, muscle mass and endurance, Dr. Robert Brashear, orthopaedic surgeon of Knoxville, Tennessee, made the following comments in his booklet on "Athletic Injuries": "Whether one is trying to rebuild a weakened muscle postoperatively or whether one is trying to develop a boy's muscles, he must strain his muscles to the ultimate if he is to build muscle mass. We develop grace and agility by handball and boxing, by fancy diving . . . and even by doing the jitterbug. We develop endurance by running up and down the stadium steps, but we never develop muscle mass except by strain."

A suggested weight-lifting program for football players is as follows:

BUILDING STRENGTH, POWER, BODY BULK

Breathe in deeply when lifting, exhale when lowering. In the first six exercises below, start with 40 to 50 pounds and increase the weight five to ten pounds per session. Athletes should build up to maximum weight, with 15 repetitions of each exercise done in three series of five each. These exercises should be done three times a week, with adequate warm-up before each exercise (running, stretching exercises, and rope-skipping).

1. To develop spring, initial charge, ankles, body balance and strength:

Calf Raises. Place a weight on back of neck, feet eight inches apart, body straight. Raise up on toes as high as possible.

2. To develop leg power and strength, back strength, explosive power, increase size of thoracic cage (good weight-gaining exercise):

Knee Bends. Place a weight on back of neck, feet 12 to 14 inches apart, heels flat on ground, toes pointed slightly outside, head up, shoulders back, buttocks low. Squat down *three-fourths* knee flexion, return to starting position. If weight is too heavy, do only a half squat. (*Do not do a deep knee bend.**)

3. To strengthen upper back muscles, pulling power, shoulder snap, fingers and wrist:

Rowing Motion. Feet 24 to 30 inches apart, head up and forward, knees straight but not stiff. Lift weight from ground to chest and return. [*This should be done carefully with no jerking motion.*]

4. To strengthen lower back, shoulders, wrist and fingers:

Stiff-Legged Dead Lifts. Bar on floor in front of feet, feet 12 to 15 inches apart, legs and arms straight. Bend at waist and grasp bar in middle of hand grip. Straighten back and lift weights up to low abdomen. Lower weights to ground in same manner as they were picked up.

5. To develop upper body, shoulders, chest, forearm and elbows:

Bench Press. Lie flat on back (on bench), with feet on ground. Grasp bar on outside edge of grip of bar. Elbows are placed wide and along line of bar. Lift weights straight up, extend elbows.

6. Best all-around strength exercises. Neck, arms, back and legs:

Place feet under bar and about 12 inches apart, toes slightly outward, head high, back and arms straight, heels down. Bend at knees and grasp bar, arms and back straight. Lift bar to low abdomen, keeping arms and back straight. Lower to ground with same body movements.

7. To build up knee and thigh:

Quadriceps Lift. Use iron boot or table. Sit on table, knee bent. Lift foot, knee straight. Use maximum weight and lift three series of ten (30 lifts total). *Hamstring Lift.* On stomach or standing, use iron boot and raise knee to right angle. Same technique as quadriceps lift.

8. To build up or prevent shoulder injury:

Bar Hang. Five chins and two minutes of hanging at arms' length.

Heavy resistance with low repetitions builds strength, and high repetitions with less resistance builds endurance.*

---

*Italics added by author.

The Ingredients of Greatness

As part of athletes' mental conditioning, the following qualities and applications can be posted in the training room.

C-oncentration
H-eart
A-ttitude
M-odesty
P-ractice
S-acrifice

Coaching

The coach himself has a responsibility in the program of prevention of injury that can be exercised by no one else. A great deal of the time and effort of the coach must be spent on fundamentals. The player must be taught to improve his agility. He must have extensive work on coordination. He must be instructed as to the proper stance. The player who is constantly alert, whose muscles are in balance and who is prepared for motion in any direction will usually not be hurt. The injury most often comes at a moment when the player is off guard and unprepared for the blow. In football training, the coach should teach him how to protect his head and neck in tackling, how to block most effectively and avoid injury to himself and how best to avoid the bruising block or the damaging tackle. The rules of sport are so designed as to minimize injuries and the coach will advise the players to obey the rules, not only because it is proper but also because if everyone obeys the regulations, there is less chance that anyone will be hurt. An illegal maneuver by one player invites retaliation by another. Proper coaching will keep this to a minimum.

Attitude

The attitude of the player is all-important from the standpoint of prevention of injuries. Here the combined efforts of the whole organization are important. The coach, the trainer, the physician, the specialist—each has his part to play. Attitude is, however, the primary responsibility of the coach and the trainer. The player's desire to play, to excel, to do a good job, will stimulate him to carry out those things needed to reach this goal. In order to play well he will recognize that he must be in good condition, and recognition is the first step toward accomplishment. The player must have confidence in his own ability. This confidence arises from his knowledge that he is in excellent condition and that he can put out maximum effort without exhaustion or injury. The player must be tough. *This does not imply that he must be mean or dirty.* It simply means that he must be physically tough so that he can take whatever physical punishment is required to accomplish the desired end. He must be physically stronger per pound than his opponent. This can come only from excellent conditioning. Given the desire to play, self-confidence, mental alertness and a tough physical condition, he must then learn to play with "carefree abandon." This does not mean he should be reckless, but that he should not be apprehensive and fearful. If the coach can inculcate this spirit in the minds of his players, he will find a sharp decrease in the number of disabling injuries among them. This is an extremely important product of physical conditioning.

ENVIRONMENT

It is also important that proper environment for athletics be available, since this can be a major deterrent to injury.

Artificial Turf Versus Natural Grass

The interest in artificial turf continues because of the advantage of having a uniform and constant playing surface. I constantly get inquiries about the relative merits of artificial turf versus natural turf and, as a matter of fact, about the various types of artificial turf. When Astroturf and other types of artificial turfs were first introduced, much was said about their importance in the prevention of injuries. I will not discuss statistical evidence because I have found, particularly in relation to the care of the athlete, that statistics are very unreliable. Without any particular change in conditions, a team may have multiple serious injuries one year and none the next. I remember one bowl game in which the promoters of the bowl had just put in artificial turf. Between halves they spoke about how it would eliminate knee injuries. Within the next quarter, the University of Oklahoma lost two of its star players by ligament injuries of the knee. My point is that artificial turf is not a revolutionary thing that should be opted for by every school. The distinction between artificial and natural turf is a subtle one and making a comparison is difficult. If you compare the best type of artificial turf with the best type of natural turf, the natural turf will probably come out ahead. But if you compare artificial turf with some of the fields that are in use, that is, converted baseball fields or fields that are shy of grass or ill-prepared, there is no question that the artificial turf will prove superior.

Certainly one can say categorically that artificial turf has not prevented injuries. As far as I can tell it has not had much effect on knee ligament injuries, although it has increased contusion-type injuries. Various foot conditions, such as first toe injuries from snubbing—including injuries to the toenail, the interphalangeal joint, etc.—seem to be more frequent (Fig. 1). The artificial turf, particularly after it gets a bit worn, becomes very hard. As a result, turf burns are almost inevitable on the elbows and on the knees and are not completely prevented by adequate padding.

I have some personal feelings about the effect of artificial turf on shoulder injuries. I have noticed, both in the teams I see regularly and in the consultations that I get, that the frequency of collapsing-type injuries of the shoulder girdle is definitely higher with the use of artificial turf. This is based on my personal experience and observation; it is not statistical data. A mechanism as to how this type of injury may occur is as follows: The player falls on his side with one shoulder down, the other shoulder obviously up, and somebody falls onto the raised shoulder. Whereas with well-maintained natural turf there is considerable "give" in this situation and the shoulder can collapse into the turf somewhat, with artificial turf no such collapse is possible. The result is an increase in collapsing-type injuries of the shoulder. Sternoclavicular injury, which in the past has been very infrequent, is showing up to a greater extent now. Acromioclavicular injury, a long-time bane of the athlete, certainly has not diminished. Contusion injuries of the rotator cuff or acromion have definitely increased.

As stated previously, it is difficult to compare artificial turf with natural turf. You would have to specify the type of natural turf. Is it a recovered baseball field with an elevated diamond and other artificial contour? Does it have very short grass? Are there bare areas? Natural turf with any of these characteristics is obviously not as good as artificial turf. However, if you compare artificial turf with a well-kept field in a climate with adequate rainfall and snow, if any, only late in the season, you will

Figure 1. Linear fracture extending obliquely into the MP joint as a result of jamming the big toe against the shoe. The shoe stopped and the toe jammed forward into the shoe. This type of injury seems more prevalent on the artificial turf.

find that natural turf will probably be better. In any event, we will continue to have both kinds of turf, and I do not think that either one has any real bearing on the incidence of major injuries.

Artificial turf has been found to be much less long-lived than had been anticipated. In many cases this is caused somewhat by the use of the same field for both practice and playing. This certainly does not occur on natural turf fields. Replacement of artificial turf should be done before it becomes like a "well-worn carpet" that can neither keep the players' feet from slipping nor protect the players from bruising. Some of the more sophisticated designs of natural turf, complete with irrigation systems, are far too expensive for most schools to obtain.

As artificial turf became popular it became a very good recruiting gimmick. Schools promoted the idea that the institutions with the more advanced programs would have artificial turf. I do not think that this concept is valid. A fine, natural turf may well be preferable to artificial turf. In our area, artificial turf is invading the high schools. This raises the question if one high school puts it in, will all the others have to? My own opinion is that there will be a gradual shift back to good, well-cared-for and well-drained natural turf. This may occur much more definitely in the southern areas of the United States where there is not a long season of cold and snow. Artificial turf may be distinctly better in some areas, although it is very cold when it gets wet and frozen. Dan Pickett, head trainer at the University of Oklahoma, has reported a definite increase in illnesses related to the extreme heat reflected off the artificial turf; temperatures often exceed 125 degrees.

The Playing Field

The university programs lay great stress on the condition of the field—not only the game field, which is often reserved for weekends, but particularly the practice field. The secondary schools do not have the advantage of adequate funds for constant supervision of their play areas. However, a little rudimentary care and common sense will accomplish the greater part of the same objectives. Each sport has its individual field requirements.

In *football,* the practice field should be level and preferably firmly sodded. At the beginning of the season, before it is used, the field should be carefully screened for all foreign material before it is used. If necessary, the squad can fan out and cover the field to remove rocks, boards, tin cans, paper and all the objects which may have accumulated on the field during the summer when it was out of use. Whoever mows the area should be instructed to remove all such foreign material, not just avoid it. Of perhaps even greater importance is the necessity for leveling the field. This does not simply mean that it should not be put on a hillside. It means that small imperfections should be filled. A person is more likely to receive an injury stepping into a gopher hole than he is running into a trench. He can avoid the larger imperfections but may fail to see the smaller ones. A few hours spent in so conditioning the field will be well worthwhile. It may be impossible to do much about the firmness of the terrain once the season starts. However, a little effort in the spring may pay dividends in the softening of the soil and obtaining cover with grass. Watering the field, if possible, helps immensely. A good playing surface is far more important than a fancy stadium, decorated goal posts, and the like, and comparatively little money spent on the field will produce gratifying results.

I do not believe anyone uses lime to mark the fields anymore. Certainly its use should be condemned. Ample room should be provided at the sidelines so that the player does not crash into obstructions such as stakes, brick piles, or fence rails if he runs out of bounds. Similarly, ample room should be provided at the ends of the fields, extending well beyond the end zone so that the pass receiver does not charge into a stone wall or fall over the curb of the running track. Safety equipment around the field is important. The markers should be nontraumatic. There should be no stakes driven into the ground as permanent markers unless they are flush with the surface. The "chain gang" should be instructed to throw their rods flat on the ground if the play approaches the sideline. Wooden benches should be kept well away from the sidelines. All these things seem quite rudimentary, but a season never passes that someone does not receive a serious injury from hazards that could have easily been removed.

Other sports, too, have their problems. The *basketball floor* should be smooth and free from splinters and not too slick. There should be ample room along the sidelines, even at the penalty of making the court narrower. Charging into a wall can result in breaking an arm, leg or skull, since the basketball player does not wear much protective equipment. The practice of hanging the goal at one end of the court just at the front of the stage is a dangerous one. There should be ample room to run under the basket at the ends. No foreign material should be allowed on the floor.

The *baseball field* presents equally important problems. Much attention is usually paid to the infield, and rightly so since irregularity of the infield causes many "bad bounces," and this is of interest to everyone. All too often the outfield is a weed patch. Grass is allowed to grow tall enough to conceal bricks, cans and stones, which are definite hazards. The sprinting fielder stepping into a hole in the ground receives the same type of injury as the football player but is less able to cope with it because he has less protective armor. The interest of the school in the baseball team can be stimulated by having the younger boys police the outfield.

In *track,* attention should be paid to the running surface. The curb should either be high enough that the runner will avoid it or else low enough that he will not flip his ankles if he hits it.

You may say that these things are not the responsibility of the physician. They are the responsibility of the physician if he feels himself responsible for the prevention of injuries.

There is little accomplished by conditioning a player well and then having him break an ankle as he steps into a hole where a dog has dug up a bone.

If it is necessary for play to take place on inadequate areas, certain precautions must be taken. There is no excuse for leaving debris around, since it can always be removed. If may be necessary, however, to play basketball on concrete or blacktop. It may be that some of the football fields are "hardpan" and cannot be remedied. In these circumstances more contact padding should be provided. Knee and elbow pads are mandatory. The wearing of full-length stockings may prevent painful abrasions on the legs. Long-sleeved shirts serve a similar purpose.

BALANCED COMPETITION

There is considerable controversy over the desirability of competitive athletics in the younger age groups. After many years of an active orthopaedic practice, it is my personal belief that the youngster is in much less danger under controlled competitive conditions than he is in ordinary backyard play. Certainly this is true from a physical standpoint. We see relatively few grade school youngsters with injuries from football. We see many with injuries from incidental things. The energy of the youngster is such that he is going to expend it doing something. He is safer under supervised athletics than he is walking along the top of a fence, climbing trees or playing in the streets. Neither do I go along with that group of my pediatric colleagues who believe that competition is dangerous for the youngster. From a practical standpoint the youngster is competitive soon after he is born. If the competition can be directed into proper channels, it can be a healthy thing and much more educational than being beaten up by the neighborhood bully. To a youngster the frustration of losing a game is no more severe than that of a baby who breaks a rattle, and it is equally short-lived. This is partcularly true if his competition has direction and understanding. He is taught to recognize that someone must lose each time someone else wins.

Competitive athletics does have a real responsibility with regard to equalization of the competitors. Most of the organized programs do this very well. The youngster is regulated not only according to age but according to size, so that the 200 pound 14 year old does not compete with the 85 pound 12 year old. This is a distinct improvement over the casual sand-lot games which are catch-as-catch-can and usually are dominated by some prematurely developed youngster.

Balanced competition is particularly necessary in the grade schools but also is important in the high schools. A small high school that is dependent upon a relatively small squad must of necessity have boys on the team who have something less than Olympic capacity. Hence, care should be taken in scheduling games that a team of immature boys does not compete with a juggernaut of excellent, well-trained athletes. This is not nearly as pertinent now as it has been in the past. Comparatively few teams now schedule a so-called "warm-up" or "breather." They usually start right out in competition with their equals. Much credit is due to the secondary school conferences, which make a real effort to match teams of equal capacity against each other. The danger of injury is thus minimized.

Many sports medicine committees which have studied the problem carefully, including the Sports Medicine Committee of the American Academy of Orthopaedic Surgeons and the American Orthopaedic Society for Sports Medicine, have stated that properly controlled competitive athletic programs not only are permissible but are desirable for the youngster. The well-organized programs will control the factors stated previously. Such programs should be particularly concerned with over-emphasis on winning, poor participation of the players, overenthusiasm by parents and over-ambition on the part of the coach.

EQUIPMENT

Athletic equipment has a great deal to do with prevention of injury. This is especially true of football, and most of our attention will be given to this sport. Good equipment is a must for a football program. We immediately run into the obstacle of an inadequate budget in many schools and for these a happy medium must be sought.

The physician must take a decisive part in directing the equipment phase of the preventive program. To do so he must inform himself, since ill-founded advice based on personal bias is a poor substitute for well-informed judgment. The first step is to determine what things are necessary and are within the budgetary capacities of the particular program. There are two somewhat competitive facets of this problem. Certain items of equipment will add to the ability of the player and so are very desirable from the standpoints of both coach and player. However, one should not allow too much emphasis to be placed upon this facet to the disadvantage of protective measures.

For convenience the items of equipment for the football player will be discussed beginning with the headgear and working down. I believe that this plan will serve our purpose better than an attempt to grade them according to necessity. Indication will be given as to the relative importance of the various pieces of equipment.

There have been vast improvements in *headgear* in recent years and these continue. The old felt headgear that fit like a skull cap did little more than dull the blow and is a far cry from the modern plastic suspension helmet of today. The most important single element of the helmet is the system of webbed suspension straps. Currently the so-called geodetic helmet is being used. It is modified by suspension strap system but has the forward anterior and posterior straps padded, which keeps the head from contacting the shell of the helmet. The player himself should be instructed about the purpose of the straps, since only he can really tell whether the fit is proper. The helmet should protect the back of the neck and should fit so that when the neck is extended, the helmet does not drive into the back of the neck but rather slides down it. The front of the helmet should protect the forehead. The ear pieces should fit well over the ears. The orifice for hearing should coincide with the external auditory canal. *It is obligatory that some sort of bar be worn to protect the face.* There has been much experimentation with these bars. One of the most effective is a single bar so placed to make it difficult for the knee or elbow to reach the eye or nose, but protecting the mouth as well. Double bars are more expensive and probably are not necessary for routine use, although they may be needed in specific circumstances. Attempts to use a wide plastic bar have failed because the player tries to see through the plastic with resultant distortion of vision. *The headgear is the most important single piece of equipment.*

The player with a fractured nose or malar bone will require a double bar or "bird cage" to more fully protect the area around the front of his face. The player with an injury to the jaw will need a bar placed lower to protect the mandible. Incidentally, the players must be sternly instructed that they must not grab the bar of their opponent. All of this is designed to protect the wearer of the helmet. Currently there is considerable agitation over the hardness of the helmet in terms of its striking the opposing player. The plastic shell is extremely hard. Its blow is cushioned somewhat by the fact that it is not at the end of a rigid pole, so that there is a certain recoil element when the head of the player hits the opponent. There is continued effort to reduce the potential for injury implicit in the headgear so that it is hard enough to protect the wearer yet resilient enough to protect the opponent (Fig. 2). The use of a mouthpiece is universally accepted as mandatory for the football player. Most of the high schools and many of the football conferences in college require it. Some of the players don't particularly like to wear a mouthpiece. I think this depends to a considerable extent on how well it is fitted. The dentists now have a very quick and accurate method of making these mouthpieces, and the mouthpiece should be made and fitted for each individual player. It used to be the mark of an athlete to have his two front teeth knocked out, but this is no longer true—nor is it necessary, since the mouthpiece should effectively prevent this.

Injuries to the *neck* are relatively common in football. Most of them are minor but may be quite distressing. Obviously the player should not play with a serious injury to his neck. After a sprain or during the recovery period, it may be desirable to protect his neck against excessive motion. This cannot be done well with adhesive, which is widely used elsewhere on the body, but quite effective use can be made of the so-called "cotton collar." This is actually a quilted pad narrower at one end than the other that is wrapped around and around the neck and fastened with suitable Velcro straps to support the chin, mandible and occiput. A very simple substitute is an ordinary turkish towel (see Fig. 2) folded lengthwise to about the width of the distance from the angle of the jaw to the shoulders and then wrapped firmly around the neck. This is quite effective for the player who occasionally gets a "pinched nerve" in the neck, since it serves to prevent the motion that causes the pinching. A resilient "horse collar" is commercially available and is also effective.

Most modern *shoulder* pads are not too effective in preventing injury to the shoulder girdle. Ideally they should be designed to protect the sternum and clavicles and particularly the acromioclavicular areas. The cap that extends over the deltoid serves to prevent painful contusions in this area. The most important attribute of any shoulder pad is that it fit the wearer. Too frequently the player picks his

Figure 2. Protective equipment—neck, face and head. Upper two rows illustrate different types of football face protection. (Courtesy of Rawlinson, "Modern Athletic Training," © 1961 by Prentice-Hall, Inc.)

1. Mouthpiece
2. Headgear snubber—protects bridge of nose
3. Oral screw

4. Tongue forceps
5. Face guards for sports other than football
6. Rolled towel

own pads out of a pile, and he is unable to judge a proper fit. Someone should see that the pad actually fits to protect the parts it is designed to cover. A common injury to the front of the arm is the so-called "blocker's spur," which may often be caused by the edge of the shoulder pad itself rather than by the opponent. If the shoulder has been injured, more adequate support can be obtained from the so-called "Big Boy," or a double cantilever pad. A properly fitted foam rubber or plastic pad may be placed judiciously to protect bruised areas. Straps and strings should all be intact (Fig. 3).

Elbow pads are usually not worn unless there is a specific indication. The person with an olecranon bursitis, abrasion over the elbow or anything else of this nature should wear a suitably fitted pad. This applies to basketball as well as football players.

Simple coaptation foam rubber or plastic splints may be used on the *arm* or *forearm* to protect an injured area (Fig. 4). No unyielding fiberboard or plastic splint may be used below the elbow.

A suitable protective pad should be applied to the *hand* over injured areas. Again, great care must be exercised. A rigid pad is not permissible. Protective wrapping of the normal hand, utilized by many professionals, is increasing in popularity among the unversity

players. However, a recently developed plastic foam pad protects the back of the hand, leaving the front of the hand free, and is much less bulky and less awkward than the larger pad.

Properly fitted shoulder pads protect the upper part of the *chest* quite adequately and we would not ordinarily recommend supplemental chest pads. Fractured ribs are best protected by circumferential strapping or a rib binder (see Fig. 4). The essential purpose of adhesive strapping of the chest is to limit the motion of the ribs on breathing. In order to accomplish this, the strap must completely encircle the chest, since taping one half of the chest will not adequately prevent motion of the ribs. This circumferential wrapping is not compatible with the deep breathing necessary for active participation in a sport. In fact, it is designed to prevent deep breathing. In the second place, the fractured rib is not well protected by a contact pad at the tender site, since pain in the ribs comes as much from compression or expansion of the chest in any diameter as it does from a direct blow. Indeed, compression injury is more likely to hurt than a blow over the tender area. Contusions, however, are troublesome, since any direct contact with them causes pain. The contusion may involve the skin or underlying bone and both can be well protected by a fiber pad, one of the most effective being the pad with a sponge

Figure 3. Protective equipment—shoulder, arm, elbow and hand. (Courtesy of Rawlinson, "Modern Athletic Training," © 1961 by Prentice-Hall, Inc.)
1. Heavy duty linebacker, big boy shoulder pads
2. Double cantilever shoulder pad (two rolls of paper denote the double cantilever)
3. Protection for under a shoulder pad
4. Home-made bruise pad—takes pressure off the shoulder
5. Shoulder harnesses (dislocations, strains and sprains)
6. All-purpose injury pad with hole cut in top

Figure 4. Protective equipment—shoulder, arm, elbow and hand (continued). (Couresty of Rawlinson, "Modern Athletic Training," © 1961 by Prentice-Hall, Inc.)

1. Elbow bruise pad
2. Fracture glove
3. Sternum or chest injury pad—lace to shoulder pads
4. Upper arm bruise pad—fiber and sponge rubber
5. Forearm pad
6. Hand pads
7. Rib belt
8. Resusitube Airway
9. Bandage scissors
10. Tape cutter
11. Handle of a spoon made into a finger splint
12. Felt thumb pads

rubber or plastic doughnut around its margin, which holds the pad away from the injured part. A supply of this type of contact pad is inexpensive, and will add to the ease and comfort of the competitor.

Although the use of a vest to hold padding in place is a longstanding practice, a recent development has been the use of a vest of very lightweight material with compartments that cushion and prevent the shock of a direct blow. Unless this vest is put on snugly, however, it does not prevent motion of the ribs upward with inspiration. It will protect against a direct blow, but the major pain from a broken rib is from motion as the chest expands on inspiration. The pain is more notable when the player is "panting" for breath. The best way to prevent this pain is to strap the *lower* ribs circumferentially to prevent elevation of the ribs and encourage diaphragmatic breathing.

Since the *abdomen* is essentially soft, there is no requirement for contact padding here. The player with deep abdominal tenderness, as from liver or spleen injury, should not compete. The back of the abdomen or flanks is best protected by pads built into the pants or a belt-type pad that incorporates two contact pads running along either side of the spine to protect the so-called "kidney area" (Fig. 5). The football pants themselves contain padding for the iliac crest and trochanters. Here again, well-arranged contact pads may protect tender areas, provided always that the underlying pathological condition is not such that competition should be prohibited. The athletic supporter is a must and no player should be allowed to practice or compete without one. The popular jockey shorts are not an adequate substitute for a well-fitted athletic supporter. If there has been injury to the genitalia, with a painful testicle, a more protective type of support may be utilized, although this type is not particularly comfortable and is awkward to wear.

Most of the football pants incorporate a quadriceps pad that covers the front and lateral aspects of the *thigh*. Many of these pads are quite inadequate. If they are built into the pants leg, the latter should fit very snugly or the pants should be strapped down with adhesive. A loose thigh pad does far more harm than good, since its edge may cause the very injury it is designed to prevent. In case of painful injury the pad may be strapped to the thigh with adhesive, preferably elastic in type. Anything constrictive around the thigh has the

Figure 5. Protective equipment—groin, pelvis, buttocks and back. (Courtesy of Rawlinson, "Modern Athletic Training," © 1961 by Prentice-Hall, Inc.)

1. Tail piece and hip pad
2. Hip injury pad
3. Low back injury pad
4. Rubber slingshot bandage
5. Hip pad
6. Pads for protection of a bruised hip
7. Back brace

potential of reducing its blood supply and causing muscle cramps. This does not occur as frequently in the thigh as in the calf, but it may occur. The strapping should be snug but not tight. The protective pad prevents contact injury only. If the muscle itself is damaged, active motion of the muscle is the danger and this is not prevented by any pad. Similarly, contact pads are useless in protecting the hamstrings against strain either at their attachment to the pelvis or at the musculotendinous junction in back of the thigh.

The normal *knee* is usually not strapped to prevent injury. Occasionally the boy who has grown rapidly to 6 feet or so but still has immature joints may feel that his knees are insecure and want to wear some type of protection. It is extremely difficult to protect the knee against the most common type of injury, namely, injury to the medial collateral ligament mechanism due to external rotation of the leg with the knee slightly flexed, with or without forcible contact against the lateral aspect of the knee. The ordinary pull-on elastic bandage is worthless protection here. It may add to the player's feeling of security, but if tight enough to do much good, it may also constrict his circulation.

If the knee has been injured, the protective wrapping becomes important. It then has some design, namely, to prevent recurrence of a particular type of stress injury. Here again, the pull-on or wrap-on elastic bandage is of little value, since it does not in any way protect against lateral or rotary stress. One must also question the value of an elastic pull-on bandage that incorporates a short metal bar or hinge either on one or both sides. The bar is not long enough to prevent leverage action of the leg and thigh. It is cumberstone and at best is inconvenient to wear. There are almost as many modifications of knee braces as there are people treating injured knees, a sure indication that not one of the braces is particularly good. Recently the aim has been to produce a corset-like brace that is longer and therefore more effective than those currently available. The present tendency is to apply a brace that is a good deal more complicated and actually does limit excess stress on the ligaments. One disadvantage is that it is difficult to wear and has to be precisely fitted. Another device, which is strictly in the developmental stage, is a brace with some sort of shock-released mechanism that will suddenly tighten the straps in the brace. In other words, when the brace is worn regularly, the straps are loose enough not to be binding, but when the player receives

a blow on the side of the leg, the straps immediately tighten. One objection to this type of brace is that not all ligament injuries are caused by direct blows, thus negating the rapid-release mechanism for ligament support.

Many players with greater or lesser knee disabilities are attached to one or another type of support. If this support gives them confidence and they feel it helps, I think it is permissible to use it. It will not prevent reinjury. If there is swelling in the knee, particularly effusion, and it is mild enough to permit the player to participate, it is proper for him to wear a pull-on or wrap-on elastic bandage in order to prevent further stretching of the suprapatellar pouch. All of these bandages have the doubtful virtue of restricting flexion of the knee and so to some extent they may prevent overstrain by the deep knee bend or duck waddle position.

If the knee actually needs protection for a weak ligament, such as the medial collateral, it can be best obtained by adhesive strapping. Cross strapping of the knee either on one or both sides as illustrated (Fig. 6) gives considerable protection against the knee's "springing open" on the injured side. Owing to the bipod nature of the femoral condyles, it is usually necessary that the condyle of the femur and the tibial plateau actually separate to put stress on the medial collateral ligament, and this can be minimized by adequate strapping. The cross-hatch strapping also to some extent restricts rotation of the leg on the thigh and so the familiar position of external rotation-abduction is prevented. We now believe that the medial collateral ligament capsular fibers can be damaged without an actual separation between femur and tibia. The taping described helps to prevent the rotation that may cause the tearing.

If the injury to the knee was caused by hyperextension, strapping to prevent hyperextension (Fig. 7) will be much more effective than any permissible brace. Each trainer has his own methods of strapping, and one who intends to do this sort of preventive strapping should familiarize himself with the various methods and practice them. Some prefer regular adhesive, others, elastic adhesive. Actually, I believe a combination of the two is probably best. The newer type of elastic tape that stretches laterally rather than lengthwise gives much firmer support than the regular elastic type and conforms well to rounded surfaces. By the very virtue of its firm support, it allows somewhat less mobility.

The knee also needs to be protected against

Figure 6. A method for strapping the knee to support the lateral collateral ligaments (x). The criss-cross straps should cross in the midline. Maximum support for this dressing is medially and laterally, but it is also effective against rotatory stress between tibia and femur, especially if both sides are taped as illustrated here.

Figure 7. Strapping of knee to prevent hyperextension. Note that the leg is positioned with the knee slightly flexed. A convenient way is to have player stand on the table with a 3 or 4 inch block under the heel.

direct contact. Most football pants have knee pads, although in most cases they are woefully inadequate. However, they are far better than nothing and I think every school should have a rigid requirement that these pads be worn. This is even more important in a secondary school. I insist on this requirement in the secondary schools because in these young people the cartilage of the patella and of the femoral condyle is more susceptible to injury, and irreparable damage may be done to these areas by direct impact. This is particularly pertinent because many of the fields of play are very hard, and the youth is likely to pay for his indiscretion not only by a ruined football season but by permanent damage to the knee. It is the responsibility of the physician, trainer or coach to insist on the wearing of proper protection of the knee against direct contact.

In most sports, *leg* protection is not necessary. The exceptions are such games as soccer and hockey. It is self-evident that athletes who play certain special positions, such as the baseball catcher, require leg protection. Painful areas in the legs may be protected by contact pads.

There has been constant debate as to the virtue of support of the *ankle* during competition. It is my considered opinion that in football every player should have his normal ankles wrapped for every practice or game session. Many players will resist this, since they feel it may diminish their agility. However, when the situation is explained to them, they will almost always accept the wraps gratefully. It is very easy to learn to put on an ankle wrap. The Louisiana wrap (Fig. 8), or some modification, is perfectly adequate. The wraps are inexpensive. They can be laundered easily, and there is no excuse for not insisting on them if the athletic administration concerned agrees they are valuable. The ankle wrap does not restrict ankle motion per se at all, since ankle motion is simply dorsal and plantar flexion. It does restrict lateral motion somewhat, but even tarsal motion is not greatly restricted. It is protective against excessive tarsal motion, however, and so will effectively reduce the danger of sprain. It is difficult to sprain an ankle that is protected by a well-placed ankle wrap unless the force is a major one, sufficient to tear the wrapping.

If the ankle has been previously injured, the ankle wrap probably will be inadequate, and one should resort to adhesive tape. One should familiarize oneself with a good standard method for taping and learn to do it well (Figs. 9 to 14). The tape has the advantage that it may be extended up as high on the leg as is desirable. The greater the protection needed, the higher the strapping should go. Since the tape is placed on the skin, there is a certain amount of "give" in the bandage, but the further the strip extends up the leg, the less the resultant play and the firmer the fixation. If the strapping is applied because of an old injury, it should vary according to the part to be protected, since different types of strapping will be required for the lateral and the medial ligaments (see Fig. 10), the arch (see Fig. 11), the metatarsal area (see Fig. 12), the tendo Achillis (see Fig. 13), and the dorsiflexors (see Fig. 14).

Which type of *shoe* is best for the football player is a debatable question. There is no doubt that a high shoe protects the ankle and foot better than a low one, but many players feel that they are much more active in a low-cut shoe. Presumably a low-cut shoe plus the ankle wrap should be adequate. However, the high shoes do not replace the ankle wrap. The player cannot be relied upon to lace his shoes tight enough to give support and yet not so tight as to be uncomfortable. I believe the ankle or foot that has been injured should be fitted with a high shoe.

So, too, there is considerable argument about the type of cleat. The value of certain types of cleats will depend a good deal upon the terrain. Many factors argue against long, pointed cleats. They have a real disadvantage on frozen surfaces as well as on hard ground, as well as on matted bermuda, which may catch the cleat. Some players feel that the hold secured by the pointed cleat on the sod will prevent injury, whereas the proponents of the opposite view believe that its fixation to the ground may encourage injury. In any event the cleat, whatever type is used, should be properly placed on the shoe and should be intact. A broken cleat is a danger not only to the opponent but also to the player himself, since it gives him insecurity when he expects security. The football shoe leaves an unprotected peg sticking out when the cleat breaks off. This is indeed a lethal weapon. Also, running on this peg concentrates force on a very small area and is likely to result in a disabling bruise of the plantar surface of the foot.

There has been much indecision about the proper shoe for artificial turf. Certainly the long, pointed cleat is not the best. The present

Figure 8. Louisiana ankle wrap. This requires a 100 inch web ankle bandage. The start of the wrap is shown in the upper left drawing and is continued at the upper right, then lower left. At 7 the starting point is reached. The wrap is continued in this same fashion, with overlapping of turns, until the bandage is exhausted. Directly to the right, one complete turn of the bandage is shown. This is not the whole wrap. The bandage may be applied over a heavy sock, as shown, but wrinkles must be avoided.

Figure 9. Taping procedure. If this taping is for a previously injured ankle, the long strips should extend higher on the leg. Views 3 and 4 are direct Gibney strapping. Views 5 and 6 add the "heel lock," View 5 to help prevent eversion and View 6 to help prevent inversion. The two combined give much better stability but also less mobility. (Courtesy of Rawlinson, "Modern Athletic Training," © 1961 by Prentice-Hall, Inc.)

A

B

C

D

Figure 10. Typical Gibney strapping. *A*, Patient holding the foot with a loop of muslin to keep it at the right angle and inverted or everted as the case may be, depending on the location of the sprain. *B*, First strip of one inch adhesive tape that begins well back on the calf, at the bulge of the calf, extending down under the heel and up the opposite side. If the sprain is a lateral sprain, the strip should start on the medial side and come to the lateral side. *C*, Other portion of the weave, a strip running from the base of the first toe around the ankle and back to the base of the fifth toe. *D*, Application of successive strips, as many as necessary to reach the front of the foot. The horizontal strips should not overlap in front. If the strapping is for a chronic case in which swelling is not a factor, it would be more secure to overlap the strips in front. The whole thing is secured by a circumferential strip around the top of the dressing and then further secured by gauze bandage. It should be emphasized again that in an acute case there should be no circumferential wrapping overlapping on the front of the foot or on the front of the ankle.

Figure 11. Drawing shows a classical arch strapping on an adult male. Strips of one inch adhesive tape are necessary. Strip 1 starts just above the lateral malleolus and passes under the heel up the inner side of the foot to above the bulge of the calf. Strips 2, 3 and 4 pass up the leg in a similar course; the number of strips used depends somewhat on the size of the leg. As strips 5, 6 and 7 reach the front of the ankle, they are then twisted across the front of the leg to the lateral side. Five or six strips are utilized with the arch strapping extending clear up and clear forward to the base of the head of the metatarsals. Strips are anchored at the calf and above the ankle with one or more circumferential strips. If the injured arch is high, a felt pad should be inserted under the arch and held in place by short strips of tape, particularly if a flat support shoe is worn. This felt pad is probably not necessary in a shoe having a heel and a good support.

Figure 12. Strapping for the metatarsal area.

Pad

Circular
bandage

Figure 13. Strapping for the Achilles tendon. This is strapping of the ankle in plantar flexion; a strip extends from the toes, under the arch of the foot and up the back of the leg. The posterior strip of two inch tape is the most important here. The other strips give added security and help fix the initial strip.

Figure 14. Strapping for the dorsiflexors. The dorsiflexion is overdone in this drawing and will interfere with running. Neutral position (right angle) is desired.

trend (1980's) is toward the soccer-type shoe with multiple, short cleats. It also makes some difference whether the field is wet or cold, or both. Sometimes in these instances a basketball-type shoe will grip better.

It is extremely important that the shoe be well fitted, since a shoe that is too tight or too loose will inevitably give trouble. This is true whether the shoe is for football, basketball, baseball or track.

The feet are extremely vulnerable to minor ailments, such as blisters, athlete's foot, stone bruise, and so forth, and the player should be instructed early in his career as to their proper care.

Although the education of the player in aspects of injury prevention may seem to be a forbiddingly comprehensive problem, it actually will require relatively little time. Much of the instruction can be given en masse to the whole squad, and a few minutes of explaining to the players that prevention is in the individual interest of each one and should be his responsibility will be of great value. This must be followed by inspection. At first this should be carried out at relatively frequent intervals. Once the season is under way, however, the routine will be so established that only an occasional inspection will suffice, and this can be done in the course of other instruction with the expenditure of little extra time. For example, a method to determine whether or not the athletes actually have their ankles wrapped properly during the practice session is to have them remove their shoes on the field while the coach is talking to them at the end of practice. The players who have their ankles properly wrapped are permitted to go on in and shower at the conclusion of the talk. Those who do not must remain for another work-out. Such measures are not unduly punitive and serve to call attention to the fact that observance of the regulations is important to the staff.

There is nothing more rewarding than to conclude a football season with the players in better condition than when they started. As in all fields of medicine, prevention is far better than cure.

part

II

GENERAL PRINCIPLES OF TREATMENT

3

Precepts and Examination

Some of the principles of treatment mentioned in the introduction merit repetition here. The basic treatment of the athlete is that of any young, healthy human. The most important consideration is that recovery be prompt and, above all, complete. Later in the book specific treatments for certain conditions will be detailed, but the same basic principles apply to each, modified according to the location and the degree of the injury.

PRECEPTS FOR THE CARE OF THE ATHLETE

THE FIVE A'S
1. ACCEPT ATHLETICS.
2. AVOID EXPEDIENCY.
3. ADOPT THE BEST METHOD.
4. ACT PROMPTLY.
5. ACHIEVE PERFECTION.

Prompt Examination Is Mandatory

Prevention is better than cure; but if injury occurs, the first step must be early recognition of the nature and the severity of the damage. There is usually no better time to determine the extent of an injury than when it happens. The practice of waiting to see is not compatible with the first principle of treatment of athletes, namely, prompt and specific care. As time passes, edema and inflammation supervene to cloud the picture. A careful, complete examination, done early, will often permit definitive treatment days or even weeks earlier than the "wait and see" method. Saturday's injuries should not be examined on Monday morning just to suit the convenience of the doctor or others. Once a decision concerning treatment is reached, it should be carried out confidently and completely. If a specialist is needed, he should be consulted early. It is disheartening

to examine a patient weeks after his injury and find that the time for proper treatment is long past.

Believe in the Value of Competitive Athletics

The physician must recognize that it is vital to this patient to be restored to athletic competition. If the patient believes that the doctor disparages the importance of athletics, a sympathetic link between patient and doctor is lost. A master violinist would not trust the treatment of his hands to one who believed fiddle playing to be unimportant.

Avoid Expediency

Too often outside influences may overbalance sound judgment. The player's desire to compete, overoptimism, failure to admit the extent of the damage, or hesitation to interfere with school attendance may lead the physician to adopt a "middle of the road" course. Strict medical evaluation, not temporary convenience, must be the deciding factor.

Adopt the Best Method of Treatment

Here too, a temporizing attitude is antithetical to good results. If you really believe the patient needs a cast, use it! If you think he should be on crutches, insist on it! If his ligament needs surgical repair, see to it! The best treatment is early treatment. Time is of the essence in obtaining a complete recovery in most injuries. It is particularly important in ligament and muscle-tendon injuries. See that the athlete understands the reasons for the proposed treatment program. Make it abundantly clear that he must accept responsibility for unauthorized departures from the treatment program. It is inexcusable for an athlete to remove a protective device during an athletic contest and then attempt to blame someone else if a complication ensues.

Above All, Treatment Must Be Prompt

Unnecessary delay is not compatible with good results in ligament, muscle-tendon and vascular injuries. "Don't hurry but don't fiddle" is as applicable here as it is in the operating room.

The Goal Must Be 100 Per Cent Recovery

It may not be possible to attain a perfect result in a given case, but if we do not try for it, we will never reach it. The young, well-conditioned athlete will tolerate whatever reasonable measures are necessary to give him complete recovery, and the doctor must resist compromise or unjustified complacency that tends to negate this goal.

The foregoing precepts will simplify the care of the athlete so that the physician, instead of dreading this responsibility, will learn to look forward to the patient who gives such prompt and gratifying results. It is an interesting fact that most of the principles set forth here are readily applicable to other aspects of medical practice.

EXAMINATION

Time

The optimum time for the first examination of the injured athlete is as soon after the injury as possible. The prevalent custom of making a superficial and hasty examination (often on the field) and then sending the player to the ice bag for several hours is certainly to be deplored. It may not be possible to examine the player at once, but the goal should be to examine him as soon as it can be done properly.

Place

Obviously, the first superficial examination of a player will be done on the field or on the sidelines. This can be little more than a cursory evaluation of the severity of the injury. If the injury is of any consequence, proper facilities must be available to make a detailed examination away from the crowd, preferably in a suitable examining room. At this time it will be possible to remove all the clothing from the part and all the protective strapping. The knee cannot be examined, for example, through a pair of football pants or over adhesive or elastic strapping. It follows that arrangements must be made to transport the player to suitable surroundings. It is highly desirable that this examination be carried out without the usual cluster of players, parents and fans gathering around and offering gratuitous advice.

Manner

In order to treat injuries to athletes successfully, one must cultivate the practice of detailed, meticulous examination. In the case of an extremity injury, an examination should first be carried out on the uninjured extremity for the purpose of comparison. This procedure also can allay the apprehensions of the injured player to some extent and prepare him for the type of examination that is to be carried out on the injured part. Then the examination itself must be performed in a tender manner, taking care to show the injured person that you have great concern for him and his injury. More detailed suggestions will be made under the appropriate headings.

History

The first step in the examination is the history. Try to obtain as accurate a story as possible from the player or other people concerned as to the mechanism of injury. Did the injury appear to be severe or did it seem mild? Was disability immediate or delayed? Was deformity originally present and later reduced either spontaneously or with help? Did the player feel something slip or tear? Obtaining a careful history may give a vital clue as to the nature of the pathological condition.

Physical Examination

By *observation* note the general appearance at the site of the injury. Observe the location of the swelling, any possible deformity, any damage to the skin or evidence of a direct blow.

By *palpation* determine the degree of underlying tension in the tissues, possible fluctuation caused by hematoma formation, and the presence of local heat, tenderness or crepitation.

By *manipulation* determine the range of pain-free motion, the location of pain on motion, significant instability or abnormal motion. For any given area it is well to develop a routine for examination designed to check all the stabilizing elements of that particular joint. For example, a knee should be checked not only for lateral stability in extension but also for lateral stability in partial flexion and for anteroposterior or rotatory stability. By overlooking any one of these, vital information may be missed in the course of the examination.

X-ray examination should be carried out both when fracture is manifest and when only suspected. In this day and age there is little excuse for failure to obtain x-ray visualization, since it is so readily available. X-ray examination is an art in itself, but it should be noted here that it is of little value to take excellent radiographs if they are not carefully studied and properly evaluated (Fig. 15). (See the following section on x-ray examination.)

With a complete examination of this nature, only the unusual case will not present a definite clue as to the proper diagnosis. If, for one reason or another, diagnosis cannot be made at the time of the first examination, repeated examinations must be made until the diagnosis is clear. Every effort should be made to make a definitive diagnosis at the first examination, since this will permit the institution of specific treatment at once. In any event, re-examination should be made from time to time in order to obtain an exact picture of the progress of the condition. Details of examination of individual parts will be given under appropriate sections. It cannot be overemphasized that successful treatment depends upon accurate diagnosis, which in turn depends upon a careful, all-inclusive, atraumatic examination of the injured part.

X-ray Examination

X-ray visualization is taken so much for granted now that one cannot justify the omission of this examination if any possibility of positive findings exists. It follows, therefore, that there will be many negative and, to some extent, useless x-ray examinations carried out. However, even if the examiner ignores the medicolegal complications (which he would indeed be bold to do), there is a good argument for generous use of x-ray visualization. The current agitation against overuse of x-ray need not apply to films made for diagnostic purposes, provided they are made under proper control with suitable equipment. The extremely rapid x-ray film in common use today entails minimal radiation exposure. A few confident words of explanation to the timorous will allay fears of over-radiation. One is justified in refusing management of a case in which x-ray visualization is not permitted.

However, it is not sufficient simply to order that a film be made of the injured part. Rou-

Figure 15. A radiograph *(A)* and a line drawing *(B)* of the shoulder showing posterior dislocation. On casual glance, no lesion is apparent. Careful inspection will reveal the head of the humerus medial to the glenoid convexity. In this case special views not routinely made will confirm the diagnosis (see Fig. 165).

Figure 16. *A,* "As is" view. Film made in an air splint reveals complete dislocation of the talus, rupture of the tibiofibular ligament, fracture of the medial and posterior malleoli of the tibia and a fracture of the fibula. Note the clarity with which all of this pathology is demonstrated. *B,* Anteroposterior view after careful positioning shows there to be a fracture of the medial malleolus and a fracture of the fibula. Although this would suggest the injury revealed in *A,* further testing is not necessary by manipulation to determine the pathology since the "as is" view demonstrates it exactly.

Figure 17. Case 1. Exostosis of tibia. Note that the lateral view (A) is negative. The anteroposterior view *(B)* is inconclusive as to the nature of the mass, whereas the oblique *(C)* reveals the tumor very distinctly.

Illustration continued on following page

Figure 17 *(Continued)*. Case 2. During blocking drill, this 22 year old football player felt something snap in his right hand. It swelled up and an x-ray was made, which was interpreted as being normal. *A,* Straight anteroposterior view shows a little change of density of the index metacarpal, as does the oblique (B). C, Special oblique view clearly reveals the nature of the pathology, the spiral, oblique fracture with displacement.

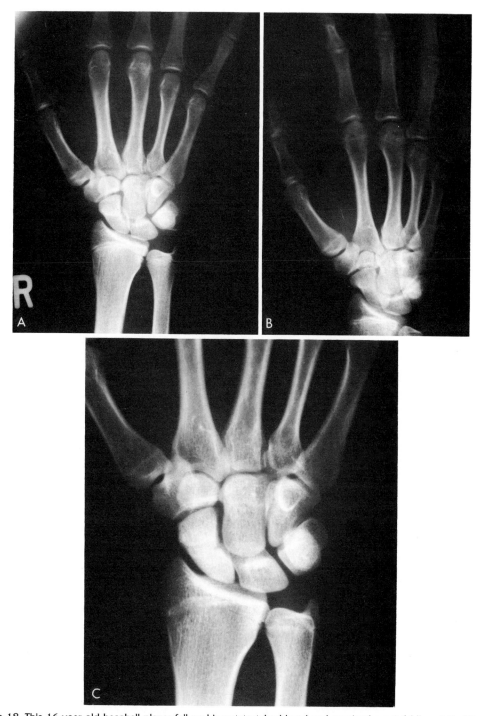

Figure 18. This 16 year old baseball player fell on his outstretched hand and received a painful "sprain" of the wrist. Radiographs *A* and *B* were interpreted as being negative. *C,* X-ray ten days later shows definite fracture through the navicular. This boy wore a protective splint during this interval. If there is any doubt about the possibility of a fractured navicular, a splint should be worn until recheck x-rays are made.

tine x-ray films, although they may be of some value, may not serve at all to rule out the presence of a lesion. The "as is" film may be extremely enlightening. Simply place the injured part over the x-ray film and take a picture of it without any positioning, holding or restraint. After this picture is made, then make the standard views. Very often the "as is" picture will be more enlightening than any other (Fig. 16).

The prevalent practice of sending a patient for radiological examination and having the film made by the technician or even the radiologist, who has no actual knowledge of the injury suspected, results in many faulty interpretations. The physician should know what he is looking for on the film and so advise the radiologist. He should himself be prepared to position the part to demonstrate the lesion he suspects. If anteroposterior and lateral views are not sufficient, other views should be made (Fig. 17). If abnormal motion is suspected, stress radiographs may be desirable. If the original films are negative, repeat films after seven to ten days may be diagnostic (Fig. 18). Once the x-ray film is made, it should be carefully studied, not only immediately but after the film is thoroughly dried and prepared for viewing. If doubt remains, views of the opposite extremity or further views of the injured part may be desirable. If the original film is inadequate technically because of over-exposure, underexposure, poor positioning or blurring due to motion, one should not hesitate to request repeat films. With such careful planning and adequate follow-up by the doctor, the x-ray examination may indeed be a valuable adjunct to the management of a given case. Definite suggestions as to positioning and the use of multiple views will be made when considering specific injuries (see Fig. 17).

Laboratory Examination

The laboratory examination has taken a larger place in athletic medicine in recent years. It is particularly important in the preliminary examination to determine whether or not the player should compete. Routine tests are not mandatory; however, it is quite simple to obtain a blood and urine evaluation. The electrocardiogram is valuable in the diagnosis of suspected heart lesions.

The laboratory may be quite valuable in the treatment of special conditions, as will be indicated in the text. The electroencephalogram and CAT scan in a head injury, cultures of infected wounds and tests for gout in severe joint inflammation are examples of tests that involve some expense and should be used only if indicated. Each should be used unsparingly, however, when a necessary part of the treatment.

4

Principles in the Management of Specific Injuries

CONTUSION

A contusion may be defined as a direct blow against the integument, causing bruising of the skin or underlying tissues. This results in capillary rupture and an infiltrative type of bleeding, followed by edema and inflammatory reaction. The result is local swelling which may be superficial or deep, depending upon the nature of the object striking the blow and the location involved. Thus the blow of the patella against the hard ground catches the skin between two hard objects and the resulting damage is to the skin and subcutaneous areas and possibly to the patella. On the other hand, the blow of a hard headgear against the unprotected thigh will catch the muscle between the headgear and the femur. The resulting damage is to the muscle, since the underlying soft tissue effectively protects the skin. The basic pathological change is the same regardless of the area involved or the type of blow.

Treatment. Proper treatment consists of limiting bleeding by application of cold and a pressure bandage in the early stages for 12 to 24 hours, together with immobilization and protection to prevent further injury. This is followed by measures to encourage healing. Local heat, rest and protection are vital at this stage. The area involved and severity of the involvement will determine the specific method utilized in a given case. Basically, the part must be protected from further damage by another direct blow or from overfunction or injudicious methods of treatment. Faradic stimulation, for example, should not be used early in a severely bruised muscle. Unless the bleeding is considerable and of major proportions, the local injection of hyaluronidase or local anesthetic is not justified. In extensive contusion, particularly of the thigh or back,

systemic medication with the various enzyme preparations may be of value.

Rehabilitation. Rehabilitation should begin slowly, within the limitations of pain, and should progress in parallel with the healing. Obviously a simple contusion may require little treatment or rehabilitation. However, when an extensive contusion occurs in a vital area, it may be difficult to restore function while continuing protection.

HEMATOMA

The athlete is particularly prone to hematoma formation, since he regularly exposes himself to the type of trauma likely to cause hematomas. For this discussion a hematoma will be defined as a collection of pooled blood within a relatively restricted area (Fig. 19A). Pooled blood is not blood which has infiltrated through soft tissues but rather blood which has collected in a localized area and has maintained its identity as blood. It can readily be appreciated that this pooling will occur in many situations, in many locations and from varying types of trauma, since the basic condition from the pathological standpoint is bleeding within the tissues. We do not ordinarily refer to bleeding within an anatomically closed space, as for example, in a joint, bursa or hollow viscus, as a hematoma. In hematoma formation, bleeding takes place into the tissues, and by virtue of pressure from the hemorrhage, the blood makes a space for itself which it wholly fills by pushing other tissues away. This may be extremely extensive, as in hematoma formation up and down the fascial planes of the back following a serious vessel rupture in the vicinity of the spine, or it may be extremely localized, as in the collection that forms be-

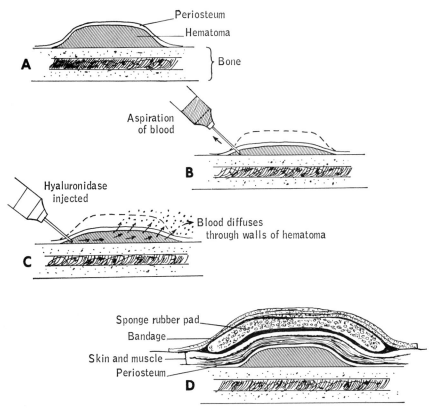

Figure 19. *A,* Cross section of a hematoma. In this instance the skin and subcutaneous tissue overlie bone and there is a collection of blood underneath the periosteum, well walled off. *B,* Needle extending into the hematoma with the blood aspirated and the walls partially collapsed. *C,* Showing hyaluronidase inserted into the hematoma with little arrows indicating the blood that then diffuses through the walls. *D,* Same hematoma with overlying pressure dressing, indicated by sponge rubber pad and bandage in cross section.

tween the skin and the periosteum over the shin.

Diagnosis. A superficial hematoma is easily recognized, but the diagnosis of a deep-seated hematoma may be difficult. The presence of fluctuation is pathognomonic, but this may indeed be difficult to determine deep in a muscle mass. In doubtful cases, diagnostic aspiration is justified.

Treatment. The treatment of hematoma must of necessity vary widely according to its location and extent. Treatment may be directed toward elimination of the hematoma itself or toward relieving pressure caused by it on an adjacent structure. The general principles of treatment consist of (1) prevention of further bleeding; (2) evacuation of the blood; (3) encouragement of absorption of the blood and (4) protection of the part until healing takes place.

During the diagnostic phase, even before definitive treatment is begun, pressure dressings should be applied to prevent further bleeding. An ice pack is used for the same purpose. Once it is determined that there is

enough blood present so that aspiration is possible, one may appreciably shorten the convalescent time by removing the blood (see Fig. 19*B*). Aspiration demands surgical aseptic technique. A large 15 or 16 gauge needle should be employed, since one could hardly expect to evacuate old blood through a 22 gauge needle. Following aspiration, the area should be infiltrated with hyaluronidase (see Fig. 19*C*), which tends to break down the confining wall and hasten the absorption of blood. Any attempt to aspirate a hematoma under any but the most aseptic conditions must be condemned. The dressing room or indeed the average training room is not the place for aspiration because the possibility of infection is particularly great in extravasated blood.

The center of a hematoma is to some extent like the center of an abscess. It may be quite avascular so that the circulating blood does not reach it, and many months may be required for absorption of the blood even in the absence of infection or other complications. The speed of absorption of the hematoma may be increased by diffusion of the hematoma, which is aided by the administration of hyaluronidase and the application of a pressure bandage (see Fig. 19*D*). These measures lead to more rapid absorption by bringing about greater exposure of the hematoma to the circulating fluids of the body, It has been said that it is unwise to aspirate a hematoma until it is certain that the bleeding has stopped because the increasing pressure of the hematoma itself will tend to discourage further bleeding. This is fallacious reasoning, since the same amount of pressure can readily be applied by external means. The hematoma should be evacuated as completely as possible, even at a very early stage, and then a pressure bandage will actually keep more pressure on the area than could intrinsic pressure from the blood alone.

Under certain circumstances, surgical evacuation of a hematoma may be justifiable. Certainly if the blood has coagulated and consequently is not aspirable, removal will shorten the recovery period. Various factors must affect the decision to operate. The extent of the surgical approach necessary, possible further damage to tissue already involved, damage to new areas by the approach and, above all, the condition of the skin should be weighed carefully against the possible benefits of evacuation. The utmost care must be taken to prevent infection. Any compromise in this area may lead to disaster.

When the area involved is an actively moving part of the body, it should be protected not only against a direct blow but also against motion, since motion tends to break down the clot within the vessels and to perpetuate the bleeding. Motion also tends to cause irritation throughout the lesion and to encourage over-reactive scar formation, calcification or ossification. Many a potential case of myositis ossificans has been aborted by careful protection of the part after proper local treatment. It is particularly important in muscle bleeding not to employ the "work it out" technique using massage, since this simply encourages further bleeding and promotes ossification. Absorption is also accelerated by the application of heat, which tends to improve the circulation of the area.

Protection against contusion should be continued as long as the area is symptomatic. However, protection against motion may be terminated much sooner. If the hematoma involves muscle, joint or a moveable part, mobility can be resumed *within the limits of pain* almost at once. Voluntary pain-free contraction will tend to aid absorption, but forcible exercise of a muscle containing a hema-

toma will only aggravate the pain. The dividing line between what is a good level of activity and what is deleterious may be very fine indeed. In many instances the athlete will be prone to minimize his symptoms in order to step up his activity, so that real acumen is required in judging how soon full activity may be permitted. Hematomas of more static areas, as under the skin, require protection during periods of bodily contact. The compression bandage should be removed whenever it is obvious that the liquid hematoma is no longer present, unless further support is needed because of circulatory embarrassment. It should be noted that following a relatively superficial hematoma there will be gross discoloration of the skin and that this may migrate a considerable distance if a pressure bandage is used. It is not at all unusual in the case of a hematoma over the shin or calf for ecchymosis of the skin to appear about the ankle or even in the foot. This occurrence is often alarming to the patient, and he should be reassured that it only represents a late stage in the absorption of the hematoma and does not indicate that his condition has grown worse or has extended. It is wise to warn the patient early that he may develop severe discoloration in the skin of the involved area and that it may take weeks to disappear.

To recapitulate:
1. Diagnosis should be prompt, with aspiration, if necessary, to make a final determination.
2. The volume of contained blood should be reduced by aspiration, hyaluronidase, pressure, cold first and then heat, and closely controlled activity.
3. Re-injury should be prevented by protection against trauma or against excessive activity.
4. Resorption should be encouraged by exposing the hematoma to a larger surface area of circulation, by improving the local circulation and by maintaining the general circulation.

Excessive scar formation, ossification or calcification can be prevented by the preceding measures.

MYOSITIS OSSIFICANS

Myositis ossificans is a frequent complication of the combination of contusion and hematoma involving the muscle near its origin on bone. The term is often used to include several conditions which may differ considerably. The name implies inflammation of a muscle followed by ossification. However, I do not think this often happens. Much more commonly there is ossification of infiltrated blood along the muscle origin on the bone. The condition may appear as a simple exostosis having a broad base with a sharp extension into the muscle and may seem to be an involvement of the periosteum rather than the muscle (Fig. 20). The muscle is merely displaced by the ossifying mass. In this type of case, the etiology is probably partial avulsion of the muscle fibers from the periosteum or a simple contusion of bone causing a subperiosteal hematoma. The mass is true bone and is firmly attached to the parent bone. In another type of so-called myositis ossificans, there is actually a plaque of bone lying within the muscle and separated from the bone by a layer of muscle. It is difficult to determine here just what causes the ossification. The most likely assumption is that some periosteal cells invade the hematoma at the time of injury and form true bone and that the condition is not a metaplasia of muscle into bone. A third condition which is also called myositis ossificans is the ossification about a traumatized joint or a fracture site. A hematoma in these locations will ossify as a result of the repeated insult to healing tissue (Fig. 21). In these instances there is no involvement of muscle whatever.

Etiology. Trauma is almost always the initiating cause of myositis ossificans. In the case of the long muscles, the cause may be repeated trauma such as occurs in the upper arm of the blocker in football as a result of the constant blows (see Fig. 20). It may be a single forceful blow, as on the quadriceps lateralis or intermedius (Figs. 22 and 23) in the anterior thigh, followed by active use of that part of the limb. It may be caused by unwise or excessive manipulation of a fractured bone (see Fig. 21). In all these conditions, one underlying factor is present, namely, repeated chronic irritation of an area already damaged. If blood infiltrates into the muscle and the muscle is put at rest, the chances are that this blood will be absorbed without further complication. If the muscle continues to be irritated by active use, by repeated blows, by unwise manipulation or by massage, these repeated insults superimpose a new injury over the early repair and the result is ossification.

Pathology. The process begins as an infiltrating hemorrhage either subjacent to bone or directly involving it. As healing progresses, instead of the orderly formation of scar to be replaced to a greater or lesser extent by normal tissue, osteogenesis occurs in the tissue and it is transformed into bone. This may be an extensive process or a very mild one, depending more upon the extent of the repeated insults than upon the original injury. This process tends to continue as long as the irritation continues. When the part is put at rest and the blood supply is improved by local heat, the ossifying process may be arrested. In

Figure 20. Myositis ossificans. *A*, Well developed but immature ossification. *B*, Completely mature ossified mass with wide base attached to the bone and spurlike projection into the muscle. *C*, One year after removal. No evidence of recurrence.

Figure 21. A year prior to the first examination, this patient dislocated his elbow and it was in a cast for nine days. One year later he dislocated his elbow again, and it was again in a cast for nine days. He returned to practice in one month and dislocated it once more. With each episode he had marked swelling. With his last injury eight days ago he had numbness of the ring and little fingers that gradually cleared up. A, X-ray from initial examination shows the ossification on the lateral side of the elbow. This is characteristic of repeated injuries with inadequate immobilization. It also shows an avulsion of the epiphysis of the medial epicondyle on the inner side. The fragment was removed and the muscle mass was secured to the epicondyle through drill holes. B, One year later. Note maturity of the ossification laterally, but with a large mass of bone. At this time he is asymptomatic except for restriciton of motion due to the lateral mass.

Figure 22. A, X-ray four months post injury, showing the definite osseous shadow along the proximal third of the femur. B, Six months later, this has almost completely regressed and disappeared.

Figure 23. *A,* Ossified mass in the quadriceps intermedius muscle overlying the anterior femur at six weeks (arrow). *B,* Six months later, following immobilization and controlled rehabilitation. Note regression of mass (arrow).

many instances the bone will be absorbed and the mass will shrink in size and disappear. In other instances, as the bone formation matures it becomes smaller (see Fig. 23) and terminates as normal bone in the form of an exostosis.

Diagnosis. Diagnosis is not difficult once the ossification has matured. It is much more important to recognize the impending pathological condition. If following a bruise on the thigh or arm a diagnosis is made of contusion with hematoma formation, and this condition does not promptly resolve, one should be on guard against formation of bone within the area. This explains why, in the discussion of contusion and hematoma, I insist that rehabilitation be carried out within the limits of pain and that reactivation of the area depend not upon any predetermined time but upon the subsidence of symptoms. X-ray films made early will be negative and should be repeated after two or three weeks if the symptoms persist. I have seen many cases in which the clinical examination demonstrated to my satisfaction a calcified mass within the muscle, but the radiograph showed only a little cloudiness (see Fig. 22). The symptoms disappear under proper management, and the result is a small flake of ossification either on the bone or in the underlying muscle. More often the result is complete resolution (Fig. 24).

Treatment. The early treatment of myositis ossificans is preventive and not surgical. *There is no place for operative treatment in the early stage of myositis ossificans.* As the impending condition is recognized, the muscle should be put at rest. Physical therapy in the form of heat is permissible but no passive manipulation should be done. Some active motion may be permitted within the restriction of the splint, but only if it is painless. So treated, the condition may well subside and become asymptomatic. Granted, there may be considerable

temporary stiffness of the part and much time will have elapsed, but a crippling condition will have been averted.

Rehabilitation. Rehabilitation should be carried out well within the limits of pain, at least for the first several months. (See Chapter 22.) Should the patient be seen after the ossification has occurred, the same treatment is instituted, namely, rest and inductive heat.

In the early stage, particularly in myositis ossificans around a long bone, the appearance is frequently that of a new growth, with characteristic laminations of ossification or sometimes the stellate sun-ray effect which may simulate osteogenic sarcoma. One should not ignore the history of trauma in a case of suspected bone tumor. There have been many cases of myositis ossificans mistakenly treated by operation for bone tumor, and major tragedies have resulted. This is particularly prone to occur because the biopsy of an early myositis ossificans will reveal actively growing young bone, very similar to callus. This may be indistinguishable from a neoplasm to the pathologist. Careful attention to the symptoms and above all to the course of the lesion is of value. Since myositis ossificans runs a relatively short course, at least in the expanding stage, a period of watchful waiting is justified in case of any doubt. In the meantime the part is put at rest and films are made at two-week intervals. In myositis there will be diminution of ossification or maturity of the margins; these characteristics are quite different from those seen in the development of an osteogenic type of tumor. Operation even for the purpose of biopsy may be disastrous (Fig. 25). A few weeks delay probably will be of little importance in the development of an osteogenic tumor.

As the healing progresses and the bone becomes more mature, more activity can be

Figure 24. *A*, Ossification in midarm that matured and disappeared within a year *(B)*. This probably represented bleeding into the periosteum.

permitted, again limited by pain. There should be no passive stretching, certainly not within the first six months, and the physiotherapist or trainer must be carefully instructed so that the patient's urge to hasten rehabilitation will be controlled. One must rigorously resist the use of surgery. Under the exigencies of sport, everyone is anxious to have the player rehabilitated and may feel that the sooner the operation is done, the quicker will be the recovery. This is one instance in which the reverse is true. Recovery will be quite prompt following removal of a mature exostosis, whereas it will be indefinitely postponed by an

attempt at removal of forming bone. See page 434 for a more detailed discussion of surgical treatment in myositis ossificans.

OPEN WOUNDS

This category of injury includes a wide range of conditions of varying severity, from a simple scratch on the skin to a compound fracture. A simple classification of breaks in the skin begins with an *abrasion*, which may be defined as a scraping and sliding injury to the skin, usually accompanied by a contusion as the

Figure 25. *A*, Early myositis ossificans. Rather typical case but operated on elsewhere when misdiagnosed as a malignancy. *B*, X-ray a few weeks postoperative showing marked increase in the size of the mass due to the meddlesome surgery. This should be left alone for at least six more months or longer if the mass does not appear to be mature. (Note two types of involvement in the first view: ossification along the periosteum and the oval mass completely separated from the periosteum.) Resection of mass after maturity resulted in good function.

integument is caught between an external object and underlying structures. In the ordinary abrasion the full continuity of the skin has not actually been broken through. A *laceration* is a wound of the skin caused by a relatively sharp object, so that the skin has actually cut through its full thickness. A *puncture wound* is one made by a penetrating object which pierces all layers of the skin. *Vesiculation* is blistering caused by mechanical, thermal or chemical burning in which the layers of the skin are separated by an exudation of fluid.

Abrasion

An abrasion, or scraping injury to the skin, may be of any grade of severity from a simple excoriation of the skin by the opponent's headgear to very extensive damage. The major abrasions occur over areas of the body where there is firm underlying tissue, particularly bone. Areas commonly injured are the shin, the knee, the iliac crest, the elbow and the back of the hand. Abrasions in themselves are not particularly serious, but their complications may indeed become a problem. The most immediate consideration, once injury to the deeper structures has been ruled out, is the prevention of infection. It cannot be overemphasized that the player should be carefully instructed to report any break in the skin that occurs on the playing field. The combination of an open wound and mother earth has very serious connotations from the standpoint of local and generalized infection.

Treatment. The first step in the management of abrasion is prevention by providing adequate playing fields. Contact sports should not be played on concrete, cinder tracks or rough irregular ground with rocks and glass in the soil. The requirements for player protection will vary directly with the nature of the terrain. Thus a player on a well-groomed, heavily sodded playing field may need but little protection, whereas one playing on hard, poorly sodded ground or on abrasive surfaces should have protection such as elbow pads, long-sleeved jerseys and long socks.

Once an abrasion occurs, it should be reported promptly and as promptly treated. When this is done, an abrasion usually is of little importance. The first step in treatment is to clean the skin, and there is no better cleansing agent than soap and water. There seems to be no real virtue in a surgical soap (such as the hexachlorophene soaps) for a single wash, since the unique value of a preparation of this type is in the build-up of the antiseptic in the skin by repeated washings. Ordinary bland white soap and water are entirely adequate, thorough cleansing being the important factor. The soap acts as a solvent for grease and embedded dirt. If necessary one can brush out ground-in dirt with a soft brush so that when the washing is complete, the wound is fresh-looking with no embedded foreign material. Some attention to detail at this first washing will save a great deal of effort later.

If a wound has been properly cleaned, the application of a topical antiseptic is of doubtful value. In the ordinary abrasion we do not recommend painting with iodine, Merthiolate or other chemicals. If the surface is not too moist, a protective spray such as tincture of benzoin may be applied in order to reduce pain. Such a spray tends to seal the wound and yet permits exudation of fluids. The application of collodion over such an area is to be condemned, since it may simply seal in the infected fluids. The use of a bland ointment with a water-soluble base is recommended if the surface is "weepy." Greasy ointments should be avoided. An antibiotic ointment, such as polysporin, may be used. It should be borne in mind that such preparations may cause sensitivity and local reaction and may even delay healing.

A suitable dressing and pad are applied to prevent re-injury, since disability from an extensive abrasion that has been repeatedly crusted over and peeled off may last for several weeks and materially impair the activity of the athlete, particularly if the abrasion is on an area such as the knee, ankle or hand. The amount of protection necessary will vary a great deal with the severity of the abrasion, its location and its extent. Protection must be (1) against direct trauma and (2) against active overuse of the skin. The latter is particularly pertinent in an abrasion over the extensor surface of a joint such as the knee. Should infection ensue, warm moist packs, rest, elevation and suitable antibiotics are indicated. Great care should be taken in the dressing room in handling the infected wound, since one infection may spread to many other players.

Laceration

As defined, a laceration is a separation of the skin with relatively sharp edges. Ordinarily in athletics it is not a cleanly incised wound as is that from a knife or razor blade; instead, it is a combination of a contusion and a lacerated wound in which the lacerated edge is jagged and irregular. These wounds, too, may be of any degree, from an extensive tearing of the skin with considerable separation of the skin edges to a fissurelike injury with but little external evidence of damage.

Treatment. After it has been determined that there is no underlying injury, the first goal in management is to obtain a clean wound. A laceration caused by a blow of a blunt object against a sharp underlying bone, as in the eyebrow, represents simply a splitting of the skin without penetration and is probably amply cleaned by the bleeding which accompanies it. On the other hand, a laceration caused by a broken cleat or the sharp equipment of the opposing player is potentially dirty and should not be closed without ample cleansing. A wound that has had direct contact with the ground must be promptly and thoroughly cleansed. The player should be taken to the dressing or treatment room and the wound should be very carefully explored for foreign material. If necessary, procaine may be injected along the wound edges to facilitate this examination. If the wound appears clean with no penetrating foreign matter, it is unwise to scrape out its interior with an abrasive—and a gauze compress qualifies as such. Simple flushing of the wound with saline or 0.5 per cent procaine solution will usually be adequate.

Next, the wound edges are carefully inspected. Often the wound does not cut cleanly through the skin at a right angle but is a slicing type with a very thin edge on one side and a thick sloping edge on the other. In this instance, careful minimal trimming of the skin margins in order to get sharp edge-to-edge contact will speed up healing and prevent excess scar formation. If it is felt essential that the player return promptly to the game, he may have a preliminary suture and then a definitive suture immediately after competition is over. From the medical standpoint this course is much inferior to proper closure of the wound in the first place, but it is preferred to leaving a jagged wound imperfectly sutured. If there are undermined edges and considerable soft tissue damage beneath the skin, the wound may require drainage. It is better to put in a small wick that permits exudation than to allow fluid to accumulate. Frequently such accumulation can be prevented by direct, suitably placed pressure on the wound. Direct pressure also serves to prevent edema of the wound edges, which may cause considerable tension on the sutures and finally disrupt them.

In suturing the wound, swelling and edema should be anticipated. Only enough sutures to obtain accurate wound approximation are used. This principle accounts for the emergency room aphorism that "the slicker the wound looks immediately after suture, the sloppier it looks the following day." This is not to imply that the repair should be careless but simply that one should not place multiple small, shallow sutures in an effort to obtain fine approximation, since these will inevitably pull out as swelling ensues.

The wound should be carefully inspected daily over a period of several days, since it is potentially infected and should be treated as such. If there is any suggestion of a collection of fluid in the wound, one or more stitches should be removed and the wound allowed to drain freely. The question of further participation in athletics before the wound has healed must depend entirely upon its location and extent. In many body areas the laceration can be adequately protected against both trauma and undue stretching of the skin and there is no reason why further participation cannot be permitted. Once there is evidence of any complication, more protection should be utilized and the inflamed wound must be treated by the usual measures of immobilization, warm wet dressings, antibiotics and general support.

Careful primary attention to the lacerated wound will give very gratifying results. A tetanus toxoid booster should be given. Antitetanic serum of human origin is now almost always available and should be used if toxoid immunity has not been developed previously. The danger of anaphylactic reaction to horse serum outweighs the importance of giving antitetanic horse serum, except in the most unusual circumstances.

Puncture Wound

This condition has been defined as a wound by a penetrating object. The object may be small, as a splinter or nail, but a rather broad object may also penetrate the skin, making a relatively small opening and continuing deeper into the soft tissues. This has the potentiality of a puncture wound and should be treated as such. Such wounds are not common in athletics but should be promptly and adequately treated when they do occur. The author recalls an incident during a track session in which one of the participants, who was kneeling on one knee with the other thigh thrust forward was struck by an errant javelin in his anterior thigh. This not only caused a puncture wound through the skin and ruptured the muscle mechanism but also split the shaft of the femur.

Of first importance are the severity of the wound, the depth of the penetration and the possibility of underlying damage to the joint or bone, but particularly to the blood vessels or nerves. A penetrating wound over a joint should be assumed to have entered the joint without proof to the contrary because the consequences of joint penetration are of major importance. A history is carefully taken as to the nature of the penetrating object, the depth of the penetration, whether or not it went through clothing, and whether the entering body was contaminated, as would be a peg of a broken cleat, a piece of wire or a nail which happened to be on the playing field. It will not suffice to wash off the skin, apply protective dressing and "wait and see." It may be necessary to wait and see, but this decision should be made only after a careful history, a thorough examination and some effort to explore the wound. If there is underlying damage which will require surgical repair, this repair should be done at once, since the wound is potentially infected. Even a few hours delay will change it from a potentially to an actually infected wound. After that, definitive surgery is extremely hazardous.

Treatment. After one has satisfied oneself that there is no underlying damage, the wound itself is treated. The skin will often be puckered and discolored around the margins, which indicates that the hole at one time was considerably larger than it is at the time of examination. The skin tends to stretch and tent inward under pressure of the blow, so that when the point does penetrate the stretched skin, it may make a fairly large hole. When the skin returns to its normal tension, this hole will shrink and appear minute. The importance of determining the nature of the object and the depth of penetration is obvious.

If the object was contaminated and has penetrated deeply, it is wise to split the skin, examine the underlying tissue, clean out the sinus tract and then decide whether or not to carry out primary closure. Primary closure may be carried out if the wound has been treated promptly and satisfactorily lavaged. The use of a drain will depend upon the degree of damage and whether or not one expects continued oozing and collection of fluid. It is much better to let the fluids seep outside through a tissue drain than to let them accumulate in the wound, where they will make an ideal medium

for infection Only if the wound seems minor, the penetrating object small and the depth not great is one justified in simply cleansing the skin and observing. If the decision is made to observe the wound, exactly that should be done—and frequently. It is not proper to wait until secondary symptoms demand attention, for by this time a definite infection will be developing. A tetanus toxoid booster should be given. (For tetanus serum, see page 50.)

Blisters

Mechanical Causes. Blisters on the skin may occur under varying circumstances, the most common being friction from an ill-fitting shoe or a wrinkle in the sock. Another frequent source is irritation by adhesive tape or by friction between the tape and the skin due to the fact that the tape was poorly applied or has been under undue tension or that the individual has perspired, causing the tape to separate from the skin in certain areas while remaining adherent in others. In any event, the resulting traction on the skin tends to separate its superficial layers from the underlying dermis, the area fills with exudate and the blister forms. Although the blister itself may be a relatively simple and apparently minor ailment, its location may be such as to make it a problem of some magnitude. A blister on the back of the heel, for example, may handicap the player throughout the season. Extensive vesiculation under the adhesive tape may render it impossible to use adhesive in that particular area of the body, and so vital protection may have to be discontinued with resultant injury to the unprotected joint or ligament beneath.

Another disabling area of vesiculation is the sole of the foot, where it is not uncommon to have a blister directly under the first toe or first metatarsal head. This is particularly common in the track man who runs in light shoes with very pointed spikes, so that he may get direct pressure in a single area of the sole. This constant sliding of the skin on itself results in blistering. The skin of the sole is thick and a very deep blister under the skin (Fig. 26) may go unrecognized and be treated as a simple contusion. I have seen such a blister enlarge until it separated a large portion of the calloused skin under the forefoot. This condition manifestly is not compatible with competition.

The best treatment of blisters is *prevention*.

Figure 26. Cross-section drawing of the vicinity of the first metatarsal head, showing the heavy epidermis of callus with a blister lying between this and the underlying dermis. A needle has been inserted to draw out the fluid. (Needle inserted away from the blister margin, through intact skin.)

Carefully fitted shoes and clean, wrinkle-free socks are extremely important. If strapping or wrapping is used, it should be carefully placed and its location changed if it begins to irritate the skin. Careful preparation of the skin before application of adhesive will often prevent irritation either by reaction to the tape or by partial slipping of the tape on the skin. A simple wrinkle in the tape in a weight-bearing area of the body may cause prompt blistering beneath it. If an irritated area develops which appears to be the prelude to a blister, careful protection should be provided either by very thin, smooth tape applied directly to the skin or by soft padding to prevent friction between the skin and the equipment. An ounce of prevention is certainly worth a pound of cure here.

Once a blister develops, proper *treatment* is of considerable importance. Here again the location of the lesion makes some difference in the type of treatment instituted. If the blister is located in an area where there ordinarily is no friction, such as the thigh or calf, the top of the blister may be removed, the area carefully cleansed and the resultant abraded area treated appropriately (with benzoin spray, for instance). This management, however, is not practicable for a blister caused by pressure from a shoe or another piece of equipment. In this instance it is quite important to protect the skin over the blister. The blister should be treated by passing a hypodermic needle through the adjacent skin and into the blister to drain the fluid and relieve the pressure. This is particularly applicable on the plantar surface of the foot so that some of the callus can be preserved until such time as the floor of the blister develops some resistance of its own. Once the roof of the blister is broken, it is

important to trim it all away and treat the floor by benzoin solution, proper protection, etc. The ragged edges of the top of the blister serve not only to irritate the lesion further but also to form peripheral pockets containing infected fluid.

Chemical Causes. Chemical blistering is not frequent, since the marking of fields with lime is no longer common practice. This type of blistering does have the added complication of irritation of the surrounding skin and should be treated by protection with bland emollients much as in a thermal burn. The *thermal burn* has no particular application to athletic injuries but occasionally occurs as a result of carelessly applied physical therapeutic measures and as such may be extremely distressing. The burn from the ultraviolet machine is of course similar to sunburn and should be treated as such. Injuries from the infrared or electric heating pad and various types of hot packs are true thermal burns and may cause vesiculation but usually remain a local reaction. These direct heat applications usually cause sufficient pain if producing a burn, so that the treatment is stopped before the burn is severe. The result is usually a first degree burn or, at the worst, a mild second degree burn with only moderate vesiculation. The deep electrical burns caused by diathermy or other inductive agents may be extremely severe. A diathermy burn should be very carefully investigated to determine whether or not the damage is limited to the skin. It may well be so, since oftentimes the burn is secondary to the condensation of fluid between the applicator and the skin; thus the burn actually is from hot water. If it is a true electrical burn, the deep tissues may indeed be burned more severely than the skin. An electrical therapeutic appliance is no plaything, and its indiscriminate use by untrained personnel should be discouraged. The patient should be instructed not to put too much faith in the dials of the machine, and he should be told to report the slightest discomfort, since it is neither safe nor desirable to have the heat reach the level of discomfort to the part being treated.

Skin Infections

Skin infections secondary to direct trauma are often the bane of the training room, because they may start in one player and spread like wildfire through the whole squad. Any skin infection, however superficial, should be very carefully washed. The surrounding skin should be cleansed, protective dressing applied and great care taken not to reinfect the skin by use of dirty clothing. It is obvious that once suppuration occurs, the pimple or boil should be opened under aseptic technique and the area of surrounding skin protected by careful cleansing with antiseptic solution and protective dressing. The dressing should be destroyed and not indiscriminately tossed to the floor. Many of the so-called eczemas are indeed skin infections, and therefore the affected player's clothes should be isolated from the remainder of the squad.

Fungus infections are particularly distressing and are prone to develop under adhesive tape applied to the feet. Occasionally on removal of the tape the whole plantar integument will peel off as a result of extensive fungus undermining. Application of proper fungicidal measures will clear up the local lesion quite adequately. The big danger is that casual handling of the socks, and contamination of the floor and common shower stalls will spread the fungus from the player who is relatively immune to his own fungus to his neighbor who has no resistance to this particular organism. Although it may be an entirely latent infection in one player, his locker mate may develop a virulent infection. Ordinary rules of cleanliness, soap and water, clean socks and some type of bath shoes will help to minimize this problem. If it becomes epidemic in a given situation, special measures will be necessary to sterilize the shower stalls and locker room floors. Enteric drugs are promising, and one of the oral fungicides should be used if the infected area is extensive or resistant to local measures.

Tetanus Prevention

In spite of its great rarity, the problem of tetanus is very important in the athletic program. It is one condition in which prevention is almost completely effective and treatment is relatively ineffective; therefore little justification exists for not employing preventive techniques.

Toxoid. Every athlete should have tetanus toxoid injections prior to his participation in sports. These injections have proved successful. They were adopted by the armed forces and have been extremely effective in eliminating the danger of tetanus from questionable wounds. There is ordinarily no reaction to toxoid injections and it is entirely feasible to insist on the series for each athlete at the beginning of the school year. If the patient has had toxoid within the year, one can relax about the ordinary skin involvement. If he sustains a particularly virulent type of puncture wound, as by a rusty nail, injection of a booster dose of toxoid can be given at that time with no danger of reaction and with complete effectiveness, since tetanus develops rather slowly and the toxoid booster can develop the antibodies much more rapidly than the organism develops its toxin.

Antitetanus Serum. If the injured player has not had toxoid, the toxoid series should be started at once. It probably will not be effective for the current lesion. Antitetanic human serum is usually available and should be used in a prophylactic dose in all penetrating wounds. *Horse serum should be used only under the most urgent necessity.* The dangers of anaphylaxis either at the time of initial administration or at a later exposure are so great and the reaction so dangerous that routine use of the antitetanic serum in horse serum is not recommended. If it is necessary to use antitetanic serum, a careful sensitivity test should be run and given at least one hour to react before the serum is injected. After injection, the patient should be carefully watched for at least 24 hours, and he should be warned that he is subject to anaphylactic reaction as long as two or three weeks following the injection. He should also be warned that another injection of horse serum may be particularly dangerous. If the wound really seems to be a dangerous one, it should be opened freely and thoroughly lavaged. Massive doses of antibiotics should also be given.

STRAIN

Injuries to the Muscle-Tendon Unit

For the purpose of this discussion it is important that we make a clear distinction between strain and sprain. The subcommittee on Athletic Nomenclature of the AMA Committee on Sports Medicine has confirmed that strain should apply to the muscle-tendon unit and sprain to the ligament injury. These structures are quite distinct; the muscle-tendon units include a motor element, whereas the ligament is primarily a stabilizer.

Strain may be defined as damage of some part of the unit (muscle, tendon or the attachment) occasioned by overuse (chronic strain) or overstress (acute strain). So we properly have mild (first degree), moderate (second degree) and severe (third degree) strain of the unit. The strain will occur at the weakest link of the muscle-tendon unit at a given time. Under a given stress the tendon may rupture, the muscle-tendon junction may give way or the damage may be to the muscle itself or to its bony attachment.

There has been a tendency to consider muscle and tendon in different categories; frequently injuries to the tendon and injuries to the muscle are described in separate chapters. More recently, however, proper emphasis has been placed on the fact that the muscle-tendon mechanism is indeed a unit which consists of a muscle arising usually from bone which terminates in a tendon, or a tendon which itself attaches to bone. Such a unit crossing a joint or joints serves a double purpose: (1) it acts to stabilize the joint, in this case combining with its antagonist to prevent motion; and (2) it serves as a motor to accomplish a certain motion. Under this conception it can be seen that functionally it is a unit. Impairment of any part of the unit affects the whole. Each part must be restored to its normal condition if normal function is to be maintained. It is bootless to speak of injury to the muscle and of injury to the tendon as separate elements. Injury to the unit is of two types: (1) strain and its consequences, and (2) contusion and its complications. (See page 39.)

Chronic Strain. Chronic strain from overfunction causes fatigue of the muscle and its sequelae—muscle spasm, myositis and ischemia. It may also result in irritation at the musculotendinous junction, tenosynovitis along the course of the tendon or inflammatory reaction at the tendinous attachment. Although these seem to be different conditions, they are basically the same and require basically the same treatment, specifically, rest, local heat, local injection and protection against strain. General measures such as antispasmodics may be of some value if the area involved is a major one such as the hip, thigh or back. In this condition, prevention is of more importance than cure. In the athlete, the whole purpose of his long training is to build up the musculotendinous unit gradually so that it is able to withstand a progressively heavier work load, thus increasing its strength, endurance and ability to avoid strain. Once the strain occurs, the problem is magnified by the fact that relief will require a sharp reversal of the activity cycle. A period of complete rest must be followed by the same gradual progressive build-up. This is very onerous to the athlete and his impatience to resume activity often results in recurrence of this injury with an even more frustrating period of disability. Prevention of recurrence is a major problem in any strain of the muscle-tendon unit. Often the anatomical or physical condition of the athlete will make him more vulnerable to overstress of the muscle. If his hamstrings are tight and short, if his calf is so short he cannot dorsiflex his foot, if his back is so tight he cannot touch his fingers to the floor, a course of stretching exercises may be very fruitful in preventing recurrence of the strain or, indeed, in preventing strain in the player who has not yet developed the condition. (See Chapter 22.)

The extent of disability and the difficulty of maintaining adequate protection will vary considerably with the unit involved and also with the type of activity to be restored. For the track man, a strain of the muscle-tendon unit of the calf may be completely disabling. To the baseball player, it may be the triceps that throws him out of action. The rower may be disabled because of strain to his back. In every instance the strain has resulted from the very activity which is important to this individual. As such it poses a major problem in rehabilitation.

The complications of such a condition may be major. The baseball pitcher, for example, may develop painful myositis which progresses to ossification and spur formation at the origin of the triceps from the glenoid (Fig. 27); it

Figure 27. Baseball pitcher who developed ossification at glenoid attachment of triceps brachii. Nonsurgical treatment consisted of patient's retirement from pitching for one season.

may continue until pitching is impossible. Tenosynovitis may develop in a tendon, particularly one which is surrounded by a sheath. The recurrent irritative strain of the biceps tendon passing through the bicipital groove is a classic example. Chronic strain may be caused by prolonged overuse or by a single episode of overactivity. It is not caused but may be initiated by an acute injury. The result is an inflammatory reaction between the tendon and the sheath, congestion with inflammation, oversecretion of fluid and increase in fibrin content, which causes sticky adhesions between the tendon and the surrounding synovium. If the strain is not eliminated in the early stages, the tenosynovitis progresses to a chronic inflammatory reaction with swelling, edema, pain and possibly painful crepitation. If the tendon continues to slide up and down its sheath, irritation is increased until a constrictive or adhesive tenosynovitis results which may completely arrest the motion in this particular tendon and sharply interfere with function of this muscle-tendon unit. Although this may seem to be a specific condition, the same thing may happen in the muscle and will require the same treatment, this time directed

to the muscle rather than to the tendon. Indeed, the treatment may finally have to be surgical resection of the tendon sheath or possibly transference of a tendon to a less constricted area. Again, the classic example is the bicipital tendon at the shoulder, which is likely to advance to adhesive or constrictive tenosynovitis. On the other hand, the tendo Achillis, lacking the specific sheath, may have the inflammatory symptoms but not the complication of constriction. Chronic strain is not likely to result in hemorrhage into the muscle. The calcification resulting from chronic strain will be in the origin of the muscle or at the insertion of the tendon.

Acute Strain. Acute strain, in distinction to chronic strain, is the result of a single violent force applied to the muscle; for example, the force of the sprinter coming out of the blocks when his muscles contract violently against the resistance of the blocks. It may be the result of resistance to a force. For example, with the muscles contracted, a violent force is applied which is greater than the unit's ability to withstand. This is exemplified by the strain to the biceps brachii resulting from trying to support a weight with the flexed forearms that is greater than the biceps unit will tolerate (Fig. 28). The injury is likely to be localized and may occur in any part of the unit. One can see that inflammation of the origin of the muscle and strain at the attachment of the tendon to bone appear to be, and indeed are, identical injuries. So also are injuries to the musculotendinous junction or injuries in the muscle belly itself. The injury occurs at a certain location simply because at this given moment it is the weakest link in the chain. It must be obvious that the amount of damage (mild [first degree], moderate [second degree] or severe [third degree]) that occurs is contingent on the violence of the force and the strength of the resistance. The pathological feature consists of disruption of some of the fibers of the unit. There may be rupture of a few muscle fibers or of the entire muscle. The tendon may be partially avulsed from the bone or completely torn away.

Whereas the treatment of chronic strain is rest and avoidance of the activity that caused the strain, the treatment of acute strain must be restoration of the integrity of the unit. This may require, in one case, simple protection against additional stress until healing occurs or, in another, surgical restoration. In the great majority of instances the injury is minimal and recovery is prompt. As the individual steps on the curb of the running track, his ankle is

Figure 28. Rupture of long head of biceps brachii caused by patient's awkward catch of partner in gymnastics. Note bunching of muscle attended by complete loss of function of long head. Condition was resolved by reattaching long head, which would no longer reach to bicipital groove, midway down shaft of humerus. Symptoms were relieved and some function was restored.

forced sharply into dorsiflexion and he has pain localized at the junction of the calf muscle and the tendo Achilles. He has sharp pain, sits down and rubs his leg, exercises his foot up and down and is able to resume walking. If he tries to sprint or to dorsiflex his foot violently, he will have discomfort. The following day the area will be sore. The muscle will be contracted and dorsiflexion will be resisted. This is caused by some degree of damage to the muscle and tendon fibers with attendant bleeding, inflammatory reaction and protective resistance to motion. The subsequent course of the injury will depend on the extent of damage and the effectiveness of treatment.

Mild (First Degree) Strain. In this degree of strain there is no appreciable disruption. Pathological changes are confined to a low-grade inflammatory process with swelling, edema and some discomfort on function of tendon or muscle. There is neither discernible loss of strength nor any restriction of motion. Early examination will elicit pain on active motion or passive stretching which is sharply confined to the area of damage. Later as muscle spasm occurs, exact localization may be difficult. Localization of the point of stress may be impor

tant in treatment. Mild strain is very distressing to the athlete. Hamstring strain may sideline the sprinter even though the injury is mild. A classic example of chronic strain of the arm, wherein the strain is not severe enough to restrict motion or strength but may sharply reduce endurance, is seen in the baseball pitcher.

Treatment of the acute strain must be rest of the unit and protection against active use. Local injection may be hyaluronidase in the muscle, lidocaine in the tendon sheath. *There is no place for steroid injection in the acute injury.* The most important treatment is protection, which must vary with the amount of damage. In one case it may consist of immobilization; in another, of simple avoidance of violent activity. Enteric acute inflammatory agents, such as aspirin or phenylbutazone, may be useful. Muscle relaxants will help control spasm.

Moderate (Second Degree) Strain. The distinction between first and second degree strain lies in the extent to which pathological development has occurred. Whereas in a mild strain there is no loss of strength but only irritation, in moderate strain there has been actual dam-

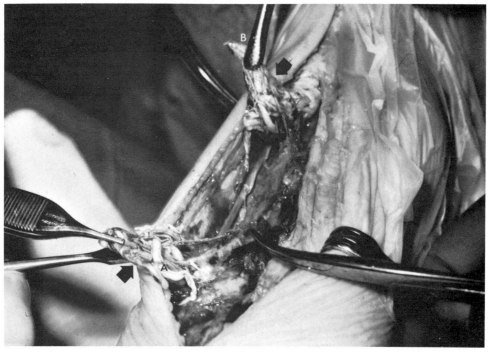

Figure 29. Professional football player injured calf six weeks prior to surgical procedure shown here. Symptoms, which subsequently subsided, included swelling, pain and tenderness at muscle-tendon junction of calf. Six weeks following initial trauma, patient, running down a ramp, slipped, heard something snap, and felt acute pain in the back of the lower leg. Loss of function of the calf was essentially complete with a defect at the muscle-tendon junction. At time of surgical repair, roughly half the tendon was found to have been torn six weeks previously, whereas the remaining half showed a fresh tear. Repair and reconstruction using the peroneus brevis was carried out with apparent success. Photograph shows earlier *(A)* and later *(B)* pathological changes at torn ends of tendon and extensive disruption of tendon with early degenerative changes (arrows).

age to the muscle, tendon or attachment which definitely compromises the strength of the unit. There is not complete disruption as in severe strain but there is definite loss of strength; whether it is 90 per cent or 10 per cent is the question. Diagnosis depends upon a careful evaluation of the unit—all symptoms are more severe than in mild strain, yet careful examination will demonstrate that the unit is intact.

Treatment of this injury must be more definitive. Whereas in mild strain the treatment is largely symptomatic, in moderate strain we predict specific weakness but no loss of continuity. Local treatment is by ice pack and injection (lidocaine). This, together with protection, will give symptomatic relief. Since there has been definite damage to some part of the unit, *protection* becomes all-important. Since protection means cessation of violent muscle activity, it follows that splinting, taping and so on are important. Tendons and muscles heal slowly, so protection must be prolonged for several weeks. If activity is resumed too soon, at best the muscle spasm recurs, at worst the unit may rupture (Fig. 29). Consequently

activity must be carefully resumed and kept within the limits of pain. The part must be protected against further injury. The situation is frustrating to the athlete, the doctor and the coach. In the final analysis, adequate treatment is largely protective and will result in complete recovery. Inadequate care will result in a chronic, more or less crippling impairment of the unit which is devastating to the athlete.

Severe (Third Degree) Strain. Rupture of any component of the unit is usually the result of violent contraction against firm resistance, that is, the irresistible force and the immovable object. It may be preceded by damage to a lesser degree which has improperly healed. The tendon may give way or separate at the muscle-tendon junction, or the muscle itself may rupture. When the forces applied are greater than the strength of the unit, something must give. In a first or second degree strain the primary treatment is *protection*. In a complete (third degree) tear it must be *restoration* of the unit.

Diagnosis depends upon recognition of the loss of function of the unit. This may be quite deceptive. On the one hand, muscle spasm may render the unit inoperative, although it is actually intact. On the other, the unit may be disrupted, a condition that may be very diffi-cult to detect. Sometimes the actual defect may be palpated in the muscle-tendon unit (Fig. 30). At other times the muscle may bunch up, as in rupture of the long head of the biceps

Figure 30. This 20 year old pole vaulter had severe pain in his groin as he thrust off the ground. He was no longer able to run or vault without immediate swelling in the area. An ice pack was applied and he was examined the following day. There was swelling in the groin, with palpable muscle separated from the pubis. When the thigh was adducted against resistance, the adductor muscle bunched up, and this mass traveled distally. A, At surgery, the incision parallels the adductor longus distal to the pubis. The tenaculum holds the avulsed tendinous end of the adductor longus muscle. B, Mattress sutures were placed in this mass allowing it to be pulled up to its origin on the pubic bone and fastened through drill holes. A plaster spica case was applied, to be worn for eight weeks, but after six weeks the patient and his local doctor removed the cast. The muscle attachment seemed firm and the cast was left off. Six months postoperatively, the adductor was intact and there was no bulging of the muscle; the patient was asymptomatic and was released for sports activity. Note: Knee to right of picture, pelvis to left.

Figure 31. While straining against opponent, professional football player felt painful snap in "groin"; swelling was massive. Patient treated for "hematoma." Bunching up of rectus femoris in front of thigh with extensor stress one year later is obvious. Condition was only mildly disabling and no treatment was recommended.

brachii, the rectus femoris or the hamstrings (Figs. 31 and 32).

If detected early, repair of the unit is quite feasible whether it is tendon or muscle, and it is even more important to repair these injuries early than those of ligament or bone. Every effort must be made to determine separation of the muscle or tendon. If it can be diagnosed early, surgical repair will give the best results (Fig. 33). If it cannot be diagnosed, treatment as for moderate strain should be carried out until the accurate pathological condition is demonstrable. Often it is then too late for repair because of muscle spasm and shortening. Athletic activities must be eliminated until healing has occurred (eight to ten weeks). Too often resumption of the activity that caused the trouble will cause recurrence. Late reconstructive procedures may be necessary and will be described in relation to specific areas. In far too many instances this will be a procedure of salvage and cannot be expected to restore normal function.

Discussion of Muscle-Tendon Injuries

Successful treatment depends upon an accurate diagnosis of the location and extent of the injury. It has been emphasized that in ligament injuries the doctor must be able to make a definitive decision concerning the best treatment based on a true recognition of the pathological process present. In muscle, early treatment is even more important than it is in the ligament or tendon. An early muscle rup-

Figure 32. Sprinter felt something "give way" in back of thigh and had to stop running. He was treated for hematoma in muscle. Figure shows bunching up of muscle under stress (six months following injury). Any stress of the hamstrings caused pain between the bunched up muscle and the fibrous band running from muscle toward ischium. Reattachment of torn muscle to adjacent hamstring muscle was required.

Figure 33. Patient fell on outstretched arm while performing gymnastic maneuvers. *A*, Avulsion of flexor pronator attachment at internal condyle occurred. *B*, Fragment of bone was removed and attachment to condyle repaired. Patient regained normal function of arm.

Figure 34. Avulsion of a portion of the flexor pronator muscle attachment to the medial epicondyle. This was an old injury resulting in disability. On exposure of the epicondyle, the detached bundle of muscle, including the flexor carpi ulnaris and portion of the flexor profundus, is shown. *A*, The tenaculum grasps the avulsed muscle end. The hemostat indicates the medial epicondyle about two inches away. *B*, The avulsed muscle is in the retractor. The larger (upper) hemostat indicates the pronator radii teres. The smaller (lower) hemostat is on the epicondyle. *C*, The pronator radii teres is mobilized but not detached from the condyle ready to shift into the space left by the avulsed muscle. *D*, The repair. The avulsed end is sutured into the angle formed by the pronator above and the flexor bundle below. The arrow indicates the end of the avulsed muscle with the pronator above it and the undamaged muscle below it. The condyle is at the right arrow. Patient has resumed his activity as a professional quarterback.

Figure 35. Three weeks before, this 16 year old boy had severe pain when hurdling. He did not fall but immediately had to stop. X-ray shows an avulsion of the ischium including the biceps and semitendinosus origin. *A*, Neutral position. *B*, In abduction showing the gross displacement. This required open reduction and internal fixation to assure good healing. Overcoming the contracture was easy because of bone fragment that permitted firm traction by the suture.

ture can be readily repaired. It may be impossible to suture a ruptured muscle after a lapse of as little as two weeks (Fig. 34). Consideration of the problem will show why this is true. The muscle-tendon unit is normally in constant tension. The tone of the muscle is such that it keeps the tendon taut and ready for function. In a normal unit, at no time is the tendon relaxed in the sense of a slack rope. Consequently when the muscle is ruptured, the fibers immediately separate. At this time, however,

no actual contracture has developed. The fibers have simply shortened and can readily be pulled back to their normal length if it is done early. By the same token, the muscle itself is in good condition. Edema and necrosis have not occurred and ordinarily successful suture can be made even in the belly of the muscle. Within a very short time the contraction of the muscle becomes a contracture and it is impossible to get the ruptured ends together; particularly since the local condition is such that the

Figure 36. Excessive ossification from untreated avulsion of hamstring muscles from the ischium. This extremely painful mass required resection and repair and caused more than one year's disability.

suture will not hold. This also applies to avulsion of the muscle from bone. However, when the muscle is avulsed from its origin, a fragment of bone, or at least periosteum, frequently is peeled away with it. This gives an additional base for retention of sutures, so that it may be possible to reattach a muscle to its origin somewhat later than it is to suture the muscle itself (Fig. 35). It still becomes increasingly difficult with the passage of time, and before many weeks, repair will become impossible (Fig. 36). In an avulsion of the tendon from bone there is considerably more leeway, since the tendon gives fixation for the suture and the muscle itself is normal and has less tendency to fibrose than if it is torn (Figs. 37 and 38). Ironically, however, it is relatively easy to diagnose rupture of the tendon or avulsion of tendon from bone, whereas it may be very difficult to diagnose muscle rupture. A little consideration will verify this observation. Frequently the tendon is in a position wherein it can readily be palpated, since the muscle is intact and its tendency to *bunch up* on contraction may be obvious. Also, this is not screened by the inflammatory reaction within the muscle itself which occurs when the muscle is damaged.

The ultimate fate of injury to the muscle-tendon unit depends upon the severity of the injury and the acuity of the diagnosis (Fig. 39). If the injury is not severe, the diagnosis may never need to be made and recovery, although incomplete, may eventually occur (Fig. 40). Unfortunately, the severe injuries may be more difficult to diagnose than the less severe ones, since the area involved will be greater and the local reaction more severe (Fig. 41). One can only urge that when the physician suspects injury to the muscle-tendon unit, he at least make those rudimentary tests which may determine whether or not the function of this unit has been changed. This may seem elementary, but the observance is often honored only in the breach. The injury occurs and there is obvious disability, diffuse tenderness and considerable pain. The involved area may be wrapped, strapped or splinted or the patient put to bed without any actual effort to determine the exact diagnosis (Fig. 42). During the examination, every effort must be made to localize the pathological condition to a specific area.

A rather common injury occurs to the thigh adductor muscle group (Figs. 43 and 44). This area may be quite difficult to examine, because

Figure 37. Avulsion of central portion of the patellar tubercle by acute trauma. X-ray shows central fragment is avulsed. The operation revealed this to be a block of bone with almost the entire patellar tendon attachment. The block was resected and the tendon attached to the underlying bone. No growth disturbance occurred. *A,* Displaced central portion of the patellar tubercle apophysis. *B,* The opposite side for comparison.

Figure 38. Patient fell between two trucks, catching himself with right arm overhead and taking his whole weight with the arm stretched up. Despite severe pain in shoulder, patient continued working. Roughly one month following initial trauma, he noticed knotting of muscle in arm upon contraction. Condition gradually worsened until he was unable to lift anything overhead and experienced weakness and pain in arm when stress was placed on arm in flexion. Examination revealed bunching up of biceps brachii in lower arm upon contraction to flex elbow. Photograph shows mass of biceps just proximal to elbow with rupture of long tendon at, roughly, level of bicipital groove. Since tendon could not be extended upward to bicipital groove, it was fastened through a hole drilled in humerus at junction of upper and middle thirds. Function improved and pain lessened, but muscle continued to bunch up. Rupture of the tendon near its attachment permitted a better result than if tendon had pulled off muscle junction or if muscle had ruptured through its own substance.

Figure 39. Six months earlier this 14 year old male jumped off a diving tower, a wet rope caught around his upper arm, and he hung by his arm. There was immediate bulging of the muscle with gross indentation. His doctor advised him to wear a sling for 12 days. *A,* At examination six months later, he had a notable indentation with bunching up in the midarm. He still favored the arm and experienced tiring on prolonged use. At surgery, there was a gross defect transversely across the medial and long heads of the triceps with retraction of both ends, the interspace being a very thick walled bursa. *B,* The gaping hole between the muscle heads, held in the tenacula. *C,* The two ends apposed, held in the tenacula. These were repaired by direct suture. Good function of the long head was restored with less definite contraction of the medial. Some of this deep furrowing in the arm persisted owing to loss of subcutaneous fat.

Figure 40. Avulsion of the lesser trochanter by the psoas tendon. It was treated by immobilization with fibrous union. Asymptomatic.

in such an injury the player tends to keep his thighs together and resist abduction, since this causes pain. A little careful persuasion will ordinarily permit manual examination, at which time a defect in the tendon can be noted, the location of tenderness may be defined, and by careful testing, interference of function of a specific muscle may often be determined.

Active contraction or passive stretching of the unit will elicit pain at the site of injury. If active adduction of the thigh causes pain along the descending ramus of the pubis or in the vicinity of the ischium, one should suspect muscle damage in this area, particularly if the injury consists of overabduction. Careful palpation may actually localize the muscle involved. After careful physical examination, x-ray examination is valuable. It should be borne in mind, however, that routine views may be very unenlightening. An anteroposterior view of the pelvis for avulsion of the semimembranosus tendon may be completely negative, whereas the flake of bone avulsed will show quite readily in the oblique or tangential views.

Treatment. Treatment of these conditions is very rewarding. It may be enough simply to put the muscle at rest in the position in which the muscle is the shortest. In rupture of the adductors, for instance, the patient could be placed with the knees together. This will not suffice if complete rupture has occurred, since the very tone of the muscle will shorten it beyond its normally relaxed position. For example, in the avulsion of the distal attachment of the biceps brachii, the arm may be placed in complete flexion so that the hand is on the shoulder and yet the avulsed tendon end will not lie in its normal position, since the shortening of the muscle will draw it away from its

Figure 41. Eighteen year old boy was water skiing four days prior to surgical treatment. He had looped the handle of the tow line around his flexed left elbow, was thrown head over heels, the rope locked around his arm, and he was dragged through the water. The following morning extensive swelling was present in the entire arm. The nerve and blood supplies in the hand were intact. A balled mass that could have been either muscle or hematoma was present just above the front of the elbow. However, unlike an ordinary muscle, the mass did not contract when the elbow was flexed. Because patient was unable to define the exact site of pain, surgical exploration was temporarily deferred. Three days following initial trauma, a defect in the upper arm in the region of the biceps brachii was detected. Surgical treatment was performed on the fourth day following injury. A, The exposed mass is the belly of the muscle with the fibers and muscle bundles running transverse to the arm at right angles to the biceps. Releasing it from below, we flipped the end up and found that the proximal end was tucked under the distal portion. Nerve and blood supplies were completely severed, accounting for inability of muscle to contract. B, Necrotic mass was removed. Note: Elbow to the right of picture, shoulder to the left.

Figure 42. Shoulder x-ray of 20 year old wrestler in whom increasingly severe disability developed over many months. *A*, X-ray film reveals calcification along margin of bicipital groove which was found at surgery to be calcification within the partially avulsed attachment of the teres minor at the lateral side of the groove. Resection of mass resulted in relief of patient's symptoms. *B*, Some postoperative recurrence with return of symptoms.

bed. In the great majority of instances, complete rupture of the tendon unit requires surgical repair for normal function. Results of early repair are extremely gratifying. The difficulties of delayed repair are enormous and such repair seldom results in complete restoration of the muscle unit. In many instances complete removal of the muscle units will be required because of functional interference by other adjacent groups.

Figure 43. Avulsion of the inferior ramus of the pubic bone by the adductor muscle attachments following a fall by patient "attempting to do splits." Cartilaginous end of pubic epiphysis was palpable under the skin. Injury was treated by open reduction and internal fixation.

SPRAIN

Injuries to the Ligament

Definition

A sprain may be defined as an injury to a ligament resulting from overstress which causes some degree of damage to the ligament fibers or their attachment. A ligament is designed to prevent abnormal motion of a joint while permitting normal functional motion. Certain ligaments may bind two bones firmly together with relatively little motion, such as the tibiofibular syndesmosis, which permits slight rotatory motion while preventing separation of the two bones. Other ligaments serve to reinforce a joint and permit a rather wide excursion of normal motion but prevent motion in an abnormal direction. Fundamentally, abnormal motion to a degree beyond the power of a ligament to withstand it will cause a sprain. This is to be contrasted with a direct blow over a ligament, which may cause a contusion. As abnormal force is applied, the ligament becomes tense and then gives way at one or the other of its attachments or at some point in the substance of the ligament (Fig. 45). If the attachment pulls loose with a fragment of bone, it is called a "sprain-fracture," but the mechanism is the same. The location of the damage will depend upon the weakest link in the chain of the ligament, which may be within the ligament itself or at one of its

Figure 44. Surgical slides show exposure of thigh of 26 year old male who, while running relay, felt something snap on back of his thigh with attendant balling of muscle. Subsequently, he experienced posterior thigh pain. Although he was able to run moderately, he experienced a catching pain in this region whenever he attempted to sprint. Although desirous of playing professional football, he was unable to engage in even ordinary athletics. The injured muscle is exposed by a longitudinal incision along the back of thigh parallel to it. (For orientation, the right side is toward the trunk, the left is toward the knee.) A, The end of the ruptured long head of biceps femoris muscle is held by two tenacula. Towel clamp in center is on conjoined raphe of the long and short heads, the short head being intact. B, The two heads opposed. Tenacula now hold ruptured long head against its tendinous insertion. C, Mattress suture placed through muscle in three layers and passed up and through aponeurosis. D, After sutures are tied, biceps is restored to its normal attachments. Suture was possible after six weeks, since tendinous fibers were present with muscle mass.

Figure 45. Various types of sprain. A, Mild (first degree) sprain, in which there is a little hematoma in a very localized area in the ligament with only a few fibers separated. B, Moderate (second degree) sprain, a more severe tear of the ligament but with at least half of the fibers remaining intact. C, Severe (third degree) sprain. Complete tear through the ligament with separation of the ends. D, Sprain-fracture. The ligament is torn off bone with a fragment of bone.

attachments, possibly at the site of an area of previous damage. The extent of the damage depends upon the amount and duration of the force. If the abnormal force is arrested or terminated promptly, there may be little actual functional loss to the ligament and only a few of its fibers may be involved. In this instance there is localized hematoma formation with prompt deposit of fibrin in the hematoma. The fibrin is invaded by fibroblasts, and as the reparative process proceeds, the final termination is restoration of a normal ligament. If the damage is more severe, so that there is actually more disruption of ligament fibers, there may be considerable functional loss. When the ligament is completely torn, all function is lost. In this case the findings will depend upon the location of the tear. Ordinarily there will be relatively extensive hematoma formation with swelling and edema. The process of repair will be much slower and much less complete and, if untreated, will result in scar formation rather than restoration of normal ligament. The ligament may heal overlong and hence be slack and be subjected to repeated stress. This will ultimately terminate in instability causing degenerative changes in the joint.

Degree

For the purpose of this discussion, sprain will be divided into three different categories according to the severity of the injury.

Mild (First Degree) (see Fig. 45A). This is a sprain in which some fibers of a ligament have been torn with a little resultant hemorrhage into the ligament but with no actual functional loss. There is no demonstrable diminution in strength in the ligament. This is of considerable importance from the standpoint of treatment, since the factor of protection is not important. The ligament is not materially weakened. Treatment is symptomatic only.

Moderate (Second Degree) (see Fig. 45B). A moderate sprain is one in which some portion of the ligament is torn and some degree of functional loss is present. The amount of damage may range from the tearing of a relatively small portion of the ligament to the almost complete avulsion—from "mild" with no functional loss to "severe" with complete functional loss of the ligament. The emphasis here must be on protection, since one may be unable to determine the actual extent of the damage. One would not expect wide retraction of the torn ligament ends in a moderate sprain.

Union can therefore proceed in an orderly manner with replacement of fibrous scar by ligament during the process of repair. If the damage is relatively severe, however, there may be considerable permanent scar formation with resultant weakness in this segment of the ligament. Obviously, protection here is mandatory to promote efficient repair and prevent permanent weakness. "Once a sprain always a sprain" is an aphorism not acceptable in the modern concept of therapy.

Yes, a sprain may heal. The greatest challenge to the physician in the treatment of sprain is in the moderate type. Many orthopaedists now accept surgical treatment as being necessary for the complete recovery of a complete ligament tear. The fact that it takes six, eight, or ten weeks for the ligament to heal after surgical treatment is readily accepted by both doctor and patient. The ligament is protected for this period.

Not so the moderate sprain. For the ligament to heal properly, the ligament ends must be apposed and held there until they have healed. In the moderate (second degree) sprain the ligament ends have not been widely separated, since the remaining portion of the ligament has prevented dislocation of the joint. Hence, the ligament ends are presumably close together. It will, however, require the same length of time to heal (namely, six, eight, or ten weeks) and probably will require four months to become secure. In the case thus treated nonsurgically, the symptoms of pain, swelling and edema subside in two or three weeks. The joint is stable. Normal motion and even stress are pain-free. Yet, the ligament is in the very early stage of healing and not really any stronger than on the day of the injury. The player returns to play. The so-called "healed ligament" is subjected to repetition of the very forces that hurt it in the first place. The injury recurs. This often happens repetitively and the joint that was stable after the first injury becomes unstable. Witness the influx of athletes with unstable joints sent in for treatment at the season's end.

The player may have had excellent treatment for the early, brief period; yet the treatment failed because protection was too short. It takes as long for a ligament to heal as it does for a bone.

Severe (Third Degree) (see Fig. 45C, D). In severe sprain there is complete loss of function of the ligament due to a force that eithers tears it completely away from one or the other of its attachments or pulls it apart somewhere within its substance. One must presume that there has been at some time wide separation of the ligament ends or else the tear would not have been complete. Since efficient repair is dependent upon apposition of the torn ends of the ligament, it becomes vitally important to replace the ligament ends in approximation. We have been able to show experimentally in the dog that if the torn ends of the ligament are placed together, the tissues heal by ligament fiber. On the other hand, ligaments which heal across a gap by scar formation never take on the characteristics of normal ligaments.

It can be seen, therefore, that in first-degree sprain, *treatment* is relatively unimportant and is designed mostly to prevent pain, and that in second-degree sprain, the critical factor in *treatment* is *protection* in order to permit repair. On the other hand, in third-degree or severe sprain the emphasis must be placed on *reapposition* of the ligament ends in order to assure that the ligament not only heals in its normal length but also heals with its normal strength. It follows that diagnostic acumen is of great importance in the management of ligament injuries, since treatment depends upon the nature of the lesion rather than upon the patient's progress following injury.

DISLOCATION

Dislocation, or luxation, may be defined as an actual displacement of the opposing contiguous surfaces making up a joint. This, of necessity, presumes loss of function of some of the ligament structures of the joint, since the ligaments are designed to prevent displacement or abnormal motion. *Subluxation* is a partial dislocation. In acute sprain when the ligament finally tears, the joint subluxates either by a slipping of the bone ends on themselves or by a separation of the bone ends. If the force continues until the joint actually is disrupted, there is a dislocation. This may be spontaneously reduced or the bones may lock in the dislocated position (Fig. 46); in either instance there is loss of function of the ligament.

It is possible to have a chronic dislocation without fresh damage to the ligament. In this case one presupposes that the ligament has been previously torn or stretched to the point that dislocation of the joint occurs within the capacity of the surviving ligament. However, in acute dislocation or acute subluxation, the ligament must tear. This is of considerable importance from the standpoint of treatment because if, in an acute dislocation, one visualizes a complete tear of one or more ligaments, the advisability of surgical repair must certainly be considered seriously.

Treatment. Since dislocation is simply the end result of a severe sprain, it can be treated as such. Thus, protection is essential until the ligament has healed, regardless of the method used to secure its repair. For example, if a shoulder dislocates, it may promptly be reduced either by a teammate, the coach or the physician. The fact that it remains out of joint 30 seconds or 30 days is no indication of the extent of ligament damage, although it may have vast effect on the end result. Even if the

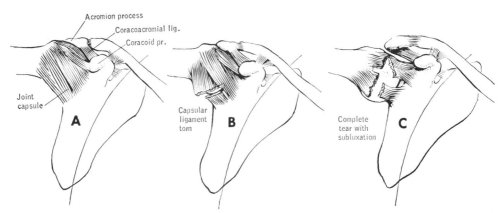

Figure 46. Complete dislocation showing attendant ligament damage. *A,* First stage of dislocation of the shoulder. The arm is externally rotated and abducted, tightening up the anterior and inferior capsular ligaments. The tuberosity hinges on the acromion. *B,* Continuation of the force with the tuberosity locked firmly against the acromion. The ligament fibers tear anteroinferiorly and the head begins to subluxate. *C,* Head subluxating downward and further away from the acromion. Complete rupture of the capsular ligaments.

joint dislocates and immediately reduces itself, there is nonetheless ligament damage and treatment must be designed to further the repair of this tear. In some instances surgical repair will be advisable, whereas in others it will not be necessary. In either event the importance of carrying out protection until the ligament completely heals cannot be overemphasized.

Dislocations as a group are vastly undertreated and as a result are notorious for poor results. The dislocated finger may be promptly reduced, but if the player continues to play or goes without medical care or without splinting of the finger, permanent disability of the involved joint almost inevitably results. Either a painful, swollen joint with restricted motion or a weak, relaxed joint with recurrent dislocation is often the consequence of a nonprotected dislocation. A minimum of six weeks is needed for a ligament to repair even under optimum circumstances. Even at six weeks the actual strength of the repaired ligament does not approach normal, so suitable protection should be continued. After the six weeks of complete immobilization of the involved joint, the finger may be fastened to the adjacent one by tape loops or other bands so that the finger flexes and extends but lateral stress is eliminated. (See Knee Dislocation, page 510.)

TENOSYNOVITIS

Tenosynovitis may be defined as inflammation of the synovium surrounding a tendon. This inflammation is usually due to strain from unaccustomed overuse but may be due to a direct blow or to infection. The result is that the normally avascular synovium reacts with increased blood supply, invasion by inflammatory cells, oversecretion of synovial fluid and increase in fibrin content, causing "sticky" adhesions between the tendon and its surroundings. The exact manifestations vary greatly, depending upon the tendon involved, and will be considered in some detail under various headings. Actually the symptoms are those which would be expected to result from irritation of inflamed tissue by motion of the tendon. The first manifestation is pain on function, which may progress to the point of constant pain even at rest. Crepitation is frequently present. As the tendon slides up and down, it adheres to the synovium, causing so-called "snowball crepitation," which can be felt by placing the fingers over the involved tendon while it slides up and down. As the

condition progresses, the adherence between the tendon and the synovium becomes more firm and may finally result in complete loss of the gliding capacity of the tendon within its sheath. This is particularly true in areas where there is a true tendon sheath (such as the long head of the biceps at the shoulder) and is not common where mesotendon is concerned, as in the tendo Achilles. *Treatment* is directed toward the pathological disorder, and the principles of treatment are rest, local heat and local injection. The specific treatment will vary according to the site of the condition. Steroids should not be used topically for acute conditions.

Sequelae of Tenosynovitis

Under ordinary circumstances and with proper care, the tenosynovitis will subside completely and normal function will result. In certain cases, however, either because of the severity of the condition or as the result of inadequate treatment or the anatomical characteristics of the area involved, complications may arise which may cause severe and permanent disability.

The first of two common sequelae of chronic tenosynovitis is *adhesive tenosynovitis*. As the name implies, the tendon and its surrounding sheath become bound in an inflammatory mass leading to actual adherence between the two, which interferes with the normal gliding motion of the tendon (Fig. 47). This restriction of motion may be complete or only partial. The degree of disability will depend upon the location of the involved tendon. If it is in an area where there is a true sheath, such adherence will prevent motion completely and the muscle-tendon unit will lose its function in regard to this particular area. On the other hand, if it is in an area not constricted by a true sheath, the adherence may simply result in traction strain and possibly some restriction of function rather than complete loss. Treatment for true adhesive tenosynovitis is difficult, since if the adhesions are trimmed away, they may promptly re-form. However, resection of the sheath or transferring the tendon to a less constricted area may be an effective remedy.

The second common sequela is *constrictive tenosynovitis* caused by thickening of the walls of the sheath with resultant narrowness of its lumen. This frequently occurs in an area where more than one tendon passes through the same tunnel or sheath. In such an instance, the

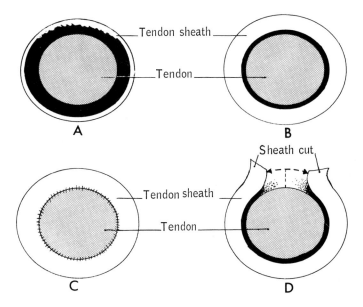

A

B

C

D

Sheath cut

Tendon sheath

Tendon

Tendon sheath

Tendon

Figure 47. Tenosynovitis. *A*, Drawing showing the tendon lying in the sheath with some irritation of the inner wall of the sheath. *B*, Same area, showing the tendon sheath and underlying tendon both swollen and the sheath very tight. *C*, Same area, showing the sheath and tendon adherent to each other. *D*, The area after sectioning of the sheath and releasing of the pressure.

tendon itself is not adherent to the sheath but the sheath is so tight that the tendon will not slide through it. This may start as an initial snapping, such as in a trigger finger, and may terminate in complete loss of gliding of the tendon through this tunnel. Whereas adhesive tenosynovitis is difficult to treat adequately, this constricting type is readily relieved by simply enlarging the tunnel surgically by resection of a part of the sheath. These conditions will be discussed in some detail in relationship to specific areas of the body.

BURSITIS

Bursitis is an inflammatory reaction within a bursa. It may vary in degree from very mild irritative synovitis with discomfort to suppurative bursitis with actual abscess formation. A bursa is specifically designed to facilitate motion between contiguous layers of the body, and the athlete with his violence of motion is particularly prone to bursal involvement resulting from repetitive local trauma due to tissue friction or from direct blows.

The examples of bursitis are legion. The bursae most frequently damaged by direct trauma are the prepatellar, lying between the patella and the skin (Fig. 48) and the olecranon, between the olecranon process of the ulna and the skin. The trauma is usually repetitious, resulting in synovial irritation with thickening of synovium and formation of excess fluid. A large sac of synovial fluid is contained within the bursa. By virtue of the increased tension in the bursa, additional direct trauma tends to further extend its walls until the bursa may reach an amazing size. *Treatment* is directed toward prevention of repeated injury and reduction of the irritation within the bursa. Aspiration of fluid, local injection of corticoids, protection against direct trauma and application of a pressure bandage to appose the walls of the sac are in order. If the condition becomes chronic and the synovitis is persistent, surgical removal of the bursa may become necessary.

Bursitis caused by friction between moving parts is exemplified by that occurring in the bursa beneath the internal hamstring tendons at the knee. Here the principal manifestations of bursitis will be pain on motion of the knee,

Patella

Prepatellar bursa

Superficial and deep infrapatellar bursae

Figure 48. The patellar bursae.

tenderness over the bursa and local inflammatory reaction. Aspiration will be of little value but local injection may reduce the inflammation. *Treatment* must consist of preventing the motion that is causing the inflammation rather than protecting it against direct trauma. Local injection of a long-acting anesthetic agent plus a corticoid, together with application of local heat and a protective splint, is of value. Here again it is important to continue protection until healing is complete because recurrence is likely if the activity that originally caused the inflammation is resumed earlier.

SYNOVIAL HERNIA (GANGLION)

Another condition involving the tendon sheath and sometimes the joint is the synovial hernia or so-called *ganglion*. This condition as a rule results from a defect in the fibrous sheath of the joint or tendon that permits a segment of underlying synovium to herniate through it. In the athlete it usually follows a mild sprain, although it may also be degenerative in nature. The irritation accompanying this herniation results in continued secretion of fluid so that the sac gradually fills up and enlarges. In some instances it may reach an alarming size.

As a rule the synovial hernia will appear as a small, discrete, sometimes extremely hard nodule lying directly over the tendon or the joint capsule. It is often impossible to tell whether the primary involvement is tendon or joint. The consistency of the tumor may vary from that of bone to that of a soft, fluctuant, obviously liquid mass. This difference in consistency is more apparent than real and is due to the degree of tension within the sac, since the sac uniformly will be found to contain a clear, gelatinous, viscous fluid which is blood-tinged only following aspiration or recent trauma. Certain areas of the body, notably the wrist, have a particular predilection for synovial hernia.

The *differential diagnosis* is that of a tumor mass and is not unduly difficult. Synovial hernia may be confused with a dislocated bone such as the semilunar at the wrist. It must be distinguished from a neoplasm. Its general location, lack of local symptoms, and consistency are all definite diagnostic leads. The mass will ordinarily be translucent on transillumination, but on occasion this may be extremely difficult to demonstrate because of unfavorable location. Pain is not a notable factor. The complaint usually is that of a sprain of an adjacent joint. There may be pain and aching on overuse. Frequently extremes of motion may cause considerable discomfort, particularly if the protrusion is recent and rather tight.

Treatment. *Treatment* of synovial hernia is essentially surgical. Although these masses do tend to come and go, and so may respond to periods of splinting and protection or snug wrapping, these measures do not usually solve the problem. They merely postpone it. I have, however, known of many cases in which the ganglion spontaneously regressed and to my knowledge never recurred. When it is symptomatic enough to interfere with athletic activity, it should be removed. In surgical excision, great care must be taken to remove the whole mass. The defect in the capsule or sheath must be repaired, since recurrence is very likely after incomplete removal. The prevalent habit of making a ½-inch incision and popping the mass out like a cyst is really no more effective than the time-honored method of beating it with the edge of a book and is doomed to failure. I well recall a romance that was blighted when I temporarily cured a ganglion over the dorsum of the lady's foot by a sharp blow with the edge of a frying pan.

Aspiration of hernia followed by injection of corticoids has been recommended. In my experience this has been unsatisfactory. However, it may serve to postpone definitive treatment until a more suitable time. To the athlete such a time is at the termination of his season of activity. Under these circumstances the joint should be carefully protected against overstrain. There is no objection to adequate strapping and continued participation, provided this can be made pain-free. Following successful surgical removal, rehabilitation should be as careful as following any joint surgery, and protective strapping should be used throughout the remainder of the season, since there is some weakness of the joint inherent in this condition.

STRESS FRACTURE*

With the increasing involvement in sports activities by nonathletes that seems to characterize the 1980's, the non-conditioned partici-

---

*Printed in part in O'Donoghue, D. H.: The Deceptive Stress Fracture. Consultant Magazine. *13*(11):106–111, 1973.

pant is exposed to the same hazards of injury as the trained athlete. Alas, he is ill-equipped physically to withstand the forces to which his weekend activities will expose him. A particular puzzling condition is the stress, or fatigue, fracture.

During World War I, many young men were put into uniform with ill-fitting shoes and a pack on their backs and were required to take long hikes over rough terrain. Metatarsal bones were not prepared for this excessive stress. The term "march fracture" was coined to describe the fracture of the metatarsal shaft that was caused not by acute injury but by repeated stress (Fig. 49). The condition is peculiarly deceptive, since even though there is no history of injury and early x-ray films are negative, the symptoms persist. "Goldbrick" is a common label applied to those injuries, and it is dispelled only by the appearance of periosteal new bone formation that develops at the site of the insult.

Nor is the appearance of this new callus a wholly unmixed blessing; it is deceptive once again because of the absence of injury, early negative x-ray films and persistent local tenderness and pain in the bone. The delayed

Figure 50. This long distance runner began to have cramping in his calf and pain in his leg that was increased by exertion. X-ray made after several weeks shows periosteal proliferation back of the tibia and a transverse line of sclerosis across the bone, indicating the original stress fracture. Because of his persistent complaint and the appearance of the x-ray he was biopsied elsewhere one week later. The biopsy report was "proliferation of new bone, probably callus." This is a rather classical instance of stress fracture that is quite common in track athletes and is frequently confused with tumor.

Figure 49. This youngster was playing football and complained of soreness in his right foot. He had no history of any specific injury. There had been three weeks of continued crippling when this x-ray was taken. Note complete absence of any fracture line as such. This is a typical "stress" fracture in that there was no definite injury and no specific moment of disability. Although his lesion was fairly mature when first seen, he was treated with a boot cast because he was still symptomatic. Uneventful recovery.

appearance of periosteal new bone formation mimics that of the dreaded bone sarcoma (Fig. 50). Biopsy is particularly misleading, since early callus is then indistinguishable from early tumor.

As this condition has become better understood, it has been recognized that a little patience will reveal the progression of early callus to mature bone with healing of the stress defect (Fig. 51). Often this may occur without

Figure 51. This 17 year old male, while running in track, started having pain in the right shin. This continued to get worse and interfered with his running. *A,* The original x-ray three weeks post onset shows early callus with bone production around the distal third of the tibia. He was advised that he had a stress fracture but there was no treatment. He continued to have trouble off and on all summer; toward the end, so severe, he could not run at all. Examination revealed tenderness of the distal third of the tibia, particularly posteriorly. *B,* Six months after the onset, x-ray shows increased maturity of the bone. Since he was still quite symptomatic, a plaster cast was applied at this time with symptomatic improvement. *C,* One year later, x-ray shows complete maturity. Patient asymptomatic.

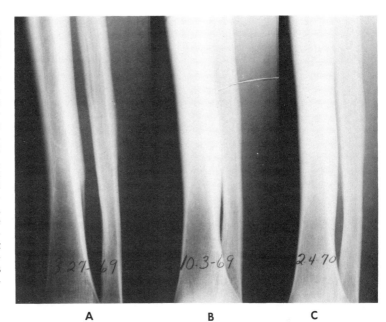

A   B   C

an actual fracture line ever appearing across the shaft.

Although this condition is very common in the foot, this stress or fatigue fracture can appear almost anywhere and under the most confusing of circumstances (Figs. 52 to 54). A high index of suspicion, plus a careful examination that reveals painful stress and tenderness over the bone occurring without specific trauma but under rather unusual stresses, adds to the diagnostic picture.

Once suspected, x-ray examination, repeated at weekly or biweekly intervals, will secure the diagnosis. I must repeat that one must resist the temptation to biopsy. An early biopsy may lead to tragedy. If the mass is really malignant, the two to four weeks of delay necessary to permit the callus to mature

Figure 52. Stress fracture of olecranon process. This 16 year old male felt pain in the elbow while pitching baseball three months earlier. He had started pitching at age eight years and had had no previous trouble with his elbow. He stopped pitching for two weeks. Afterwards he was unable to throw hard. He noticed pain with snap extension of his elbow. *A,* Anteroposterior view is noncontributory. *B,* Lateral x-ray shows stress fracture of the olecranon process, with some sclerosis on either side, as it has been several months since the original injury. Arm placed in plaster cast for six weeks. X-ray three weeks later showed solid union. Three years later he is a scholarship baseball player and continues to pitch.

A   B

Figure 53. This 18 year old male injured his left fibula in the middle third six months before. X-ray negative. No treatment. The leg improved and apparently healed. Three months later he started running and began to have increasing pain so that finally he could not run. Examination revealed tenderness over the distal third of the shaft of the fibula with some thickening of tissue and some enlargement around the bone. A, X-ray six months subsequent to the injury reveals a typical stress fracture at the junction of the middle and lower thirds. B, Two months later, x-ray shows the resolution and maturity of the callus.

Figure 54. Several weeks before, this 19 year old male strained his back playing football. X-ray findings were reported negative. He continued to have a painful low back that was relieved some by a brace. One week later he tried to play, collapsed, and had to be helped from the field because of severe right lumbar muscle spasm. Routine anteroposterior and lateral x-ray film findings were negative. A, Right oblique view shows stress fracture of the pars interarticularis of L-3 Right. B, Uneventful recovery following conservative treatment. If routine x-ray films do not reveal the pathology, special views should be made. (Standard anteroposterior or posteroanterior oblique views will illustrate this whereas usual anteroposterior and lateral films will not.)

Figure 55. This 56 year old female took an unaccustomed long hike. Toward the end of the day she noted increasing pain on the top of the foot, more severe during the night. Examination revealed tenderness over the second metatarsal with swelling. Clinical diagnosis was stress fracture. *A,* Radiographic findings were negative. She was placed in a walking case for six weeks. *B,* X-ray six months later shows minimal mature callus. Uneventful recovery. I believe the early immobilization accounts for the minimal callus formation.

will not adversely affect the progress of the tumor. It may well prevent a diagnostic and therapeutic error. If biopsy is carried out, the pathologist will be faced with a real dilemma. It may not be possible for him to differentiate between early callus and new growth of a tumor. Recommendations for amputation have been made and, indeed, carried out when it seems, in retrospect, that the pathological condition was probably a stress fracture rather than a malignancy.

No age is spared. While the condition is common in young athletes, it may occur at any age (Fig. 55). Only very occasionally will stress fracture progress to actual separation of the fragments. Stress fracture is not the same condition as the incomplete fracture occurring after an acute injury. In the acute injury, the fracture line may not be immediately recognizable and the patient may be treated for sprain. The history of the acute injury, however, renders the problem less confusing and subsequent x-ray films will confirm the diagnosis. The uncertainty about the diagnosis of a true stress fracture is in the absence of a history of acute injury.

Treatment. The treatment is protection against stress until the lesion has solidly healed, followed by gradual resumption of activities in order to build up strength and resistance in the involved area. Since weight-bearing bones, i.e., foot, tibia, fibula (Fig. 56), femur, pelvis and back (Fig. 57), are subject to the most stress, prevention of weight-bearing may be necessary. A walking cast may not

suffice to protect leg bones from stress. Pain is the indicator. If it hurts to walk, walking must be interdicted until it becomes pain-free as the healing progresses. Since the diagnosis may not be confirmed for two or three weeks, treatment of the painful extremity—one that has a possible history of some unusual activity followed by aching pain, which becomes more severe, remains localized and is accompanied by tenderness on the bone—should include non–weight-bearing and whatever degree of immobilization is necessary to relieve the pain. There is no reason to postpone the initiation of treatment until the radiographic findings are positive, since this only prolongs the period of disability. Surgery has no place in the diagnosis or treatment of this condition. Spare the scalpel!

FRACTURES

Treatment. There is nothing particularly unique in the *treatment* of fractures of the athlete. The general principles previously mentioned must be constantly borne in mind, for although one should always attempt to get the best result in the quickest time with a minimum of interference of activity, this is particularly pertinent in the athlete. By and large, a definite fracture is usually adequately treated, since the injury is severe enough to make the diagnosis obvious. The use of x-ray examination is so universal now that the ordinary fracture is recognized early.

Figure 56. Fatigue fracture. This fracture may be mistaken for myositis ossificans or a tumor. *A,* Early film shows periosteal proliferation suggestive of tumor. *B,* There is increased periosteal proliferation but the fracture line is now appearing. *C,* Healing stage. The fracture line is disappearing. Notice consolidation of callus.

Figure 57. This 16 year old male pulled a muscle in his back while wrestling. It did not seem too severe and he was treated by the usual heat modalities. He had some improvement. Almost six weeks later, he was running and had recurrence of severe intractable pain in the back with muscle spasm in the back extending into either hip. Examination revealed pain in the right lumbar muscle mass with spasm. *A,* X-ray reveals a fracture across the pars intercularis over L-5 on the right. *B,* Two months later his cast was removed and he had solid union. Asymptomatic.

Certain exceptions to the previous statement will be discussed in detail under proper headings. I should like to mention specifically fracture of the navicular at the wrist, "march" fracture of the metatarsals (see Fig. 49) and fatigue fracture of the fibula (see Fig. 56). These conditions are all too frequently overlooked because the immediate symptoms may be chronic in nature. Invaluable time is lost, during which the crippled athlete believes he has a strain or a sprain. The ideal time for treatment has frequently passed when the condition is finally recognized.

Another type of fracture that may easily be overlooked is the avulsion fracture. The athlete is subject to sudden spurts of violent activity that may forcibly avulse a fragment of bone either at a tendon or at a muscle attachment (Fig. 58). The condition is primarily one of muscle-tendon injury, the bone fragment being incidental. Its treatment should be that of the primary condition. Neglect or oversight may cause long periods of chronic disability. This is particularly true because this fracture is very prone to calcification or ossification of the accompanying hematoma.

The optimal treatment of fractures depends upon prompt and definitive diagnosis. Since these patients are in good health and in splendid physical condition, one may almost always use the best method of treatment for the fracture without that compromise so often necessitated in regular practice by patients in poor condition. Hence, we are more prone to carry out open reduction of the various fractures when indicated, not only because the

Figure 58. Fresh injury of the neck showing avulsion fracture of the tip of the seventh cervical spinous process.

general condition of the patient will permit it but also because by firm internal fixation we are often able to start rehabilitation at once. We may even be able to entirely avoid external fixation involving the adjacent joints.

Rehabilitation. The great importance of maintaining the athlete in good physical condition, if he intends to resume his athletic activity in the near future, must be borne in mind. If we presume in the case of a certain fracture that the patient will be able to resume athletic activity in four weeks, he will be wholly unable to do this if he has not in the meantime continued his rigorous training. For example, a minimal fracture of a malleolus without displacement may require fixation in a cast for four weeks. Throughout this interval the patient should be actively exercising his opposite extremity and his upper extremities. He should keep up exercises vigorous enough to maintain his endurance to some extent and keep on his training diet in order to avoid gaining weight. It is important also that the muscles of the involved extremity be actively exercised. In this instance the boot cast itself can serve as a weight to permit exercise of the quadriceps, hamstrings, hip, abdomen and back. It is not so commonly recognized that by isometric contractions of the muscles within the cast, he may also keep the muscles of the lower leg and foot in tone.

Again depending upon the location of the fracture, it may be possible to apply protective splints or a protective dressing in such a way that the athlete can resume competition. With judicious application of proper equipment, participation, even in football, may be permitted.

It can be seen that the whole success of such a program depends upon prompt, definitive diagnosis so that healing may progress rapidly and efficiently. Adequate protection must be maintained to minimize irritation at the fracture line, which may result in overcalcification or delayed union. A prompt return to athletic competition will be hastened by early diagnosis, accurate repositioning, firm fixation, either internal or external, continuing rehabilitation and protective dressing. The doctor who is capable of treating fractures should have sufficient ingenuity to devise a specific program for each definite condition.

This book will make no attempt to cover the whole field of fractures but some that are more common to athletes will be discussed in considerable detail. An effort will be made to point out methods of treatment which have stood the test of time in regard to acceleration of physical activity following particular fractures.

CHONDRAL AND OSTEOCHONDRAL FRACTURES*

Although to a large extent chondral and osteochondral fractures have been overlooked in the management of those injuries involving the joint, more attention has been paid to them in the last few years. This is particularly pertinent in regard to the knee and ankle, since by far the greatest number of injuries occur in these two joints. Since the initial symptoms of the injury are often obscure and the immediate disability slight, an early definitive diagnosis may be difficult. By the time a proper diagnosis is made, the condition may have advanced from an acute injury to a chronic condition. Indeed, the initial injury may have been or may be completely overlooked or its significance minimized.

This whole question of separation of cartilage from bone with or without a bony fragment has been buried in a morass of contradiction. Osteochondritis dissecans, chondromalacia (particularly of the patella), joint mouse, idiopathic synovitis with effusion, chronic sprain and, in fact, many other lesions of the knee not initially diagnosed may well have originated as chondral fractures. The diagnosis is frequently so delayed that the

*Printed in part in O'Donoghue, D. H.: Chondral and Osteochondral Fractures, Journal of Trauma 6:469–480 © 1966. The Williams & Wilkins Co., Baltimore.

original injury may have been forgotten, particularly by the young athlete who is subject to multiple injuries and whose memory for them, at best, is none too good (Fig. 59). Many cases of so-called osteochondritis dissecans lesions originate as chondral or osteochondral fractures. The chondral or osteochondral fracture may be an avulsion fracture caused by traction of the posterior cruciate ligament at its femoral attachment (Fig. 60, Case 1). They may be caused by the direct contusion of a blow driving the patella against the femur (Fig. 61). They may be shearing fractures (Fig. 62) which occur in the patella or in the lateral femoral condyle as the patella is dislocated over the lateral condyle. These injuries often cause relatively few early symptoms. The x-ray films may well be entirely negative. There is too great a tendency for the x-ray film to be considered the ultimate diagnostic instrument (Fig. 63). As a result, the patient goes along for weeks or months, his injury classified under various diagnoses indicated previously. Yet, there has been no real recognition of the true nature of his lesion nor any effort to determine the exact etiology.

This subject naturally divides itself into two categories: the *acute fracture* and the *late manifestations*. The former must be differentiated from acute injuries to the ligaments, to the menisci, to the synovium or to the periarticular structures of the knee. The latter must be distinguished from other chronic intrinsic conditions of the knee.

No such simple division can properly be made, however, since it is apparent that the two groups are one and the same, the latter being the logical sequela of the former.

Figure 59. Fourteen year old girl seen with swelling of the ankle and persistent pain and disability, especially after prolonged standing. A fall, two years before, had been treated as a slight sprain. A, Shows osteochondral fracture at the dome of the talus, laterally. B, Normal ankle. C, Inversion view demonstrating fragment. D, Two months after surgical removal of fragment. No resultant instability but some persistent discomfort.

Figure 60. Comparison of acute and chronic chondral fractures of the femoral condyle. Case 1 (top). Injury to the knee at four weeks with continued disability and hemarthrosis. Surgery reveals a large osteochondral fragment containing two thirds of the femoral attachment of the posterior cruciate ligament. There is relatively fresh granulation tissue on both the fragment and the bed. A, Typical appearance of osteochondritis dissecans. B, The fragment with its vascular bed. Treatment was removal of the fragments and repair of the ligament into the bed by drill holes. Uneventful recovery. This is a chondral fracture, sub-acute.

Case 2 (bottom). Similar case at 18 months with intermittent effusion and moderate disability, and showing increasing synovitis. C, Surgery reveals fragments at the same location as in A, Case 1. Fragments and bed are quite sclerotic. The posterior cruciate ligament attaches to the fragments. D, Removal of the fragment and repair of the ligament through drill holes. This is a typical osteochondritis dissecans and would seem to have the same etiology as the Case 1 fracture. (From O'Donoghue, The Journal of Trauma, Vol. 6, 1966.)

Figure 61. *A,* Acute injury by direct fall on the flexed knee with bloody effusion. Negative x-ray film findings. *B,* The defect after removal of the fragment showing the fresh vascular bed with blood that has infiltrated the cartilage. (From O'Donoghue, The Journal of Trauma, Vol. 6, 1966.)

Figure 62. Patient was blocked from behind in football, dislocating the patella; reduced by doctor, no support. Examination four weeks later revealed gross swelling, hemarthrosis and pain. Patella not loose or malaligned. *A,* The obviously fresh injury with fresh granulating bed caused by shearing force of the patella against the femoral condyle. *B,* Silhouette showing the osteochondral fragment (arrow). (From O'Donoghue, The Journal of Trauma, Vol. 6, 1966.)

Figure 63. *A,* Acute injury in baseball from sliding into second base with direct contusion of the knee. Note fresh vascular bed and mosaic of blood through the avulsed fragment. Negative x-ray film findings. *B,* A similar older injury in which the fracture bed is sclerotic and the fragments of cartilage are necrosed. This would be called osteochondritis dissecans. If fragments were completely loose, it would be called a joint mouse. Negative x-ray. (From O'Donoghue, The Journal of Trauma, Vol. 6, 1966.)

Figure 64. *A,* One year after direct fall on the knee, with chronic patellar symptoms since the fall. Note central area with degenerative cartilage similar to Figure 61*A*, *B,* "Shaving brush" protrusion of the cartilage. Note similarity of the lesion shown here with that in Figure 61: Both are chondral fractures, the one acute, the other chronic. (From O'Donoghue. The Journal of Trauma, Vol. 6, 1966.)

Whether or not the acute fracture results in the chronic condition often depends directly upon the treatment or lack of treatment given the original condition. Chronic chondral fractures do not occur as such. They must evolve from an acute injury.

Once the chronic condition develops, it may be classified under a wholly different category. The acute fracture of the patellar cartilage becomes patellar malacia (Fig. 64). Avulsion of the femoral articular cartilage by the posterior cruciate ligament attachment becomes osteochondritis dissecans (Fig. 60, Case 2). The displaced chondral fragment becomes the joint mouse (Fig. 65). Indeed, I believe that many, if not the majority, of cases of joint mouse, patellar malacia and osteochondritis dissecans occurring in young people are really chondral fractures.

Acute Chondral Fracture

Mechanism of Chondral Fractures
1. Compaction
   A. Patella—direct trauma
   B. Tibial plateau—by femoral condyle
   C. Patellar groove of femur—by patella
2. Shearing force
   A. Patella—over femoral condyle
   B. Femoral condyle—by patella
   C. Condylar margin—by direct trauma
3. Avulsion
   A. Upper tibia—by anterior cruciate ligament
   B. Medial femoral condyle—by posterior cruciate ligament
   C. Patella—by quadriceps tendon, by medial retinaculum, and by patellar tendon

Acute chondral fractures result from three main types of trauma: compaction, shearing and avulsion. *Compaction* fractures result from direct force applied vertically to the joint surface. The mechanism of the compaction fracture is exemplified by the direct blow over the patella, crushing the patellar cartilage against the femoral cartilage. Because it is convex, the femoral cartilage is better able to withstand the injury, and the cartilage under the patella is compressed or compacted (Fig. 66). Similarly, the same type of injury which may cause a plateau fracture of the tibia may be limited in its force and cause compaction of the tibial cartilage as the convex femoral condyle crushes

Figure 65. Acute traumatic dislocated patella. Note the acute chondral fracture in the middle third of the patella resulting from the forceful blow of the patella against the femur. (From O'Donoghue, The Journal of Trauma, Vol. 6, 1966.)

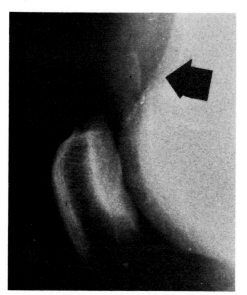

Figure 66. While running cross-country one year before, the patient stepped on a board at the edge of the track, fell and injured the knee. (Previous hyperextension injury three years before.) Immediate pain and swelling ensued. Patient was operated upon elsewhere but no pathological condition was found. No postoperative support. Two weeks postoperatively the patient kicked a football and the knee became swollen; subsequently, with continued trouble, a palpable mass was noticed, sometimes medially, sometimes laterally. At the second operation in November 1963, a large osteochondral fragment was removed. The defect in the femoral condyle was represented by a small amount of dishing of the cartilage that was proceeding to complete obliteration. (From O'Donoghue, The Journal of Trauma, Vol. 6, 1966.)

into it. The femoral condyle itself may be damaged by either the patella or the tibia by the same mechanism.

Shearing fractures are the result of a glancing blow almost tangential or parallel to the articular surface. Such a fracture is exemplified by the shearing force of the patella against the lateral femoral condyle as the patella forcibly dislocates across it. The cartilage of the patella may be sheared off (see Fig. 62) or the articular cartilage over the femoral condyle may be knocked off with or without a segment of bone (Fig. 67).

Avulsion fractures of the cartilage, often with a shell of bone, in many ways are the most intriguing because of the disability which may result from loss of function of the avulsing agent. A well-recognized example is the fracture caused by the traction of the anterior cruciate ligament on the upper end of the tibia (Fig. 68). Similarly, avulsion of the portion of the cartilage by the quadriceps tendon (Fig. 69) or by the medial retinaculum of the patella is frequently seen (Fig. 70). Much less recognized is avulsion of the articular cartilage from the lateral side of the medial femoral condyle at the attachment of the posterior cruciate ligament (see Fig. 60). Significantly, this is also a common place for so-called osteochondritis dissecans, which is neither a chondritis nor a dissecting lesion.

Although this pathological condition results

Figure 67. *A,* Twisting injury of knee causing osteochondral fracture, x-ray showing the fragment lodged in the intercondylar notch. *B,* Defect left by the osteochondral fracture of the lateral femoral condyle caused by the subluxating patella as the medial retinaculum ruptured. Inset shows fragment. (From O'Donoghue, The Journal of Trauma, Vol. 6, 1966.)

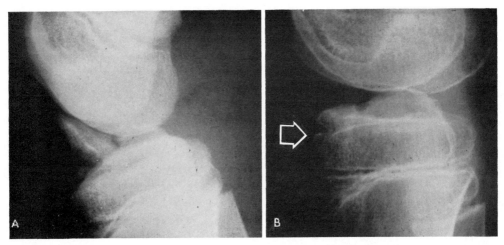

Figure 68. Young girl with injury to the knee from a bicycle accident, six months previously. Marked restriction of both extension and flexion. *A,* Osteochondral fracture caused by the anterior cruciate ligament pulling from the top of the tibia. *B,* Replaced and held by internal fixation through drill holes (arrow). (From O'Donoghue, The Journal of Trauma, Vol. 6, 1966.)

from an acute injury, it can readily be seen that each of these types of trauma can under certain circumstances result in the chronic conditions previously mentioned, such as patellar malacia, osteochondritic foreign body and os-

Figure 69. X-ray revealing osteochondral fragment avulsed by the quadriceps tendon. This fragment includes the whole attachment of the quadriceps mechanism. There was substantially more cartilage with the fragment than is indicated by the shell of bone seen in the x-ray picture. (From O'Donoghue, The Journal of Trauma, Vol. 6, 1966.)

teochondritis dissecans. Thus a fall on the patella may well cause a stellate type of fracture of the patella with or without compression of the subchondral bone. Early operation makes this abundantly clear (see Fig. 61). Delayed observation reveals malacia (Figs. 64 and 71).

Avulsion of the osteochondral fragment by the posterior cruciate ligament is quite obvious if the patient is operated on early (Fig. 60, Case 1). Operation in the chronic stage reveals osteochondritis dissecans (Fig. 60, Case 2). The fragment sheared from the femoral condyle by the dislocating patella is obvious if enough bone goes with it to throw a shadow on a radiograph (see Fig. 67). If, on the contrary, a dislocation shears off the undersurface of the patella, so-called patellar malacia may result. If the cartilage alone is sheared off, early surgery reveals the fresh fragment separated from a fresh bleeding bed like coconut meat from its shell. Yet, if this is not surgically treated until chronic symptoms supervene, we find a cartilaginous foreign body, often without an obvious defect in the articular cartilage (Fig. 72).

It is difficult to describe osteochondritis dissecans of the femoral condyle as a vascular defect, since it occurs in an area which is so well vascularized. If infarction is the cause of the lesion, why does it not happen in the femoral head, for example, where circulation may be regarded as poor, or possibly in the head of the talus or even more likely in the lunate or other carpal bones? We rarely see osteochondritis dissecans in these areas, but

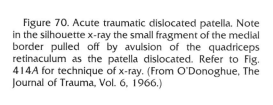

Figure 70. Acute traumatic dislocated patella. Note in the silhouette x-ray the small fragment of the medial border pulled off by avulsion of the quadriceps retinaculum as the patella dislocated. Refer to Fig. 414A for technique of x-ray. (From O'Donoghue, The Journal of Trauma, Vol. 6, 1966.)

we frequently see it where the circulation is very good. The etiology must be trauma and not aseptic necrosis from a primary vascular defect.

The same type of pathological change may occur in virtually any other location, the exact findings varying according to the nature of the injury. It must be agreed that at least some of the cases which are illustrated here are the direct result of acute trauma. Many others could be shown in which this seems equally acceptable but in which the definitive diagnosis was so late that they were labeled patellar malacia, osteochondritis dissecans, osteochondral foreign bodies and so forth. The patient is entitled to a meticulous examination at the

time of his original injury. If at all possible a definite diagnosis should be made before the ideal time for treatment has passed. Most of these cases of osteochondral fractures that are recognized early and treated properly will have an entirely acceptable result. The old concept that hyaline cartilage does not regenerate must be abandoned. I personally have seen many cases in which a large defect from an acute osteochondral fracture has filled in completely. Many cases are seen in which there is a large osteochondral foreign body in the knee without any recognizable defect in the joint cartilage or with a defect which is essentially obliterated.

Ironically, the more severe injuries are rec-

Figure 71. Radiograph of a patient with chronic recurring effusion of the knee. A, Note the dishing out of the central portion of the patella (arrow). B, Normal patella. (From ODonoghue, The Journal of Trauma, Vol. 6, 1966.)

Figure 72. A 28 year old woman who had knee symptoms at age 16 and who has had occasional trouble since. Note the large osteochondritic fragment just below the femoral articular surface (arrow). Careful inspection of all the articular surfaces of the knee failed to reveal any defect from which this fragment was avulsed. The defect had completely filled in during the 12 years. (From O'Donoghue, The Journal of Trauma, Vol. 6, 1966.)

ognized early and treated adequately. Therefore, better results are obtained in these than in the lesser injuries in which the treatment is delayed or inadequate. Thus, the severe injury recognized and treated promptly not only spares the patient the physical, mental and economic trauma of the prolonged period of disability but usually leaves a lesser degree of permanent disability.

Diagnosis. These cases may be quite difficult or even impossible to diagnose early. This certainly should not be used as an excuse not to try. In any case in which the symptoms (i.e., pain under the patella, bloody effusion, tenderness along the condyles of the femur or pain on anterior or posterior stress of the flexed tibia) seem worse than the recognizable findings, one should suspect chondral damage. If the patient does not respond to treatment, he should not be called uncooperative or a nonconformist. *It is just possible that the treatment is at fault rather than the patient.*

In any acute injury of the joint, it behooves us to try to make a definitive diagnosis as soon as possible. A very worthwhile extra dividend may be received from early diagnosis. Thus, if a meniscus rupture is diagnosed promptly and operated on at once, it may be possible to recognize associated chondral damage early.

Early diagnosis and prompt surgical treatment of an acute dislocation of the patella is the best treatment. Exposure reveals the medial retinaculum to be torn and gaping apart. Unrepaired, it can only heal with redundancy and in many cases with insecurity. Prompt surgical repair obviates this danger. Early surgery may reveal undiagnosable chondral fracture of the patella or femur, which should be treated surgically if treatment is to be successful. The reason for procrastination has often been an unwillingness to accept the responsibility for making a definitive diagnosis and then acting upon it. If you believe that the acute rupture of the meniscus should be treated surgically, how much better it would be to initiate this treatment early and so be able to handle other pathological conditions in which the treatment must be carried out early if it is to be successful. The percentage of meniscus ruptures that completely heal is not large enough to justify waiting for the second, third or fourth episode before surgical treatment is recommended.

I have urged that the best results can be obtained only by prompt, definitive diagnosis. This may present very serious problems in the acute injury. Of first importance is the fact that the surgeon is cognizant of this injury. If he has a high index of suspicion in cases in which chondral fracture may have occurred, he will be much more likely to make the definitive diagnosis. Careful examination of the patient who presents following a fall on the patella, for example, may reveal tenderness around the margin of the patella. There may be evidence of a retinacular tear. Aspiration of the joint may reveal bloody fluid with fat globules. Very careful search of repeated radiographs may give some clue as to the lesion. The fact that these lesions often accompany other injuries to the knee is of great importance. One might hesitate to explore a knee simply on the suspicion of infraction of the patella. On the other hand, if the injury accompanies a retinacular tear, a double dividend may be awarded by permitting early treatment of both lesions. In my practice of early surgical treatment of ligament and meniscus injuries to the knee, I have many times been rewarded by recognition of an associated chondral fracture. Repeated examinations from day to day, not from week to week, and an objective analysis of the positive findings may lead to the proper conclusion. Once reached, the conclusion should be acted upon.

Treatment. Once the diagnosis is made, treatment becomes easy. If the patellar retinaculum is torn, it should be repaired. If either cruciate ligament is pulled away, it can be sutured. Not so well defined is the treatment of the chondral fracture. I have not been a proponent of replacement and pinning of the displaced chondral fragment. If it is an osteochondral fragment and is of fairly good size, such as a fragment of the femoral condyle, replacement and internal fixation may indeed result in union. So, too, if the fragment which is pulled off by the anterior cruciate ligament is large, such as a portion of the upper tibia, it may be easily replaced with appropriate suture and firmly held to its bed (Fig. 68). The osteochondral fragment pulled away by the posterior cruciate ligament also may be replaced surgically. If the fragment is small or is mostly cartilage, it should be removed and the ligament repaired to the raw bed. In each of these circumstances, the accompanying lesion demands some period of immobilization so that replacement of the fragment does not entail additional morbidity.

On the other hand, the purely chondral fragment, whether or not it is entirely loose or simply knocked loose and attached in some portion of its surface, poses a different problem. Regeneration of articular cartilage is encouraged by active function. Pinning of the fragment requires not only immobilization but also non–weight-bearing. This is not conducive to cartilage regeneration. My own preference in these instances is to remove the fragment, including all of the margin which is detached from the bone, and to trephine the defect by cutting the cartilage vertical to the articular surface until all of the fragmented or undermined cartilage is removed. This leaves a defect in the cartilage like a pit rather than like a saucer.

In acute injury, the bed is vascular and should be left alone. The defect should not be saucerized. To taper the cartilage down to the bed simply enlarges the defect. Whether regeneration comes from the bony bed below or whether it grows in from the margin is immaterial, since in either case the defect to be filled will be less in a trephined hole than in a tapered or shaved one. The patient is then encouraged to undertake active function, including weight-bearing. Articular cartilage does regenerate. Whether or not it is true hyaline cartilage is beside the point, since it so resembles hyaline cartilage that it cannot be distinguished by observation, palpation, microscopic examination or even by chemical analysis. Certainly, if an acute defect is found in the cartilage, diligent search must be made in the joint to find and remove the fragment.

Chronic Chondral Fracture

It is not the purpose here to discuss in detail the treatment of the chronic chondral or osteochondral fracture. This will be discussed under the specific joint concerned. As has been indicated, these fractures often cannot be distinguished from malacia, from osteochondritis dissecans, from cartilaginous foreign body and so forth. The treatment of each of these may be quite different. I repeat that there is little rationale for shaving of the defect in weight-bearing bone. I frequently do shave the patella, particularly since the lesion is often quite diffuse.

Treatment in the chronic case becomes a matter of salvage. The best judgment must be used, adjusted strictly to the circumstances present. The relatively small, well-defined malacic area should be trephined, not shaved. After trephining, the sclerotic bed should be drilled in order to improve vascularity and to make a more suitable bed in which the new cartilage may develop. Diffuse areas of malacia in the patella, femoral condyle or patellar groove must be shaved until firm cartilage is found, even though bare bone is exposed. If severe enough, patellectomy may be indicated. Patellectomy should be avoided in the young child until clinical trial of other measures is carried out.

In an old avulsion fracture the sclerotic fragment should be removed and the ligament repaired to the freshened bed. I see no purpose in replacing a necrotic fragment. So also, in the old shearing fracture, no attempt should be made to replace the fragment, which at best fits imperfectly into the old sclerotic bed. The fragment should be removed and appropriate treatment applied to the bed. If sclerotic, it should be drilled or curetted; if filled with unorganized debris, it should be curetted; if filled in well with organizing tissue, it should be left alone.

Early treatment is often rewarded by complete recovery. Procrastination might be successful only in the case of a patient without a disabling injury.

OSTEOCHONDRITIS DISSECANS

Osteochondritis dissecans is an articular cartilage involvement occurring most frequently in the knee. There is considerable disagreement concerning the exact etiology; some believe that the condition results from spontaneous ischemic necrosis due to faulty circulation in the epiphyseal vessels, whereas others believe that it is due to trauma, with a fissure-type chondral fracture down to the subchondral bone. As in so many conditions in which there is disagreement about the exact cause, it is probable that in certain instances, more than one factor may be present and that in others there is a disparate etiology. Thus, it may be that repeated trauma precedes the ischemic necrosis. Or, it may be that the necrosis develops spontaneously, and the actual dislodging of the fragment may be due to trauma superimposed on a pathological area. It seems probable, however, that localized trauma is the most frequent cause.

In any event, the pathological condition consists of the separation of a fragment of cartilage from the underlying matrix. This line of separation fills with granulation tissue. The separated fragment necroses because of poor circulation and, in effect, becomes a sequestrum. Since the articular cartilage of this fragment is nourished primarily by synovial fluid, the cartilage does not necrose at this stage but remains intact. In fact, the whole cycle of separation, necrosis and regeneration may occur without any defect in the articular cartilage and may terminate in spontaneous healing of the condition. On the other hand, if enough of the fragment is absorbed to permit it to depress into the crater in the epiphyseal bone, fissuring of the cartilage and ultimate separation may occur. It may be that in some cases, trauma is the factor that ultimately breaks the fragment loose. So, in some cases the fragment may never separate and spontaneous recovery ensues. In other cases the fragment may become entirely free in the joint and then is a foreign body. The age incidence coincides with the age of active athletics, namely, adolescence and early adulthood. Thus, this condition is frequently seen in athletes. There is no preventive measure of any value.

The condition may be completely asymptomatic and may be discovered only by incidental radiographs. More commonly there will be discomfort in the joint, sometimes accompanied by effusion, with symptoms of internal derangement. This may go on until there is actual locking of the joint if the fragment becomes free or if a flap of cartilage turns up and interposes between the articular surfaces. Many patients will present themselves with the complaint of chronic nonspecific joint pain with very few localizing symptoms.

The *management* varies from no treatment to operative excision of the fragment and will be discussed in detail under the various joint categories. In general it may be said that in the very young, treatment should be conservative, since spontaneous regression will be seen in many cases if the part is protected (Fig. 73). In a non–weight-bearing joint, surgery is less frequently required than in a weight-bearing joint. If the fragment completely separates (Fig. 74) or forms a flap interfering with motion of a joint, surgical treatment is mandatory and includes removing the fragment and trephining the cartilaginous margins of the crater. Further measures will depend upon the extent and location of the lesion, since function may need to be restricted. Drilling of the sclerotic crater may help reconstitution of the cartilage.

MUSCLE CRAMPING

Muscle spasm or cramping is a very frequent complaint in the athlete. I am sure that there are many causes for this condition. I am equally sure that there are many things which are called muscle spasm or cramping that are due to some other pathological state. Actually, the etiological and the pathological features seem to be inextricably confused. Many common injuries will cause spasm of the muscle. Some of the more common are a blow to the muscle causing slight infiltration of blood, overstretch of the muscle causing rupture of some of the fibers, and strain by overcontraction of the muscle against resistance. Each of these causes the same type of injury to the muscle-tendon unit.

Frequently the muscle cramp or spasm appears to be an entity in itself. One of the most common and dramatic examples is the severe cramping that occurs in the calf of the apparently normal athlete. While going at full speed, he suddenly gets a violent contraction of the calf which pulls the foot down into equinus and causes severe cramping pain. Indeed, this may come on when actual exertion is at a minimum, at least with respect to any overuse or overstretching. There are several causes of this condition, some remediable and some not. There appears to be no doubt that reduction of the quantity of salt by excessive perspiration will cause a condition in which the muscles of the body are quite subject to cramping. Changes in temperature, sudden chilling or

Figure 73. Osteochondritis dissecans in a 12 year old athlete. *A,* Note the fragment on the medial femoral condyle, not detached. *B,* Five months later the mass is resolving with no treatment.

even sudden overheating may also be responsible. Dietary considerations are sometimes important. Many of these factors can be obviated in an adequate training program. Such metabolic causes will require more emphasis on prevention than on cure.

In another category are those cases in which there is definite local impairment of circulation to the part, as when the cuff of the pants is too tight around the calf or the calf muscle has been strapped circumferentially in such a way as to interfere with its blood supply. There is no actual pathological change in the muscle other than rapid build-up of muscle waste products and diminution of oxygen supply. Overfatigue may cause cramping for much the same reasons that constriction does. In this area I think the spasm is basically due to build-up of CO_2 and diminution of oxygen, which would indicate that increased oxygenation might help. It has been my observation that individual muscle cramping, not necessarily

Figure 74. Osteochondritis dissecans with free fragment. On removal, this fragment was found to be attached to a portion of the posterior cruciate ligament.

under violent activity, can often be alleviated by deep breathing. This seems to be further supported by the fact that most of the isolated cramping occurs at night during sleep when oxygen exchange is at a minimum.

Ruling out all these potential causes for cramping, there still remains a group of cases in which there is no specifically recognizable cause for the condition. In most instances the player has had no preliminary symptoms, the muscle jumps into intractable spasm and the player is rendered helpless both by the pain and by the restriction of motion. Examination will elicit nothing other than the contracted muscle. The muscle is not particularly tender. There is no swelling or edema. One should suspect muscle spasm when sudden severe pain occurs in any muscular area of the body. It is particularly prevalent in the neck, in the back, in the hamstrings and in the calves. The fact that the cramping is common in weight-bearing portions of the anatomy but relatively infrequent in the upper extremities may be of some significance.

Treatment. The _treatment_ of muscle cramping is usually simple and in the majority of instances can be administered by the player himself. His immediate instinct is to apply local pressure to the spastic muscle and to try to force it through a normal range of motion. The player will sit on the ground and grab his calf firmly with one hand while he dorsiflexes his foot with the other—an expedient that is often amazingly effective. The cramp may be released by simple contraction of the opposing muscle, so that if there is a cramp in one flank, stretching the muscle by leaning to the opposite side will frequently relieve the tension.

If the player needs help in relaxing his spasm, the same principles apply. Steady, even, firm but atraumatic local pressure will often give dramatic relief. So also will simple stretching of the muscle. The combination of the two appears to be even more effective. One should constantly bear in mind that he is trying to restore only a normal range of motion; he must not overstretch the muscle. In the contracted hamstring, the knee should be extended, but forceful straight leg raising should not be carried out. If the calf is involved, the foot should be pushed up to 90 degrees but not forced into extreme dorsal flexion. For this reason these manipulations should be carefully controlled. Passive manipulation should be applied steadily and smoothly with no jerk or swing. To apply massive force with leverage against a muscle

in spasm may result in rupture of the muscle fibers or even avulsion of the tendon, in which case a relatively simple condition is replaced by one much more serious. I know of no place in the treatment of any acute injury where this type of excessive manipulative force is desirable. It certainly is not desirable in the treatment of muscle spasm.

The same thing can be said about massage. Massage directed toward restoring circulation to the muscle is quite acceptable, whereas deep kneading, pounding or pummeling of a muscle that is already insufficiently supplied with metabolites can result only in harm. As the muscle spasm relaxes, relatively gentle massage toward the direction of the venous flow may be useful. The muscle may be tapped gently from side to side by the two hands with a rolling manipulation of the muscle between the two palms. Usually this cramp is relatively short-lived, and the player may continue to compete, although the condition is quite prone to recur within the immediate future. If the cramping is more persistent, it will require further treatment. This consists of rest of the part and application of local heat. This can be done by whirlpool baths, warm packs, infrared rays or diathermy or in fact any heat modality. Inductive heat appears to be more effective than radiant heat. Massage is valuable in restoring circulation to the muscle.

A patient who has had persistent muscle spasm may have residual soreness and aching in the muscle, and during this period he should avoid forceful activity. A carefully planned regimen of physical therapy with gradually increasing resistive exercises within his tolerance and short of pain-producing stimuli should be carried out. It may well be that these persistent symptoms following cramp are actually due to ruptured muscle fibers with edema and blood infiltration and should be treated as such. The duration of treatment will depend upon the symptoms. I cannot agree that the best treatment for torn muscle fibers with hematoma into the muscles is immediate active use in spite of pain and muscle spasm. Until one is absolutely sure that there has been no damage to the muscle itself in the nature of hemorrhage, edema or separated muscle fibers, there is no place for stretching, massage or active exercise.

In these conditions, in so far as medication is concerned, there is a general feeling that the possibility of the occurrence of cramping can be reduced by adequate salt intake. However, this theory is currently somewhat under fire.

Certainly, in severe cases, injection of intravenous saline solution seems to relieve cramping. A time-honored remedy, which I have not encountered recently in any medical text, is the use of quinine sulfate. It seems to be amazingly successful and, even when taken orally, may give relief of the cramping in as little as 10 or 15 minutes. It is difficult to verify its effectiveness, as the patient may have been relieved in that time without any medication. If the cramping occurs at night in bed, it is comforting to have some quinine sulfate on hand. A 5 milligram tablet can be taken, followed by another in two or three hours if necessary.

PHLEBITIS

Phlebitis is not a common condition in the athlete, at least as a definite clinical entity. There is, of course, a certain amount of phlebitis accompanying contusions, sprains or strains, but this is a secondary local reaction and is quite amenable to the measures taken for relief of the specific injury. In the treatment of any local inflammatory condition, one should be on the alert to detect signs of phlebitis. This is particularly pertinent in the lower extremities, where the saphenous vein is quite susceptible to inflammation. The symptoms of developing phlebitis may be lost in the symptoms of the original lesion.

There is some conflict of opinion in regard to the best therapy, once phlebitis is imminent. Certainly, the best therapy is to *prevent* phlebitis by encouraging actual activity of the muscle that is affected, thus accelerating the flow of blood. Once the phlebitis is definite, one must consider whether it still remains just an inflammatory reaction or whether there is actually clot formation in the vein. If the phlebitis is local and of little consequence, rest of the part and support by a snugly fitting elastic bandage may suffice. If it is more generalized and there is considerable febrile reaction, anticoagulant therapy should be instituted. This will require hospitalization. If there is clot formation, complete immobilization of the affected area is advised. This is contrary to the general concept of preventing phlebitis. Good judgment must be exercised in this regard. If the phlebitis seems to be of serious consequence, the aid of some physician who is schooled in its treatment should be sought. The main factor here is to be on the alert for developing phlebitis so that it can be treated before it becomes a problem.

LYMPHADENITIS AND LYMPHANGITIS

Lymphadenitis and lymphangitis frequently accompany infection and are particularly prevalent following abrasions of the hands or infection around the feet, such as an ingrown toenail or severe athlete's foot. The involvement of the lymph system is due to the drainage from the infection. The symptoms are increasing pain in the local lesion, followed by the appearance of red streaks extending toward the neighboring lymph glands (lymphangitis). If one is familiar with the distribution of the lymph system, he will not expect to find glands at the back of the knee involved in an infection in an area of the foot that drains directly to the groin. These red streaks will have local heat and tenderness but are not particularly painful. Soreness will develop in the regional lymph glands, which may become swollen and inflamed (lymphadenitis). Only occasionally will they go on to suppuration.

Treatment. The development of lymphadenitis demands more adequate treatment of the local lesion, such as adequate drainage of the infection, elevation of the part and application of heat locally. Antibiotics should be used and one of the broad-spectrum type will usually be adequate. If it is possible to get a culture and determine which antibiotic is most effective, this should be done. This will require 24 to 48 hours, and the antibiotic therapy should not be postponed while awaiting a report from the laboratory. If the local lesion is handled well, the secondary involvement of the lymph system will usually promptly subside. Needless to say, active athletics should not be permitted during the period of inflammation, not only to protect the affected player but also to protect his fellows from contamination. This player should not participate in athletics until the condition has entirely subsided and there is no longer inflammation in the glands.

NERVE INJURY

Contusion

Fortunately, the nervous system is not too commonly involved in injuries to the athlete because the player is usually in excellent condition, with strong muscles to protect the nerves from overstress. In only a few areas of the body are the nerves particularly exposed to trauma, and these will be considered in the discussion of specific areas. The peripheral nerves most frequently involved are the ulnar nerve at the elbow, the peroneal nerve behind the fibular head, the radial nerve in the midarm and the axillary nerve at the shoulder. The injury is usually from a direct blow on the nerve, causing a contusion. There is an immediate "shocking" sensation followed by numbness and pain. The condition may be entirely transient. The player may "shake it off" in a few minutes and be none the worse for the experience. If the injury is more severe, there will be persistent aching pain along the distribution of the nerve, the result of swelling and edema and congestion within the nerve and nerve sheath. The treatment of this degree of contusion should depend upon the area involved and the severity of the symptoms. In general, as long as the symptoms are relatively acute, the part should be protected against overuse. The nerve should be protected by all means against further contusion.

In the isolated case there may be paralysis of the muscles supplied by the nerve. This may be immediate owing to direct damage to the nerve fibers. In this instance, one should seriously consider whether the nerve may actually have been crushed by the blow. Usually the early symptoms of numbness, aching and pain will be followed by disability of the muscle involved, which may progress to complete loss of function. If the peroneal nerve is involved, there will be a foot drop. If it is the ulnar nerve, there will be weakness and loss of function of the intrinsic muscles of the hand. There may be hypesthesia or sensory loss throughout the sensory distribution of these mixed nerves. As long as this weakness or paralysis continues, the muscle should be supported by cast or brace. Physical therapy should be instituted to encourage return of function in the muscles. Recovery is almost always complete and usually is fairly rapid. The need for further protection after recovery from the paralysis will depend upon the condition of the muscle. The muscle should be protected as long as it is weak. Its strength should be improved by appropriate physical therapy.

Stretch Injury

Another type of injury to the nervous system is caused by overstretch of the nerve, for example, overstretching of the peroneal nerve

after rupture of the lateral collateral ligaments of the knee. A recent case was seen eight months following an injury in which the patient "sprained" the lateral ligament of the knee. Examination revealed peroneal paralysis with a positive Tinel sign just above the head of the fibula. There was instability of the lateral collateral ligament. Exploration revealed a badly scarred peroneal nerve, tightly bound down with scar from torn lateral collateral ligament. The nerve was carefully dissected out with separation of the fibers by neurolysis entirely across the 1½ inch scarred-in area. The lateral collateral ligament was advanced on its femoral attachment. The patient was in splints for eight weeks and wore a drop-foot brace most of the time for one year. At the end of this period he had active but not complete dorsiflexion, with complete recovery from his sensory paralysis except for a little hypesthesia over the top of the foot. His knee was stable. It was three months before he got any return of function and over a year before the return was complete. He is now a college scholarship football player.

In such a case the severity of the ligament injury may screen the nerve condition so that it is not recognized until later. The symptoms will vary with the severity of the injury. If there is a complete avulsion of the nerve, there will be immediate and complete loss of function, whereas if the nerve is stretched but not torn, there will be hemorrhage and shock to the fibers but function will be more slowly and less completely lost. Whenever there has been complete loss of function of a nerve, one must decide whether or not surgical exploration is justified. The examining physician is responsible for the early detection of these injuries. Any statement by the patient about numbness, weakness or loss of motion should be carefully investigated. It is very important to determine the function of the nerve before definitive treatment is undertaken. A classic example is the dislocated elbow. If one discovers some hours, days or even weeks later that there is paralysis of the median nerve, it may be impossible to determine definitely whether this injury was athletic or iatrogenic. It is of particular importance to note carefully any sensory loss, since the diminution or increase of such an area may well be the determining factor in selecting the proper treatment.

Treatment. From the surgical standpoint, one should be quite conservative in treatment of an injury to the nerve. In a great majority of cases, gradual recovery will take place as the weeks go by. Such recovery will ordinarily be well advanced at the end of three months if it is likely to be complete. On the other hand, late surgical suture of the nerve may be quite successful and one can afford to delay exploration for a reasonable period of time (three months). Most surgeons agree that if nerve repair is to be done, it should be done within the first three months if at all possible. I should like to repeat that a well-regulated, faithfully adhered-to physical therapy program is of extreme importance. It serves to prevent deformity by contracture of the muscles during the period of complete paralysis and serves to build up the strength of the muscles as the nerve function returns.

The subject of nerve involvement in conditions of the neck and spine includes some rather special problems and will be discussed in detail under these headings.

III
THE TREATMENT OF INJURIES IN SPECIFIC AREAS

5

Injuries to the Cranium and Central Nervous System During Athletics

BOB J. RUTLEDGE

Injuries to the head in sports events account for more fatalities than injuries to any other part of the body. There have been no significant changes in the treatment of athletic injuries to the cranium or to the central nervous system in recent years. Controlled respiration and intracranial pressure monitoring are being done in patients who are comatose; this may result in less permanent residual damage in athletes sustaining these severe injuries. The perfection of computerized axial tomography (CAT) scan has had the same diagnostic impact on cranial injuries as it has had on neurosurgery in general. Nuclear magnetic resonance (NMR) imaging is a newer procedure that may be even more valuable than the CT scan in the diagnosis of intracranial injuries. Dural hematomas are diagnosed earlier and intracerebral hematomas are being diagnosed more frequently since the development of this special procedure.

Football is now the most popular contact sport in the United States and close to one million young men are participating in organized football throughout the country. There has been a renewed emphasis on the evaluation and investigation of head injuries, using the football field as the main research laboratory. During this period of time, changes have been made in the headgear, so that for the most part it offers more protection to the player's head; however, lack of unanimity among physicians, coaches and manufacturers concerning helmets still remains a problem. Continued attention to the modification of the face guards seems to be both prevalent and important; nevertheless, there are some who are inclined to do away with face guards altogether.

With the improvement of the helmet, there has been a tendency for players to use their heads as "battering rams," which has resulted in frequent cervical spinal cord injuries. Severe head injuries, on the other hand, have decreased in frequency. There is and has been a collective effort by neurological and orthopaedic surgeons, as well as by other physicians, to educate coaches, players and officials concerning the dangers of "spearing" or stick tackling. This resulted in the outlawing of "spearing" by the National College Athletic Association (NCAA) Rules Committee. Neurological surgeons are increasingly practicing preventive medicine by advising coaches and team physicians of practices that are dangerous to the head and central nervous system. It is obvious that neurological and orthopaedic surgeons, team physicians, coaches, officials and manufacturers of sporting goods must work together to lessen the danger of injuries to the head and central nervous system of the athlete.

Professional boxing is the only sport in which a participant's objective is to render his opponent helpless. A resolution "opposing professional, collegiate, and amateur boxing in its present form" was adopted by the Southern Neurosurgical Society in 1970. Although professional boxers may receive injuries to the brain, it is the less adept fighters who are injured more frequently and severely. Death usually occurs from severe acute injury to the brain, most commonly caused by acceleration or, to a lesser degree, by deceleration of the head. "Punch drunk" is still the best term used to describe an individual whose symptoms result from chronic, repetitive insults to the brain.

With the increase in participation in noncontact sporting events, there has been a corresponding increase in less serious injuries, such as those caused by being struck in the head by a golf club, ball bat or ball, as well as those unique injuries from sports such as snowmobiling.

The most common cause of death in craniocerebral acceleration injuries is an acute subdural hematoma. Physicians who attend athletes should be taught how to recognize this condition and neurosurgical facilities must be close by. Military Assistance Safety Transportation (MAST) as well as air ambulance service has become more accessible and sophisticated since the last revision of this book. Air evacuation makes early neurosurgical evaluation and surgical intervention possible in those athletes with signs of increasing intracranial pressure, thereby lessening morbidity and mortality. Computerized tomography (CT) scan is the ideal adjunct for the early diagnosis of surgical lesions created by trauma to the head. Steroids and dehydrating agents such as intravenous mannitol remain useful in managing severe injuries to the brain. Preventive medicine is still the most important factor in the handling of cervical spinal cord injuries. A prompt application of skeletal traction is paramount in lessening the severity and permanency of quadriparesis in athletes who have an impaired cervical spinal cord. Traction can be easily instituted by the application of tongs with spring pressure pins. These pins are screwed into the skull while the patient is under local anesthesia; incision of the scalp is not necessary. The tongs that are most commonly used today are the Gardner-Wells tongs. The early administration of large doses of cortisone intravenously is still important in the management of spinal cord injuries. Last, but not least, the conduct and attitude of the individual athletes are of great importance in decreasing the price paid for participation in contact sports.

PREVENTION OF HEAD INJURIES

It is just as important in the prevention of craniocerebral injuries as it is in the prevention of other injuries that athletes be in excellent physical and mental condition. Preseason health questionnaires and physical examinations are mandatory before beginning practice in contact sports. A clear line of authority must be established by the team physician—he must make the final decision as to a player's ability to participate in a sport. Coaches and instructors must teach participants how to avoid injury. Continued research and early adoption of definite improvements in protective gear, such as helmets and face guards, are necessary. A collective effort is necessary to change the rules in boxing to award the bout to the opponent of any exhausted fighter. A boxer in such a state cannot bring his neck muscles into play and is therefore extremely vulnerable to severe brain injury.

The following conditions should usually disqualify an athlete from participation in contact sports:

1. Neurological sequelae from injury to the head or from organic brain disease.

2. Uncontrolled episodes of impaired consciousness.

3. Temporary paralysis of a limb from any cause.

4. Spontaneous subarachnoid hemorrhage.

5. Recurring cerebral concussion.

Finally, a player should not re-enter a game after he has been "dinged" (had a blow to the head that affects his memory) or after a concussion until he is perfectly normal.

ANATOMY OF THE HEAD

The *scalp* consists of five layers: the hair and skin, the galea, two layers of connective tissue, and the pericranium. The scalp serves as a protective covering for the skull and tends to lessen impact to deeper structures in the cranium.

The *skull* is divided into the cranium and the facial bones. The cranium houses the brain, its coverings, blood and cerebral spinal fluid. The foramen magnum is an opening at the base of the cranium for the passage of the spinal cord. The middle meningeal artery makes an impression in the skull and is of practical clinical significance in craniocerebral injuries, particularly in skull fractures.

The most important of the *brain coverings,* or meninges, is the dura mater, a tough fibrous tissue that serves as the inner lining of the skull and gives protection to the brain. It also provides a firm structure for venous sinuses, which return blood from the brain to the heart. There are two extensions of the dura mater.

One, the falx, divides the cranium into a right and left half; the other, a horizontal portion called the tentorium, separates the base of the brain from the superior portions. The connections from the brain to the spinal cord go through an opening in the tentorium called the incisura.

The middle of the three meninges is the arachnoid; the inner, which is intimately associated with the surface of the brain, is the pia mater. Between the arachnoid and the pia mater is the subarachnoid space, which contains cerebral spinal fluid. This space is traversed by blood vessels.

The brain itself is similar to gelatin in consistency and its average weight is $1\frac{1}{3}$ pounds. It occupies irregular recesses formed by the cranium and the dura partitions. The falx separates the two large cerebral hemispheres, which are in turn divided into frontal, temporal, parietal and occipital lobes. The anterior parts of the frontal and temporal lobes are the frontal and temporal poles, and the posterior portion of the occipital lobe is the occipital pole. The main function of the two cerebral hemispheres is controlling movement of the body, perception of sensation and the higher cerebral functions such as speech, learning, memory and emotion. Each hemisphere controls function of the opposite side of the body.

The cerebral hemispheres are connected with the brain stem, which passes through the incisura of the tentorium down to the level of the foramen magnum at the base of the skull where it becomes the spinal cord. The important function of the brain stem, in addition to transmitting information between the cerebral hemispheres and the spinal cord, is its control of the vital functions of the body, such as blood pressure, heart rate and respiration.

Also located under the tentorium and connected to the brain stem are the two cerebellar hemispheres, whose main function is the coordination of movements initiated by the cerebral hemispheres.

Within each cerebral hemisphere is a cavity called a lateral ventricle. The brain stem has two such cavities, the anterior being the third ventricle and the one near the spinal cord the fourth ventricle. They are interconnected by small ducts or foramina.

Spinal fluid is found mainly in the lateral ventricles and circulates from there through the third and fourth ventricles. It flows out of the brain through openings in the fourth ventricle, known as the foramen of Magendie and the foramen of Luschka, and then circulates and bathes the brain and spinal cord. The main purpose of spinal fluid is to serve as a cushion between the rigid skull and soft brain.

The blood supply to the brain comes from the two carotid arteries and two vertebral arteries. The latter join to form the basilar artery, which then connects with the carotids through smaller branches, forming the circle of Willis at the base of the brain. Venous blood is drained by the internal and external jugular veins.

ASPECTS OF CEREBRAL PHYSIOLOGY ATTENDED BY TRAUMA

Cerebral Edema

Significant head trauma results in two categories of brain injury. The first is only a transient alteration of brain function without any structural damage, the classic example being concussion. The other category includes injuries that are more serious in that there is structural damage to the brain coverings or to the brain itself. This damage may result in the development of an expanding mass, such as a blood clot within the rigid cranial vault, causing brain compression. Also, serious alterations in cerebral physiology may result in increased pressure on the brain. Either the development of an expanding intracranial mass or a physiological disturbance can result in increased intracranial pressure, which if not relieved promptly will cause permanent brain damage or death.

In structural injuries the brain cells (neurons) usually are damaged to some degree. This alters their physiology in such a way that they accumulate H_2O within themselves; this condition, known as *cerebral edema,* usually takes 24 to 36 hours to develop after an injury. Such an accumulation of mass (in this instance H_2O) within the skull acts in a manner identical to a blood clot and causes increased intracranial pressure.

The brain receives 15 per cent of the body's blood circulation and consumes 25 per cent of its oxygen. Any process impairing the delivery of oxygen to the brain or the removal of carbon dioxide from it results in similar physiological alterations at the cellular level in the brain. Hence, neurons may be damaged and cerebral edema may result from anoxia or hypercarbia alone. Causes of poor cerebral oxygenation include obstruction to pulmonary ventilation, such as from nose and face injuries, neck injuries, rib fractures with lung collapse, and shock in which blood pressure is too low to adequately perfuse the brain. It should be emphasized that *shock is rarely associated with head injuries alone,* and when it is present, one should always suspect an associated injury such as a ruptured spleen with intra-abdominal hemorrhage.

The effect of retained carbon dioxide should be elaborated upon. Not only is elevated carbon dioxide directly toxic to nerve cells, producing cerebral edema, but it is also a potent cerebral blood vessel dilator, resulting in the increased flow of blood and fluids to the brain, where they accumulate in the injured cells, further elevating intracranial pressure.

A vicious cycle develops in unrelieved cerebral edema. The brain becomes swollen with H_2O, causing elevated intracranial pressure, which compresses and interferes with the veins draining blood from the brain. The result is that more blood is pumped into the brain than can escape through the veins, and intracranial pressure is further elevated. These problems are compounded if a blood clot is also accumulating at the same time from a vessel ruptured at the time of injury.

With severe increased intracranial pressure, blood pressure is elevated, the pulse is slow and there are respiratory changes. When pressure is generalized, such as with edema, decreased consciousness is the most prominent sign. Usually there are no lateralizing signs. In contrast, with an extradural hemorrhage the pupil is dilated and fixed on the ipsilateral side and there is contralateral hemiparesis. When the brain stem is involved, the temperature regulatory mechanism falters and there is frequently hyperthermia. Decerebrate rigidity is a sign of brain stem dysfunction and is usually bilateral. In this phenomenon the extremities are in extensor rigidity and the upper extremities tend to internal rotation. The rigidity is enhanced by stimulation of the patient, and Babinski's sign is present bilaterally. In increased intracranial pressure caused by chronic subdural hematoma, the pupil is frequently dilated on the side opposite the hematoma owing to compression of the third cranial nerve against the edge of the tentorium.

Skull Fractures

Skull fractures are not common in football. They are more common in sports played on a harder surface and in those utilizing a ball and club. Skull fractures are classified into the following types: (1) closed, or simple, fractures, which do not involve a break in the overlying skin or membranes; and (2) open, or compound, fractures, which involve a tear in the covering adjacent to the fracture.

Linear skull fractures may be simple or compound. Signs of a simple linear fracture are pain, swelling over the fracture line and discoloration. X-ray studies will reveal a "crack" in the skull. This can be of particular importance if it crosses the groove of the middle meningeal artery, which will be considered in the discussion of extradural hematomas. The simple linear fracture demonstrates that the patient has sustained a physical blow with sufficient force to crack the skull. The fracture itself ordinarily does not require any treatment other than observation in a hospital for 24 hours to be sure that intracranial structures have not been concomitantly damaged. Compound linear skull fractures require early, careful debridement and the administration of the appropriate antibiotics.

Depressed skull fractures usually occur when the head is struck by an object such as a golf club and the skull is pushed onto the brain (Fig. 75). These fractures can be compound or simple. When compounded, emergency surgery is indicated for debridement and elevation of bone fragments from the brain. In comminuted fractures I always replace the fragments in the defect, even in a mosaic pattern, if necessary. This is of particular importance in athletes so that they will retain a solid cranium without a skull defect that could require a subsequent cranioplasty with foreign material. Simple depressed fractures can be elevated as an elective surgical procedure.

Skull fractures in the bones at the base of the skull cause discoloration around the eyes and nose or over the mastoid and may be accompanied by leakage of cerebral spinal fluid into the ear (otorrhea) or the nose (rhinorrhea). They are not usually visible on x-ray films. This is a special type of compound fracture that should always be managed by a neurological surgeon.

Cerebral Concussion

Concussion is a syndrome in which there is an immediate impairment of neural function following a blow to the head. This deficit is usually noticeable in the degree of conscious-

COMMINUTED FRACTURE OF VAULT OF
SKULL WITH TEAR OF SAGITTAL SINUS
PLUGGED BY BONE SPICULE

LINEAR FRACTURE OF FRONTAL
BONE WITH DIASTASIS OF
CORONAL SUTURE

HEMATOMA WITH HARD, CREPITATING EDGE
SIMULATING FRACTURE TO PALPATING FINGER

FRACTURE OF BASE

Figure 75. Fractures of the skull. (© Copyright 1953, 1972 CIBA Pharmaceutical Company, Division of CIBA-Geigy Corporation. Reproduced with permission from The CIBA Collection of Medical Illustrations by Frank H. Netter, M. D. All rights reserved.)

ness but may also involve memory, visual disturbances or equilibrium problems. In third degree concussions there is unconsciousness for more than five minutes and moderate retrograde amnesia. No treatment is required because there is no permanent deficit, although a decision does have to be made concerning a participant's ability to return to play. Multiple concussive episodes may result in permanent sequelae, and individuals reflecting this pattern need to be evaluated by a neurological surgeon to determine whether they should continue in athletics. Multiple concussive blows to the head, as those received in boxing, can result in a combination of symptoms from involvement of the pyramidal, extrapyramidal and cerebellar pathways. The common symptoms are slurred speech, dull face, slowness of movement and mentality, and tremor. Slang terms to describe an individual with such symptoms are punch drunk, goofy, slaphappy, stumblebum and slugnutty.

Cerebral Contusion

Cerebral contusion is a bruising of the brain. When a small area of the brain is involved, a contusion is difficult to distinguish from a concussion and no permanent effects occur. In more severe contusions, cerebral edema with brain swelling results in increased intracranial pressure. If a generalized contusion with bruising of the brain stem occurs, decerebrate rigidity follows and the patient may die or have permanent deficit after a long illness. The usual treatment is medical and is aimed at reducing increased intracranial pressure with good oxygenation, dexamethasone and mannitol. The usual supportive nursing care must also be provided. Diagnostic studies such as angiography and echoencephalography are utilized to help determine whether surgical intervention may be warranted. A decrease in the level of consciousness is the single most important sign in determining the need for surgery. Subtemporal decompression can be a lifesaving procedure for a patient with this condition.

Extradural Hematoma

This hemorrhage usually results when a fracture tears the middle meningeal artery (Fig. 76). Typically the patient is unconscious for a short period of time and then returns to normal. Drowsiness and headache ensue an hour or more later, followed by vomiting, dilation of the ipsilateral pupil and contralateral hemiparesis. Time is of the essence at this point because if the pressure is not relieved, respiration decreases, both pupils dilate, decerebrate rigidity occurs and finally respiratory paralysis and death result. Surgical treatment is mandatory. In the emergency room, if necessary, a burr hole is placed on the side of the dilated pupil. After evacuation of some of the blood clot, a craniectomy is done and the remaining clot removed; bleeding is then controlled. Recovery should be complete if the clot is removed before there is bilateral brain stem compression.

Acute Subdural Hematoma

This entity is the most frequent cause of death from trauma in contact sports. The patient usually remains unconscious following the injury and shows signs of rapidly increasing intracranial pressure. This condition is usually caused by contrecoup movement with contusion and laceration of the brain and tearing of vessels. The mortality rate is extremely high and many patients succumb without the benefit of neurosurgical consultation or surgery. The treatment is appropriate craniotomy with removal of the blood clot and control of hemorrhage by coagulation, metal clips, suturing, Gelfoam and Avitene. In those patients who do survive, morbidity is severe.

Chronic Subdural Hematoma

Fortunately in my practice I have not had any patients with acute subdural hematomas from participation in football. I have had several patients with chronic subdural hematomas who, in all instances, completely recovered (Fig. 77). One boy was playing for his coach-father and he continued to play football the following year against my advice.

Chronic subdural hematomas are always caused by trauma. Usually the trauma to the head is considered insignificant and is sometimes completely forgotten. The pathophysiological manifestation is bleeding in the subdural space from a torn bridging vein from the brain to the superior sagittal sinus. The subdural space is developed by the blood from a potential space from which absorption does not occur. In about a week a neomembrane surrounds the blood and the hematoma grad-

LINEAR FRACTURE OF SKULL CAUSING
MIDDLE MENINGEAL HEMORRHAGE

EXTRADURAL HEMATOMA DUE TO TEAR OF MIDDLE
MENINGEAL ARTERY AT THE FORAMEN SPINOSUM
BY FRACTURE OF THE BASE OF THE SKULL

CLOT EXPOSED ON SKULL BASE
BY REFLECTION OF DURA

Figure 76. Extradural hematoma. (© Copyright 1953, 1972 CIBA Pharmaceutical Company, Division of CIBA-Geigy Corporation. Reproduced with permission from The CIBA Collection of Medical Illustrations by Frank H. Netter, M.D. all rights reserved.)

DRAINAGE OF DARK, FLUID BLOOD

SUBDURAL HEMATOMA COMPRESSING AND DISTORTING BRAIN — DEVIATION OF VENTRICLES

DURA

HEMATOMA ENCASED IN MEMBRANE

Figure 77. Subdural hematoma. (© Copyright 1953, 1972 CIBA Pharmaceutical Company, Division of CIBA-Geigy Corporation. Reproduced with permission from The CIBA Collection of Medical Illustrations by Frank H. Netter, M.D. All rights reserved.)

ually increases in size by osmosis through a semipermeable membrane and by further bleeding from stretched, small vessels.

Symptoms are initially mild to nonexistent and, if present, usually disappear in a few days. A patient harboring a chronic subdural hematoma will feel normal for several weeks and then will complain of headache. The headache becomes more severe and is unrelenting. Other symptoms include loss of appetite and vomiting, drowsiness, personality change, blurred vision and gait disturbance. Approximately 50 per cent of patients have bilateral hematomata; 40 per cent have papilledema. The diagnosis may be confirmed by a nucleide brain scan or CT scan. Arteriograms will show the hematoma in 95 per cent of the cases.

Treatment is removal of the hematoma through trephine openings in the skull. Occasionally a large osteoplastic flap is warranted. These patients are prone to have convulsions temporarily following surgery and should be treated with intravenous sodium Dilantin. The symptoms disappear quickly following surgery and recovery is complete. I do not recommend that athletes continue to participate in contact sports after having a subdural hematoma.

Intracerebral Hematoma

The computerized brain scan has shown that this condition occurs more frequently than previously thought. The size and location of the clot are well delineated; however, since causes of intracerebral hematoma other than trauma need to be considered, arteriography is still necessary in some cases. Intracerebral hematomata may be treated medically or surgically, with surgical intervention becoming more frequent in the treatment of larger hematomas. The prognosis is variable and depends on the location and size of the hematoma.

Combined Intracranial Injuries

I had a patient who was involved in an auto racing accident. He was reported to be confused immediately following the accident and was conscious when I saw him about three hours later. He had some tenderness on the left side of his head and was dysphasic, but otherwise he had no complaints, was alert and had no other abnormalities.

A skull series revealed a linear fracture across the groove of the left middle meningeal artery. He was therefore admitted to the In-

tensive Care Unit of the Oklahoma Neurological Surgery Institute for observation.

The following morning he was the same neurologically. About 4:00 A.M. on the third day I was called and told that he was very somnolent. When I examined him he had a dilated, fixed pupil on the left side and was semicomatose. His respirations were full at the rate of eight per minute, his pulse was 56 beats per minute and his blood pressure had risen to 190/110 mm Hg. He also had a slight weakness of the right extremities and a positive Babinski sign on the right. A left carotid arteriogram was immediately obtained, which showed elevation of the middle cerebral artery such as that seen with an intracerebral hematoma; the angiogram also revealed a subdural hematoma.

The patient was taken to the operating room and a perforator and burr opening revealed an extradural hematoma. A subtemporal decompression was performed and the hematoma was evacuated. The dura was discolored and when it was opened a large subdural hematoma and a swollen, contused temporal lobe were revealed. It was necessary to make an osteoplastic flap to remove all of the "currant jelly–like" subdural hematoma. A portion of the contused and softened temporal lobe was also removed.

On the following morning the patient appeared as he did on the day of his admission. He was discharged from the hospital in six days and was asymptomatic at the time of my examination one month later.

DIAGNOSIS AND EMERGENCY TREATMENT OF HEAD INJURIES

Any blow to the head is potentially serious and should be so considered. Coaches, teammates and trainers may receive the first warning that an injury to the head has occurred by watching the game itself and the reactions of the individual players.

The first thing to do for a player with a suspected head injury is to render lifesaving measures such as establishing an airway and maintaining blood circulation. Closed-heart massage or defibrillation may be necessary. The player should not be moved.

A bolt cutter should be available for rapid removal of the face guard; headgear should not be removed except for a specific reason, since concomitant neck injuries are always suspected in players who sustain injuries to the head. Next a thorough, unhurried examination should be made. After the general examination, the head should be palpated and a brief neurological examination should be made, including examination of the pupils and movement of facial muscles and extremities. A decision must then be made as to the method of moving the patient. If there is any suggestion of a neck injury, such as pain or tenderness in the neck or weakness in the extremities, great care should be taken to keep the patient's head in a neutral position while moving him to a firm stretcher where his head can be kept immobilized to avoid further injury. Any player who was unconscious, even if only for a few minutes, must not re-enter the game.

A decision must be made on the playing field as to who should be sent to the hospital for further evaluation. In general, only the athlete with a "ding" or concussion lasting a minute or two with rapid recovery of all senses should be allowed to pass without further examination. All those with other injuries, including possible neck injuries, should rapidly be taken to a hospital with neurosurgical facilities.

At the hospital, x-ray films of the skull should be obtained as well as of cervical spine, since head and neck injuries are frequently associated and a comatose patient is unable to complain of neck pain.

All patients with concussions lasting more than five minutes or those associated with posttraumatic amnesia should be admitted to the hospital for observation for the development of symptoms of increased intracranial pressure. Likewise linear skull fractures without neurological deficit should be observed for 24 hours, especially if the fracture line crosses the middle meningeal artery groove or a venous sinus.

All other injuries demand neurosurgical consultation. The neurosurgeon can usually decide on the basis of the history and neurological examination whether the patient can be managed medically or if he will require surgery. If there are any doubts, further studies may be necessary. By far the most important test in the evaluation of intracranial injury is cranial tomography. Arteriography and nucleide brain scans are being used less frequently. The electroencephalogram (EEG) may still be useful in evaluating chronic and subacute conditions.

MEDICAL MANAGEMENT OF HEAD INJURIES

The patient's vital signs, pupils and ability to move extremities should be recorded every hour to detect signs of the development of increased intracranial pressure. The head should be elevated 30 degrees to assist venous drainage of the brain. In order to prevent hypoxia or hypercarbia, the airway must be kept clear by turning the patient from side to side frequently and by nasopharyngeal suctioning. Tracheostomy may be necessary if indicated by measurements of the patient's blood oxygen and carbon dioxide. Because of cerebral edema, dexamethasone, a steroid, is frequently given intravenously to stabilize cell membranes and to help prevent the accumulation of fluid. Mild dehydration is also useful in treating cerebral edema; therefore, the patient's intake of fluids is restricted and 20 per cent mannitol may be given intravenously to further dehydrate the brain. Since the patient's level of consciousness is the most sensitive clinical indicator of intracranial pressure, sedation is avoided. For analgesia, codeine is preferred because of its minimal sedative effects and because it does not change pupillary signs as other morphine derivatives can.

SURGICAL MANAGEMENT OF HEAD INJURIES

The surgical treatment of head injuries has been discussed largely under the specific conditions. Usually dexamethasone (Decadron) and mannitol are used preoperatively in all conditions. Decadron is usually continued in decreasing doses for several days postoperatively, depending on the patient's condition. Mannitol may be continued if postoperative cerebral edema is a problem. Usually this subsides in five to seven days. Uncontrollable cerebral edema may require a decompressive procedure involving removal of a portion of the cranial vault to allow the swollen brain to expand. Some medical centers place devices between the skull and the brain at the time of surgery to monitor intracranial pressure and to help determine the best therapy.

REHABILITATION

The importance of rehabilitation has long been recognized in sports injuries. Emphasis has been placed on athletes' returning to active participation in sports; trainers have been the stalwarts in this cause. Although this approach is important in head injuries, serious brain injuries require a prolonged, sophisticated team approach to return the patient to a normal active life and, if possible, to continued athletic endeavors. Sequelae from brain injuries are very complex and can cause mental deficiency, sensory or motor aphasia, pain, paralysis, sensory loss, disturbance of balance and incontinence of the bladder and bowel. One or more of these symptoms can tax the energy of teammates, coaches, relatives, trainers and physicians.

In addition to the need for many medical specialists, paramedical personnel such as speech therapists, psychologists, physical therapists and visiting nurses are important. Most communities do not have the necessary medical talent to deal with and rehabilitate players suffering from severe head injuries. Initially, these individuals should be in a general hospital with an active neurosurgery service and ancillary programs for rehabilitation. Fortunately, prolonged symptoms from brain injury are not as common in athletic trauma as those following a spinal cord injury. However, when they do occur, there are cities that have excellent rehabilitative facilities and those should be utilized by athletes suffering from neurological deficit to aid in their maximum recovery.

Every coach and team physician should be familiar with the nearest appropriate rehabilitation center.

REFERENCES

Anderson, B. D., Kraus, J. F., and Mueller, C. R.: The effectiveness of a special ice hockey helmet to reduce head injuries in college intramural hockey. Med. Sci. Sports, 2:162–164, 1970.

Beedle, C. W., Kovacic, C. R., and Moon, D. W.: Peak head acceleration of athletes during competition—football. Med. Sci. Sports. 3:44–50, 1971.

Karleen, C. I.: Snowmobiling with associated maxillofacial injuries. Minn. Med. 56:975–979, 1973.

Lavine, S. A.: Field diagnosis of athletic injuries. Md. State Med. J., 20:45–47, 1971.

Lynch, S., and Yarnell, P. R.: The "ding": amnestic states in football trauma. Neurology. 23:196–197, 1973.

Norrell, H.: The neurosurgeon's responsibility in the prevention of sports injuries. Clin. Neurosurg. 19:208–219, 1972.

Schneider, R. C.: Head and Neck Injuries in Football. Baltimore, Williams and Wilkins Co., 1973.

Unterharnscheidt, F. J.: Head injury after boxing. Scand. J. Rehabil. Med. 4:77–84, 1972.

Injuries of the Face

6

ANATOMICAL CONSIDERATIONS

A brief discussion of some of the anatomical characteristics of the face is pertinent, since they relate specifically to the type of injury to be expected and the treatment recommended. Practically the entire face is subcutaneous. The skin extending from the hairline above to the neck below is stretched over subcutaneous bone with relatively few areas protected by any intervening structures. In the upper face, the hard bone of the skull is separated from the skin only by the very thin muscles of the scalp and the aponeurosis connecting these muscles. The bony structures of this portion of the face are entirely immobile and serve as protection for the brain. At the supraorbital margins, the layers of the cranium separate to form the frontal sinus, which may be of almost any size. The characteristic "beetling brow" does not necessarily imply any change in contour of the cranial cavity but rather a large frontal sinus. This portion of the face is essentially part of the skull. Moving laterally from the midline in front, one finds the temporal fossae filled with the fanlike temporal muscles. The muscle layer here is considerably thicker than it is directly in front. The supraorbital nerves pass out of the orbital cavity through the supraorbital foramen at the junction of the inner and middle thirds of the superior orbital margin and pass subcutaneously up over the forehead. The essential injury in this area is contusion and its complications rather than strain or sprain.

The central portion of the face, that is, the area between the supraorbital ridges and the bottom of the superior maxilla, presents a complicated maze of anatomical structures, some of which will be considered in more detail later in the description of injuries to the various organs. The facial bones, which in the infant are separated by suture lines, become fused relatively early, but the very irregular suture lines persist and may well be confused with fracture lines. The orbit, for example, is a complete bony socket, open only anteriorly and posteriorly, yet it is made up of five or six different bones fitted together as in a jigsaw puzzle. The central portion of the face also has no motion between its bony structures. However, it is involved in the motion of the lower jaw, since many of the muscles attached to the lower jaw have their origin on the fixed bones of the face. The lower portion of the face, the mandibular portion, consists of the horseshoe-shaped mandible, which has bony contact with the rest of the skull only at the temporal articulations and the teeth.

Injuries to the face are not nearly so frequent now as they have been in the past. The football headgear and the various other helmets worn serve to protect not only the skull but also the upper portion of the face. With the addition of a bar of some type extending across the front of the face, the incidence of injuries to the supraorbital ridge, the zygomatic process, the malar bone, the nose, the teeth and the jaw has been greatly reduced. Almost all of the professional and university teams now require some sort of facial protection. Many of the high schools and junior high schools are rapidly following suit (see Chapter 2, Prevention of Injuries). I will not attempt in this section to give the detailed treatment of injuries of each of the areas of the face but rather will discuss those injuries that are likely to fall under the aegis of one treating athletic injuries.

LACERATION OF THE FACE

The broad expanse of facial skin with underlying subcutaneous bone is subject to contusion, abrasion and laceration more than any other type of injury. Treatment of abrasion and laceration of the face should be the same

105

as it is elsewhere on the body. One should bear in mind, however, that an intervening aponeurotic layer is present between the skin and bone on the forehead. It is important in laceration of the *forehead* or of the *scalp* to determine whether the underlying muscle or galea has been damaged. Each laceration should be carefully cleaned and the wound margins separated sufficiently to explore the depths of the wound. There is no substitute for irrigation with copious quantities of clean water. This water is not necessarily sterile. Running water from the tap of the city water system is adequate and is always available. If it is possible to hook up a tube or hose, the procedure is simplified. Under hospital conditions it is better to use sterile saline. It should be emphasized that it is the force of the flowing water that cleans out the contaminants. If nothing else is available, an ordinary shower may be utilized in the preliminary cleansing.

Usually in athletics the wound is through the skin only and is in the nature of a crushing, tearing injury rather than a direct cut. Such a wound extends deep enough to expose but not damage the galea. It should be thoroughly cleansed and hemostasis secured either by direct pressure or by injection of the skin edges with procaine plus epinephrine. The use of procaine is advisable in any event, since it will make the repair of the wound much less painful. Once the skin edges are anesthetized, they can be retracted gently and the area underneath investigated. Since the skin over the forehead is quite loose, the defect in the underlying structures may be some distance above or below the split in the skin itself. The skin can be readily shifted, and with a small curved forceps, any underlying defect can be explored. If there is a defect in the galea, careful palpation will determine whether or not it extends downward to include the skull. Only after careful exploration of the wound should the skin be closed. Here, as anywhere in the face, it is extremely important to appose the skin edges accurately. Whether you are a believer in multiple, very small sutures or favor fewer but more widely spaced ones, the end result will depend greatly upon how accurately the edges of the skin are apposed. The skin cannot accommodate for overlapping or a vertical shift of its edges and a troublesome and unsightly ridge will remain if the original suture is sloppy. If the galea has been damaged and the wound can be thoroughly cleansed, the galea can be closed with one or two interrupted sutures. The wound should be carefully inspected daily for any accumulation of fluid under the skin or under the galea. This is a relatively silent area from the standpoint of sensitivity and a tremendous abscess may develop with relatively few symptoms. The abscess may spread under the skin or under the galea over the whole top of the head. After a laceration of the area is carefully protected by a contact pad, athletic participation may be permitted. A special foam rubber pad in the football helmet may be necessary. In other sports an appropriate protective pad may be molded to form a cup over the involved area.

Laceration of the *eyebrow* is a relatively common injury and requires the same treatment as indicated above. If the laceration is in the region of the supraorbital nerve, this nerve may be severed. In such an instance repair of the nerve should be carried out to avoid subsequent troublesome anesthesia, tenderness or itching on this side of the forehead.

In the *central portion* of the face, laceration is also quite frequent and here again one must determine carefully whether or not there is damage to the underlying structures. This is quite obvious in lacerations about the eye. Lacerations about the face require meticulous handling and one must condemn the prevalent custom of rushing the player to the dressing room, where someone places several stitches to close the wound with scant reference to either asepsis or accurate apposition. The emergency is not that great. If it is absolutely necessary for the player to compete throughout the remainder of the game, a suitable pad should be applied as a temporary expedient, with the definite understanding that a complete repair will be done at the earliest possible moment. Although this course is not recommended, it certainly is better than to accept a less than perfect apposition of the wound edges. The definitive treatment should be carried out directly after the completion of the game and not the next day. If a delay of a few hours is unavoidable, the application of pressure and cold to the wound will help to control the swelling. By the next day it will be virtually impossible to carry out actual plastic closure of the laceration. Ideally, the suture should be done at once. It will never be as easy again. If the laceration is at all extensive, it is preferable to anesthetize the wound edges, preferably by infiltration of procaine plus epinephrine as indicated previously. It is particularly important that laceration of the *eyelids* receive very accurate closure in an effort to match up the skin creases. This is even more important if the laceration crosses the skin creases, since an irregular scar will disfigure the eyelid and interfere with its motion.

So also laceration through the *ala of the nose* should be carefully closed, great care being taken to secure accurate apposition of the edges of the nostril. Similarly, laceration involving the *ear* requires accurate repositioning of the skin. In fact, there is no area of the face where meticulous handling is not essential. It is extremely distressing to have a scar across the face with one edge of the skin higher than the other. This is disfiguring in the female and is very distressing to the male, since it interferes with shaving. It also is often a source of unsightly ingrown hairs.

CONTUSION OF THE FACE

By far the most common injury to the face is contusion. This may involve damage to the skin when it is caught between the hard, underlying bone and the force of the blow. The skin over the face is loose, and an area of areolar tissue is present between it and the underlying structures. In the forehead there is an areolar space between the skin and the galea or the frontalis, offering ample room for local swelling with hematoma formation. A blow to the forehead is likely to be followed immediately by extensive swelling, which may be diffuse, having the shape of an egg transected on its long axis, or local, with simply a rounded area of local swelling. One should be sure that there is no serious underlying pathological condition by close attention to the general symptoms of the patient as well as by local and general physical examination. Immediate application of cold and pressure will minimize the local swelling and to a great extent may prevent the infiltration of blood. It is debatable whether or not the local swelling should be aspirated. Very frequently the swelling is more in the nature of bloody edema than hematoma, and in such an instance aspiration will be unrewarding. Only when the area feels distinctly fluctuant is aspiration indicated to expedite recovery. After the area is aspirated under careful aseptic conditions, it should be infiltrated with hyaluronidase and then cold and pressure applied. The latter can be done quite simply by a circumferential wrap around the head. If it causes distressing headache after a few hours, it is too tight and will need to be released and rewrapped. The ordinary elastic bandage makes a very adequate pressure bandage. If there are no complications, there is no contraindication to athletic participation following such a contusion.

Complications of Contusion

Injury to the Brain

The most critical complication of contusion of the forehead is injury to the brain, and this has been discussed previously (see Chapter 5). I believe it should be emphasized here, however, that if the patient has actually been knocked unconscious by such a blow, he should be kept under very careful observation for at least 24 hours and resumption of athletic competition should not be permitted within that time. This is because of the danger of delayed intracranial hemorrhage or edema.

Fracture of the Skull

If the blow was so forceful as to fracture the skull, the patient should be immediately removed to a hospital and kept under constant observation. The most important consideration here is damage to the brain, and this should take precedence over any attempt at correction of the deformity. There may be a fracture of the frontal bone, which will involve the frontal sinus and will not actually break into the cranial cavity. In such a case the deformity is usually minimal and requires no treatment. If the whole anterior wall of the frontal sinus is collapsed, advice should be sought from a competent otolaryngologist to determine whether or not the fragment should be elevated.

Supraorbital Nerve Damage

Contusion of the supraorbital ridge may cause damage to the supraorbital nerve as it passes over the ridge in the subcutaneous tissue. Expectant treatment is usually adopted here because in contusion the nerve is rarely severed and complete recovery follows. This is particularly true because this is a sensory nerve and tends to regenerate quite promptly.

INJURY IN THE VICINITY OF THE EAR

Injury to the external ear is not common in amateur athletics. Professional prizefighters are frequently injured in this area, but in the amateur ranks the athlete usually wears a protective pad. In football the ear is protected by the helmet.

In the simple contusion in which the ear is smashed against the mastoid, prompt care may often prevent seriously deforming sequelae. The ear should be carefully examined. Any hemorrhage between the perichondrium and cartilage should be aspirated under the most aseptic conditions. If early hemorrhage is not present, an ice pack should be used to reduce the local edema. If edema persists and there appears to be fluid in the soft tissues that irons out the wrinkles and crevices of the ear, one might seriously consider release of the pressure of this fluid by multiple small incisions. These should be made under the most aseptic conditions, since infection in this area may be very serious.

A chronic infection may well supervene when contamination develops as a complication of the treatment of contusion and hematoma or when the initial injury breaks the skin. This causes local swelling and edema but has little or no systemic reaction. When the cartilage is involved, there may be either dissecting infection along the perichondrium or an aseptic necrosis of the cartilage. This type of infection is very difficult to manage, and the team physician would do well to seek specialized care from the plastic surgeon.

The resulting scar from contusion with infiltration of blood through the soft tissues results in some thickening of subcutaneous tissue and perichondrium, so that each subsequent injury is more serious than the previous one, and the final result is the well-known cauliflower ear, which defies any definitive treatment. Careful release of tissue tension by pressure bandage and application of ice are excellent preventive measures.

A laceration of the ear may occur from a sharp instrument. Much more common is the avulsion in which the ear is partially torn away. Such an injury occurs when the ear is forcibly pulled forward and the skin fold between the scalp and the ear is split. As the ear falls back into its normal position, this split may be completely concealed and infection may supervene because of contamination of the wound. Given a history of such an injury, a careful inspection of the ear should be made. If there is a laceration it should be carefully cleansed and sutured. Any tear in the external ear itself must be meticulously apposed, particularly if the auricular cartilage is torn; otherwise, an unsightly notch will appear at the suture line.

Injury to the *internal ear* is not frequent. The possible exception is the ruptured ear drum. The history of a blow across the side of the head with pain, slight hemorrhage from the ear and a feeling of fullness in the ear demands investigation of the drum. These ruptures of the drum usually heal spontaneously, but in the young athlete, if there is any question at all as to damage of the drum or inner or middle ear, the service of a competent otologist should be provided. Perhaps the most dangerous sequela is infection.

INJURY IN THE VICINITY OF THE EYE

by C. P. WILKINSON

The eye and its surrounding structures are occasionally seriously injured in athletic competition. Although severe injuries of the lids and the globe should be managed by an ophthalmologist, most cases are initially seen by the team physician, and the importance of a routine examination of the eye in any case in which trauma has occurred in or around the orbit cannot be overemphasized. The team physician is not expected to handle severe ocular injuries, but it is quite important that he develop an awareness of the types of injuries that can occur as well as a practical knowledge of their management.

Orbit. The orbit is constructed to give protection to the eye. The supraorbital ridge above, the infraorbital margin below, the malar bone on the temporal side, and the nasal bone on the inside all serve to form a recess protecting the eye from a blow from a large object.

A direct blow to the anterior orbit is typically followed by the rapid passage of serum and blood into the soft tissues of the lids, frequently resulting in their closure. Hemorrhage can also occur more posteriorly in the orbit, and swelling in this area will usually result in a significant degree of proptosis and ophthalmoplegia. In addition there may be subcutaneous or subconjunctival emphysema from fractures of sinuses. Focal anesthesia of the skin may occur if the nerves supplying such areas are damaged by fractures of the bones upon which they lie. The immediate concern of the primary physician should be to rule out severe intraocular trauma. The eyelids must be separated, utilizing lid retractors if necessary. (These can usually be more easily used if an anesthetic drop is first placed between the lids and on the cornea.) Movement of the eye should be observed both to assess the function of the respective eye muscles and to view more effectively the conjunctiva and sclera. Severe limitation of movement in any direction may be due to a blow-out fracture of the orbit or to neuromuscular damage, and this finding should prompt referral to an ophthalmologist, as should severe ocular trauma of any kind. The lids should be carefully examined for lacerations. Any question regarding facial fractures should be followed up with x-ray studies. (It should be noted that routine films frequently do not detect orbital blow-out fractures.) If one is satisfied that there is no underlying ocular complication, the patient should be promptly treated. The most important measure in this early stage is an adequate ice pack. It should consist of crushed ice folded in a soft cloth such as a towel rather than an ice bag. The ice bag is heavy and cumbersome, and it is generally poorly tolerated by the patient. It should be noted that if the patient has an intraocular injury, an ice pack or any other device increasing pressure upon the eye should *not* be applied to the lids.

Lids. As in the case of orbital trauma, the first step in caring for an injury of the lid is to carefully examine the eye. The general management of lid trauma is the same as for lacerations and avulsions elsewhere. Lacerations of the lid involving the lid margin or severe avulsions of the lid should prompt referral to an ophthalmologist or a plastic surgeon. Of special importance are injuries to the lacrimal apparatus. Any laceration near the medial canthus should prompt a detailed examination of the puncta and canaliculi leading into the lacrimal sac, and any laceration extending through these structures should be referred to an ophthalmologist for meticulous repair.

Globe. The cornea is the most exposed portion of the eye, and one of the most common eye injuries in sports is abrasion of the cornea by either a fingernail or a rough foreign body. A patient typically complains of significant pain and a sensation of having a foreign body in his eye, even when the offending agent is no longer present. A drop of a topical anesthetic will temporarily make the patient quite comfortable in most cases. The cornea should be inspected with a bright light using oblique illumination. If no foreign body is seen on the cornea, the upper lid should be everted and the patient instructed to look down. Frequently a foreign body will lie on the tarsal conjunctiva. Foreign bodies in both of these

locations can usually be easily removed with a moist cotton applicator following the instillation of a topical anesthetic drop. If no foreign body is found and no corneal abrasion noted, commercially available fluorescein dye may be instilled into the eye to outline the area of epithelial damage. Corneal abrasions are usually managed with mydriatic drops, antibiotic drops and patching. Mild abrasions usually heal quite quickly. If any doubt exists about the severity of the injury, ophthalmological consultation is necessary.

For a rupture or laceration of either the cornea or the sclera, prompt consultation must be obtained. As noted previously, it is extremely important for the team physician to be aware of these possibilities in any case in which severe blunt trauma has occurred around the eye. Once detected, such eyes should no longer be manipulated. Corneal lacerations frequently are complicated by incarceration of the iris, which distorts the pupil. Similarly, anterior scleral lacerations or ruptures are frequently complicated by uveal prolapse, and a very dark tissue is typically observed between the edges of the white scleral wound.

Blunt trauma to either the cornea or the sclera frequently results in the presence of intraocular hemorrhage, and the term hyphema refers to blood in the anterior chamber. This is quite frequently associated with other severe intraocular injuries, and the detection of any blood in the anterior chamber or vitreous cavity should result in the referral of the patient to an ophthalmologist. Blunt trauma to the eye is generally followed by inflammation of the iris and ciliary body. Such eyes frequently exhibit either a dilation or a constriction of the pupil, which may persist for days or even permanently.

Other Injuries Affecting the Eye. Mild injuries to the eye may cause varying amounts of irritation associated with mild changes in vision and lacrimation, and transient diplopia may occur after apparently minimal head injuries. Any of the symptoms that do not quickly clear should lead to an ophthalmological consultation.

INJURY IN THE VICINITY OF THE NOSE

As has been recorded in song and story, contusion of the nose presents many fascinating aspects. However, it is not particularly funny to the recipient of the blow. Here again,

Figure 78. Fracture of zygomatic arch and malar bone bilaterally. Note the good view of the nasal arch. (For technique of x-ray, see Fig. 79.)

careful attention to the possible complicating factors is most important. If the patient is seen before swelling occurs, a very adequate examination can be made digitally from the nasal bone to the infraorbital margin. A simple speculum and a flashlight will enable one to examine the inside of the nose fairly well in the early stages. Careful observation of the face may also reveal telltale deformity, particularly lateral deviation of the nose. I think it is of some advantage to have the patient look at himself in the mirror and also for the doctor to study the patient's physiognomy in the mirror. A tangential view of the nose is extremely important. With the patient lying supine, the doctor can look across the forehead, down the bridge of the nose to the tip and observe a deviation that may not have been noticed otherwise. Palpation of the two nasal bones between the fingers will be rewarding, since one can outline the exact area of pain on pressure. This may have some significance, particularly if the pain is at the junction of the nasal bones with the frontal process or at their junction with each other in the midline. Careful palpation may determine a difference in the angle of the ridge of the nose. One side may seem flat and the other bulging. Sometimes actual crepitation can be felt. All this is much more effective if done early. In the later stages, swelling is very likely to be unilateral or at least worse on one side than on the other, and one will be convinced there is gross deformity of the nose when there is simply uni-

laterally increased swelling. X-ray study, although important, may be quite unsatisfactory. Tangential x-ray studies of the nose may reveal variation of the angle of the bones with each other or possibly a defect or fracture line (Figs. 78 and 79). Again, one must be very wary not to interpret a suture line as a fracture line.

If there appears to be a fracture of the nose, the patient should be referred promptly to a surgeon skilled in such cases. It will be his responsibility to decide upon the proper time for reduction of the fracture. It is unwise for the untrained physician to attempt reduction of the displaced nasal bones. The nose is an extremely prominent feature and may deviate from normal if the correction is imperfect. This crooked proboscis may haunt the unwary. Additionally, the internal mechanism of the nose with the intricate arrangement of the septum and various turbinates requires especial skill to prevent persistent intranasal symptoms.

Bleeding from the nose is a very common accompaniment of a blow, owing to the extremely copious blood supply of the nasal mucosa. Fortunately, bleeding from the nose is usually readily controlled without resorting to any major procedure. The patient should hold himself upright if possible rather than lie down or hold the head low. The nasal area should be covered with cold cloths or ice to constrict the vessels. Under ordinary circumstances if the patient is kept quiet and semi-erect and if cold cloths or ice is applied, the

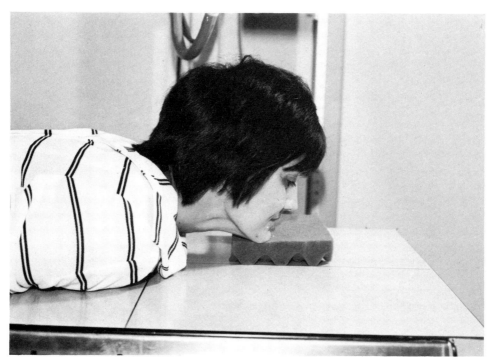

Figure 79. Exaggerated Water's position. The nasal arch, the zygomatic arches and malar bones are well visualized in this variation of the routine Water's position. Place the patient's head so that a line from the external auditory meatus to the symphysis menti is perpendicular to the table. The chin may need to be elevated by a sponge to assume this angle. Center cassette to outer canthi, and the central ray perpendicular to the cassette.

bleeding should stop promptly. If the bleeding is profuse and not easily arrested, careful packing of the anterior nares may reach the area of bleeding and control it. A tampon soaked in thrombin will be of help. It should be emphasized that the packing should not be forced deep into the nose or placed under pressure. Pressure is not required with this type of pack. If it becomes necessary to pack the posterior nares, the equipment of the emergency room and the skill of one accustomed to working in this area are required.

Nasal packing should not be left in place for a long time, since it may force an infection backward through the cribriform plate and cause dangerous meningitis. Because the trauma of removing the pack will sometimes reinitiate the bleeding, various measures have been suggested to permit its easy removal. The pack may be inserted within a very thin film of rubber, such as a condom, packing the rubber ahead of the gauze so as to make a finger-like pouch. Vaseline gauze may be used. However, this last method does lessen the effectiveness of the pack, and gauze directly against the area, particularly if impregnated with thrombin, will be much more effective.

INJURY IN THE VICINITY OF THE MALAR BONE AND SUPERIOR MAXILLA

Injuries to the malar bones, zygomas and orbits used to be extremely common in football, particularly from the opponent's helmet or knee. The almost universal use of the face bar has very materially reduced this type of injury so that whereas we used to see many fractured zygomas, orbits and noses, we seldom see them anymore—another evidence that we are constantly striving to handle injuries by prevention rather than by treatment. This is true for the most part and is particularly in relation to the use of the face bar and the mouthpiece.

Contusion over a malar bone or superior maxilla extending back to the zygomatic arch may well cause a fracture in this area (Figs. 78 to 81). Fracture of the malar bone extends into the maxillary sinus. So too, on frequent occasions, does fracture of the superior maxilla, and then it should be considered to be an open fracture. A blow of sufficient severity will justify investigation to determine whether or not a fracture exists. Here again, as in the

Figure 80. Typical fracture of zygomatic arch on the right. Note normal arch on the left. (For technique of x-ray see Fig. 81.)

Figure 81. Zygomatic arches. Both zygomas may be shown on one cassette in a position that is comfortably assumed by the injured patient. With the patient supine on the table, elevate the shoulders with sandbags so the chin can be elevated. Align a cassette at a 30 to 45 degree angle at the vertex of the head. The central ray should bisect the orbitomeatal line at an angle of 120 degrees to the cassette.

case of the nose and orbit, early examination is extremely important, since the next day the face will simply be a mass of tense, swollen edematous skin that will prevent any pretense of adequate physical examination. Since the maxilla is important for attachment of the upper teeth, and the zygoma and malar bone are concerned with protection, and since all these bones are related to the orbit, the teeth and the mandible, a careful attempt should be made to evaluate any deformity. The maxillo-facial surgeon should be consulted in case of serious injury. Expectant treatment should be carried out while awaiting consultation, since it is important to control the swelling as much as possible.

Contusion around the mouth may cause damage to the teeth, and this is usually accompanied by laceration of the lip. One should examine the inside of the lip, since there may be an extensive laceration here that does not extend through the skin. A cursory examination of the teeth may fail to reveal the entire damage. A tooth that in breaking has included a portion of the alveolar process may not appear to be loose or broken. Direct pressure over each tooth will usually determine whether or not the attachment of that tooth is damaged. In many cases if a tooth is broken with a portion of the alveolar process, healing will occur if it is properly replaced and held, whereas if it is overlooked, a subsequent blow, although relatively minor, may knock the tooth out completely. Careful examination is the watchword here. A massive fracture of the face is uncommon in ordinary sports, but if it occurs it should be readily recognized. The injury most likely to be overlooked is the one that seems relatively inconsequential.

A fractured alveolar process that includes one or more teeth should be very carefully reduced and kept reduced by interdental wiring. In some instances, simply wiring the upper teeth to a molded arch wire will be adequate. In others, it may be necessary to wire the two jaws together. A good deal of expensive dental reparative work may be avoided by adequate early care in these cases. It is important to remember that any open wound about the mouth is subject to infection. Although the patient may be relatively immune to his own organisms, one cannot assume this to be the case. Any fracture of the alveolar process, into the sinus, into the nose or into the mouth should be considered an open fracture. Antibiotics are recommended and prompt attention must be given to any developing abscess. This applies to fractures of the lower as well as the upper jaw. For prevention of injury to the teeth, the molded mouthpiece is extremely effective. It should be required equipment. The day when an athlete is identified by having lost his upper front teeth should be in the past.

INJURY IN THE VICINITY OF THE LOWER JAW

Dislocation of the Temporomandibular Joint. Such injuries are infrequent in the athlete who is not subject to the forces that ordinarily cause them. In the ordinary process of mastication, the condyle of the mandible swings forward out of the cotyloid fossa and subluxates each time the mouth is opened. The force that causes dislocation is the one that forces the mandible to open wider than its normal range on either or both sides. Dislocation may occur as the result of yawning, at which time the jaw is actively opened beyond its normal capacity and the condyle slips forward in front of the fossa and locks in this position. Conceivably it could be caused by forcible opening of the mouth, but the immediate response of muscular resistance to this motion will usually prevent the dislocation. The dislocation usually occurs at a time when the muscles that pull the teeth into occlusion are relaxed in a synergistic manner as the muscles that open the jaw contract. An attempt to open the mouth widely, as to bite a large apple or to insert a billiard ball, may result in dislocation and locking of the temporomandibular joint. Once the condyle slips forward and locks, muscle spasm occurs and contraction of the masseter and temporals firmly locks the jaw in the dislocated position. This may be a habitual condition and result much as any habitual dislocation either from an abnormally relaxed joint or from stretching the capsule by repeated episodes of dislocation.

The dislocated jaw can be readily reduced if the patient can be made to relax. Before an attempt is made at reduction, the patient should be relaxed somewhat by sedation. In a cooperative patient, the operator's thumbs may be inserted onto the posterior inferior molars while the index fingers are locked under the point of the chin. Pressure downward on the thumb will unlock the condyles and rotatory pressure forward on the fingers will reduce the forward displacement. If the patient cannot relax, a light anesthetic may be necessary and

Figure 82. Barton's bandage. A single turn. Many more turns make a firm, compact dressing.

will make the reduction easy. Forcible traumatic manipulation is neither necessary nor advisable.

If this has been the first episode, the jaw should be prevented from opening widely for a considerable period of time. Preliminary treatment by a Barton's bandage (Fig. 82) for a week or ten days will usually be adequate if the patient is cooperative enough to avoid overopenings of the jaw, as in yawning. In recurrent habitual dislocation there probably is little value in temporary immobilization. I have seen many cases of habitual dislocation that were extremely distressing, particularly because of an almost irresistible impulse to yawn and so cause a recurrence. These cases have been relieved by wiring the teeth in

apposition for four to six weeks. The threat of wiring the teeth together has in many instances been effective in preventing overopenings of the jaw.

Fracture of the Mandible. The mandible is much more susceptible to damage than is the superior maxilla or the temporomandibular joint. Since fracture of the mandible is usually caused by a direct blow, a contusion may be the first thing that calls attention to the injury. Any contusion involving the mandible should be carefully examined. The entire inferior margin of the mandible is subcutaneous, and by palpating carefully along the subcutaneous border, one can determine areas of tenderness, areas of local swelling or any irregularity of this margin. If the injury is major, the fracture of the mandible may be quite obvious. The jaw will hang open and the lips may be badly swollen. There will be hemorrhage in the mouth where the gum is torn as the jaw fragments separate. These cases are readily diagnosed. Of greater difficulty is the case with little or minimal displacement. After careful observation and palpation, the patient should be asked to open and close his mouth and to appose his teeth. Since most athletes with these injuries are young individuals, they usually have a complete set of molars. These should properly occlude without discomfort if there is no displacement. This is the best single test of the accuracy of reduction of any deformity following fracture. It is not advisable to attempt to produce motion at the fracture site. If motion is observed, however, it is quite obvious that a fracture is present. Roentgen-

Figure 83. Incomplete fracture of angle of mandible on the left. This should be treated by immobilization of the jaw with interdental wiring.

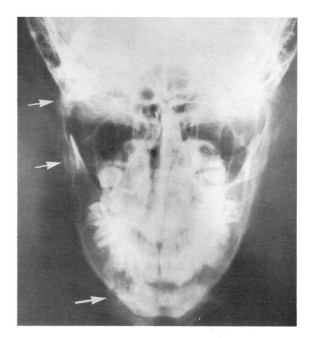

Figure 84. Fracture of the neck of the condyle on the right with fracture through the mandible on the same side. Whenever one fracture is shown in the mandible, search carefully for the second.

ographic examination in both anteroposterior and lateral planes should be made and should be carefully interpreted.

Fracture of the tooth-bearing area of the mandible is more readily determined than is fracture posteriorly where it may cross through the angle of the jaw (Fig. 83), through the condyle or through the condylar neck (Figs. 84 and 85). Here again, careful palpation is important. Have the patient open and close

his jaw and observe whether or not the chin swings to one side or the other. Palpate the condyle as it comes forward out of the glenoid. Both of these signs are valuable. If the teeth appose properly and there is some question as to whether or not the jaw has been broken, a supportive bandage such as Barton's bandage (see Fig. 82) should be applied to the mandible to hold it to the maxilla until a more detailed examination is made. If the mandibular frac-

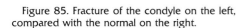

Figure 85. Fracture of the condyle on the left, compared with the normal on the right.

ture is undisplaced or can be readily reduced, interdental wiring to fasten the upper and lower teeth firmly together should be carried out. If perfect reduction cannot be obtained and one cannot be assured of perfect occlusion, consultation should be sought as early as possible. If there is any question about the occlusion, the patient's dentist may be able to provide a valuable hint as to any change in the position of the jaw. Frequently malocclusion predates the injury, so it is wise to consult with the patient and with his parents to determine whether or not the patient previously had an overbite, underbite or irregular occlusion. I well recall spending an inordinate amount of time one humid Sunday morning in an attempt to get good occlusion in a man who had been more than slightly inebriated the night before. His truculence had been rewarded by a blow to the chin. In confiding to his wife that we were unable to get good occlusion, she examined his mouth and said it had never been better than that. This proved to be the case. A little foreknowledge of this patient would have prevented a good deal of needless, painful and arduous manipulation.

The management of the patient with his teeth wired together can be difficult, particularly if he is a young and impatient athlete. Actually it is more difficult when his teeth fit well than when they do not, since it is easier for him to eat through the interstices of the teeth if they do not fit perfectly or if one is knocked out. We do not recommend knocking out a tooth to permit eating, however. It is important that the patient have adequate caloric and vitamin intake during the period when he cannot chew. Rich soups, whipped potatoes and gravy, and ground meat can be handled quite well. These will be much more acceptable to the youth than a constant diet of malted milks and sweet drinks.

INTERRUPTION OF THE AIRWAY

Interruption of the airway is one of the unusual complications of fracture of the face that occurs particularly with fracture of the mandible but that may also occur with fracture of the maxilla. This complication is, of course, first in order of importance in any injury, taking priority over hemorrhage, contamination, unconsciousness or any other complication. The patient cannot long survive without adequate respiration. Occasionally in fractures of the superior maxilla, edema may be severe enough in the back of the soft palate and in the throat to seriously interfere with respiration. It is the rule for nasal obstruction to occur in almost all of these injuries, hence breathing must be through the mouth. Swelling of the back of the tongue that presses the tongue against the pharynx is a very real hazard. Whoever is to care for the person with this type of injury should be warned of the urgency of an adequate airway. Holding the tongue forward by insertion of an anesthetist's airway is of value.

In fracture of the lower jaw, hemorrhage from the external maxillary artery may cause sufficient swelling at the base of the tongue and front of the neck to seriously interfere with breathing. Although this is not common, it is extremely distressing when it occurs. At Children's Memorial Hospital a case of fracture of the mandible was accompanied by considerable bleeding. It was felt permissible to proceed with reduction of the fracture and apposition of the teeth by interdental wiring. In subsequent hours these measures compounded the problem rather than improved it. The swelling increased and a tracheotomy was necessary to permit breathing. Following this, the surgeon had to tie off the carotid before the hemorrhage could be adequately controlled. It follows that any fracture of the mandible should be carefully observed and not left unattended until the critical period is past, that is, for 12 to 24 hours.

PENETRATING INJURIES

Occasionally there may be an injury to the face by a penetrating sharp object and the complications of such an injury, particularly injury to the eye, demand immediate hospitalization and definitive care. An injury to the *mouth* with damage to the hard or soft palate or with severe intraoral bleeding may be easily overlooked. In case of any suspected penetrating wound, the patient should be questioned as to the nature of the injury and carefully examined to determine the depth of penetration and any possible damage to the underlying structures. Another area of the face that is rather frequently injured is the *tongue*. The most common injury of the tongue occurs when it is caught between the upper and lower teeth as the teeth are forcibly apposed in response to some external force. This is a painful injury but usually is not severe. If the laceration goes completely through the tongue, it should be carefully sutured, apposing the edges exactly. Overlapping of the edges will give troublesome irregularity, which may require the service of a plastic surgeon at a later date.

It should be evident that the importance of this chapter could be greatly minimized by the mandatory use of mouthpieces and face guards. It has been my observation over the years that these facial injuries have been reduced very drastically, and I attribute most of this to prevention by protection. The basis of adequate protection is a well-fitted helmet to which face bars can be attached. Many times the young athlete is impatient of anything that smacks of undue protection. It should be recalled that although he may be extremely smart, he has not yet developed much common sense and so it is necessary to think for him by strict requirements concerning the mouthpiece and the face bars. In the university programs, fractures of the malar bone, zygoma and nose used to occur frequently and, along with knocked-out teeth, were in fact among the most common injuries in sports. These have been essentially eliminated from football by teams that insist on the wearing of the mouthpiece and the face bars.

Injuries of the Shoulder Girdle

7

In contrast to the pelvis, which is a solid bony ring that provides great stability for transmitting the body weight from the trunk to the lower extremities, the shoulder girdle is a very loosely constructed, highly mobile complex of bones, muscles and ligaments designed to give great mobility to the upper extremity, with only sufficient stability to provide a proper foundation for the muscular activity of the upper extremity (Fig. 86). The skeletal connection of the shoulder girdle to the trunk is extremely tenuous and consists only of the relatively insecure articulation of the inner end of the clavicle against the sternum and the first rib (Fig. 87). I will discuss only those details of anatomy that are needed to orient the reader in regard to the various areas of injury, since a full anatomical study of this region would of necessity be voluminous.

Briefly, then, the *clavicle* acts as a strut or crane arm to prevent the shoulder from dropping forward across the chest. It is a rigid long bone, with its inner end apposed to the sternum and its outer end apposed to the acromial process of the scapula. Thus it maintains a constant distance between the upper end of the arm and the midline of the chest. The shoulder may move forward, backward, upward or downward, but so long as the clavicle maintains its integrity, the shoulder will not approximate the sternum. Thus, it may be seen that the clavicle has a vital role in shoulder function. The various muscles and ligaments about the thorax and neck tend to stabilize the clavicle in this position. Its function is well illustrated by the forward displacement of the shoulder, which results when the clavicle is completely broken.

The *scapula* is a broad membranous bone designed primarily for muscle attachment (see Fig. 87 and Fig. 128). It has no bony connection to the thorax. Its concave undersurface lies over the muscles of the posterolateral thoracic cage. On motions of the arm and shoulder, the scapula glides over the muscles of the chest wall through a wide range of motion, which may be inward, outward, upward, downward, rotatory or any combination of these movements. Its range of motion is subject to the limitations of the clavicular strut and the excursion of the various muscles that control its motion. These muscles have both synergistic and antagonistic actions, which under normal circumstances permit very smooth movement of the scapula over the trunk. The scapula also serves as the origin of many of the muscles that move the arm. This motion of the arm may be carried out by various mechanisms. For example, the scapula may be fixed by synergistic contraction of antagonists, and the arm then moves in relation to the rigid scapula. In this instance the muscles extending from the scapula to the trunk are in tonic contraction, and the muscles extending from the scapula and trunk to the upper extremity move the upper extremity on this firm base. On the other hand, the muscles attaching the arm to the scapula may be fixed, and the upper extremity is then moved by the gliding of the scapula over the chest wall. Obviously, neither of these situations exists in the pure state under ordinary circumstances. Usually the movement is a synchronous one of the upper arm on the scapula and the scapula on the trunk. This makes for extremely smooth and coordinated action and permits precise motions of the upper extremity, where controlled mobility is a good deal more important than stability. One of the early signs of a lesion about the shoulder girdle is a disturbance of this coordinated movement. Various clues may be obtained as to the character of the lesion by careful study of the motion of the arm and shoulder girdle, noting any disturbance of scapulohumeral rhythm.

A discussion of the various injuries to the shoulder in relation to specific areas follows. It should always be borne in mind, however, that the shoulder is an extremely complex mechanism and that anything affecting one

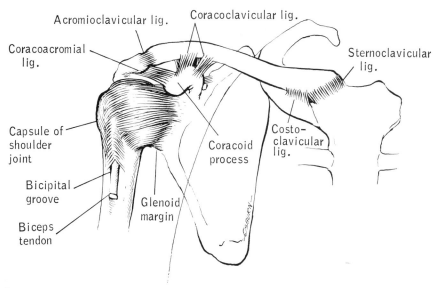

Figure 86. Anatomical drawing showing the ligamentous structures about the shoulder girdle.

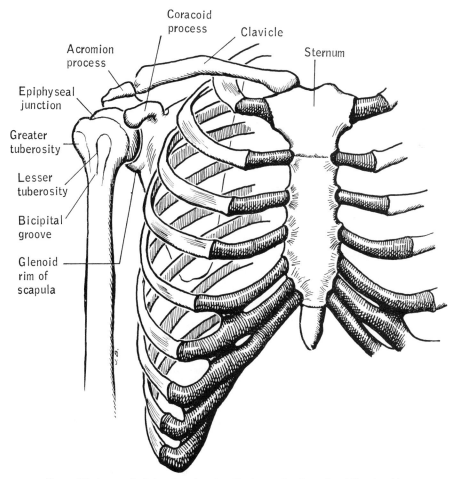

Figure 87. Anatomical drawing showing the bony structure about the shoulder.

portion is bound to have an effect on the other components of the girdle. This is particularly pertinent in relation to the function of the upper extremities and, more particularly, in relation to the throwing arm. Affections of the shoulder girdle have been the ruin of many a budding athlete whose major forte was throwing, such as a baseball pitcher, a football quarterback, a basketball player, a tennis player and even a horseshoe pitcher. Rehabilitation is of utmost importance, and often the complete recovery of function depends upon the effort applied to the rehabilitation of the injured part (see Chapter 22).

REGION OF THE STERNAL END OF THE CLAVICLE

Anatomical Considerations

The integrity of the sternoclavicular joint is maintained by the ligamentous structures that bind the inner end of the clavicle to the sternum and the first rib (Fig. 88). There is little inherent bony stability in this articulation. Indeed, the articulation is notably insecure. The inner end of the clavicle resting against the oblique outer angle of the manubrium is in contact with not more than one half of the surface area of the end of the clavicle. It is secured by the *sternoclavicular* ligament, a circumferential band of capsular tissue passing

from the head of the clavicle to the sternum. This ligament serves to hold the clavicle against the sternum rather than to hold it down. The major structure holding the inner end of the clavicle down is the *costoclavicular ligament.* This is a broad band arising on the proximal one fourth of the inferior margin of the clavicle and extending in an oblique manner downward and inward to attach to the first rib. This ligament is analogous to the coracoclavicular ligament at the outer end of the clavicle. These two ligaments together prevent the clavicle from displacing upward at either end.

It seems strange that this joint is not injured more frequently, considering that it does have rotatory motion and has little anatomical security.

Contusion

Contusion in this area is not frequent, since the athlete has been trained to protect the anterior part of the neck and chest by tucking his chin down. In football the shoulder pads protect the area fairly adequately. Contusion here is treated as it is elsewhere. Disability is slight unless hemorrhage is extensive.

Sprain

The most common injury to the sternoclavicular joint is sprain (Fig. 89A). The force

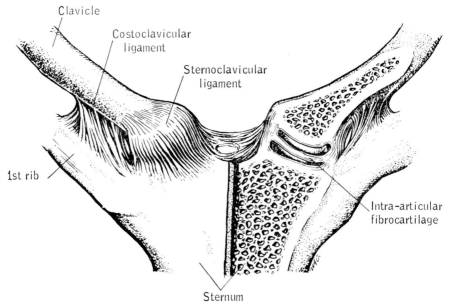

Figure 88. Detail of inner end of the clavicle showing (left) the sternoclavicular area with ligaments intact and (right) a cross section of the area. (Redrawn from Spalteholz, Hand Atlas of Anatomy, published by J. B. Lippincott Co.)

A

B

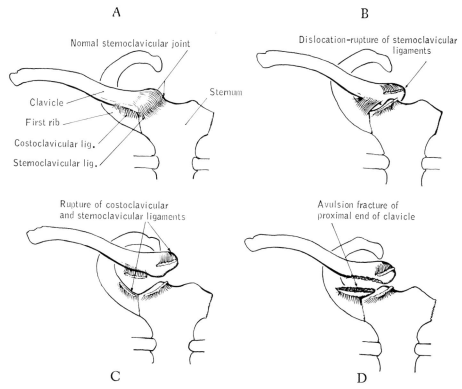

C

D

Figure 89. *A*, Normal sternoclavicular joint. *B*, Dislocation with rupture of sternoclavicular ligaments. The inner end of the clavicle is caught behind the sternum. *C*, Similar injury with rupture of both the costoclavicular and sternoclavicular ligaments, with the end of the clavicle free. *D*, Avulsion fracture of proximal end of clavicle, with rupture of sternoclavicular ligament.

applied to cause this injury is one which thrusts the shoulder sharply forward. As the shoulder girdle moves forward and inward, force is applied along the long axis of the clavicle, and the clavicle may be disrupted anywhere along its length. On reaching the sternoclavicular joint, this force will tend to impel the inner end of the clavicle medially, upward and forward. The leverage may be such, however, that the clavicle is impelled medially, upward and backward. In either instance the major strain will be upon the costoclavicular ligament. If this gives way, the inner end of the clavicle slips upward and medially as the sternoclavicular ligament gives way. If the force is arrested after minimal damage, the result is a mild (first degree) sprain of these ligaments. Stronger application of the force may rupture the sternoclavicular capsular ligament while the costoclavicular ligament remains relatively intact. In this case the inner end of the clavicle may snap in front of or behind the sternum and be held firmly in position by the intact costoclavicular ligament (Fig. 89*B*). The treatment of this latter condition may be relatively simple if recognized early. Simple traction ap-

plied to the shoulder to pull it backward and outward, with simultaneous direct pressure on the inner end of the clavicle, will usually snap the bone back into place. If the costoclavicular ligament is intact, a simple yoke or sling may be adequate for fixation.

If the driving force continues and the costoclavicular ligament is torn, dislocation or subluxation of the inner end of the clavicle takes place, causing severe (third degree) sprain. In this instance the proximal end of the clavicle is much more free and may ride upward over the sternum toward the midline (Fig. 89*C*). Another modification of the same type of injury consists of a fracture-dislocation in which some part of the inferior portion of the proximal end of the clavicle remains fixed by the ligament, whereas the upper portion of the clavicle breaks away and dislocates. This undisplaced fragment may include the whole costoclavicular attachment as well as the inferior portion of the head of the clavicle (Fig. 89*D*). In this instance outcome of treatment is much more favorable, since open reduction and fixation of the main portion of the clavicle to the undetached inferior segment is relatively simple. Careful internal fixation should result in complete recovery (Fig. 90). Even if treatment for this condition is delayed, the prognosis remains much more favorable because there is a firm base to which the displaced portion of the clavicle can be attached. In this instance, open operation and fixation should be recommended at any time and at any stage of the injury (see Figs. 91 to 93).

The *treatment* of a mild or moderate (first or second degree) sprain of the sternoclavicular or the costoclavicular ligaments is the same as treatment of sprain in other areas. The local treatment consists of application of cold, then heat, compression, local injection and protection. Protection consists of immobilization of the shoulder or application of a figure 8 yoke, which tends to hold the shoulder girdle backward, combined with adhesive strapping of the local area. Strapping of the inner end of the clavicle is ineffective, since it does not prevent the motion that causes stress on the ligament.

Dislocation

If the ligament tear is complete (third degree) and the inner end of the clavicle dislocates, prompt reduction and operative repair of the ligaments will give very good results. Unfortunately, the condition is usually not recognized in its early stages, and chronic upward displacement results (Fig. 94). This delay in diagnosis is caused in part by the fact that the deformity is not dramatic and that local swelling obscures observation or palpation of the displacement. Added to this is the problem that good x-ray visualization is extremely difficult to obtain, and errors in interpretation of the films are relatively common (see Fig. 93). The result is that several weeks will often have elapsed after swelling has subsided before persistence of discomfort calls attention to the deformity and instability present. At this time the injury is difficult to treat.

Treatment. Various measures designed for

Figure 90. This patient was struck by a car and examined two weeks post-injury. X-rays were taken, but no fracture was found. His complaint was that he could not lift the right arm, and it was painful at the inner end of the collarbone; it hurt to turn his head, with pain in the chest. Examination revealed marked prominence of the inner end of the right clavicle, the clavicle being set forward on the sternum. *A,* X-ray showing the inner end of the clavicle was anterior and superior to the sternum. Under anesthetic this was not reducible. Open operation showed the mass of healing debris beneath the clavicular head. On cleaning this out there was found to be a gutter of bone, which consisted of the section of inferior cortex of the clavicle as shown in Figure 89*b. B,* This was reduced and held by fixation wires, one through the sternum and one through the clavicular fragment. There was good recovery.

Figure 91. Fracture of the inner end of the clavicle (arrow). Clinically the patient, a boy, appeared to have sternoclavicular dislocation. His injury, which was actually a fracture-dislocation, consisted of approximately the upper one third of the inner end of the clavicle together with the shaft breaking off from the lower two thirds, which remained attached to the sternum and to the first rib. Repair was readily made by suture to the undisplaced fragment, which simplified the whole procedure. The displacement was primarily forward and therefore was not well revealed in the film. The x-rays are posteroanterior views.

Figure 92. X-ray of the chest for lung disease revealed abnormality of the sternum. Clinical examination then revealed dislocation of the inner end of the clavicle, riding above and behind the sternum (left). (For technique of x-ray, see Fig. 93.)

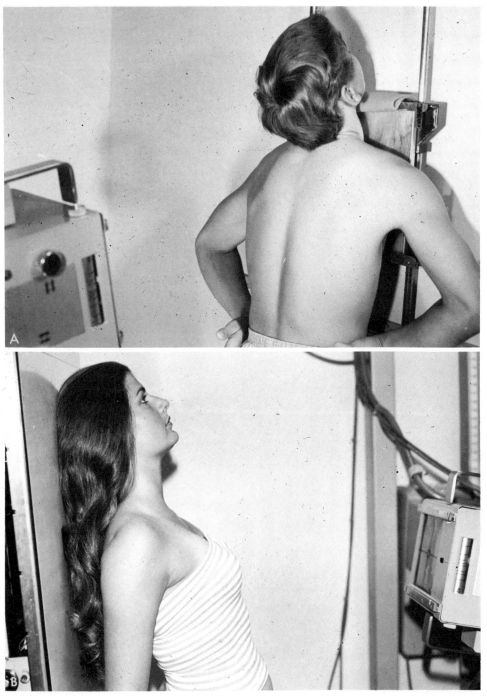

Figure 93. Dislocation of the inner end of the clavicle. Radiographs of sternoclavicular articulations made in routine positions are frequently difficult to interpret. The view in Figure 92 was obtained by a routine examination for apices of the lungs. A, With the patient in a posteroanterior position for lungs, shoulders depressed and touching the cassette, the central ray should be directed 10 to 15 degrees to the head and centered to the third thoracic vertebra. B, The patient may be more comfortable in an anteroposterior position. In this view the patient should stand slightly away from the table in order to lean back in a slightly lordotic position. The shoulders should be depressed and touching the table. The central ray should be directed to the sternoclavicular joints at a 15 to 20 degree cephalad angle. Note: Technical factors for ribs or cervical spine give better visualizaiton.

Figure 94. *A*, Showing original displacement of sternal end of clavicle. *B*, Removal of sternal end. Too much of the bone has been removed, since the major portion of the costoclavicular attachment has been lost.

reconstruction of the costoclavicular ligament are not particularly successful, certainly not to the point that athletic participation should be encouraged after a procedure. It is unwise to fuse the sternoclavicular joint because motion in this joint occurs with almost any motion of the shoulder girdle. Usually one must be reconciled to accept the deformity and advise enough restriction of activity to minimize the discomfort. At this time local measures, such as corticoid injections, are palliative only. This is not to say that operative reconstruction should never be attempted. However, we usually reserve reconstruction for those cases marked by disabling pain as a result of the displacement. One of the most successful procedures to relieve pain in frank dislocation is resection of the inner end of the clavicle proximal to the costoclavicular attachment (Figs. 95 and 96). If the costoclavicular ligament is torn or redundant, an attempt should be made to reconstruct it.

REGION OF THE CLAVICULAR SHAFT

Contusion

The portion of the clavicle lying between the coracoclavicular ligament attachment, which coincides with the beginning of the distal flat portion of the clavicle, and the proximal expansion leading to the sternoclavicular joint is designated as the shaft of the clavicle. Since the clavicular shaft is subcutaneous, it is subject to contusion. This occurs when the skin and periosteum over the clavicle are impinged between the hard bone and a striking object. The injury is ordinarily readily recognizable because of local swelling. Hematoma formation may occur, but it is not common in this area. Infiltration of blood into the skin and the subcutaneous tissue usually occurs. Following a severe contusion, the possibility of an injury

Figure 95. This 19 year old boy had a recurrent dislocation of the inner end of the right clavicle which lasted for two years. He was a champion swimmer and had increasing trouble with his backstroke. *A,* Standard anteroposterior view not specific for dislocation. *B,* The oblique view shows the gross dislocation superoposterior, as in Figure 89c.

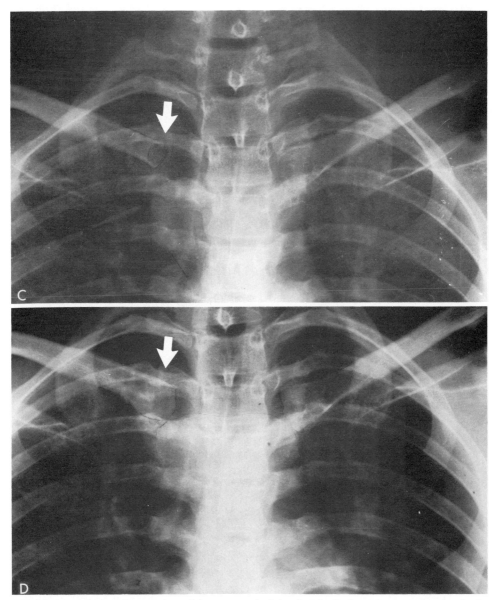

Figure 95 *(Continued). C,* After resection of the inner end of the clavicle. *D,* One year postoperative. In this young person the inner end of the clavicle has regenerated with minimal displacement. He has no complaint of the shoulder and is swimming without difficulty.

Figure 96. A, Wrestling injury one year before, diagnosed by an orthopaedic surgeon as dislocation of the inner end of the clavicle. There was no definitive treatment. The patient had persistent pain localized in the sternoclavicular joint, and reconstruction was not feasible this long post-injury. B, Resection of the inner end of the clavicle was carried out. The acute pain was somewhat relieved in the sternoclavicular area, but the patient still had gross complaint in the cervical spine, the glenohumeral joint, and the acromioclavicular joint.

to the underlying bone must always be considered. This can be determined fairly well by physical examination, since fracture of the clavicle usually will result in considerable pain on any attempt to move the shoulder, whereas simple contusion will not be painful on motion. Later, when there is diffuse swelling and blood infiltration, there may be pain on motion and the exact diagnosis will be more difficult. In case of doubt, x-ray examination will help to confirm the diagnosis.

There is nothing out of the ordinary about the *treatment* of contusion in this area. The usual measures are local injection, compression, and application of cold and, later, heat. Simple contusion will require relatively little immobilization of the shoulder, and with proper padding, athletic participation can be continued. Continuation of pain on use of the shoulder should arouse suspicion of a more serious injury, and x-ray examination 10 to 14 days subsequent to the injury will often show a fracture, even if earlier films were interpreted as negative. Incomplete fractures may be revealed by early callus formation or by signs of absorption at the fracture line.

Fracture

Fracture of the clavicle is a frequent athletic injury. It is much more likely to occur in the preadolescent or adolescent youngster than in the adult (Fig. 97). However, ligament injury at either the inner or the outer end of the clavicle is more likely to occur in the adult than in the youngster. A detailed description of the various types of fractures of the clavicle will not be given here, but a few generalities peculiar to athletic injury will be stated.

Treatment. One of the most common injuries in childhood is fracture of the shaft of the clavicle. The bone is subcutaneous, and it is fully exposed anteriorly as it arches forward. A direct blow against the outer point of the shoulder jams the shoulder inward. In the preadolescent or adolescent, the most vulnerable area of the clavicle is the shaft. Because of the forward bowing, the end-to-end stress increases the arc, and at some point, the anterosuperior cortex of the bone gives way. As the bone bows forward, it angulates at the fracture site (Fig. 98). In most cases the fracture of the anterior cortex permits the elastic posteroinferior cortex to bend. The result is a greenstick fracture with or without angulation, but always with good apposition. Further stress

may complete the fracture, and loss of apposition occurs (Fig. 99). Torsion force does not ordinarily fracture the shaft. A direct blow may cause a fracture, but this is much more likely after adolescence, when the bone becomes more brittle. One must be particularly wary of the greenstick fracture without displacement, because if it is unprotected it may progress into a fracture with angulation or even with complete displacement.

If the young patient has a painful injury of the shoulder that is causing tenderness directly over the shaft of the clavicle, one should suspect greenstick fracture without displacement (see Fig. 98). Early x-rays may be interpreted as negative, and the first convincing sign of a fracture may be palpable callus formation, which later (10 to 14 days) may show up on the repeat x-rays. One should always obtain a vertical view of the clavicle as well as the standard anteroposterior view (Fig. 100). If there is any doubt as to the diagnosis, the child should wear a yoke, or at least a sling, to hold the shoulder back. My own preference is for an elastic yoke made of stockinet in which cotton or soft felt pads have been placed.

The fracture of the clavicle in a child (male up to age 12, female up to age 10) is relatively easy to treat. Open operation is seldom, if ever, indicated in a child of this age; however, the fracture should not be ignored. If there is no deformity a simple yoke will suffice. In children, considerable deformity will be corrected by modeling, so that the fracture which is offset or angulated, or both, may terminate with a normal appearing bone. True enough, the youngster has great compensatory capacity, and the physician may accept positions that would be intolerable in the adult. This should not be taken as an excuse for sloppy care, and every effort should be made to restore the alignment and length of the clavicle to normal, even though this requires anesthesia. The fracture will not ordinarily require open reduction, since it is not necessary to have end-to-end apposition so long as length is reasonably well maintained. It should be emphasized that the preceding statements apply to children and that the term children refers to bone age rather than to chronological age. The 13 year old female with a fractured clavicle should be treated as an adult, since her bone growth may well be complete. The husky 6 foot male of 14 years may have bones quite comparable with those of the average male of 16 or 17 years. The physician only deludes

Figure 97. *A*, Eight year old child with complete fracture of the shaft of the clavicle, with upward angulation and offset held in yoke (arrow). *B*, Note modeling, which developed during a two month interval.

Figure 98. *A*, Child age 10, with greenstick fracture of the clavicle. Excessive upward and forward angulation was manipulated to break the greenstick. *B*, Position in yoke. *C*, Union at six weeks. Note modeling.

Figure 99. *A*, Twelve year old child held in yoke, with overriding and angulation. Massive callus has developed beneath clavicle. *B*, Note the modeling and disappearance of excessive callus. Also note that the general alignment of the clavicle remained good with no excessive forward bowing or any excessive upward displacement of the proximal fragment.

Figure 100. Frequently malposition or nonunion of the clavicle can best be determined by a vertical view of the clavicle (axial projection). With the patient in a supine position, elevate shoulders about 5 cm. Turn the patient's head to the unaffected side as far as possible. Place a cassette in a vertical position at the top of the shoulder, pressing it into the neck in order to view as much of the clavicle as possible. Depress the shoulders and pull the arms downward. Tilt the tube so the central ray is as horizontal as possible as it bisects the clavicle. Extreme expiration helps to depress the chest. If the fracture is medial, also angle the tube outward about 10 or 15 degrees.

himself if he expects compensatory correction of a deformity in a person whose bone growth is relatively complete (Fig. 101). I have no hesitation in advising open reduction of a fractured clavicle in a teenager if he is approaching the end of his growth period.

It should also be pointed out that in the treatment of an athlete certain important considerations must be kept in mind. In the first place, the athlete is healthy and strong. In the second place, his skeletal structures must be restored to normal if possible. In the third place, his healing time is vitally important. These factors must be considered in selecting the method of treatment of fracture of the shaft of the clavicle. My own preference in athletes of high school age or older is open reduction, with internal fixation by intramedullary pinning, which is later removed (Fig. 102). This permits early mobility of the shoulder and prevents atrophy of the muscles and stiffness of the joints. It does demand the ultimate in surgical technique and asepsis. One must have a strong, healthy patient with intact, uninfected skin; a qualified anesthetist; a first class surgical facility; proper tools; and last but

not least a capable surgeon. Lacking any one of these, conservative treatment is preferable.

On occasion, comminution at the fracture site will make it advisable to support the intramedullary rod by wire sutures looped around the fragment. The wire sutures alone are usually not secure enough to permit the free use of the arm that is possible with the intramedullary rod (Fig. 103). In any event, the arm should be immobilized in a sling with a swathe (Fig. 104) for at least a couple of weeks to permit the local reaction to subside. The patient is encouraged to wear the sling alone for another two weeks and is given permission to take it off ad lib. He should wear the sling while carrying out ordinary activities.

REGION OF THE OUTER END OF THE CLAVICLE

Anatomical Considerations

At the outer end of the clavicle an ingenious arrangement of bone and ligament promotes stability between the clavicle and the scapula

Figure 101. *See legend on the opposite page.*

Figure 101. Young adult with an oblique fracture of the middle third of the clavicle, with butterfly fragment. *A,* Original anteroposterior view. *B,* Position in yoke. *C,* One week post-injury. *D* and *E,* Eighteen months post injury, essentially same position as original, with nonunion. Note: Anteroposterior and vertical views. (For technique of this vertical view, See Fig. 100)

Figure 102. *A,* The fracture proximal to the coracoclavicular ligaments is shown. Note particularly the upward riding of the proximal fragment and the normal relationship between the distal fragment and the scapula. It is virtually impossible to reduce and hold this fracture without internal fixation, since the shoulder tends to fall downward and the proximal fragment to ride upward. *B,* In this case fixation was intramedullary, with the partially threaded pin left protruding under the skin proximally. This permits better motion of the shoulder than if the pin protrudes distally. The pin is removed after union is complete. The open epiphysis of the humerus indicates that the patient is an adolescent. Nonetheless, open reduction was indicated.

Figure 103. Fracture at the junction of the outer and middle third of the clavicle proximal to the coracoclavicular ligament, held by intramedullary wire fixation. Comminuted butterfly fragments were held by two stainless steel wire loops. There was no damage to the ligaments of the shoulder.

Figure 104. Sling and swathe. General utility dressing for shoulder fixation. This does not give adequate support for acromioclavicular sprain or dislocation. It is ideal for more moderate injuries, for postoperative care and the like. Note the hand is supported in the triangular sling, yet the sling allows for movement of the elbow and utilization of the fingers. The circular adhesive strip is of double thickness and is placed over the gauze to avoid irritating the skin of the chest wall. This circular swathe limits external rotation and abduction to any desired amount, depending upon its tightness.

and prevents the clavicle from displacing upward but at the same time permits a wide range of motion of the upper extremity (see Fig. 86). The outer end of the clavicle butts against the anteromedial aspect of the acromion and is firmly bound to the acromion by the *acromioclavicular* ligaments (capsular ligaments). A wedge-shaped fibrocartilaginous articular disc formed by a thickening of the anterosuperior part of the capsular ligament extends downward into the joint. It lies between the upper portion of the outer end of the clavicle and the acromion. This is sometimes referred to as the semilunar cartilage of the shoulder. The top of the shoulder presents a U-shaped bony subcutaneous surface, the anterior wing of the "U" beginning as the flat outer end of the clavicle, crossing the acromioclavicular joint and extending to the flat anterior process of the acromion which makes the bottom of the "U" directed laterally. The posterior wing of the "U" is the spine of the scapula, which extends from the acromion transversely across the broadest portion of the scapula to blend into its vertebral border. This whole bony "U" is subcutaneous (Fig. 105).

The acromioclavicular ligaments surround the joint but run in an almost horizontal direction in the anatomical position, so that they are well designed to prevent distraction of the

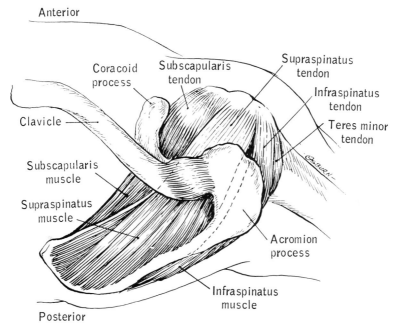

Figure 105. Top view of the shoulder joint.

two bones but are poorly designed to prevent upward displacement of the clavicle on the acromion. The ligaments between the clavicle and the coracoid process of the scapula make up for this deficiency. The coracoid process extends forward from the scapula much like a pointing finger crooked slightly laterally. It lies directly underneath the clavicle, being separated from it by approximately 1½ cm. The long axes of the two bones are at right angles. The ligaments arising along the superior surface of the coracoid twist approximately 90 degrees to attach along the undersurface of the clavicle as a broad, flat band with different divisions, the trapezoid attaching most distally, the conoid proximally. Actually, these divisions are usually indistinguishable after an injury. These ligaments have a much more vertical course than the acromioclavicular ligaments and effectively hold the clavicle down to the scapula.

From the anterior portion of the coracoid, the *coraco-acromial* ligament extends upward and laterally to attach to the top of the acromion in front. This ligament plays no part in acromioclavicular stability but actually serves to reinforce the glenohumeral joint in front. The section of the clavicle from the conoid portion of the coracoclavicular ligament to its distal end is called the *interligamentary* portion. In this region it is a broad, flat bone with no medullary canal. Proximal to this, the cla-

vicle becomes rounded and takes on the typical characteristics of a long bone. The upper surfaces of the clavicle and the acromion, together with the spine of the scapula, form the superior portion of the shoulder and are subcutaneous.

Contusion

The top of the shoulder is frequently contused. Because of the subcutaneous character of the bone, there is often a subperiosteal hematoma and even more frequently rather severe damage to the skin. Contusion here is treated as in other areas. The major problem is to determine whether or not there is more serious injury to the underlying structures. One should accurately locate the area of contusion and, by careful examination, determine whether or not there is involvement of the acromioclavicular joint. In such a case the contusion may be entirely incidental.

Strain

Since the deltoid muscle attachment encompasses the entire outer clavicle and the acromion, strain may be a problem. However, contusion of the deltoid is much more common than strain. The deltoid has a broad attachment without any particularly well-localized area of stress. If muscle tendon injury occurs, it is usually in the muscle belly. The most common site of this in the whole deltoid mechanism is at the attachment of the deltoid muscle to the shaft of the humerus.

Treatment should be that of muscle strain elsewhere, i.e., rest, application of heat, protection and gradual resumption of active motion, with no passive stretching. Complete rupture of a segment of the deltoid is unusual in the athlete.

Occasionally the deltoid of the throwing arm may be subject to chronic strain and may require treatment. This is much more common around the glenohumeral joint, in the biceps, in the rotator cuff or in the attachment of the triceps to the glenoid. This will be discussed in relation to the glenohumeral areas.

Sprain-Subluxation-Dislocation

Since there is no "built-in" bony stability between the acromion and the clavicle, it follows that the entire integrity of this joint is maintained by ligamentous support. A sprain of these ligaments is caused by anything that forces the acromioclavicular joint through a range of motion beyond its normal capacity. Normally this joint has but little excursion. The acromioclavicular ligaments completely surrounding the joint permit only a certain degree of rocking motion but allow no actual flexion or extension.

Various forces may cause injury to the acromioclavicular joint. The most common is a downward blow against the outer end of the shoulder, driving the acromion downward, the clavicle remaining upward. Another is traction on the arm, pulling the shoulder away from the chest wall and causing true lateral displacement of the acromion. Neither of these, however, can adequately account for the instances of injury to this area caused by falling on the out-stretched arm or on the point of the elbow. The football player is well protected by shoulder pads from a downward blow against the top of the shoulder. The sport in which this type of force most commonly occurs is polo, in which the horseman falls and lands on the unprotected point of the shoulder. I believe the majority of these injuries in football result from a fall on the outstretched hand or flexed elbow, with the arm flexed forward 90 degrees and in a neutral lateral position. In this position the humerus drives against the glenoid

and acromion, pushing them forcibly backward. The clavicle, however, remains forward, so that stress is applied to the acromioclavicular and also the coracoclavicular ligaments. This same mechanism could well cause an isolated injury to the acromioclavicular ligament by rotation of the scapula to permit the acromion to move backward while the coracoid either remains in normal relationship to the clavicle or actually rotates forward. As these various forces occur, stress is applied to the acromioclavicular ligament, which permits a certain amount of upward displacement of the outer end of the clavicle. The tension is then taken on the coracoclavicular ligaments. Either of these ligaments may be injured to a variable degree.

Mild (First Degree) Ligament Sprain

In a mild sprain the force is contained before any real damage is done. There is slight tearing of the fibers of the acromioclavicular or coracoclavicular ligament. In this case there is little or no disability of the shoulder. There is localized pain over the area of injury. This pain may be directly over the acromioclavicular joint or may be medial to it, just in front of the clavicle in the sulcus between the clavicle and the coracoid. In the well-muscled individual this pain may be difficult to elicit by palpation. The differentiation between a mild sprain and a contusion is extremely difficult, since a mild sprain does not entail any hypermobility, and indeed, ordinary motions of the shoulder girdle will elicit no pain.

Treatment here is relatively unimportant, and actually, treatment of contusion and sprain may be quite similar, that is, local injection of Xylocaine or Marcaine (no corticoid is used in an acute injury) into the tender area, application of cold followed by heat, and the use of padding to protect from a blow rather than to restrict motion.

Moderate (Second Degree) Ligament Sprain

In a moderate sprain of these ligaments I project relatively severe damage to the fibers of the ligament, and in this case, the symptoms will be more pronounced. Since there has been tearing of some of the ligament fibers, there will be pain on forced motion of the shoulder, even though there is no actual hypermobility of the clavicle on the acromion. In such a case I do not expect the clavicle to be riding high.

There will be pain, swelling and tenderness, with the pain increased by an attempt to separate the acromion and clavicle by pulling on the arm. There is also pain on depressing the acromion in relation to the clavicle by pulling straight down on the arm, with the arm against the side. This case can be distinguished from contusion by the severity of the symptoms and their aggravation when the ligament is placed under stress. Within a short time there will be local swelling at the joint that may simulate upward displacement of the clavicle.

Treatment of a moderate sprain of the acromioclavicular or coracoclavicular ligament should be local and general. Local treatment is the same as for mild sprain, i.e., local injection of procaine, application of cold followed by heat, and use of a pressure dressing in case of swelling. Protective treatment here is all-important, since it is vital to prevent subsequent injury. One must visualize that a definite portion of the ligament is torn or avulsed and that the remaining portion is substantially weakened. If athletic participation is permitted in contact sports, the next blow may well complete the tear.

It is important that the arm be strapped to the side in such a way as to push it upward and the clavicle downward. This can be done by various methods. One of the simplest and

best for this type of injury is as follows: With the arm at the side and the elbow flexed to 90 degrees, the midpoint of a long strip of 3 in. tape is placed under the forearm about 2 in. distal to the elbow and carried forward up over the shoulder, proximal to the acromioclavicular joint, and then down the back, crossing toward the opposite side. The posterior portion of the long strip should go up the back of the arm, cross over the shoulder from back to front, and then diagonally across the chest again, medial to the acromioclavicular joint (Fig. 106A). The dressing is completed by a circumferential strip of protective tape placed around the arm and the chest to hold the arm to the side (Fig. 106B). These are the key straps of the dressing. The dressing is made more comfortable by supporting the forearm loosely in a choker-type sling made of elastic stockinet, which is suspended from the neck and looped around the wrist (Fig. 106C). Additional adhesive strapping can be applied for compression directly over the shoulder if desirable. The principle of this support is that, as the weight of the forearm and hand drops distally, the lever fulcrum is at the broad band of the tape under the proximal forearm, and the short posterior arm of the lever tends to thrust the humerus upward as the hand drops downward. There are obviously many modifi-

Figure 106. Strapping to support the acromioclavicular joint in acromioclavicular sprain. *A,* The vertical strip holds the humerus upward and the clavicle downward. Note particularly the length of the strip, since it extends from the waistline in back to the waistline in front as a single strip. Note the leverage action as the hand and forearm drop downward at the waist, the short lever of the inner end of the ulna pushing the humerus upward. *B,* The application of a tape swathe to hold the elbow to the side. This strip should not be tight. Before this strip is applied, a powdered abdominal (ABD) pad is placed in the axilla. *C,* Choker sling of stockinet is added. This sling is loose and may be changed from the hand to the wrist or eliminated altogether, as the patient wishes. Some of the details to note are the felt pads (here dark felt used for contrast) to protect the skin at the pressure areas. There are also the felt pads within the stockinet behind the neck and under the hand.

Figure 107. Modification of dressing shown in Figure 106, which is often used postoperatively. In this instance the initial application is of the pressure dressing over the wound and top of the shoulder using Elastoplast. The second step is the application of a triangular sling carefully pinned around the elbow. Step three is the application of a swathe around the body to hold the arm to the side. The dressing is stabilized then by the vertical strip, applied as in Figure 106, only over the dressing rather than over the skin.

cations of this type of support, and any one that effectively holds the clavicle down and the arm up is satisfactory (Fig. 107).

This type of support is continued for a minimum of six weeks in order to permit the ligaments to unite and become relatively strong. It should be borne in mind that the simple force of the weight of the arm hanging at the side may be sufficient to distract the ligament ends. A period of rehabilitation will be required to mobilize the shoulder and improve the muscle tone in the upper extremity before participation in sports is advisable (see Fig. 163). Such a plan carefully followed will result in complete recovery from a rather severe injury; however, if continued function is permitted the ligaments will gradually stretch and a loose acromioclavicular joint, which is subject to either chronic disability or repeated injury, will result.

Severe (Third Degree) Ligament Sprain (Subluxation-Dislocation)

Severe (third degree) ligament sprain is one in which one or more of the ligaments have been completely torn. It can be classified roughly into two categories: (1) a complete tear of the acromioclavicular ligament with the coracoclavicular ligament intact and (2) a complete tear of the coracoclavicular and acromioclavicular ligaments.

Severe (Third Degree) Sprain of the Acromioclavicular Ligament. It is possible for a complete tear of the acromioclavicular ligament to occur along with an incomplete tear of the coracoclavicular ligament. The force applied here is downward on the acromion and it usually has an outward component, so that the acromion is forced outward and downward away from the clavicle. This causes rupture of the horizontal fibers extending from the clavicle to the acromion. The resulting symptoms· depend to some extent on the degree of injury to the coracoclavicular ligaments. If this is slight and largely of the distal component, the symptoms will be those of moderate sprain, that is, local pain, swelling and tenderness in the acromioclavicular joint. There will be pain on any effort to distract this joint or on downward pull on the arm or on manipulation of the shoulder toward wide abduction. There will frequently be a mild degree of instability between the outer end of the clavicle and the acromion, with the clavicle appearing to be slightly higher than the acromion. The space between the clavicle and the acromion may well be widened in comparison with that of the normal or the opposite shoulder. There will not be extensive upward riding of the clavicle in relation to the acromion. This cannot take place with intact coracoclavicular ligaments. One may visualize that there has been complete rupture of some of the fibers of the acromioclavicular ligament but that the scapula has rotated downward rather than been displaced downward. The coracoclavicular ligament is still effective in holding the clavicle in its normal position in relation to the acromion.

Treatment. Treatment of this type of acromioclavicular injury taxes the best judgment. Far too often the injury is treated by the so-called conservative method, with resulting chronic relaxation of the acromioclavicular joint, arthritic changes and disability that may later require surgery eventuating in less than a complete recovery. On the other hand, one hesitates to perform an open repair in the absence of upward displacement of the clavicle. Local treatment consists of the usual measures: aspiration, injection, application of cold then heat. The subluxation should be reduced by downward pressure on the clavicle and upward pressure on the arm. The temptation then is to maintain this reduction by external fixation, and this is usually done by the method previously described (see Fig. 106). The fact that this is often ineffectual is indicated by the wide variety of methods suggested as improvements, i.e., support in a plaster jacket with straps over the clavicle to hold it down and various other lever actions designed to hold the acromion and clavicle together. In the final analysis I think that internal fixation is probably desirable in the majority of cases in the young athlete. If one can obtain complete reduction manually, it indicates that there is no interposing tissue between the two bones. It is justifiable then to attempt skeletal fixation by pins across the acromion and the joint into the clavicle, without open reduction. Proper positioning of the pins is extremely difficult, and this method is not for the uninitiated. However, the operator who has repeatedly inserted these pins at open reduction may be able to place two pins in a position adequate to hold the bones together. This is much easier to do under fluoroscopic control. Since it is important to prevent distraction of the acromion from the clavicle as well as to hold the clavicle down, the use of a smooth pin with a 1 in. overlay screw thread at one end is desirable.

Complete Rupture of the Acromioclavicular and Coracoclavicular Ligaments. The second type of third degree sprain presumes a com-

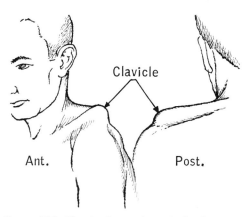

Figure 109. Sketch shows dramatically the upward displacement of the outer end of the clavicle in complete acromioclavicular dislocation. (From DePalma, *Fractures and Dislocations—An Atlas,* Vol. 1, p. 227.)

plete rupture of both the acromioclavicular and the coracoclavicular ligaments (Fig. 108). In this injury there is more swelling and tenderness, and pain is elicited on any manipulation of the shoulder. The characteristic finding, however, is marked upward riding of the outer end of the clavicle in relation to the scapula (Fig. 109). This may be quite obvious in clinical examination of the patient. If the patient is examined sitting up and if swelling is not severe, the outer end of the clavicle can be felt and be seen pushing up under the skin while the acromion remains down. This finding may be completely obscured when the patient is supine, but when he stands (Figs. 110 and 111), particularly with some weight in the hand, it becomes quite obvious. Comparable pictures of the two shoulders, with the patient in the standing position, will reveal the displacement. In this instance the displacement of the clavicle is primarily upward, whereas in the other type of subluxation the acromion pulls away from the outer end of the clavicle rather than downward. However, both types of displacement may well be present.

Treatment. Although this dislocation is usually readily reduced, it is virtually impossible to hold reduction in a manner that will allow primary repair of the torn ligaments at their normal length. When one recalls the pathological changes, this is apparent. In order for the clavicle to displace upward, the distance between the clavicle and the coracoid must be increased (Fig. 108). The coracoclavicular and acromioclavicular ligaments are avulsed or torn, and unless the clavicle is held in the anatomical position until healing is complete, subluxation will inevitably recur, and a painful, weak shoulder may be the result. For this

Figure 108. Complete acromioclavicular dislocation with obvious tearing of both coracoclavicular and acromioclavicular ligaments. Note particularly the wide space between the coracoid and the clavicle, with the clavicle riding high above the acromion. The x-ray was made with the patient standing but with no weight.

Figure 110. A, With the patient supine, no dislocation is noted. B, Standing with 4 pounds suspended from the wrist. Note particularly the widening at the acromioclavicular joint and also the difference in distance between the clavicle and the coracoid. This is not as dramatic as Figure 108, but comparison with the supine position makes the dislocation quite obvious. C, Lateral view of the acromioclavicular joint, made as shown in Figure 111, showing the complete separation.

reason it is my opinion that in the athlete a complete tear of these ligaments should be treated by surgical repair.

Again, we are faced with two alternatives. Once surgery has been decided upon, one must resolve whether the operation should be designed merely to hold the clavicle in position or to repair the torn ligaments as well. It is my belief that if one is going to the trouble to perform an open operation to fix the clavicle in position, he should take advantage of this opportunity to appose and suture the torn ends of the coracoclavicular ligaments. In the ordinary case this can readily be accomplished because after the skin is divided and the outer end of the clavicle is freed from its muscle attachments, the outer end may readily be displaced upward. Ready access can be had to the area of the injury between the clavicle and the coracoid, and in most instances sutures can be placed in the coracoclavicular ligaments while the clavicle is displaced upward and can be tied after replacement of the clavicle and fixation in its normal position.

Of vital importance is firm fixation of the clavicle to the scapula. This can be done by various methods, depending upon the choice of the surgeon. Basically the methods of fixation are either by transfixion of the acromion and clavicle, or by fixation of the clavicle to the coracoid, or by both. A good method for fixing the clavicle to the acromion is the use of transfixion pins, preferably threaded in part, passing through the acromion, across the joint

Figure 111. To demonstrate the separation shown in Figure 110c, a lateral projection may be made. Instruct the patient to place the hand of the affected arm under the opposite axilla, allowing the injured shoulder to hang as relaxed as possible. The acromioclavicular joint should be positioned to the center of the table. The unaffected side should be rotated about 45 degrees away from the table. The tube is angled downward 20 to 25 degrees, and the central ray is directed to the acromioclavicular joint. The cassette should be centered to the central ray.

and into the clavicle. It is necessary to use two pins, since one may not give sufficient fixation (Fig. 112). If this is done, no fixation is needed between the coracoid and the clavicle other than the ligament repair.

Another method of holding the coracoid and clavicle together involves the use of the lag (Bosworth) screw, which transfixes the clavicle (Fig. 113), and extends into the coracoid; still another is the use of sutures around the cora-

Figure 112. Illustration of fixation across the acromioclavicular joint with two partially threaded pins. This is an old case as indicated by the calcification about the clavicle, and it was felt advisable to resect 1 cm. of the outer end of the clavicle. Wider resection than this is neither necessary nor desirable. Note the close approximation of the clavicle and coracoid. These pins should be removed after eight to ten weeks.

Figure 113. Twenty-two year old college athlete with acromioclavicular dislocation on the right side. *A,* x-ray shows marked upward dislocation of the clavicle, with separation between the clavicle and the acromion. The patient was treated elsewhere in a Kenny Howard sling for six weeks, but the deformity persisted. I saw him three months post-injury, at which time the outer end of the clavicle was resected. Reconstruction of the acromioclavicular ligament by the conjoined tendon of the biceps and coracobrachialis was performed. Half of this tendon was dissected free, reflected upward and fastened to the outer end of the clavicle through drill holes. This was also supported by the clavicular acromial ligament, which was detached from the acromion, left attached to the coracoid process and fastened to the clavicle. Position was secured with Bosworth screw. *B,* X-ray six weeks postoperative shows the Bosworth screw holding in position. *C,* X-ray three months postoperative following removal of the Bosworth screw. Position is secure although there is considerable reaction around the joint. He is playing basketball with no complaint of the shoulder.

coid and clavicle with fascia, braided silk or wire. There are some disadvantages to each method. Previously I have expressed a preference for double pin fixation across the acromioclavicular joint. Because of the many complications resulting from this method of fixation, my present choice is the use of a Bosworth screw. Since it is necessary to expose the coracoid process to repair the coracoclavicular ligaments, the insertion of the screw is somewhat simplified. However, it is a technical exercise and may at times be quite frustrating.

It is of absolute importance that the thread of the screw engage completely through the coracoid or else the fixation will be lost (Fig. 114). A few hints follow as to the performance of this method: The Bosworth screw is specifically designed to permit up and down motion of the clavicle on the neck of the screw. Therefore, the hole in the clavicle should be slightly larger than the shaft of the screw. It must not be unduly large or the screw head may erode through it more readily. Since the coracoid process has no specific function in regard to its

Figure 114. This 22 year old male dislocated the coracoclavicular joint ten days before being examined. He is judo instructor and was unable to use his shoulder. Examination revealed upward riding of the outer end of the clavicle, with instability, tenderness, and pain on abduction. *A,* X-ray shows the wide separation at the coracoclavicular level. Note the degenerative change at the outer end of the clavicle just two weeks post-injury. *B,* Open reduction and repair of the coracoclavicular ligaments carried out with resection of the distal tip of the clavicle. The Bosworth screw is holding the clavicle reduced. *C,* Five months later after removal of the screw. Note some regeneration of the outer end of the clavicle and no upward displacement.

position, there is naturally a great deal of variation between individuals in the exact course of the coracoid. This points out the validity of my statement that exposure of the coracoid helps in the success of the procedure because the physician can actually make sure that the screw fixation penetrates through both cortices. After this screw is placed, it should be possible to move the clavicle up and down on the screw a millimeter or so. My reason for adopting this method is that it permits relatively rapid resumption of athletic activity, although it would be wise to protect the shoulder by forbidding football for eight weeks. I have, however, permitted an occasional college athlete to return to play after carefully explaining to him the risk of damage. So far not one of them has broken the screw, although in two instances the screw was slightly bent. I would like to emphasize again that any

Figure 115. *A,* Fixation of outer end clavicle by braided silk through drill hole in clavicle is shown (arrow). This is a late postoperative picture and is suggestive of erosion of the suture. *B,* Complete erosion through the clavicle with pathological fracture (arrow). *C,* After removal of the outer end of the clavicle. Some disability persists.

type of nonabsorbable fixation should be removed after eight or ten weeks, when one must assume that the ligament has united but not wholly healed.

After threaded pin fixation is completed, the acromioclavicular ligament should be carefully repaired. Strong internal fixation permits rapid mobilization of the shoulder joint and so shortens the period of disability. It is advisable for the arm to be held in a sling for several weeks. This will permit active motion but will protect against unguarded activity. Any type of metal-

lic internal fixation should be removed after eight weeks. This includes the Bosworth screw, which may work loose and break; the circumferential suture or wire, which may erode through the clavicle (Fig. 115); and the transfixion pins, which, after a certain period, may migrate (Fig. 116). Following successful repair with a good functional result, the patient may resume unlimited activity. When participating in sports, it would be wise for him to wear particularly well-designed shoulder pads after such an injury. However, the best the shoulder

Figure 116. *A,* Acromioclavicular joint fixed by single nonthreaded pin. *B,* Migration of this pin— fortunately after healing of the ligaments. This could have been prevented by having a portion of the pin threaded. It is inadvisable to have the threaded part of the pin across the joint because it may break through the threaded area. Migration can also be prevented by bending the end of the pin.

pad can do is to protect the shoulder against a direct blow. It has no effect on forces that are transmitted through the arm.

Chronic Lesions of the Acromioclavicular Joint

A chronic irritative lesion of the acromio-clavicular joint can be the consequence of repeated injuries which cause the acromion and clavicle to impinge forcibly (Fig. 117). Repeated minor sprains of the capsular liga-ment that result in thickening of the ligament and local swelling in the joint also cause this condition. It may result in calcific or osseous deposits within the ligament or joint. Since calcific deposits are basically degenerative and osseous deposits are basically reparative, ossi-fication of the coracoclavicular ligament does not seem to impair its function. I have seen many patients with what appeared to be com-plete ossification of the ligament, yet the con-dition was completely asymptomatic (Fig. 118). I would strongly urge against removal of an osseous deposit in the ligament, since this may substantially weaken the ligament. There

may be involvement of the intra-articular fi-brocartilage, even with ossification or fragmen-tation of the cartilage (Fig. 119). The result is pain and tenderness elicited particularly by abduction of the arm, since this movement forces the acromion and clavicle together.

Treatment. This condition is basically a trau-matic arthritis and may be treated as such by application of heat locally, rest and injection of a long-acting local anesthetic and a corticoid preparation (not more than three steroid in-jections should be used). A chronic lesion of the acromioclavicular joint may be quite dis-tressing because it is magnified by athletic act vities such as throwing, falling on the out-stretched hand or, in fact, any forceful activity of the shoulder girdle. If it does not respond adequately to nonsurgical treatment, surgery is justified. At this time the fibrocartilaginous disc should be removed and the joint carefully inspected. If there are definite irreversible changes in the articular cartilage, it is wise to resect 1 or 2 cm. of the outer end of the clavicle (Figs. 120 and 121). Care should be taken to stay distal to the coracoclavicular ligament. This procedure usually will give ex-cellent results, with good function of the shoul-

Figure 117. *A,* Irritative lesion. Degenerative changes and chronic arthritis from dislocation of the clavicle upward, although the space between the coracoid and clavicle seems quite narrow. *B,* Shows resection of the outer end of the clavicle distal to the coracoclavicular ligaments. Note upward displacement of the clavicle, which persists owing to elongation of the coracoclavicular ligaments.

Figure 118. Patient injured shoulder three months before. Radiograph shows almost complete ossification of the coracoclavicular ligament, with dislocation of the outer end of the clavicle at the acromioclavicular joint. The pain was at the acromioclavicular joint. The clavicle seemed quite stable in the position it was in, and we just resected the outer end of the clavicle and did not disturb the ossified ligament. Uneventful recovery but with upward riding of the distal clavicle.

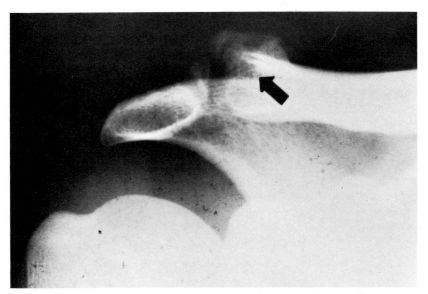

Figure 119. Soft tissue x-ray film of the acromioclavicular joint showing ossification of the capsule and cartilage (arrow).

Figure 120. This 16 year old male has had chronic acromioclavicular dislocation for the last two years following a football injury. After three weeks with his arm at his side he was operated on elsewhere; a screw was put in the shoulder, and the arm was bound down for four weeks. After the screw was removed, his symptoms recurred, and the knot recurred on the shoulder. He had a second reconstruction with the screw being removed at ten weeks. Two months later the shoulder began to bother him again with pain at night, pain on lifting and a feeling of something slipping in the shoulder. My examination two years post-injury revealed a painful shoulder at the outer end of the clavicle with upward riding, and pain particularly on abduction. *A,* X-ray shows upward riding of the clavicle, with separation between the coracoid and the clavicle. Preoperative diagnosis: Degenerative arthritis with instability. At surgery the large, thick scar was excised. The acromioclavicular ligament was divided lineally and 1 cm. of the distal end of the clavicle was removed, since the outer end of the clavicle impinged on the acromion from pressure, especially in abduction of the arm. *B,* Postoperative x-ray film shows no evidence of reossification. No upward riding of the clavicle. No complaints.

Figure 121. *A*, Chronic degenerative arthritis with production of bone around the clavicle. *B*, Illustration of resection of the outer end of the clavicle, two months postoperative.

der, although sometimes there is persistent pain or tenderness. Recognizable weakness may persist.

Fracture

When I say "outer end of the clavicle," I am referring to that area distal to the coracoclavicular ligaments. This part of the clavicle is a broad, flat bone without a distinct medullary canal. The forces likely to cause a fracture of the clavicle in this area may be the same as those causing ligament injury. As the acromion is driven downward in relation to the clavicle, the coracoclavicular as well as the acromioclavicular ligaments may remain intact, and the bone will break proximal to the coracoclavicular ligaments. This will be a fracture of the shaft of the clavicle (see Fig. 102), usually

in the outer part of the middle third of the bone. In this instance, the distal fragment will remain in normal relationship to the scapula while the proximal fragment rides upward. Although this fracture is not actually one of the outer end of the clavicle, it does require mention here because it is virtually impossible to reduce and hold without some form of internal fixation. In the previous discussion of dislocation of the outer end of the clavicle, mention was made of the difficulty of holding the clavicle down for the application of direct pressure downward, in spite of the fact that its entire length is intact. When the fracture is just proximal to the coracoclavicular ligaments, the sharp distal end of the proximal fragment not only is short but also lies close to the neck and is not amenable to fixation by direct pressure. This type of fracture is best treated by intramedullary fixation following

Figure 122. Comminuted fracture of the outer end of the clavicle in adult female. Note the distal portion is fragmented and remains intact to the acromion, whereas the proximal portion just rides upward. There must be rupture of the coracoclavicular ligament.

open reduction. To some extent these same principles apply to any fracture of the middle third of the clavicle, but they are particularly pertinent as the ligamentous area is approached.

Another combination of forces may cause the fracture to be distal (Figs. 122 and 123) to the coracoclavicular ligaments and so be an *interligamentary* fracture. In this instance, as the acromion is driven downward, the acromioclavicular ligaments remain intact, but the coracoclavicular ligaments rupture. The fracture occurs within the flat distal portion of the clavicle. The distal fragment accompanies the acromion and is displaced downward; the proximal fragment is displaced upward. In the fracture proximal to the coracoclavicular liga-

ments, described previously, the coracoclavicular ligaments remain intact, and so the outer end of the clavicle remains securely fastened to the scapula. After reduction or internal fixation of the two fragments, the acromioclavicular area is secure. In the fracture distal to the coracoclavicular ligaments, the coracoclavicular ligaments are ruptured, and fixation of the clavicle to the scapula is impaired.

This type of injury also requires open reduction, at which time the coracoclavicular ligaments should be sutured. The fracture line may be at any level between the two ligaments. If the distal fragment is small and involves only the outer 2 cm. of the clavicle, it is preferable to remove the fragment, repair the coracoclavicular ligaments and thus shorten the healing

Figure 123. A, Anteroposterior view of outer end of the clavicle, showing no evidence of injury. Clinical diagnosis of fracture led to vertical x-ray B, which revealed interligamentary fracture of the clavicle.

period and diminish the probability of pain at the acromioclavicular joint following recovery. This is particularly pertinent if a comminuted fracture involves the articular portion of the outer end of the clavicle. In many instances a small fragment will remain attached to the acromioclavicular ligament. This should by all means be removed. The surgeon must rely upon his good judgment as to whether in a given case it would be better to obtain bony fixation or to remove the fragments. As a rule of thumb, one might say that if adequate surgical repair of the coracoclavicular ligaments can be obtained, there will be less necessity for bony union between the two fragments, and thus the distal fragment might well be removed. Similarly, if the distal fragment is small or comminuted, bony security between the two fragments is not readily obtainable anyway, and these fragments would best be removed. On the other hand, if ligament repair seems insecure, the additional security of bony union in order to take advantage of the stability of the acromioclavicular ligament is important, and it is preferable to leave the fragment in.

An interligamentary fracture may also be the result of a direct blow. In such a case the fracture line may be of any character. It may be comminuted, oblique, spiral or transverse, but is most frequently either oblique from above, downward and inward, or comminuted. Since both the acromioclavicular and coracoclavicular ligaments are intact, any extensive degree of displacement is unusual in this fracture. Treatment is primarily supportive. A loop of 3 in. tape is passed beneath the flexed elbow and then crossed over the outer end of the clavicle. Felt pads should be placed over the top of the shoulder to provide some degree of downward pressure. The arm should be in a sling (see Fig. 106).

From the standpoint of treatment it is quite important to distinguish between an interligamentary fracture caused by direct trauma of the bone and one caused by disrupting forces applied indirectly. In those caused by direct trauma, treatment requires only a relatively short period of external fixation, whereas in the other types with ligament damage, open reduction is the treatment of choice. If open reduction cannot be carried out for some reason, then the same type of fixation should be used as was mentioned in relation to dislocations of the outer end of the clavicle, namely, the type of support that is designed to push the humerus upward and the clavicle downward (see Fig. 106).

Rehabilitation is extremely important in these injuries (see Fig. 163), and it will proceed much faster if there is good internal fixation of the bones. Needless to say, athletic competition should not be permitted until healing is complete. In the case of torn ligaments, this will require eight weeks; in the case of fractures, the period depends upon the progress of healing as checked by x-ray examination.

It should be remembered in any discussion of injuries about the shoulder that a ligament attachment in tearing away may include a fragment of bone, a so-called *avulsion* fracture. It should be treated basically as a ligament injury. The coracoid may be pulled off by the coracoclavicular ligament (Fig. 184), the small fragment of the proximal end of the clavicle may be torn off by the sternoclavicular ligament, or a segment of the acromion or distal end of the clavicle may be avulsed by the acromioclavicular ligament. In each instance, the treatment is basically the same as that for ligament injury. In the majority of instances it is advisable to remove the fragment unless it is large enough to allow its fixation to the parent bone, in which case the additional stability provided by the fragment may be of considerable value. This is particularly pertinent at the inner end of the clavicle, where it is difficult to hold the clavicle down by ordinary suture through the ligament, and a firmly fixed proximal fragment may be utilized to fasten the clavicle down.

Fracture of the Acromion

Many of the same forces that fracture the outer end of the clavicle may also fracture the acromial process. By far the most frequent force is direct trauma, which simply breaks off the end of the bone at any point distal to its attachment to the body of the scapula through the spine of the scapula. These fractures are usually without gross displacement and require little treatment in themselves. It is important to recognize such a fracture. A fracture without displacement may not be well visualized on the ordinary x-ray view, and it may be necessary to take a vertical view through the distal end of the acromion to show it (Figs. 124 to 126). If there is any question, repeated x-ray pictures are important. Many of these cases will be diagnosed as a contusion, and the fracture is recognized only after the "contusion" has failed to heal within a reasonable period of time.

Treatment. In the unusual case in which there is nonunion of the fracture of the acromi-

Figure 124. Transverse fracture across the acromial process by direct downward force against the acromion. *A*, Note anteroposterior view is negative. *B*, Vertical view shows fracture clearly.

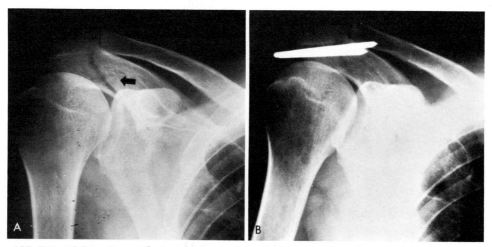

Figure 125. Patient fell, landing on the back of his shoulder. *A*, Note the oblique fracture of the acromion with some displacement. *B*, After internal fixation because of instability of the fragment, which involved the acromioclavicular joint. (For technique of x-ray, see Fig. 126.)

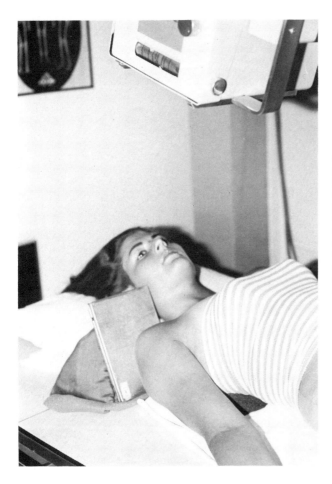

Figure 126. Positioning for acromion. Several views are often necessary to demonstrate fractures of the acromion. View *A* in Figure 125 is obtained by placing the patient supine on the table. A cassette angled about 10 degrees should be supported at the top of the shoulder. Supinate the elbow and depress the shoulder. With the tube angled about 10 degrees cephalad, direct the central ray to the acromioclavicular joint. View *B* of Figure 124 is a projection similar to a standard arteroposterior view of the shoulder, except the arm is elevated above the head to rotate the acromion posteriorly. A lateral view of the scapula (see Fig. 132*B*) with the body also rotated slightly to bring the acromion into view or an axillary view of the shoulder may be necessary.

on, the distal fragment can generally be removed without serious disability to the shoulder if the deltoid muscle is sutured to the remaining bone. Indeed, if the acute fracture involves as little as 1 cm. of the distal end of the acromion, the best treatment will be excision of the fragment, since healing will be much more rapid and with much less likelihood of any residual complication.

Occasionally the acromion may be fractured by an indirect force caused by upward dislocation of the humerus against the acromial process (Fig. 127). This usually is a major injury and will require specialized treatment. Frequently open reduction is necessary because of the probability of soft tissue interposition preventing reduction of the dislocation. More frequently the force will cause subluxation only. The fracture will be incomplete. Again treatment is dependent on recognition of the injury and requires some degree of protection of the arm against wide abduction. If displacement is gross, open reduction is advisable. At operation, the fragment may be removed if small. If it is large, open reduction and threaded pin fixation may be carried out.

Figure 127. Dislocation of the glenohumeral joint with fractured acromion. It is unusual to get this picture, since the dislocation is usually spontaneously reduced and the severity of injury may well be overlooked. (From McLaughlin, Trauma, p. 263.)

REGION OF THE BODY OF THE SCAPULA

Contusion

The only area of the scapula that is commonly subject to contusion is its spine from the vertebral border to the tip of the acromion. This area is entirely subcutaneous, and the skin may be severely contused between the underlying bone and the external blow. There may be a contusion of the bone. The diagnosis is readily made on the basis of the reaction to the lesion, with tenderness directly along the bone, usually sharply localized. Ordinary motions of the shoulder or scapula will not be painful in simple contusion. In case of a severe injury, x-ray visualization may be necessary to eliminate the possibility of a fracture of the spine of the scapula (see Fig. 132). It may be necessary to get tangential views in order to visualize the fracture line. In contact sports, such as football, this area is very adequately protected by shoulder pads and so is infre-

quently hurt. *Treatment* consists of application of cold then heat, local injection and use of protective padding. With adequate padding, this type of injury need not interrupt participation in competitive sports.

The muscles overlying the scapula may be subject to contusion by a direct blow catching the muscle between the hard underlying bone and the striking force. This may be distinguished from other injuries by the localization of the tenderness plus pain on active contraction or passive stretching of the involved muscle. *Treatment* consists of application of cold followed by heat, local injection and rest. It is unusual for ossification to occur following contusion of the muscles about the scapula.

Strain

The area of the scapula is quite subject to strain, since the entire bone serves for the origin or insertion of many muscles (see page 118). In many instances, extremely powerful

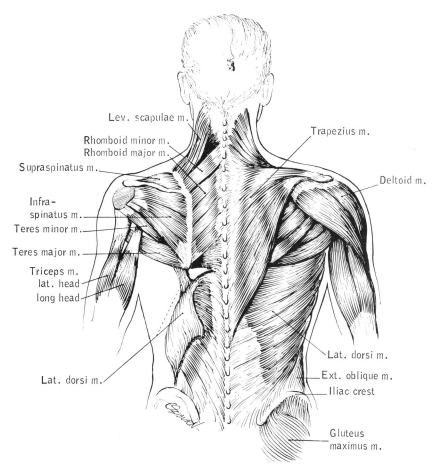

Figure 128. *A,* Muscle attachments about the shoulder.

Illustration and legend continued on the following page.

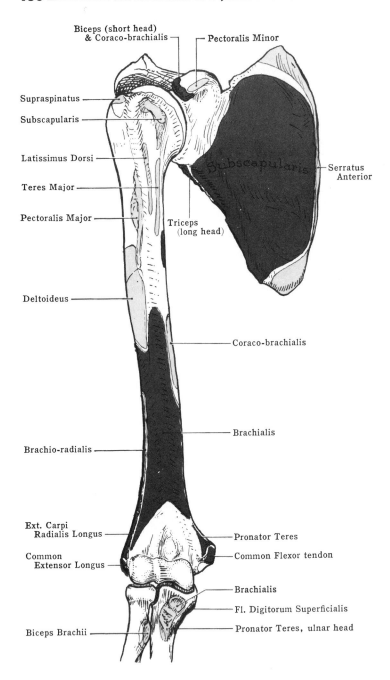

Figure 128 *(Continued). B,* The anterior view of the shoulder is shown clearly revealing the multiple muscle attachments of the scapula. The whole undersurface of the scapula is occupied by the subscapularis, and the serrati muscles attach along the vertebral border. The biceps and pectoralis minor attach to the coracoid.

muscles may attach throughout a relatively small area (Fig. 128). Thus, it may be possible for the powerful latissimus dorsi muscle to avulse its attachment from the inferior angle. This may cause avulsion of the bone but more commonly results in a simple strain with rupture of some of the fibers at their attachment to the bone. A similar injury may occur at the superior angle of the scapula, where the levator scapulae and rhomboideus minor may be subject to the same type of injury. Less frequently there may be injury in the region of the trapezius along the spine of the scapula or of the teres minor or triceps. Similarly, there may be damage to the rhomboideus major at its attachment along the vertebral border.

Acute Strain

All these injuries are caused by violent muscle action, and for this reason, treatment must provide restriction of function of the muscle

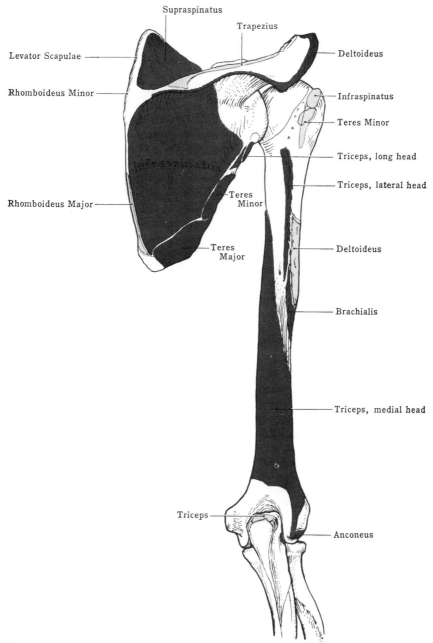

Figure 128 *(Continued). C,* The dorsal view is even more significant. Note the spinatae, the supra above and the infra below the spine and the trapezius and the deltoid on the spine. Along the border are the teres major, the teres minor and the triceps. Stability of the shoulder is increased by attachment of the rotator cuff muscles to the humeral head and also between the subscapularis by the pectoralis major coming across and attaching to the humerus without a specific scapular attachment. (*B* and *C* reproduced by permission from: J. B. Grant. An Atlas of Anatomy. Sixth Ed. © 1972. The Williams and Wilkins Company, Baltimore.)

involved. In an acute injury, *treatment* consists of local application of cold, followed later by heat, injection of a local anesthetic, aspiration of the hematoma and restriction of function of the muscle that has been damaged. The last can be carried out by placing the arm in a sling, which moderately restricts the activity of the arm. If the injury is severe, athletic competition is interdicted. Healing usually takes place without major definitive treatment. However, if a detectable fragment of bone is avulsed an appreciable distance, one should seriously consider early removal of the fragment of bone and suture of the muscle to the fracture bed. Although this may seem a little radical in a situation in which spontaneous healing will probably take place, one must bear in mind that situations involving actual separation of an avulsed fragment of bone frequently lead to nonunion with persistent pain. The athlete may respond better to surgical treatment, entailing a few weeks of early complete disability but offering the opportunity for more complete recovery than to nonsurgical treatment, involving months or years of disability of a lower grade. This is particularly pertinent when one considers that the best nonsurgical treatment should also entail complete rest.

Chronic Strain

These same areas in the scapula may be involved in chronic irritative lesions, with chronic strain of the various muscle attachments. In this situation, ordinary function of the muscle is usually pain-free. Violent exercise, particularly against resistance, causes recurrence of the symptoms of pain, muscle spasm and restriction of motion. This is the same type of chronic strain that may occur at the attachment of the tendo Achilles or at the epicondyles of the elbow or in the hamstrings. *Treatment* may be extremely discouraging, since resumption of forceful activity will often cause recurrence of symptoms. Fortunately, this is uncommon around the scapula as opposed to the glenohumeral joint. A period of complete rest may be rewarding if continued over a long enough period. In chronic cases this may be supplemented by two or three injections of local anesthetic plus a corticoid preparation. Careful! Great care must be taken to insure that function is actually restricted to that tolerated by the muscle without increasing the irritation.

In the type of case just described, the general plan of treatment is as follows: Every effort is made to pinpoint exactly the location of the lesion. This area is then injected with a local anesthetic. If this completely relieves the pain during the effective period of the anesthetic, the physician may feel confident that he has reached the area involved. If the condition is chronic, he may then proceed with local injection of a corticoid preparation. Following these measures, local inductive heat, as by diathermy or ultrasound, should be applied once or twice daily for 20 minutes. The injection may actually increase the pain immediately after the effect of the anesthetic is lost. There then may be 12 to 36 hours of acute

exacerbation of pain, often to the extent that sedation is required. The pain and other symptoms should then gradually subside until marked improvement is obtained. If this improvement persists for several days but the symptoms then gradually recur, the injection should be repeated before the symptoms become too severe again. This may be done three times, so long as gradual overall improvement is taking place. A course of treatment consists of three injections, no less than one week apart. As activity is resumed, great care should be taken to insure that rehabilitation progresses below the level of irritative activity. Several months of pain-free activity should elapse before violent exercise of the involved muscle is permitted.

This recommendation for treatment of the chronic condition should not be extrapolated into treatment for an acute strain. *There is no indication for the use of any corticoid in the acute injury.* Also, muscle strain is being discussed here, not tendon strain. A good basic principle is that a corticoid should never be injected into the tendon itself, although it may be proper to inject it into the tendon sheath or peritendinous tissue. The danger of penetration of the tendon itself should be very well recognized. One may get some idea as to whether or not the needle is in the tendon by the amount of resistance to injection, since the tendon is a dense structure and ordinarily does not accept local injection without considerable pressure, which may, indeed, increase the necrosis.

Bursitis

There are many bursae around the body of the scapula (Fig. 129), since bursae are found in any area where friction would otherwise develop between layers of tissue. One can readily appreciate their frequency in this area of excessive motion between the various muscles attaching to the scapula. Probably the most constant bursa, other than those in direct relationship to the glenohumeral joint, is that one lying between the body of the scapula and the muscles of the chest wall. This bursa is not frequently described anatomically and may indeed develop as a result of irritation between the scapula and the muscles following some type of injury. A bursa may be high up under the supraspinous portion of the scapula or may be lower, lying beneath the infraspinous part. Symptoms of bursitis in this area are related particularly to motion of the scapula against the chest wall, so that approximating the sca-

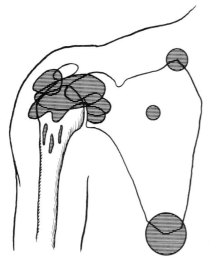

Figure 129. The multitude of bursae around the shoulder, particularly around the glenohumeral joint, are shown. (Redrawn from Codman.)

pulae posteriorly or crossing the arm across the chest anteriorly will elicit pain and, frequently, when this motion is carried out under tension, crepitation.

Treatment of this condition is by rest, application of heat and local injection. The general plan should be to determine as accurately as possible the exact location of the bursa involved. In subscapular bursitis, since the scapula overlies the bursa, it may be quite difficult to actually localize this area. It is easier to get a needle into the area under the scapula with the scapula rotated forward. The test of the accuracy of the localization of injection is the prompt relief of pain, which continues while the local anesthetic is effective. For this reason it is important to use a long-acting local anesthetic. After each location is injected, one should wait a few minutes to see if the symptoms are relieved. By this means it may be possible to spot the exact area of the inflammation. This area should then be injected with a long-acting local anesthetic, mixed with a corticoid preparation. Immediate relief should ensue. If it does not, the procedure may not be successful. The patient should be warned that the pain may be more severe for 12 to 36 hours. If after this preliminary period complete relief is obtained and then the symptoms begin to recur, the injection should be repeated within another seven to ten days. This series may be continued three to five times at gradually increasing intervals. More injections than this probably will not be effective and may actually cause damage. Any of these inflam-

matory conditions should have anti-inflammatory medication.

Fracture

Fracture of the body of the scapula is not a common athletic injury because of the protection given the bone by overlying and underlying cushions of muscle. Usually, only a violent force will cause fracture. Mention was made earlier of avulsion injury and fracture of the spine of the scapula. The body of the scapula can be fractured by muscle contraction, but this is extremely unusual. Symptoms will be those of a severe contusion, and the diagnosis must be made by x-ray examination.

Treatment. Reduction of a fracture of the body of the scapula (Figs. 130 to 134) is rarely necessary. In fact, it is virtually impossible to reduce the fragments short of open operation. Since the body of the scapula is primarily for muscle attachments, the only indication for internal fixation of the fragments would be their actual overlapping with a resulting roughness of the undersurface of the bone, extreme enough to interfere with motion of the scapula over the chest wall. This rarely occurs, and I have never seen it as a result of athletic injury.

Treatment, therefore, is local, consisting of aspiration and Marcaine injection (not a corticoid) of the hematoma, early application of cold followed by heat, and protection against extremes of motion. It is probably advisable to use a firm compression bandage for from 24 to 48 hours, strapping the scapula snugly against the chest wall. The arm is then placed in a sling. This retentive dressing should be removed after 7 to 14 days and motion of the shoulder and scapula encouraged within the limits of pain. It should be emphasized that it is inadvisable to immobilize the shoulder for more than a few days. The protective sling which is utilized will permit pendulum exercises, which should gradually increase both in range and in frequency as the pain and tenderness subside. Active function will return promptly, but it may be many months before forceful use of the extremity is pain-free.

REGION OF THE SHOULDER JOINT (GLENOHUMERAL JOINT)

Anatomical Considerations

The functional anatomy of the shoulder joint defies brief description. The student is referred

Figure 130. Comminuted fracture of scapula caused by fall on the outer aspect of the shoulder. Humeral head drove against the glenoid, fracturing the neck with comminuted fracture lines extending throughout the body of the scapula. No treatment is required other than support.

Figure 131. Fractured scapula caused by a direct fall on the blade of the scapula. Comminuted fracture without displacement. (For x-ray positioning of anteroposterior and lateral views, see Fig. 132.)

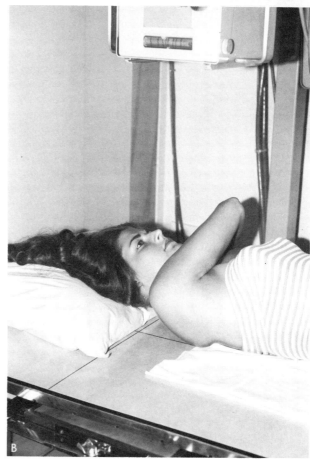

Figure 132. *A*, Body of the scapula. Position the patient in a supine position with the affected scapula in the center of the table. Abduct the arm, pulling the scapula away from the body. Supinate the forearm and immobilize if necessary. Direct the central ray to the center of the scapula. Exposure should be made at full expiration. *B*, Lateral projection of scapula. The patient should be positioned as for the anteroposterior projection in view *A* except that the affected arm should be drawn across the chest as far as possible. Adjust the position of the arm until the scapula is drawn away from the rib cage and can be felt at right angles to the table. The central ray should be directed to the center of the scapula and center of the cassette. Frequently, positioning for a lateral view of the dorsal spine will show a good lateral projection of the scapula.

Figure 133. Fracture of the body of the scapula revealed by radiograph made with the arm in wide abduction.

to the classic book *The Shoulder* by E. A. Codman, whose narrative description of the functional motion of the shoulder joint in 1934 has not been improved upon. Only a few essentials of functional anatomy can be touched upon here.

The shoulder is an extremely complex joint, owing to the fact that not only the glenohumeral joint itself but the structures making up the foundation for the glenohumeral joint are extremely mobile, so that many of the muscles and indeed even the ligaments may have separate functions under different circumstances. In describing motions of the shoulder, one had best proceed from the position of the body with the arm at the side, the palm against the thigh and the scapula snugly against the chest wall. Because of the complexity of motion of the shoulder, it has become desirable to have some sort of standard that can be universally adopted to describe the motions of the shoulder. A study of these motions was carried out by the American Orthopaedic Association and shown in their *Manual of Orthopaedic Surgery,* as illustrated in Figure 135. In Part I of these illustrations it should be understood that with the patient supine or standing with the arm at the side, and the palm against the thigh, the

shoulder is in neutral position and all motion of the shoulder relates to this position. This will aid in understanding the description of restriction of motion. Structurally, the joint is a modified ball and socket, without bony stability. Whereas the acetabulum is designed to give maximum stability to the hip and yet maintain some degree of motion, the shoulder joint sacrifices stability for extreme mobility.

The glenohumeral joint itself consists of a small, shallow, saucer-like structure on the neck of the scapula (glenoid fossa) (see Fig. 87). The humeral head rests against the glenoid and is so much larger than the glenoid that the latter serves not so much as a receptacle for the head as it does as a base against which the head may be stabilized in its circumduction motions. The capsule of the joint is somewhat redundant but is reinforced in front by capsular thickenings, which give some degree of stability anteriorly. These bands, which consist of the superior, medial and inferior glenohumeral ligaments, are tight when the humerus is placed in external rotation and abduction. It can be appreciated that from the standpoint of ligament stability, they are not sufficient to hold the head against the glenoid but simply tend to prevent anterior displacement as the head rotates into abduction-external rotation.

These deficiencies in ligament structure are counterbalanced by the muscles of the rotator cuff (Fig. 136). These muscles pass from the scapula anteriorly, superiorly and posteriorly, over the humeral head, attaching around the periphery of the head to the greater and lesser tuberosities. Together they form sort of a hood (see Fig. 105). By a tonic contraction of these muscles, the head is supported snugly against the glenoid (Fig. 137). The various tendons of the rotator cuff are indistinguishable as they reach their attachments, and they form a continuous cuff around the neck of the humerus. In addition to these muscles, namely, the supraspinatus, infraspinatus and teres minor, anterior support is given by the extremely strong subscapularis tendon, which passes directly in front of the humeral head in the anatomical position, covering approximately its inferior two thirds (Fig. 138*B*). These muscles acting individually cause rotation of the humeral head, the exact rotation depending upon the position from which the movement starts. From the anatomical position, the subscapularis is an internal rotator. In a similar manner the teres minor supports the shoulder posteriorly and acts as an external rotator from the anatomical position.

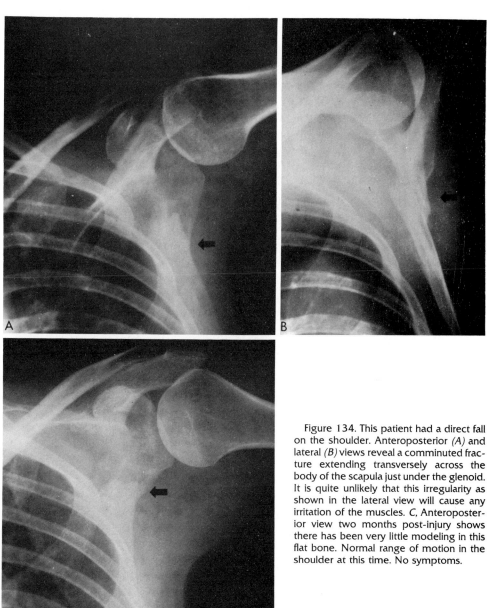

Figure 134. This patient had a direct fall on the shoulder. Anteroposterior *(A)* and lateral *(B)* views reveal a comminuted fracture extending transversely across the body of the scapula just under the glenoid. It is quite unlikely that this irregularity as shown in the lateral view will cause any irritation of the muscles. *C,* Anteroposterior view two months post-injury shows there has been very little modeling in this flat bone. Normal range of motion in the shoulder at this time. No symptoms.

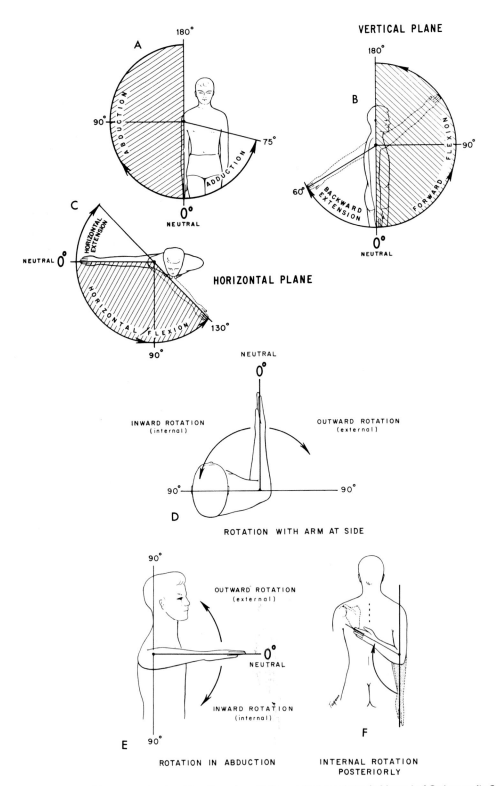

Figure 135. Motion of the arm at the shoulder. (American Orthopaedic Association's Manual of Orthopaedic Surgery.)

FLEXION

0°

EXTENSION

G

180°

90°

I   0°

NEUTRAL

180°

90°

J   0°

RANGE OF TRUE
GLENOHUMERAL MOTION

ELEVATION

H   0°

DEPRESSION

K

180°

90°

"COMBINED" GLENOHUMERAL
AND SCAPULOTHORACIC
MOTION

0°

Figure 135 (Continued).

Figure 136. Drawing of the rotator cuff, showing the relationships of the rotator cuff muscles with each other and with the capsules of the joint and the long head of the biceps which traverses between the subscapularis and the supraspinatus. (Redrawn from Codman.)

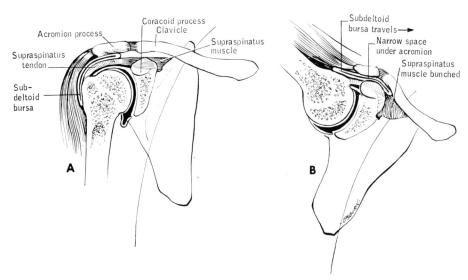

Figure 137. Sketch of the relationships between the various components of the rotator cuff and the subacromial bursa. Note that the bursa underlies the acromion and the deltoid, with more of it under the deltoid with the arm at the side. A, Relationships with the arm at the side. B, With the arm widely abducted, showing "travel" of the bursa. Also narrow space for rotator cuff as it passes under acromion.

Figure 138. Anatomical drawings of anterior region of shoulder with the anterior muscles removed. A, With the subscapularis in situ, the nerve supply to the deltoid muscle by the circumflex (axillary) nerve passing behind the humerus is shown as are the relationships of the bursae. B, Detail of the subscapularis and supraspinatus with the overlying structures removed. Note tendon of the long head of the biceps passing into the tunnel to become intracapsular.

Although one is likely to think of the main function of the rotator cuff as being abduction and rotation of the arm, a more essential function is that of holding the humeral head against the glenoid to permit abduction of the arm by the deltoid and other muscles without subluxation of the humeral head downward, since the socket of the glenoid is not sufficient to maintain stability (see Fig. 137). Without the suspending action of the rotator cuff muscles, the head of the humerus would subluxate inferiorly as the arm is abducted. To further complicate the picture of the tendons situated about the shoulder, the long head of the biceps passes through the bicipital groove, or tunnel, in front of the humeral head to pass over the head of the humerus, becoming intracapsular and finally reaching its attachment at the top of the glenoid (see Fig. 138).

This entire layer of muscle and tendon lies beneath the acromion. The more superficial covering of the shoulder joint consists of the bony acromial process, which is reinforced in front by the coraco-acromial ligament and acts as a roof over the medial part of the humeral head. The lateral continuation of this roof is the deltoid muscle, which arises along the spine of the scapula, the acromion and the clavicle to extend down over the shoulder joint. Its fibers converge at their attachment at the deltoid tubercle about two fifths of the way down the shaft of the humerus laterally. It can be seen that the shoulder joint proper is protected from external violence by the acromion and the deltoid.

Contusion

The most common contusion about the shoulder has already been described in the discussion of the acromion. The deltoid is subject to contusion, lying as it does in its exposed position over the humeral head. The deltoid is a thick resilient muscle and can stand considerable trauma. In competitive athletics it is protected well by shoulder pads, so that contusion here is not common even in major trauma. The *treatment* is that of contusion anywhere else: application of cold, compression, use of heat, local aspiration, injection, rest. The duration of treatment depends upon the severity of the injury. Anti-inflammatory medication should help.

Axillary Nerve Damage

Contusion over the front of the shoulder may result in damage to the axillary nerve. This nerve comes off the brachial plexus as a branch of the posterior cord at about the level of the coracoid process, leaves the posterior cord at a rather acute angle and proceeds sharply laterally and a little forward before it swings backward and continues laterally behind the shaft of the humerus. A direct blow striking just between the coracoid and the head of the humerus may contuse this nerve (see Fig. 138).

The principal symptom of axillary nerve damage is a severe, numbing pain in the arm, which causes the player to feel that the arm is useless. He may believe that his shoulder has been broken or that his arm has been "numbed." Examination at this time will reveal hypesthesia and reluctant function of the muscles of the upper arm. This rapidly disappears. Notable also is the inability to abduct the arm actively in the early stages. In a simple contusion this promptly clears, and sometimes within a few minutes or at the most a few hours active function will reappear. Recovery is often so rapid that the player is able to return to the same game after a brief period of rest. In this instance one can visualize that the nerve has received a sufficient blow to cause temporary numbness, as when the ulnar nerve receives a blow at the elbow.

In the occasional case there will be persistent paralysis of the deltoid, with an area of hypesthesia in the sensory distribution of the axillary nerve. If the patient is examined early, the findings will be basically negative, that is, there will be no true paralysis of the hand or sensory loss, but the arm will feel "asleep." There will usually be tenderness deep in front of the shoulder, just lateral to the coracoid process. If the symptoms persist for 24 to 48 hours, the pattern of loss of function of the axillary nerve becomes clearer. Much more frequently there will be a period of apparent complete recovery with only occasional aching pain. This is followed by the onset of loss of function of the deltoid and development of anesthesia in the sensory distribution.

Treatment. In the case marked by continuous and severe loss of function of the axillary nerve from the time of the accident, one is hard put to decide whether to recommend early exploration of the nerve or to wait for return of function. As a general rule, a period of watchful waiting is justified, the exact time depending upon the completeness of the loss or signs of possible recovery and function.

In the case that develops gradually over several weeks, we may visualize a contusion and hematoma, with scar formation about the nerve that finally becomes constrictive. This lesion is usually incomplete, but weakness in the deltoid and loss of strength of abduction may be extremely distressing to the athlete. In many instances he is unable to raise his arm over his head. In other instances a complete paralysis of the nerve follows. I believe that if there is progressively increasing loss, exploration should not be delayed. In any event, I see little reason to wait beyond three months unless there is some sign of improvement in the meantime. During this period, physical therapeutic measures are of great value in maintaining the muscle tone, and electrical stimulation of the deltoid is permissible if administered by a professional. Care should be taken to prevent contracture of the shoulder with shortening of the abductors, which results in an arm that cannot be passively elevated.

At operation, if the blow has been frontal, the axillary nerve should be exposed through the anterior incision. By an approach along the deltopectoral interval and with reflection of the deltoid laterally, the brachial plexus may be exposed medial to the coracoid, the incision extending up under the clavicle. Access to this area is markedly facilitated by detaching the distal 1 in. of the coracoid and reflecting the biceps, coracobrachialis and pectoralis minor. The plexus can now be examined from the clavicle to the superior axillary fold.

Nerve operations in this area and, in fact, in any other, require special technique and are not for the occasional surgeon. One practical approach to the problem is combined surgery by the orthopaedist and neurosurgeon. This is an area frequently entered by the orthopaedist during shoulder reconstruction. He may be better prepared for the exposure, whereas the exact decision as to what to do with the nerve may require the specialized knowledge of the neurosurgeon. The author has participated in several such cases with good success. One patient had a neuroma just distal to the separation of the axillary nerve from the posterior cord. This was resected, the nerve was repaired, and good function returned. The patient went on to a stellar career as a football player, with no restriction of abduction of the shoulder. Two recent cases revealed rather minimal findings at operation, but in both there were definite adhesions about the nerve that caused it to assume a more acute angle as it left the cord. This was aggravated by certain positions of the arm. In these two instances, the injury responded well to simple neurolysis and freeing of the adhesions. Several months may be needed for complete recovery.

It should be emphasized that the great majority of these cases are transient and probably of little true significance. Their recurrence may be avoided by an adjustment of the shoulder pad to protect this area a little more adequately. I believe the shoulder pad itself may often be the offender. As the arm is thrown up sharply and the shoulder pad comes forward its narrow edge is driven against the front of the shoulder and it penetrates the sulcus between the muscles, reaching the nerve.

Strain

Although contusion is a relatively minor problem about the shoulder, strain is an extremely major one. There may be some damage to the muscle or musculotendinous structures in any muscle that attaches at the shoulder. Since these muscles are many and the forces to which they are subject are legion, it is difficult to encompass this whole subject in a few short paragraphs.

The injury may be anything from a mild (first degree) strain with some inflammation to complete avulsion of the tendon (third degree) or of the tendon plus a fragment of bone. The symptoms will be similar but will vary considerably in degree. So, too, there are considerable differences between the symptoms of an acute (third degree) strain and those of a chronic strain. These differences have been discussed at some length elsewhere (page 51).

Some grouping of the muscles involved will aid in understanding the pathological changes present. The major internal rotators of the humerus are the subscapularis, attaching to the lesser tuberosity, the latissimus dorsi and the teres major inserting into the internal lip of the intertubercular (bicipital) groove; and the pectoralis major inserting at the outer lip of the intertubercular groove. Injuries to these attachments will be caused by forceful external

rotation of the humerus against the resistance of these muscles or on active internal rotation of the humerus by their violent contraction. These muscles are opposed in external rotation by the muscles of the rotator cuff, particularly the infraspinatus, supraspinatus and teres minor. Both internal and external rotation are supported by the anterior and posterior fibers of the deltoid, respectively.

The symptoms of an injury to these muscles are local tenderness at the site of their insertion and pain elicited by their active contraction or passive stretching. Thus, in an injury to the subscapularis, internal rotation of the arm against resistance or external rotation of the arm passively should cause pain in the same area, namely, over the lesser tuberosity.

Adduction of the arm is also carried out by many muscles. The internal and external rotators acting synchronously serve to adduct the arm against the chest wall. However, injury to the adductors of the arm is infrequent without some rotational component, so that, ordinarily, adduction and internal rotation or adduction and external rotation will be the forces involved. The injury will probably be confined to either the internal or the external rotators rather than to both.

In abduction of the shoulder the muscles of the rotator cuff fix the humerus against the glenoid, and the deltoid raises the arm from the side (Fig. 139). True enough, the supraspinatus muscles have an abduction component, but this has very little leverage, and much more important than their ability to initiate abduction of the arm is their stabilization of the humeral head.

Lesions of the Rotator Cuff

Rotator cuff lesions are common in the adult, their frequency becoming greater as age advances. They are initiated by degenerative change in the tendons of the rotator cuff (see Fig. 139). In the athlete such lesions are probably due mainly to attrition as the cuff passes under the acromial process. The isolated rupture of a portion of the cuff is an incident in the degenerative process and not the result of acute ligament or tendon rupture, as in the case of the characteristic avulsions of the athlete. Whereas in the adult so-called "subdeltoid bursitis" is usually a sign of degenerative change in the rotator cuff in the young athlete true bursitis occurs as a result of friction between the two walls of the subdeltoid bursa as they are impinged between the acromion and

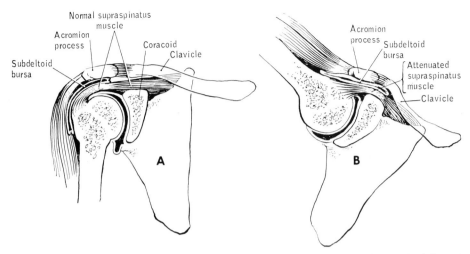

Figure 139. Drawings demonstrating the attenuation of the supraspinatus as the arm is abducted.

the cuff. This will be described later. The occasional case of calcification seen in the young athlete is probably in the bursa itself.

I do not recall having seen an acute rupture of the rotator cuff in the athlete unless it was accompanied by dislocation of the shoulder. Classic rotator cuff rupture, or supraspinatus rupture, is usually the result of active abduction of the arm against resistance and is not often a minor injury. On the other hand, the acute rupture of the cuff seen in combination with strain, sprain, subluxation or dislocation is due to a passive force, with the humeral head forcibly jammed against the components of the cuff or with the elements of the cuff ruptured as the head dislocates and slips downward in relation to the glenoid.

The forceful motion of the shoulder in throwing or in tackling or wrestling subjects the rotator mechanism to strain. In such an injury the tenderness will be along the greater tuberosity, and the pain will be in the shoulder or at the deltoid insertion. It may or may not be localized, depending upon the promptness of examination, since the pain very rapidly becomes diffuse. There may be considerable difficulty in determining just what muscle action causes pain in the tendons of the rotator cuff, and this condition is readily confused with subacromial bursitis. Actually, abduction of the shoulder, particularly against some resistance, will usually cause pain. If this strain is accompanied by some swelling and inflammatory reaction over the tendon, it may well cause symptoms of accompanying bursitis.

Strain and Tenosynovitis of the Long Head of the Biceps

Another tendon quite subject to strain at the shoulder is the long head of the biceps (see Fig. 138). This tendon passes through the tunnel formed by the intertubular groove plus a thick fibrous roof, so that the tendon is in effect a sheath throughout an area of 2 cm. in front of the humeral shaft. It passes through the groove, becomes intracapsular and traverses the shoulder to attach on the superior lip of the glenoid above the humeral head (see Figure 144 *A*). Motion of the shoulder with the elbow fixed, particularly in extension, causes this tendon to slide up and down forcibly through the groove. It may be subject to strain at its attachment to the glenoid but is more likely to develop tenosynovitis where it passes through the tunnel. The irritation of constant motion increases the inflammatory reaction until the tendon slides reluctantly through the tunnel, and finally it may cease to slide altogether. This tenosynovitis of the biceps tendon is extremely distressing from the standpoint of function of the shoulder, since with the restriction of motion and pain, many of the motions of the shoulder joint become quite limited. This is particularly true of abduction and external rotation, so that rotation at the glenohumeral joint becomes virtually impossible. Snap extension of the elbow increases this pain.

Diagnostic signs of this condition are localization of tenderness along the bicipital groove and pain on rotation of the shoulder. The location of the tenderness moves with the humeral head as it rotates. There is pain on active contraction or passive stretching of the biceps with its distal attachment fixed. A test for this motion is to extend the elbow and posteriorly flex the arm at the shoulder. This causes the tendon to slide through the groove. So also, active function by pulling the arm forward across the chest with the forearm extended and with resistance against the hand, will cause pain. In checking this motion one should be sure that the scapula does not simply rotate forward and so simulate glenohumeral motion when the motion is actually between the scapula and the chest wall.

Treatment of this condition is with local measures. The extremity should be put at rest. The tender area should be injected with local anesthetic and inductive heat should be utilized to reduce inflammatory reaction. If the condition is relatively chronic, injection of a corticoid will often be quite effective. The same precaution should be used here as mentioned elsewhere. The injection should not be into the tendon but into the bicipital tunnel. Injection of the tendon may well cause degenerative changes and accelerate rupture. The same serial injections that are used in similar conditions elsewhere are effective here.

If the condition is intractable and does not respond to local treatment, surgical treatment may be highly successful (see Surgical Technique, page 173). In this instance the shoulder is approached anteriorly, the bicipital groove is opened throughout its length and the tendon is dislocated from the groove and detached from its glenoid attachment so that it no longer crosses the shoulder joint. It may then be replaced into the bicipital groove and sutured snugly.

Tenosynovitis in the bicipital groove may go on to complete adherence of the tendon. This interdicts any extensive range of motion of the shoulder, and one of two things occurs. Either the shoulder motion is restricted or the biceps ruptures proximal to the groove. In many instances there will be restriction of motion and then a sudden painful snap, after which it is noted that the shoulder motion is less restricted. This condition is not frequent in athletic injuries because it usually predicates some pre-existing degenerative change in the tendon itself. If it occurs it usually demands surgical treatment, with removal of the remaining portion of the tendon from the glenohumeral joint and fixation of the proximal stump to the groove.

Figure 140. Drawing showing biceps lesion; biceps bunching. Long head of biceps has given way, permitting the muscle to retract toward the elbow.

Acute Rupture of the Long Head of the Biceps Tendon

Acute rupture of the biceps tendon (Fig. 140) occurs as a result of forceful contraction of the biceps muscle or forceful movement of the arm with the biceps muscle contracted. The injury may be avulsion of the tendon from the muscle belly or the tendon may rupture anywhere along its course or be pulled free from its attachment to the glenoid. The patient's history is of immediate, sharp pain, followed by tenderness along the course of the long head of the biceps. Diagnosis is made by having the patient contract the biceps, with the arm abducted and externally rotated and with the elbow at 90 degrees (see Fig. 140). If the tear is complete, it will be noted that the muscle belly moves away from the rupture and bunches up.

If acute rupture is diagnosed, the *treatment* is surgical. No attempt should be made to restore the attachment to the glenoid. The long head of the biceps should be fastened into the bicipital groove (see Surgical Technique, page 173). Prompt recovery follows surgical treatment. Unrepaired rupture usually results in some weakness of the arm and frequently in pain, depending upon the location of the tear.

Subluxation of the Biceps Tendon

Another traumatic condition about the tendon of the biceps is a rupture or stretching of the fascial covering of the bicipital groove that

Figure 141. *A,* Young female with recurrent attacks of severe shoulder pain. Careful history elicited the fact that each attack started with a snap in front of the shoulder. The findings were that of bicipital tendinitis during an attack. Between attacks she was completely relieved. Rotation of the arm at 90 degree abduction caused extreme pain. Her diffuse shoulder tenderness was localized at the bicipital groove. At surgery the shallow groove was noted with a redundant roof, so that the tendon could slide out of the groove. The glenoid attachment of the biceps tendon was transferred to the bicipital groove with relief of symptoms. *B,* A normal bicipital tunnel for comparison. (For technique of x-ray positioning for bicipital tunnel, see Fig. 142.)

permits the tendon to subluxate from the groove. This may occur as an acute injury. The predisposing factor for this condition is a congenitally shallow bicipital groove. The intertubular groove not only may be shallow but also may be broader than normal, which per-

mits the tendon to flatten out and slide back and forth within the groove itself (Figs. 141 to 143). The patient complains of a snap anteriorly in the shoulder, with pain followed by residual soreness along the bicipital groove elicited by the same motions that cause pain

Figure 142. Positioning for bicipital tunnel. Place the patient in a supine position near the edge of the table. Extend the arm, palm up, alongside the body. Place a cassette above the shoulder in a vertical position. Adjust the tube in a horizontal position slightly external to the elbow so that the central ray may be directed along the shaft of the humerus through the groove. Palpation of the groove aids in determining the angulation of the tube, usually 20 degrees medially.

Figure 143. Old avulsion injury of lesser tuberosity by the subscapularis tendon. *A*, Absence of bicipital groove (arrow). *B*, Normal groove for comparison (arrow).

on tenosynovitis. Indeed, this condition may be indistinguishable from tenosynovitis. In the muscular athlete it may be difficult to palpate the subluxating tendon. If the condition becomes chronic as the result of a defect of the roof of the groove with redundant tissue, a chronic synovitis usually occurs. On motion of the shoulder there is painful snapping as the tendon slips back and forth out of the groove, particularly on rotation of the arm. This condition also should be treated by surgical fixation of the tendon into the groove after detaching the tendon from the glenoid.

Surgical Technique. The surgical technique for transference of the long head of the biceps into the bicipital groove is as follows: The shoulder is approached anteriorly, with the arm draped free to permit manipulation. It is not necessary to reflect the anterior one-third of the deltoid from the clavicle. By palpation, locate the raphe between the anterior and the middle thirds of the deltoid. The longitudinal incision from the edge of the acromion extends distally along this raphe for about 7.5 cm. The fibers of the deltoid can be separated along this line with but little trauma. This exposes the roof of the subacromial bursa. Care should be taken not to extend this dissection more than 7 cm. distally from the edge of the acromion lest there be damage done to the axillary nerve, which extends forward on the deep surface of the deltoid to supply its anterior one third. By rotation of the arm the bicipital groove can readily be palpated and exposed.

A silver probe should be passed up along the tendon from below the bicipital groove through the groove. This will give some indication as to the degree of constriction present. The roof of the tunnel is now split along the tendon up to the insertion of the rotator cuff. This will expose the pathological condition, which might be constrictive tenosynovitis, fraying of the tendon, adhesions to the tendon sheath or possibly dislocation of the tendon from the groove (Fig. 144*A* to *D*).

If any of the aforesaid conditions are present, the tendon should be transferred. Incision in the tunnel is extended proximally and the rotator cuff incised to permit a finger to be passed into the joint. The finger passes along the tendon of the biceps to its attachment to the rim of the glenoid. With a long scissors or a tenotome, the tendon is detached as near as possible to its attachment to the glenoid. The tendon is then pulled down into the wound and may be securely sutured into the bicipital groove, using drill holes along the margin of the groove as necessary. Exploration of the joint is carried out through the split in the rotator cuff to reveal any disease of the articular cartilage on the humeral head. If this is present and needs treatment, the incision through the rotator cuff may be extended to permit more thorough exploration of the joint. The rotator cuff is then carefully repaired, inverting the knot into the substance of the cuff. Suitable wound closure using intracutaneous wire suture is carried out.

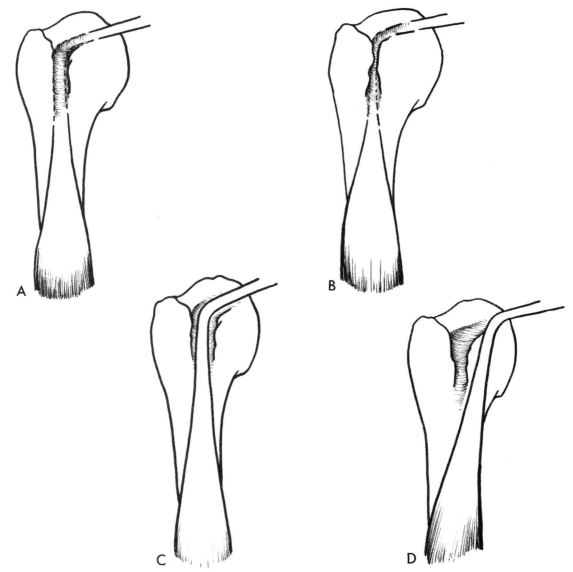

Figure 144. Drawings summarizing conditions of the bicipital groove. *A,* Normal groove with the biceps tendon in place. *B,* An unduly narrow groove with attendant adhesive tenosynovitis. *C,* An abnormally wide and shallow groove; however the episodically subluxated tendon is now in place, as will often be the case on physical examination. *D,* Another abnormally shallow groove; however, the tendon in this case is actually dislocated from the groove onto the lesser tuberosity of the humerus.

Postoperatively a sling and swathe are applied to the shoulder, and pendulum exercises, limited in range, may be initiated almost immediately after the operation (see Fig. 163). After two weeks the stitches are removed and the sling is replaced without the swathe, and activity of the arm is increased. At the end of four weeks, all fixation should be removed and rehabilitative exercises continued.

Injuries involving the bicipital tendon and bicipital groove are particularly pertinent to the athlete, since many sports involve the throwing motion of the arm. Athletes who are most affected include baseball pitchers, football quarterbacks, batters and tennis players. The throwing motion is particularly inhibited by bicipital tendon problems. It is especially pertinent to recognize this because correction of the defect, whether it is adhesive tenosynovitis, fraying the tendon, or subluxation or dislocation of the tendon, is the same, namely, transference of the attachment of the biceps tendon from the top of the glenoid into the bicipital tunnel (Fig. 145). Following this, the

Figure 145. This professional baseball player had increasing trouble with the left shoulder all through the season. He is left-handed. Finally, by the end of the season he could no longer pitch. He felt something "roll over" in his shoulder when he threw. Examination revealed pain over the anterior shoulder and the bicipital groove, traveling with the groove on rotation of the arm. A snap was noted when the arm moved from external rotation to internal rotation. *A,* Shows relatively normal groove on the left as compared with the right. Note, however, the angle is distinctly more acute than average (60 to 75 degrees). This is a little more clear in the postoperative view (upper right). *B,* The deltoid splitting incision with the bicipital tendon retracted to the left. The extreme width of the tunnel is seen by the span of the Kelly forceps across the incision. The tendon was removed from its attachment and sutured into the groove. He returned to baseball pitching.

long head of the biceps is no longer involved in shoulder motion, and recovery can be very prompt and complete. This condition has characteristic symptoms; hence, the diagnosis can be quite secure, often confirmed by x-rays profiling the bicipital tunnel. The remedy is a relatively nontraumatic operation that removes the biceps tendon from the shoulder and fastens it into the bicipital groove. To take the young athlete who can no longer throw and by a procedure of short morbidity permit him to throw without inhibition is very gratifying to both the patient and the physician. I urge definitive diagnosis of shoulder lesions in the young athlete.

Bursitis

Acute Subacromial (Subdeltoid) Bursitis

The major bursae about the shoulder are the subacromial, the subcoracoid and the subscapular (see Fig. 138). The subacromial bursa lies underneath the acromial process and extends out under the deltoid muscle to lie between the acromial process and the deltoid and between the humeral head and the rotator cuff. The bursa is separate and distinct from the glenohumeral joint and has no connection with it. It permits the tendons surrounding the humeral head to slide freely under the acromial process (see Fig. 137). This bursa is frequently involved in injuries about the shoulder, since any irritative lesion involving the rotator cuff will cause inflammatory reaction within the bursa, so that the symptoms of bursitis may well obscure the primary lesion. Subacromial bursitis may be caused by excessive friction between the cuff and the acromion. As the irritation increases the thickness of the bursal lining, the pressure increases, and the rolled-up synovium may form a fold that will at first snap as it slips under the glenoid (Fig. 146). Later it may check abduction at the point of impingement. The condition may also be caused by a direct blow over the shoulder, which causes an inflammatory reaction that is

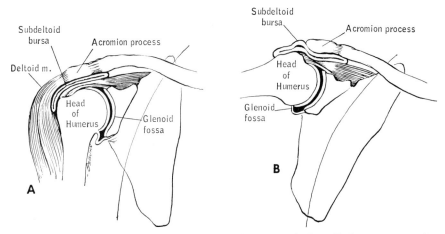

Figure 146. Chronic subacromial bursitis. *A,* Note subacromial bursa stretched out flat between acromion and deltoid above and rotator cuff and humeral head below. *B,* On abduction of the arm the thickened bursal wall cannot slide under acromion and so bunches up and checks motion.

aggravated by further motion. Primary subacromial bursitis is not common in the athlete. The bursitis is usually a secondary reaction, so one should search for the primary lesion before commencing treatment.

Symptoms of acute subacromial bursitis are pain on motion of the shoulder, particularly abduction, tenderness over the tuberosity just distal to the acromial process and pain on rotation of the shoulder, particularly internal rotation. Rotation forces the inflamed walls of the bursa into tight approximation, so that manipulation of the arm into wide abduction, as in the throwing motion or reaching behind the back, will elicit major pain.

Treatment. Acute bursitis is treated by rest and application of heat locally, using wet packs, a radiant lamp or diathermy. It usually subsides fairly rapidly. The condition is particularly annoying to the athlete, and almost inevitably he will start active use of the shoulder before the inflammation has subsided. This results in renewed irritation of the bursa. It should be emphasized that comprehensive treatment of acute bursitis will prevent repeated recurrence of the acute bursitis or a resultant chronic synovitis, adhesions and a chronic subacromial bursitis.

Chronic Subacromial Bursitis

Chronic subacromial bursitis causes subacute or recurrent pain around the subacromial bursa. This may be due to chronic inflammation within the bursa itself but is much more likely due to irregularity of the bursal walls caused by adhesion between the two layers of

the bursa or by irregularity and thickening of the rotator cuff, which may be the result of a minor tear of the tendons. Symptoms of such a condition are pain on extremes of motion, particularly abduction, crepitation on rotation and occasionally "snapping" of the shoulder when the roll of thickened synovium at the edge of the acromion finally snaps beneath it with a palpable painful click (see Fig. 146).

In chronic bursitis the *treatment* is injection of a local anesthetic and a corticoid into the bursa in serial fashion (see page 68). If this fails, surgical intervention should be carried out. The surgeon should be warned against excising the walls of the bursa if roughened surfaces are left to rub together. In case of an irregularity of the distal portion of the acromion, this portion may be excised. Indeed, up to 1 in. of the acromion may be excised in the presence of irreversible irregularity of the rotator cuff, with little resultant disability (Fig. 147). Occasionally the coraco-acromial ligament may be involved, and it too should be excised if necessary.

Subscapularis Bursitis

The subscapularis bursa is a further extension of the sac surrounding the subscapularis tendon (see Fig. 138). It usually has a direct connection with the joint. True bursitis here is not frequent. Usually there is more complicated involvement of the glenohumeral joint itself. There may, however, be a separate *subcoracoid* bursa that is a further extension of this same sac. Pain and tenderness in the area of the coracoid, aggravated by external

Figure 147. *A,* Retouched preoperative x-ray showing normal acromial process. *B,* After resection of the distal portion of the acromion, which delays the impingement of the bursa under the acromial margin.

rotation of the arm against resistance or active internal rotation, should make one suspect involvement in this area. Local treatment is of value. Physical therapy and local injection will usually give good relief.

Any of these bursae can give rise to prolonged disability. This is particularly true if the athlete is unwilling to rest the shoulder for a sufficient time to permit the inflammation to subside. Too early resumption of activity leads inevitably to recurrence of symptoms. Every time the symptoms recur they are more resistant to treatment. Finally irreversible disability ensues. All these inflammatory conditions will merit anti-inflammtory medication.

Sprain

It has been noted previously that the ligaments or capsule contributes but little to the stability of the shoulder joint. The shoulder is pressed into the glenoid by the rotator cuff, which consists of tendons. There is little inherent stability of the shoulder provided by the capsular ligaments. As a result, the only sprain which commonly occurs in the glenohumeral joint is that occurring from external rotation–abduction of the shoulder. As the shoulder is abducted and externally rotated, tension is placed upon the anterior capsule with its ligament reinforcements (Fig. 148*A*). The head

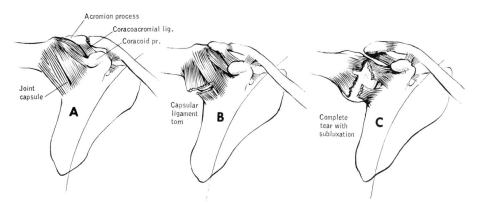

Figure 148. Various degrees of sprain of the shoulder caused by abduction—external rotation. *A,* Normal abduction—external rotation showing the anterior inferior portion of the capsule taut. *B,* Forced external rotation combined with posterior flexion causes capsule tear—moderate (second degree). *C,* Continuation of this motion rotates the anterior and inferior fibers to be superior and anterior, respectively. The head emerges through the rent in the capsule and will dislocate if the movement continues—severe (third degree).

tends to slide forward against the coraco-acromial ligament and against the capsule inferior to it. The coraco-acromial ligament, being an extremely strong structure, forces the head downward, and tension is exerted on the anterior capsule and the capsular ligaments. As the abduction–external rotation force continues (as with the arm in the overhand throwing position), the capsular ligament may tear partially or completely (see Fig. 148*B*). This may occur at the attachment of the capsule along the labrum of the glenoid or indeed anywhere in the anterior capsule. If the tear is incomplete, the shoulder does not subluxate or dislocate. The motion is arrested short of dislocation.

Diagnosis. One of the symptoms of such a condition is pain at the time of the injury. The player will usually relate that his arm was forced backward and upward. For example, in an attempt by the athlete to tackle another player as he runs by, the arm is carried forcibly backward and externally rotated (see Fig. 176). The pain is promptly relieved as the arm is placed at the side, and there may be relatively little discomfort as long as the arm remains in this relaxed position. If the sprain is more severe, there will be aching pain, which is particularly aggravated by external rotation of the humerus. The player prefers to hold the arm to his side.

On examination there will be resistance to external rotation–abduction and pain on this motion. Marked muscle spasm of the adductors and internal rotators is stimulated by any attempt to externally rotate or abduct the arm. This motion will be more or less restricted, depending upon the severity of the injury. On palpation there is tenderness in front of the shoulder joint, not along the bicipital groove but medial to it, and down to the anterior portion of the humeral head and glenoid. This area may be difficult to palpate in the muscular athlete. Owing to the multiplicity of structures subject to injury in this area it may be extremely difficult to differentiate the condition from such things as a strain of the subscapularis attachment, strain of the rotator cuff and involvement of the pectoralis major, all of which give similar symptoms.

Since the treatment is basically the same for all these conditions, the exact diagnosis may not be essential. However, there is one distinguishing characteristic. With a sprain of the ligament there should be no pain on active adduction or internal rotation of the shoulder within certain limits, such as would be elicited with strain of the rotators or adductors. This

is true particularly if the patient is examined early.

The injury may be mild (first degree), moderate (second degree) or severe (third degree). This depends upon the point at which the abnormal motion of the shoulder is arrested. Since the shoulder capsule is well relaxed with the arm at the side and internally rotated, it is usually considered that rest in this position with a sling and swathe (see Fig. 104) will be adequate because the tendency is for the fibers of the torn capsule to fold together. It is, however, vitally important to know how severe the tear is in order to regulate the period of protection and the degree of activity to be permitted.

If the sprain is mild and the shoulder has not subluxated, it may be necessary to prevent abduction and external rotation for only a few days. If the lesion has been more extensive (moderate) and the head has been partially subluxated, a longer period is necessary. The arm should be two weeks in a sling and swathe. Use of a restraining strap to prevent abduction and external rotation should follow (Fig. 149). The protection should be continued for six to eight weeks, even if the patient is entirely symptom-free. If the sprain has been severe and the capsule completely torn and the head dislocated with or without spontaneous reduction, it is much more important to prolong the immobilization. In athletes most recurrent dislocations are caused by faulty healing of the ligaments, so that redundancy of the ligament is present. This is usually caused by too early stress before the fibers have actually healed. In the severe sprain the immobilization should be by sling and swathe for four weeks and after this by the use of the restraining strap for three or four months. Only in this way is there a reasonable chance that the ligaments and capsule may heal short enough to prevent recurrent slipping.

In the preceding paragraph on treatment following second or third degree sprain or dislocation of the shoulder, it is emphasized that protection should continue for a long period of time, although the symptoms may completely disappear within two weeks or so. There has been a great deal of discussion concerning this matter, and I have made the categorical statement that the injury could result in dislocation just because of inadequate immobilization. I still believe that this is true, but I have been unable to document this. Actually, according to very exhaustive studies of this proposition, the length of time that immobilization is maintained does not really

Figure 149. Type of chain restraint popular with football players. Note the heavy leather strap around the chest not tight enough to interfere with respiration and the wide leather band around the arm. In most instances now the chain between the two bands is replaced by a leather strap as indicated here. This does not prevent external rotation but does check abduction to some degree, depending upon the tightness of the connecting strap.

seem to make too much difference. This finding relates particularly to treatment of dislocation of the shoulder. The rate of recurrence of dislocation of the shoulder is so high that there have been many studies of this particular problem. Results depend somewhat on the series, but it has been reported that somewhere between 70 and 90 per cent of complete dislocations of the shoulder that require reduction will recur. In checking out the various series, it appears that the duration of immobilization does not seem to affect the results. Although most of those studied were immobilized for two to three weeks, many of those whose dislocations recurred were immobilized for six to eight weeks. Putting the arm in a sling without restricting its motion further does not really immobilize the area. To my knowledge, there has not been a series check to determine whether the arm has actually been bound down to the chest to prevent external rotation and abduction. It is still my recommendation to sharply limit the activities of the patient with an acute dislocation for six weeks. This will be discussed further in the following paragraphs.

Treatment. Since in sprain the capsule is completely relaxed with the arm in adduction and internal rotation, it is not necessary to immobilize the shoulder completely. Treatment should involve immobilization of the arm, using a sling, preferably worn under the shirt so that the arm is supported at the side and external rotation and abduction are prevented. A simple swathe over the chest and around the arm will accomplish the same result (see Fig. 104). The patient should be instructed that any active use of the hand and forearm that does not cause discomfort is desirable. If the sprain is severe, six weeks of protection in a sling is necessary. In a less severe case (second degree), the wearing of a simple restraining chain (see Fig. 149) may permit active participation in sports. A belt is placed around the chest and another around the arm, and the two are connected by a strap or chain of a length suitable to restrict abduction at the desired angle. This treatment is based on the fact that strain is not applied to this torn structure until the arm is in wide abduction and external rotation.

Subluxation

Anterior Subluxation

Subluxation of the shoulder is caused by the same basic mechanism that causes a sprain. This is particularly true of the anterior-inferior subluxation, which is the most frequent type of athletic injury to the shoulder. As the arm comes up into external rotation–abduction, the superior portion of the rotator cuff becomes posterior whereas the anterior-inferior ligaments become anterior. In this position the humeral head is thrust forcibly against the glenohumeral ligaments in front, the rotator cuff being used as a sling around which the head rotates against the anterior capsule (see Fig. 148C). This causes tearing of the anterior capsule, and if this tearing is relatively complete, the humeral head will actually subluxate forward and ride over the rim of the glenoid. The force being arrested, the movement reverses and the head promptly slips back into its normal position without ever having completely dislocated from the glenoid. It can readily be seen that this type of subluxation is actually a third degree sprain that has caused disruption of the anterior capsule, since in a normal shoulder, the head cannot slide over the glenoid rim without loss of integrity of some portion of the shoulder capsule. In the young adult this is almost always the anterior thickening of the capsule.

Symptoms. The patient's history is important in this condition. The history is of the arm being thrown up into external rotation and abduction and the feeling that the shoulder is slipping out of position, accompanied by severe pain in the anterior portion of the joint. Immediate relief is obtained as the arm slips back into neutral position, and there may be very little discomfort so long as the arm is supported at the side. The symptoms will be identical to those of a second degree sprain, only more severe. Any attempt at abduction–external rotation will cause muscle spasm and pain and, in many cases, the feeling of imminent dislocation. The patient often volunteers the statement that his shoulder was out of joint but slipped back in. Indeed, it is often impossible to determine whether the injury has been a subluxation or a spontaneously reduced dislocation.

Treatment. Treatment is based on the assumption that there is actual structural damage to the shoulder. I cannot overemphasize the importance of adequate treatment for subluxation or spontaneously reduced dislocation of the shoulder. This condition frequently occurs in the shoulder predisposed toward dislocation, because of flattening of the glenoid or a defect on the humeral head. It also occurs in an anatomically normal joint. If the torn ligaments are protected in the relaxed position, there is every expectation that they will heal completely without undue lengthening. If con-

stant irritation and stretching are permitted, the ligaments will heal not only with overlength but also with scar rather than ligament structure, and potential weakness remains. This invites recurrence of subluxation, and finally dislocation and often recurrent dislocation. External rotation–abduction of the arm must not be permitted during the healing period.

The treatment of third degree sprain is basically the same as that for second degree sprain, namely, fixation of the arm at the side in a sling with the arm enclosed in either the shirt or a circumferential swathe (see Fig. 104). Meddlesome manipulation of the shoulder to determine the progress of the repair is to be avoided. Ligament structures heal slowly, and the initial anastomosis between the torn ligament ends is extremely insecure. One single motion in external rotation–abduction is enough to disrupt the infant union, and successive motions constantly separate the edges. The patient, the coach and indeed the physician must restrain their curiosity as to the progress of this repair and assume that short of three weeks there is no union and that it takes six weeks for union to be secure, even under favorable circumstances. Careful treatment of this initial lesion may result in complete recovery. Unwise manipulation may result in a recurrent condition of the shoulder.

Inferior Subluxation

Whereas the common subluxation of the shoulder is anterior, there is another type of subluxation of the humeral head that should be mentioned, although it is not common in the athlete. I refer to the inferior subluxation in which the humeral head actually hangs out of the glenoid, the head riding over the inferior rim. This is, of course, a frequent occurrence in paralytic conditions of the shoulder and as a result of overheavy traction by a hanging cast. As such it is readily explained by the antecedent history and is not particularly related to athletic injuries. It is possible, however, to have acute subluxation of the shoulder as a result of injury to the rotator cuff. It is to be recalled that the rotator cuff suspends the humeral head against the glenoid by the tonic action of the rotator muscles (see Figs. 136 and 137). A rupture of any one of these muscles, such as the supraspinatus or teres minor, will not result in any actual subluxation of the humeral head. However, if the whole rotator cuff is avulsed, the suspensory action of the cuff is lost and the humerus can be held in proper position only by strong contraction of the deltoid and other extrinsic muscles of the shoulder. This is a major injury and may have extremely distressing sequelae.

The writer recalls a recent case in which a young adult fell from a truck; his glove caught on the sideboard and his fall was sharply arrested by his arm extending directly upward. The sudden suspension of his relaxed arm resulted in extreme pain and disability in the shoulder. His early examination and treatment were unfortunately superficial, consisting of application of a sling for a couple of weeks and then encouragement to return to work. When this patient was examined nine weeks after his injury, he wore a very snug sling which caused pressure under his elbow. He was extremely apprehensive on removal of the sling, and when he was persuaded to permit his extrinsic muscles to relax, he had pain in the shoulder and the feeling that the shoulder had slipped out of place. Examination revealed a definite interval between the acromion and the head, and it was possible to slip the head in and out of the shoulder joint inferiorly. This finding was confirmed by both examination and x-rays (Fig. 150). This patient was extremely apprehensive because he had learned that whenever he would relax the shoulder, the head would fall out of joint. It would not actually dislocate but would subluxate inferiorly.

This patient's *treatment* was by open operation, at which time the whole rotator cuff was found to be detached and the whole area scarred in, with resultant increase in length of the rotator cuff tendons. In the operation the entire cuff was pulled downward like a hood over the tuberosity and sutured there. This immediately produced an extremely stable shoulder. Snug support was continued to prevent re-stress for eight weeks. The result was complete stability of the shoulder but considerable restriction of motion, which could be attributed to the long immobilization—nine weeks preoperative, six weeks postoperative.

Admittedly this was an unusual injury, but I believe it could have been diagnosed early by careful history and physical examination supported by x-ray examination. For this degree of subluxation I do not believe nonsurgical treatment is appropriate. However, if nonsurgical treatment is elected, the arm should be supported at the side with downward pressure on the clavicle and acromion and upward pressure on the humerus in an effort to induce the rotator cuff to resume its normal position. The inadequacy of this treatment becomes apparent when it is recognized that this is a tendon avulsion and that the tone of the involved muscles, particulary as they go into spasm with the injury, will inevitably pull the tendon away from its attachment. The primary treatment should be surgical, with repair of the rotator cuff down to the humerus.

Luxatio Erecta. A sprain or subluxation of the humeral head inferiorly *by abduction* is possible, but infrequent. At the height of abduction the humeral head levers against the tip of the acromion, and the posterior portion

Figure 150. Complete rupture of the rotator cuff. *A,* Shoulder with the arm in a tight sling. *B,* After removal of the sling and with no added weight; note wide separation between the acromion and the head, with the head hanging downward over the glenoid rim.

A   B

C   D

Figure 151. Drawing illustrating various stages in the inferior sprain-subluxation-dislocation of the shoulder. *A,* Arm in complete abduction with the scapula rotated, the tuberosity serving as a fulcrum for the acromion; stress is applied to the inferior glenohumeral ligaments. *B,* The force continues, the ligaments rupture, the head subluxates. *C,* As the force continues further, the head goes into typical position of luxatio erecta and completely dislocates. The inferior capsule is completely torn. *D,* After the arm drops back toward the anatomical position, the head remains subglenoid or may slip further and become subcoracoid. (From DePalma, Surgery of the Shoulder, J. B. Lippincott Co.)

of the head drives against the structures inferiorly (Fig. 151*A*). This results in the tearing of the capsule and ligament, and if the tear is complete, the humeral head may ride out on the inferior glenoid rim (Fig. 151*B*). This is an extremely severe injury, and if the force continues, a complete inferior dislocation of the humerus results (Fig. 151*C*). If the dislocation is not complete, the arm drops promptly to the side and is resolutely held in place by the patient, since he feels any attempt to abduct it will cause it to slip out of place. The history of the type of injury plus the fact that the tenderness is deep in the axilla up against the inferior portion of the humeral head will serve as a key to the diagnosis. Active abduction per se is not painful, because if there is any strain on the internal structures, muscle spasm will force the arm to the side before the movement is extensive enough to be painful.

Treatment is by immobilization using a sling with the arm at the side. Since only complete abduction will put strain on this redundant inferior capsule, athletic participation may be allowed in a few weeks, provided that abduction of the arm is prevented. The degree of restriction of abduction necessary can be determined by steadily abducting the arm to the point at which pain is elicited. Abduction beyond this point should be prevented by a suitable apparatus. The familiar chain restraint, with a wide band around the chest and a band around the arm and the two connected with a chain or strap is adequate (see Fig. 149).

Posterior Subluxation

Posterior subluxation of the shoulder, meaning an incomplete posterior dislocation, presumably may occur (Figs. 152 and 153). The force involved usually is a direct backward thrust of the humerus, with the arm flexed forward. This drives the head posteriorly from beneath the acromion. The posterior portion of the rotator cuff is damaged in this instance, and the humeral head slides posteriorly. Owing to the muscular character of the posterior structures, the subluxation is immediately reduced spontaneously, and in my opinion it is virtually impossible to diagnose it with any degree of certainty. The symptoms are those of strain of the posterior structures, pain on reproduction of the force causing dislocation so that with the humerus flexed forward and pushed backward there is a feeling of discomfort, and pain posteriorly in the shoulder. Attempts to internally rotate and flex the arm across the chest will also elicit pain. On examination tenderness is posterior and about the humeral head; indeed, the symptoms are identical with those of strain or partial avulsion of the external rotators of the shoulder.

Treatment. Treatment is by immobilization with the arm at the side. Ordinary internal rotation to the extent of placing the forearm across the chest is not forbidden, particularly if it is not painful. If this results in painful strain posteriorly, the arm may be immobilized at the side in a plaster spica in the anatomical position, with the elbow flexed to 90 degrees and the forearm extended directly forward—a position similar to that used in certain fractures about the elbow. The duration of immobilization will depend upon the degree of symptoms and the amount of damage. The shoulder should be protected for about six weeks. It is an unusual force that causes this injury, and it

Figure 152. Posterior subluxation of the shoulder, axillary view. *A,* The arm swung forward toward the midline. As the head rotates it slips out of the glenoid posteriorly. This required posterior reconstruction of the capsule. *B,* The horizontal position. (For positioning of patient for x-ray, see Fig. 153.)

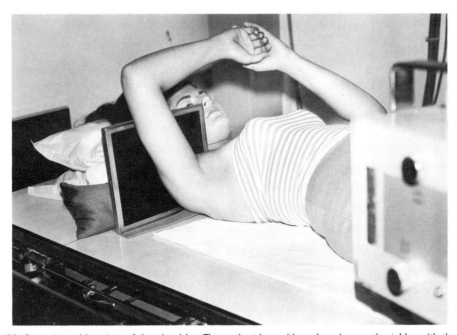

Figure 153. Posterior subluxation of the shoulder. The patient is positioned supine on the table, with the shoulders elevated by a pad. The arm is positioned as for an axillary view except that it is brought up and rotated toward the midline. The cassette is supported in a vertical position behind the shoulder. The central ray is directed horizontally to the head of the humerus. The tube usually needs to be rotated medially about 10 degrees.

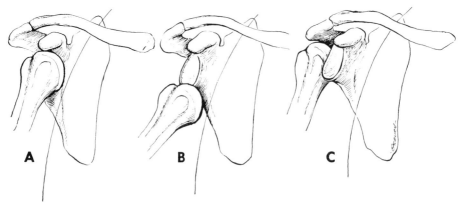

Figure 154. Dislocations of the shoulder. *A*, Typical subcoracoid dislocation. *B*, Subglenoid dislocation. *C*, Posterior dislocation.

is not likely to be recurrent. This explains the more rapid rehabilitation in this condition than in anterior subluxation, in which the position of external rotation–abduction in athletic activities is very frequent and so needed to be guarded against for a longer time.

Dislocation

Anterior Dislocation

Dislocation of the shoulder follows the loss of function of the restraining structures about the shoulder and is a result of the same mechanism that causes the subluxations described previously. By far the most common type of dislocation of the shoulder in young individuals of athletic age is the anterior–inferior dislocation (Fig. 154*A*). This is a pure dislocation, unaccompanied by fracture, in young individuals. As age advances, the ligaments become firmer and the bone less strong, so the dislocation may be accompanied by an avulsion fracture rather than a tear of the ligament. In the young athlete it is almost always the ligament or muscle that gives way. As the arm is

Figure 155. Subcoracoid dislocation of shoulder. In this case the head may well have displaced inferiorly and then swung around to anteroinferior and so subglenoid. Note head is proximal to inferior glenoid rim and caught between glenoid and coracoid process.

forced into abduction and external rotation, the humeral head is thrust against the anterior portion of the glenohumeral joint, the coracoacromial ligament serves to force it downward, and it then emerges anteriorly and inferiorly into the redundant area of the capsule, which is protected by the glenohumeral ligaments (see Fig. 86). These give way when they are torn from the glenoid labrum or because of avulsion of the labrum or actual disruption of the ligaments. The head of the humerus slips over the glenoid rim, immediately slides forward to lodge between the rim of the glenoid and the coracoid process, and the arm drops toward the side but not against it. This is the classic dislocation of the shoulder in young people (Figs. 155 and 156). The damage to the ligament may be a transverse tear across the capsule, and in addition, the capsular reinforcements known as the glenohumeral ligaments may split, with one passing above the humeral head and one below it. In some instances they actually grasp the humeral head in such a way as to impede reduction.

Symptoms. Although diagnosing the dislocated shoulder by appearance alone may be difficult in an extremely well-muscled or heavy individual, it is usually easy. The acromion is prominent, with a definite defect below it rather than the usual rounding out of the deltoid muscle (Fig. 157). The arm tends to be held away from the side and rotated slightly externally, so that it is virtually impossible to move the forearm across the chest or abdomen in front of the body or to bring the elbow to the side. On examination the defect below the

Figure 156. Twenty-six year old wrestler. The arm was forcibly jerked, dislocating the shoulder anteriorly. Anterior-posterior view illustrating subcoracoid dislocation.

acromion is, in early cases, readily palpable, and the roundness of the humeral head as it rests against the coracoid is also readily felt anteriorly. An attempt to manipulate the arm or to force the elbow to the side causes pain. The patient will usually permit some increase in abduction and external rotation but will resist adduction and internal rotation. At the time of this examination a careful neurological examination should be made, since an injury to the brachial plexus occurs quite often in dislocation of the shoulder. Neurological examination to determine the integrity of the nerves should be done before an attempt is

Figure 157. Photograph of subcoracoid dislocation of the shoulder. Note the prominent acromion, the arm held away from the side, the flat deltoid. (From McLaughlin, Trauma, p. 246.)

made at reduction. If this is not done one may wonder whether a neurological deficit discovered later was caused by the injury itself or by the trauma of the reduction.

Treatment. Dislocation of the shoulder is an acute emergency, and it should be reduced as soon as adequate facilities are available. On occasion it may readily be reduced directly after the injury, before pain and muscle spasm have developed. However, this is not to be attempted by the uninitiated, since irreparable damage may be done to the bone or capsule and particularly to the nerve structures about the shoulder by unwise manipulation. Under no circumstances should force be used. The major obstacle to reduction is general spasm of the muscles about the shoulder, so that the humeral head is firmly fixed against the coracoid and under the glenoid rim. Any attempt to move it from this position will only increase the spasm. I cannot too severely condemn forcible manipulation of the shoulder, which will not accomplish the purpose of the reduction and will increase spastic fixation.

The first prerequisite for reduction of the dislocation is complete relaxation of the shoulder. This may be possible without general anesthesia, but once the dislocation has persisted beyond the first few minutes, it becomes extremely difficult to obtain relaxation without use of a general anesthetic. This is particularly true in the athlete who is very muscular, extremely apprehensive and at the age at which he has not yet developed sufficient equanimity to permit voluntary relaxation of these painful structures.

If the doctor sees the player at the time of his injury and is skilled in manipulation of the shoulder, he may attempt immediate reduction on the field without anesthesia. This is accomplished by laying the patient flat on his back on the ground, grasping his arm securely either by the wrist or with the elbow flexed and exerting direct traction distally. The traction should be gentle and not accompanied by any attempt at lateral motion (Fig. 158). In certain instances the humeral head will slip quietly into position. The time-honored method of placing the foot in the axilla is fraught with danger. Its only justification is to permit the operator to steady himself, not to permit him to use excessive force or traction. The unshod foot should be used and great care taken not to put direct pressure against the humeral head (Fig. 159); rather, the foot should be against the chest wall. Careless use of the foot in the axilla may well result in damage to the structures of the brachial plexus, since they may be tightly caught against the humeral head.

If, after a reasonable trial of traction (60 seconds), the head does not reduce, the attempt should be abandoned. The player should be taken from the field to a place suitable for more adequate treatment. Preferably he should be taken promptly to the infirmary or hospital, and x-rays should be made of the shoulder to confirm the diagnosis and to reveal any accompanying bony abnormalities. Even if the dislocation is promptly reduced by traction, x-ray study should be made to eliminate the possibility of accompanying bony injury.

After the x-ray examination, a second and more comprehensive effort may be made to obtain reduction by simple traction. Detailed description of the various methods of reduction is not appropriate here, but a few deserve mention. The simplest one is to exert traction directly on the line of the trunk or possibly in slight abduction, with the patient flat on his back (See Fig. 158). It must be emphasized

Figure 158. Reduction of the dislocated shoulder by steady, even pull on the arm with patient in the supine position. The padded strap through the axilla is for mild countertraction and is often not necessary. This may be done with or without anesthesia.

Figure 159. *A,* The improper method of reduction. Note the foot is directly in the axilla, impinging the brachial plexus against the dislocated humeral head while the arm is levered over the foot. This can cause serious damage to the brachial plexus and is quite painful. *B,* The proper position is with the foot against the axillary wall for pressure while steady, even traction is made at about a 45 degree angle.

that this traction must be pain-free or it will not accomplish its purpose. In another method the patient lies prone on the table, with the involved arm hanging over the edge either with or without a weight suspended from the wrist (Fig. 160). Similar reduction may be carried out with the patient sitting, the arm hanging over a suitably padded back of a chair (Fig. 161). In all instances care must be taken that there is no pressure on the axillary structures. If these methods do not suffice for reduction, the patient should be given an anesthetic and an extremely atraumatic reduction carried out, preferably by traction as in Figure 158. If this fails, reduction may be accomplished by the Kocher maneuver (Fig. 162), or by whatever careful manipulation will bring the humeral head into proper relation with the glenoid. Anesthesia must be given to the patient before the physician performs the Kocher maneuver. I cannot overemphasize the importance of atraumatic, careful, gentle manipulation. Irreparable damage can be caused by forceful manipulation. Force is not required to reduce the dislocated shoulder. Relaxation is imperative either with or without general anesthesia. Following reduction, x-ray examination should be made to confirm the position and again check for possible bony abnormalities or injuries.

Attendant fractures about the shoulder are

not common in this age group. However, they may occur and as such will require definitive treatment. Avulsion of the greater or lesser tuberosity, fracture of the glenoid, fracture of

Figure 160. Pendulant method of reduction without anesthesia. The weight must be suspended by the wrist, not grasped by the hand, since complete relaxation is essential. The shoulder should swing free, and the patient should be comfortable or else he will not relax.

Figure 161. Pendulant method of reduction without anesthesia. Note the pad in the axilla, the weight suspended from the wrist, not grasped by the hand. This method is not as safe or as satisfactory as the method shown in Figure 160.

the acromion, and involvement of the biceps tendon are complications that will demand the best care of the skilled orthopaedist. If the shoulder does not readily and completely reduce, repeated attempts at manipulation are not justified, and open reduction should be done.

The occasional damage to the nerves that accompanies injury to the brachial plexus may be the cause of considerable concern. Competent neurosurgical consultation is advisable in such cases of nerve injury. Ordinary watchful waiting will be the treatment of choice. A gradual return of function should be anticipated, since this damage is usually peripheral—a contusion to the nerve—and the patient will probably recover promptly. If recovery does not occur, exploration of the nerve is advisable, and considerable judgment is required to determine the best time for it. Since recovery will occur in many cases without exploration, this avenue is usually postponed several months. Once the indications are clear, however, exploration should be recommended and carried out without delay.

Following successful reduction, the after-treatment consists of immobilization of the arm in a sling providing support under the elbow, with an added swathe around the chest to prevent abduction of the arm (see Fig. 107).

It should be emphasized that for an acute complete dislocation to occur, there must be serious damage to the ligaments and capsule of the joint. Thus, continued immobilization is required until they attain some degree of healing in direct apposition. The arm should be held in a sling for a minimum of three weeks and then mobilized only within the limits of pain. Active participation in sports without protection should not be permitted in less than six weeks after injury. I fear that this regimen is usually not carried out, since in most cases following reduction, the player usually recovers promptly and within two weeks his arm feels very good to him. Overoptimism may persuade him to participate in sports, whereupon the dislocation promptly recurs. The patient should be encouraged to exercise within the limits of pain and the restriction of his dressing (Fig. 163). After three weeks of immobilization, rehabilitative measures may be stepped up sharply, particularly active motion against resistance to develop the muscles of the shoulder. Even during the time the arm is suspended in a sling and swathe, active use of the hand and the forearm and tonic contraction of the muscles about the upper arm and shoulder will permit the player to keep his

Figure 162. The Kocher maneuver. A, Abduction—external rotation. B, Adduction—external rotation. C, The completed maneuver with internal rotation of the adducted arm. Complete relaxation is essential for this maneuver to be effective. It cannot be successfully carried out if the patient resists, either consciously or unconsciously.

Figure 163. Typical exercises for reconstruction of shoulder muscles. (From Cave, Fractures and Other Injuries, Year Book Publishers.)

arm in relatively good condition. It is extremely important that the musculature of the shoulder is in good condition before unprotected use of the arm is permitted, since so much of the stability of the shoulder depends upon the strength of the muscles involved.

One need not fear restriction of motion as the result of immobilization of the arm at the side in this age group; however, this is an ever-present danger in the elderly.

The standard and appropriate methods of treatment for dislocation of the shoulder have been discussed in the previous paragraphs. However, as indicated on page 178, the results of dislocation of the shoulder have been ex-

ceedingly poor, no matter what method of reduction was used. In fact the results have been so poor that one is tempted to seriously consider surgical treatment of the acute dislocation. Since 70 to 90 per cent of the injuries recur, there must be structures present that are not properly opposed. Hence, it would seem that open reduction and repair of the injured tissue would be the treatment of choice. I have not yet persuaded myself to do this in the "simple" dislocated shoulder. However, I have opened a good many shoulders with other injuries, such as a ruptured rotator cuff, a ruptured biceps tendon and various fractures around the shoulder, and I always find that the anterior capsule is completely disrupted. Maybe the aim of the orthopaedists of the eighties should be to get their courage in hand and operate on acute dislocations. This should be done as part of a definitely planned program involving sufficient cases so that data are substantial enough to determine which method is better, open or closed reduction. The *recurrent* anterior dislocation and its surgical treatment are discussed in detail on page 191.

Posterior Dislocation

Posterior dislocation of the shoulder is uncommon as an athletic injury. However, I have seen many late cases, and the majority of them were unrecognized primarily. The cause is a direct driving force against the lower end of the humerus with the arm flexed forward. This force transmitted up the arm drives the head out posteriorly. No gross deformity of the shoulder is evident. The patient resists any motion of the shoulder, and upon careful palpation, less fullness of the humeral head in front and some increased fullness behind are felt. There is increased prominence of the coracoid. This is readily determined only very early, since within a short time, swelling about the shoulder from this extremely disabling injury will screen any visible physical findings. Motion of the shoulder is sharply restricted by muscle spasm. X-ray examination is extremely important but difficult to interpret. In the late cases I have seen, x-rays had uniformly been taken but were as uniformly misinterpreted. The pertinent finding in the x-ray, as noted by comparison with the opposite shoulder, is not any actual displacement of the humeral head backward but an overlapping of the head of the humerus and glenoid (Fig. 164). This overlapping is not visible in a straight anteroposterior view of the normal shoulder, and it is extremely easy to overlook in any case. It indicates that the humeral head is posterior to and slightly medial to its normal position, so that the convexity of the humeral head does not fit against the concavity of the glenoid but appears medial to it (Figs. 164 and 165).

Special x-ray views in posterior dislocation are often necessary. The axillary view (see Fig. 166), if possible technically, is especially useful. Other views at various angles can be composed by a roentgenologist and should be useful if uncertainly persists.

Treatment. If seen early, reduction of the dislocation is done by traction forward and pressure forward on the humeral head. The head usually will slip into place with an audible click. If the patient is seen later, an anesthetic may be required. If he is seen very late, the dislocation may be impossible to reduce nonsurgically. (The *recurrent* posterior dislocation and its surgical treatment are discussed on page 198.) It is frequently accompanied by fracture of the posterior portion of the glenoid, which

Figure 164. Radiograph of the shoulder, showing posterior dislocation. At a casual glance no lesion is apparent. Careful inspection will reveal the head of the humerus medial to the glenoid convexity.

Figure 165. Recurrent posterior dislocation of both shoulders, which was gradually getting worse and becoming painful. Posterior reconstruction was carried on one shoulder and then, about six months later, on the other. One year later there was no trouble in either shoulder, no feeling of slipping, and no activity forbidden except football. *A*, Axillary view shows the coracoid process anterior and the head posterior to the glenoid. *B*, Similar view but with less dislocation.

may include as much as half of the entire glenoid. If this fragment does not replace into good position, surgical resection or internal fixation should be carried out. If the dislocation is seen late and is accompanied by this fracture, it is necessary at open reduction to remove the fragment and to replace by suture the capsule to the remaining rim. If the fragment is large, it should be replaced and supported by a bone graft.

Inferior Dislocation

Inferior dislocation of the shoulder occurs as the arm is forced into straight abduction. As the lateral part of the neck of the humerus impinges against the acromion, the head is forced laterally against the inferior portion of the capsule and the capsular ligaments (see Fig. 151). As the ligaments rupture or tear

away from the lower glenoid margin, the humeral head displaces laterally and slips downward over the inferior lip of the glenoid. As the arm is lowered to the side, the head slides anteriorly and the dislocation becomes a subcoracoid dislocation (see Figs. 151*D* and 155). The significance of this series of events is that the dislocation may be particularly resistant to any type of manipulative reduction other than straight traction. Indeed, many of the cases which reduce readily by straight traction along the long axis of the body may well be those in which the head has come out almost directly inferiorly. At the time of the examination it may be impossible to determine whether or not the head has come primarily forward or has gone directly inferiorly. Careful x-ray study should be made to determine the exact position of the head and whether there has been bony damage.

If the straight abduction force continues and the arm is forced over the head toward the midline of the body, a much more serious injury occurs. The humeral head is literally stripped of its attachments, so that the capsule and rotator cuff have completely lost their integrity. In this instance the head locks in a position under the glenoid with the shaft of the humerus pointing directly upward, so that the arm is held high over the head (*luxatio erecta*) (Fig. 167). This does not often occur as the result of an athletic injury. It is an extremely major injury. It is likely to be accompanied by nerve damage and will probably demand surgical intervention, even if primary reduction can be obtained. In such an instance, repair of the rotator cuff may be indicated. This may well have been the injury to which I referred on page 181 of this chapter. In such a case there will be so much damage to the whole mechanism that the humeral head actually hangs out of the glenoid. At the time of the reduction of luxatio erecta, extreme care should be taken to avoid forceful manipulation, since it may well add to the damage to the muscles, blood vessels and nerves. Under no circumstances should forcible reduction be attempted without anesthesia, and under no circumstances should any force be used in repositioning the arm with the patient anesthetized.

Recurrent Dislocation

Recurrent Anterior Dislocation. By far the most common recurrent dislocation of the shoulder is anterior dislocation. This occurs

Figure 166. This 22 year old college athlete injured his shoulder at age 16 playing football and has had constant trouble with the right shoulder since. He soon was able to slip it in and out of the socket. A, Shows normal relationship of the glenoid on forward pressure. B, Shows the shoulder displaced out of the glenoid posteriorly on backward pressure. This was treated by posterior reconstruciton. At two years postoperative he still feels some instability of the shoulder, but it doesn't bother him.

basically in two categories: first, a recurrent dislocation as the result of repeated episodes of acute traumatic dislocation in a normal shoulder and, second, a recurrent dislocation as the result of congenital deviations about the glenohumeral joint. It is of some importance to distinguish between these two conditions, since the latter is likely to be bilateral and will demand surgical correction. If the deformity is severe enough, athletic competition should be interdicted until satisfactory stability has been obtained.

The first variety of recurrent dislocation, that following an acute dislocation, is particularly distressing. Dislocation will recur in 70 to 90 per cent of patients following primary dis-

location. I think these figures depend somewhat on the demographical situation, such as whether the patients are young or old people; however, it is true that about 70 to 90 per cent of young athletes do get a second dislocation. It is not fair to say that the second dislocation is the result of poor treatment of the first one. There seems to be little difference in the recurrence of dislocation whether or not immobilization has been respected. In fact, most series that have been reported show that the type of treatment has little effect on the outcome, that is, the die is cast when the dislocation occurs the first time, and as a result if athletic activity is continued, the dislocation will probably recur. Because of the extremely

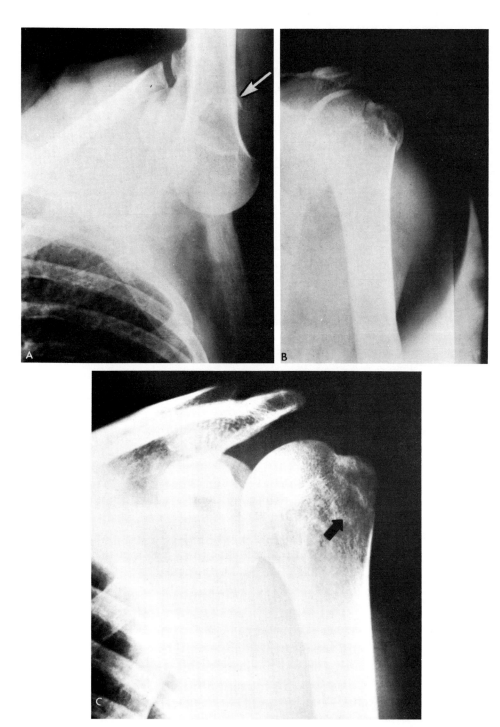

Figure 167. *A,* Case of luxatio erecta. Arrow indicates avulsed tuberosity, indicating the severe disruption of the rotator cuff. It is extremely unusual to get an x-ray in this position, since ordinarily the arm drops back to the side and the dislocation becomes subcoracoid. *B,* Following open reduction, internal fixation of the rotator cuff, which was found to be completely avulsed off the humerus, was done. *C,* One year later, excellent function. (Courtesy, Dr. Sam Moore.)

high rate of recurrence, perhaps the acute dislocation should be treated surgically. The capsule fails to heal or heals too long, and the next dislocation tears it a little bit more. With each successive dislocation, less force will be required for the dislocation, and it reduces more easily. Finally the condition develops in which the shoulder dislocates by simple abduction–external rotation without actual trauma. This type of case is readily amenable to surgical treatment. In some instances the shoulder may be improved by a long period of immobilization, provided there have not been too many episodes of displacement. I doubt that it makes any particular difference whether the first dislocation was poorly treated or whether there were successive dislocations. Nevertheless, I do not think there is any justification for tying up a patient's arm and binding it to his side for 8 weeks so that he cannot use it in external rotation and abduction, in the hope that this might prevent recurrent dislocation. However, if, for example it is the third episode and the shoulder has previously been inadequately immobilized, one might be justified in putting the arm at rest at the side for eight weeks, in the hope that union and shortening of the ligament will occur. If this fails and if the recurrent episodes of subluxation or dislocation interfere with necessary activity, operative reconstruction of the shoulder can be carried out very successfully. I have operated upon many dislocations in this category and have rarely seen recurrence in an athlete.

There are various methods for reconstruction of the recurrent anterior dislocation of the shoulder. Many of these methods seem to be entirely successful. My own preference, described in more detail in the following section, is for a modification of the Putti-Platt procedure, including meticulous repair of any lesion found in the shoulder joint. The essence of this method is to reinforce the anterior capsule with the very massive subscapularis tendon. This should be entirely adequate in most cases. Since this method provides exposure that is quite good, the detached labrum should be trimmed away, leaving no cartilaginous bodies. If the capsule and periosteum are stripped off the anterior margin of the glenoid, they should be replaced and fastened through drill holes to the glenoid rim. If there is a large Bankhart type of pouch, it should be eliminated by plication of the capsule.

Technique for Modified Anterior Putti-Platt Reconstruction Utilizing the Subscapularis. A skin incision is made to expose the anterior area of the shoulder. The axillary incision, of recent popularity, begins at the clavicle and continues down across the coracoid and into the axilla, mobilizing a lot of muscle to reach the area. Personally, I prefer an incision beginning at the clavicle, just above the coracoid and extending downward in a slight curve toward the shoulder joint. The incision is shaped like a question mark because it passes over the clavicle, down the arm beyond the coracoid and then swings laterally to go down along the anterior edge of the axilla (Fig. 168A). The skin flap is not slipped off the deltoid muscle. It is dissected off the deltoid muscle for a short distance, and as the deltoid muscle is exposed, the deltopectoral interval is located. Retraction of the deltoid and pectoralis major usually will expose the cephalic vein. This is ligated distally and proximally, and then removed.

At this point the anterior quarter of the deltoid is dissected from the clavicle to about the level of the acromioclavicular joint. This muscle, together with the skin flap, is reflected laterally (see Fig. 168B). This provides adequate exposure of the coracoid process.

A drill hole is made beginning at the distal end of the coracoid process, extending up its shaft about 4 cm. This hole is threaded with a screw of appropriate size ($\frac{7}{64}$ in.) so that the entire tract is threaded. The screw is then removed.

The coracoid is then transected at about the proximal edge of the coraco-acromial ligament and slightly distal to the anterior edge of the pectoralis minor muscle, which may be partially detached from the coracoid at this point. Reflecting this flap takes the pectoralis minor, the coracobrachialis and the short head of the biceps distally and medially (see Fig. 168C). This exposes the subscapularis tendon as it passes over to the lesser tuberosity of the humerus. The tendon is lifted, using a large curved Kelly forceps beneath the tendon at its upper margin, proceeding distally to exit below the distal margin of the tendon. This defines the broad expanse of tendon (see Fig. 168D). Sometimes it will be necessary to go through the capsule in this approach. In any event, the capsule should be divided at the same level as the tendon.

The tendon is transected transversely at a distance sufficient to let the attached end of the tendon reach the rim of the glenoid, usually about 1½ in. (4 cm.). A good deal of muscle is encountered in the tendon at this point. Stay sutures are placed in the proximal edge of the capsule, through the distal cut edge of the capsule, and also into the distal end of the tendon to the subscapularis muscle. The sub-scapularis muscle is then retracted laterally, and the whole space is defined between the subscapularis muscle and the scapula (see Fig. 168*E*). The muscle may be quite adherent to the scapula and must be freed to develop the space outside the glenoid.

The shoulder is explored at this time for any pathological conditions, such as foreign bodies. If there is a Bankhart lesion with the capsule reflected off the labrum, the lateral portion of the labrum is denuded with a curette so that the capsule can be pulled up against it. Previously I have fastened a staple here, but I do not believe this is necessary since re-suture of the capsular flap pulls it tight against the glenoid.

At this point, the subscapularis muscle is carefully dissected from the capsule so that the margin of the glenoid is palpable and visible in the area between the reflected portion of the muscle and the scapula. Stay sutures are placed in the subscapularis muscle. This exposes the area where the repair will start. Beginning below and exterior to the glenoid rim, a heavy cotton No. 1 suture using a No. 34 needle is passed from outside the joint, through the labrum area (the labrum having been denuded with a curette during exploration of the shoulder) and into the joint. Mattress sutures are then placed through the end of the subscapularis tendon and passed back out through the capsular flap, right on the rim of the glenoid (see Fig. 168*F*). This is a difficult suture to place because of the retracted structures. From then on, the suture placement is relatively easy. Four or five sutures are placed, going from outside the capsule into the joint, through the subscapularis tendon, and then back out through the capsule and tendon to the outside. The sutures are tied on the outside of the glenoid. Once these sutures are in place, they are pulled taut, and motion is checked to see how much external rotation will be permitted. It is preferable to have 15 to 20 degrees external rotation of the arm with the elbow at the side. It is not necessary to keep the arm externally rotated during this repair. The arm is allowed to fall into internal rotation, and the sutures are tied.

The reflected end of the capsule, then, lies over the tendon graft. This capsule is sutured over the tendon. From this point the arm is placed in the neutral position, and the capsular flap is pulled up and sutured to the subscapularis tendon and muscle (see Fig. 168*G*). The stay sutures in the subscapularis muscle will pull it forward, and the muscle is then sutured

to the capsular tendinous mass in front of the shoulder, at about the level of the lesser tuberosity (see Fig. 168*H*). This provides three very competent structures in front of the anterior distal portion of the glenoid to prevent dislocation: the first layer is the tendon of the subscapularis, which is a very heavy structure; the next layer is the capsule, which is pulled up tight; and the third layer is the subscapularis muscle. This step completes the reconstruction.

The fragment of the coracoid process is replaced. An appropriate length screw (1½ in. or 4 cm.) is threaded through the hole previously made in the coracoid (see Fig. 168*I*). I cannot emphasize too much that this hole should be made before the coracoid is cut off, since it is very difficult to drill through the small, movable flap of bone. The screw is readily set in place at the drill-hole site in the body of the coracoid, and this secures the detached segment. The deltoid muscle is reattached to the clavicle (see Fig. 168*J*). Ordinary mattress sutures in the soft tissue and periosteum are adequate. If this is insecure, drill holes can be made in the anterior edge of the clavicle to secure fixation. I find it less and less necessary to use the drill holes if I am careful about the way the muscle is stripped off the bone. When closure of the skin flap is carried out, one should remember that the skin flap tends to migrate off the shoulder; therefore, the subcutaneous sutures should be very secure.

The arm is placed in a sling with just enough swathe around the body to keep the forearm from externally rotating (see Fig. 107). The arm should not be bound tightly to the shoulder as in the old Velpeau dressing because this results in a position that is exceedingly uncomfortable and therefore difficult to maintain.

The aftercare is routine. Sutures are removed after two weeks, and pendulum exercises of the shoulder started (see Fig. 163), with the patient keeping the arm in the sling when standing. It is important that the forearm be released several times a day while the patient lies supine in order to extend the elbow, since the elbow does get stiff very easily. At the end of four weeks, all apparatus is left off and normal function permitted, not including athletics. Ordinary, normal use of the arm is encouraged so that external rotation and abduction, which are quite resistant at first, gradually return.

As an end result, the patient with the arm at 90 degrees abduction can externally rotate a few degrees beyond vertical. With the arm

Figure 168. Sequential drawings illustrating the anterior reconstruction of the shoulder joint using the modified Putti-Platt method. *A*, Skin incision with its characteristic question-mark shape. *B*, Dissection of the deltoid off the clavicle, followed by its lateral reflection, revealing the coracoid structures underneath. *C*, Transection of the coracoid process, and medial reflection of the coracoid muscle group. Note that this step is performed after a screw hole is made in the coracoid. *D*, Dashes indicate where transection of the subscapularis near its musculotendinous junction will be made. Care is taken to leave the tendon end sufficiently long to reach the rim of the glenoid. *E*, Retraction of the subscapularis and underlying capsule, exposing the shoulder joint. At this stage the shoulder is explored and attention is directed toward any damage encountered. *F*, Suturing of the subscapularis tendon to the anterior rim of the glenoid; this is the crucial step in this reconstruciton. *G*, Attachment of the capsular flap to the body of the subscapularis tendon, thus constructing a second layer of anterior protection for the shoulder joint. *H*, Placement of the subscapularis muscle over the capsular flap and into the body of the subscapularis tendon, thereby creating yet a third layer and completing the anterior reconstruction of the joint. *I*, Restoration of the coracoid process by inserting a screw in the hole previously made in the coracoid. *J*, Reattachment of the deltoid, which is followed by closure of the skin flap, including secure placement of the subcutaneous sutures so that the tendency of the skin flap to migrate off the shoulder is reduced.

Illustration continued on opposite page

Figure 168 *(Continued)*.

at the side, he can externally rotate it from 45 to 60 degrees. Without the rotation, the arm can be elevated to the side of the head, without obstruction to straight-out abduction.

My reason for recommending this more extensive procedure is that many recurrent dislocations of the shoulder of the athlete are, in fact, dislocations of a normal shoulder. Hence, if a normal shoulder succumbs to dislocation under the forces applied to it by the athlete, the shoulder must be made stronger, anteriorly, than it was prior to the injury. I prefer this type of operation in athletes because of the excess stress applied to the shoulder when

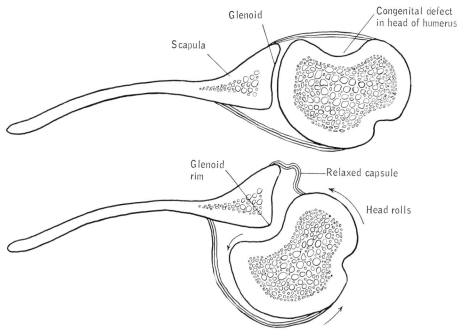

Figure 169. Schematic drawing showing relaxation of the capsule as the glenoid rim drops into the congenital notch in the humeral head. This relaxation permits the head to slip out of the glenohumeral joint. (H. Osmond Clark, Journal of Bone & Joint Surgery, Vol. 30-B.)

they return to sports activity. The restriction has not bothered quarterbacks. However, the restriction is somewhat notable in baseball pitchers because when they cock the arm, they go back into external rotation, which is not desirable after shoulder dislocations. At eight weeks, unlimited activity is possible but no sports are permitted before four months. Our recurrence rate has been one per cent in a large series. (Of the patients whose injuries recurred, one was an epileptic who had bilateral repair with recurrence in one arm. Another was inducted into the army and was required to walk across an overhead horizontal ladder, his hands gripping the rungs and his body suspended.)

In the second category of recurrent anterior dislocation, that of congenital malformations of the shoulder, reconstruction may be necessary and may be wholly successful (Figs. 169 and 170). In these cases dislocations may occur without any serious trauma. Study of the opposite shoulder should always be made.

Recurrent Posterior Dislocation. Recurrent posterior dislocation of the shoulder is not frequently encountered, since the primary condition itself is infrequent. I have personally seen more unreduced than recurrent posterior dislocations. One of the latter was in a swimmer who had the feeling his arm would subluxate at a certain point of his back stroke,

and as a result, the dislocation interfered markedly with the success of his swimming. Examination in these cases usually will not elicit pain, and it is infrequently possible to demonstrate the subluxation clinically. One may depend almost entirely on the story of the

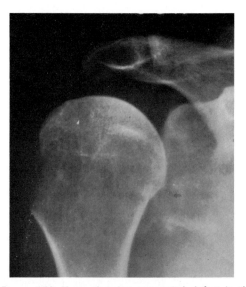

Figure 170. X-ray showing congenital defect in the humeral head. As the flat portion of the head is opposed to the glenoid, the diameter of the head is markedly shortened and the capsule relaxed, predisposing to dislocation.

patient that he has the feeling that the shoulder slips out posteriorly. Note carefully the position of the arm at which the head tends to slip. Often the history of falling on the outstretched arm or falling on the elbow with the arm forward will be a guide. In the case of the aforementioned swimmer, the arm was repaired posteriorly. A defect in the posterior capsule was found and we were able to plicate it with good support. He went on to be a champion Olympic swimmer, with complete recovery from his instability. A procedure similar to the Putti-Platt in front may be carried out, using the infraspinatus muscle-tendon to prevent posterior displacement of the head.

Technique of Reconstruction for Recurrent Posterior Dislocation of the Shoulder. Posterior reconstruction of the shoulder is not frequently done for two reasons: (1) there is no particular technique that has enjoyed great popularity or that has been universally used, and (2) there are just not that many recurrent posterior dislocations to reconstruct.

I have tried one or two of the proposed methods of reconstruction, such as osteotomy of the posterior rim of the glenoid. I do not like this method, possibly because of poor experience with the use of a bone block to stop instability, such as the use of the posterior block from the calcaneus for drop foot and the use of a coracoid block on the glenoid rim for anterior shoulder dislocation. Basically, a block requires a relatively stable joint or else the block is absorbed or is pushed off.

The method I like is called the *reverse Putti-Platt,* utilizing the strong tendinous capsular band of the infraspinatus muscle to provide stability for the head of the humerus. The patient is positioned prone, with the involved shoulder in 90 degrees abduction–external rotation and the arm resting on a suitable support. The incision commences at the back rim of the acromion and extends along the entire length of the spine of the scapula (Fig. 171*A*). One must recall that the deltoid muscle attachment is to the edge of the spine and is almost aponeurotic, with no deep attachment of the muscle fibers to the spine. The skin is not stripped off the deltoid; rather, the deltoid is folded back with the skin attached to it (see Fig. 171*B*). Great care is taken when detaching the deltoid muscle not to penetrate too deeply into the muscle and invade the fibers of the infraspinatus muscle, where a maze of muscle fibers is present without good delineation of the proper spaces. Once the deltoid is detached rather superficially, finger dissection can separate the deltoid and the infraspinatus muscles.

As the deltoid muscle and skin flap are reflected forward (laterally), the infraspinatus muscle is exposed. At this point the upper end of the tendon which attaches the infraspinatus muscle to the humerus is defined, and the tendon is separated from the muscle, leaving a long strip of tendon still attached to the humerus (just as was done with the subscapularis in front) (see Fig. 171*C*). As the tendon is freed, the capsule of the shoulder joint is also opened at the same level as the end of the tendon, so that the tendon and the posterior flap of the capsule are reflected as a unit.

The capsule is now reflected and the glenoid exposed (see Fig. 171*D*). Sometimes this capsule will be pulled away from the glenoid. In other instances the rim of the glenoid will be rough and irregular, with loose fragments of bone. In any event, the glenoid edge is denuded down to raw bone. Stay sutures are placed in the posterior flap of the capsule and also in the capsular tendon flap laterally. The shoulder joint is carefully inspected for other abnormalities, such as foreign bodies, and any spurring is removed.

Using relatively heavy No. 1 cotton and a relatively heavy swedged-on needle No. 34, the sutures are begun posterior to the glenoid and are passed through the posterior flap of the capsule at the edge of the glenoid and into the shoulder joint; they are continued into the infraspinatus tendon flap at the lateral portion of the capsular edges. Mattress sutures are then placed through this unit and back through the joint, again passing out right on top of the glenoid and out through the posterior portion of the capsule. Three or four of these sutures are placed. When they are drawn taut, they should pull the tendinous flap (consisting of the tendon and the lateral segment of the capsule) down over the humeral head and against the denuded glenoid (see Fig. 171*E*). The flap of the capsule remaining (which is really the posterior flap) is pulled up over the anterior segment and the tendon and securely sutured to the capsular tendinous mass (see Fig. 171*F*). The infraspinatus muscle is pulled up over this mass (see Fig. 171*G*). At this point, the tendon of the infraspinatus, the two limbs of the capsule and the infraspinatus muscle are placed snugly across the posterior part of the humeral head. This is done with the arm in external rotation of approximately 90 degrees. The external rotation should then be reduced to approximately 60 degrees so that the repair is not made too tight.

The deltoid is replaced and routine closure is carried out with meticulous care (see Fig.

Figure 171. Series of figures depicting the posterior reconstruction of the shoulder joint employing the reverse Putti-Platt technique. *A,* Skin incision beginning at the back of the acromion and then following the spine of the scapula. *B,* Lateral reflection of the deltoid, exposing the underlying infraspinatus, which is then transected near its musculotendinous junction. Note that the dissection should not go below the teres minor (denoted here by the letter "T"). *C,* Dashes indicate where transection of the posterior capsule will be made after the infraspinatus has been transected and reflected in both directions. *D,* Reflection of the posterior capsule, revealing the shoulder joint underneath. A search is now made for abnormalities within the joint, which if found are corrected or removed. *E,* Attachment of the infraspinatus tendon and the lateral capsular flap to the posterior rim of the glenoid, thereby creating the strongest element of the reconstruction. *F,* Construction of a second layer of posterior protection for the shoulder joint by suturing the medial capsular flap into the now underlying mass of infraspinatus tendon and lateral capsule. *G,* The third tier of the reconstruction is completed by pulling the infraspinatus muscle over the medial capsular flap and attaching it to the body of the infraspinatus tendon. *H,* Repair of the aponeurotic attachment of the deltoid to the spine of the scapula. After this step the skin incision is closed and the arm is placed in a splint in the "call a taxi" position.

Illustration continued on opposite page

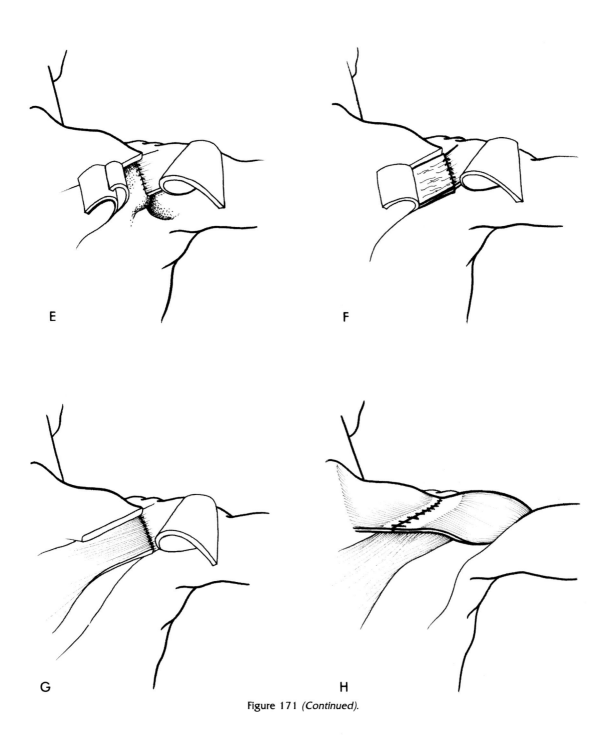

E

F

G

H

Figure 171 *(Continued)*.

171*H*). The arm is placed in a previously prepared splint, so that it is at 80 to 90 degrees abduction and at 60 degrees external rotation, the "call a taxi" position. This splint is constructed so that the position can be changed as the arm is brought down into less external rotation and against the side of the body. In about 6 weeks the external rotation should reach the neutral position, with the arm against the side. In another two to three weeks, the forearm can be passed over in front of the body, with the palm of the hand against the chest. The patient usually regains a satisfactory range of rotation within eight weeks, although it may take longer than that.

A few precautions are necessary:
1. Do not penetrate too deeply when detaching the deltoid from the spine of the scapula.
2. Do not perform any dissection below the teres minor tendon.
3. A meticulous technique pays dividends.

Recent studies have indicated more and more that there is a very great tendency for acute *subcoracoid* dislocation of the shoulder to recur. Some series put the rate of recurrence as high as 85 per cent. According to these series, the type of primary treatment does not really make much difference. Our experience has shown us in other situations that when ligaments are torn, acute surgical repair is the best way to obtain normal function. Combining discouraging high percentages of recurrences after primary dislocations with the demonstrated fact that torn ligaments heal best when their ends are put together, the question immediately arises: Why not do a primary surgical repair on an acute dislocation? I do not know of any of my colleagues who subscribe to this method or who really have even tried it, but we have gradually learned that ankle dislocations need to have ligament repairs, acromioclavicular dislocations do better with ligament repairs and certainly sternoclavicular dislocations do better with ligament repairs. Therefore I think there might be a valid case made for recommending early operation with a reconstructive type of repair in the acute case of dislocation in order to avoid the long periods of morbidity—the first one at the acute injury, then the intervening morbidity when the shoulder keeps slipping out of place and finally the morbidity involved in the reconstruction. My prediction is that in the relatively near future surgical treatment of acute dislocation will become an accepted policy. Certainly it is not accepted at the present time, and as stated previously, I know of no one who actually recommends this treatment, including myself.

Fracture

Fractures about the upper end of the humerus are not common in athletes, and those that do occur are often the result of a dislocation of the shoulder, a frequent injury in this age group.

Avulsion Fracture

This uncommon type of fracture in athletes occurs about the glenohumeral areas as a result of the traction of a tendon or ligament on a bony process, as in dislocation of the shoulder, which accounts for the majority of cases. The most frequent of the avulsion fractures involves the greater tuberosity.

Avulsion of the Greater Tuberosity. In anterior dislocation of the shoulder, as the arm rotates up and out and the humeral head slips forward, the extremely strong pull of the muscles of the rotator cuff may fix the tuberosity in situ. This results in separation of the tuberosity from the shaft. This may occur as an avulsion of the rotator cuff, an avulsion of a thin shell of bone or an avulsion of the entire tuberosity (Fig. 172). The symptoms will be those of a severe injury to the shoulder. The dislocation may or may not have been spontaneously reduced, but the player will usually relate that his shoulder has slipped out of the joint. It may have been reduced by a spectator or fellow player, or possibly the player's own motion will have reduced it spontaneously.

If the shoulder is dislocated, great care should be taken in interpreting x-rays made before and after reduction to rule out such a fracture. If spontaneous reduction has occurred, careful palpation will reveal tenderness over the greater tuberosity. There will be pain on an attempt to actively abduct or to externally rotate the arm. Given these findings, careful x-ray study should be made with the head in various positions of rotation, since in some positions the fracture may seem to be reduced and in others it may appear to be displaced (Fig. 173). The fracture in the tuberosity may be visualized well in some cases and poorly in others (Figs. 174 and 175).

Treatment. If the fracture is an incomplete one and if the tuberosity remains in place in all positions of the humeral head, treatment may be nonsurgical. Simple immobilization of the arm in a sling will usually suffice. If this does not serve to relieve the pain, the addition of a swathe around the chest may. There is no need for a plaster spica in the ordinary case. If there is persistent displacement in any position of the humeral head, surgical intervention is desirable. Although healing in malposition may be acceptable in older people with sedentary habits, deformity of the head is not well tolerated by a person who has to use the arm in violent exercise, such as throwing or swinging a tennis racket or many of the other

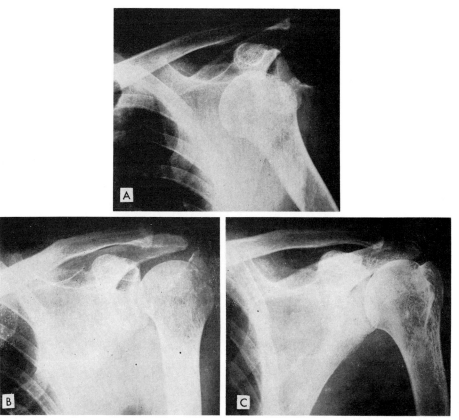

Figure 172. Residual displacement of tuberosity fragment. *A*, Original dislocation. *B*, Following reduction by simple traction. *C*, Following cuff repair and reattachment of the tuberosity fragment. Result was excellent. (From McLaughlin, Trauma, p. 252.)

Figure 173. Positioning for internal and external rotation views of the shoulder. With the patient in a supine position, center the affected shoulder over a 25.5 cm. by 30.5 cm. cassette. Direct the central ray to the midpoint of the shoulder joint. *A*, For internal rotation, position the upper arm close to the body. Bend the elbow at 90 degrees and place the hand, palm down on the chest. *B*, For external rotation, keep the upper arm close to the body and rotate it externally as much as possible or until the thumb touches the table top.

Figure 174. *A*, Radiograph showing avulsion of the greater tuberosity of the humerus. It does not reveal the displacement well, but careful study will indicate that the top of the fragment is well above the rim of the head, whereas in the reduction film it is replaced below the margin of the head. *B*, Post-reduction film.

things required of the athlete. The tuberosity can be readily exposed by a muscle-splitting operation through the upper portion of the anterior third of the deltoid, and fixation should be by suture, staple, screw or whatever method seems best. If the entire tuberosity is detached, it should be replaced and held by internal fixation (see Fig. 174*B*). If a shell of bone has been torn away, this shell should be surgically excised and the tendon repaired to the avulsed bed. If extremely secure internal fixation of the fragment is not obtainable, removal of the fragment is advisable.

Following repair, rehabilitation will depend somewhat upon the security of the fixation. If fixation is very secure, either by a screw or a staple through a firm bony fragment or by adequate suture of the tendon through drill holes, motion can be started just as soon as the operative reaction subsides, provided it does not include active abduction of the arm. If the arm is abducted against gravity, the humeral head is forced against the glenoid, and the rotator cuff takes up its function of suspending the head to prevent the slipping downward due to the leverage of the deltoid. This puts unusual stress on the tuberosity and must not be permitted. Pendulum movements against gravity, however, are acceptable on the first day (see Fig. 163). Such active abduc-

Figure 175. *A*, Avulsion fracture of tuberosity, the tuberosity remaining near its situs and not elevated. *B*, Nonsurgical treatment permitted solid union.

tion-contraction movement with the arm at the side does not have the leverage disadvantage of abduction against gravity. It may be permitted up to 45 degrees and should not be against resistance until union is progressing well.

Avulsion of the Lesser Tuberosity. The subscapularis muscle, which is attached to the lesser tuberosity, is a very massive muscle and is a strong adductor and internal rotator of the arm. Violent external rotation and abduction of the arm against the resistance of the subscapularis may cause rupture of the subscapularis tendon or avulsion of the tuberosity. The patient's history will usually be of violent and rapid external rotation of the arm, as in attempting to tackle a player as he is going by (Fig. 176). The symptoms will be identical to those of sprain of the subscapularis tendon, with tenderness at the lesser tuberosity. There is pain on active internal rotation and on passive external rotation or abduction of the arm. Diagnosis of avulsion fracture must be made by x-ray examination. Here again one should try to determine whether the avulsion is complete or incomplete. It is necessary to take pictures with the arm in various positions and at various angles to demonstrate that the tuberosity is indeed firmly fixed in all positions (see Figs. 142 and 173). If it is separated, it will be pulled medially toward the coracoid. This is most readily demonstrated by x-ray, in a view with the arm abducted. The tunnel view along the bicipital groove may be quite enlightening. Figure 176B illustrates the end result of unrecognized or incomplete avulsion of the lesser tuberosity.

Treatment. Definitive treatment of this avulsion fracture is necessary in the young athlete. If separation of the fragment in any position of the humeral head can be demonstrated, surgical repair should be carried out. The same principles of fixation are used as noted previously (greater tuberosity). If the fragment is large, it may be secured by metallic fixation. If it is small, it should be removed and the tendon repaired to the bone. The latter procedure is probably the method of choice, since it expedites the recovery. The approach is made by using the first stage of the Putti-Platt or Magnuson method of shoulder reconstruction. The approach is along the deltopectoral groove. The anterior one third of the deltoid attachment is reflected from the clavicle, after which the injured area is readily exposed. Following repair, the arm should be immobilized at the side in a sling, with a swathe around the chest. The duration of immobilization will depend upon the degree of fixation obtained. Four weeks should be the minimum, and throughout this period active rehabilitation of the arm may be carried out short of abduction or external rotation.

Fracture by Direct Trauma

In the young athlete the humeral head, which is strong and resilient at this age, is not frequently broken by direct trauma. If fracture does occur, it is a stellate fracture, usually without displacement, and hence it is very difficult to recognize. In fact, it may be recognized only by repeat films after two weeks, which show absorption around the fissures. The history is of a direct blow, as from a fall on the shoulder or by a blunt object directly against the humeral head. The cartilage of the humeral head is somewhat less resilient than the other joints, but there is no doubt that a direct blow to the head may cause chondral fracture with either fissuring of the cartilage or the actual dislodging of the fragments of cartilage. Fracture of the subchondral bone may lead to later chondromalacia of the bone or osteochondritis dissecans. None of these injuries is particularly disabling when it involves the head of the humerus. This is not a weight-bearing joint, and there is only a relatively small proportion of the head in contact with the glenoid at any one time. A little irregularity is well tolerated. By the time the fracture is recognized, the necessity for any immobilization will probably be past, since the only immobilization indicated would be to suspend the arm in a sling and encourage motion within the limits of pain. In certain cases the humeral head may be pushed in much as a side of a ping-pong ball can be. Probably both are injured in the same way, that is by direct trauma over a relatively localized area. This may be caused by driving the ball of the humerus against the posterior lip of the glenoid or conceivably against the acromion.

This condition will have the same symptoms as contusion of the shoulder, but they are more severe. Pain is out of proportion to that of ordinary contusion of the deltoid. Careful x-ray study with the humeral head rotated in various positions will reveal the defect (Fig. 177). A posterior defect in such a position that the posterior edge of the glenoid may drop into it as the arm is abducted and externally rotated will predispose toward dislocation in the same manner as a congenital defect does.

A

B

Figure 176. *A,* Typical position causing avulsion of the subscapularis. The arm is forcefully externally rotated but not widely abducted. *B,* This patient injured his arm several years ago and received no treatment. He is now asymptomatic except for slight restriction of external rotation. Left, external rotation view shows a large lesser tuberosity. This is much more specific in the tunnel view (right). Note the tremendous overgrowth of the lesser tuberosity with nonunion of the fracture. (For technique of tunnel view, see Fig. 142, and for technique of external rotation view, see Fig. 173.)

Figure 177. *A,* X-ray of the humeral head following "contusion." Careful study will reveal two lines at the periphery of the head, indicating a large segment of it has been displaced (arrows). *B,* The displacement was reduced and bone-bank bone packed into the defect. This is done by drilling a hole through the opposite side of the head. The fragment was driven back in position by an impactor.

Treatment. We have in at least one instance been able to reduce this deformity by drilling through the humeral head from the opposite side and actually pushing the cartilage upward by gently passing a punch through a drill hole made at the opposite side of the head. The defect was then packed with cancellous bone (see Fig. 177). If the defect does not appear to be too severe, expectant treatment may be carried out, and if subluxation occurs, anterior plication may be done as in the repair of recurrent dislocation of the shoulder.

Fracture by Indirect Violence

This type of fracture is not common as a result of athletic endeavor, but occasionally fractures through the surgical neck of the humerus will occur instead of a dislocation of the shoulder (Fig. 178). In the adolescent this fracture may be through the proximal epiphysis (Fig. 179). In such a case a history of a violent injury followed by severe pain, localized swelling and tenderness, together with resistance to any motion of the glenohumeral joint, will

Figure 178. Fracture of the surgical neck of the humerous, without displacement (arrow). Treated by sling, without the necessity for cast.

suggest this serious injury. If the fracture is complete, x-rays will definitely confirm the diagnosis, and appropriate measures can be carried out for treatment. It should be borne in mind that if the injury involves the epiphyses, it is advisable to get as good reduction that may be obtained by atraumatic manipulation. If atraumatic closed manipulation is unsatisfactory, open surgery should be carried out.

The chief diagnostic problem will arise with the incomplete fracture in which the displacement is slight. Here again x-rays will be confirmatory and treatment should be of the nonmeddlesome variety. It will be adequate to apply a sling with the arm to the side and to permit pendulant and pain-free movement from the beginning or at least as soon as the immediate reaction has subsided. Many weeks and months of rehabilitation may be spared if motion is initiated early in these shoulder injuries.

Fracture of the Glenoid

Avulsion Fracture. An avulsion fracture of the lip of the glenoid may occur in combination with a complete or an incomplete dislocation of the shoulder, either anteriorly, posteriorly or inferiorly. In these instances the rim of the glenoid is avulsed by the capsular attachment rather than broken off by the humeral head, since the humeral head is round and traverses the same arch as the glenoid. As the head slides over the glenoid rim, the capsule becomes very taut and may break off a fragment of bone rather than separate the capsule. Thus, the anterior dislocation will pull off the antero-inferior margin (Fig. 180), the posterior dislocation, the posterior margin (Fig. 181), and the straight inferior dislocation (luxatio erecta), the inferior margin of the glenoid. The clinical pathological change is not so much a fracture of the glenoid as a capsular tear. In most instances nonsurgical treatment will suffice, and either bony or firm fibrous union will result. It is unusual for a single injury to cause enough relaxation of the ligament or capsule

Figure 179. Fracture adjacent to proximal epiphysis of the humerus, with only moderate displacement. Treatment by simple sling and swathe fixation.

Figure 180. Avulsion of anteroinferior margin of the glenoid in the course of a dislocation of the shoulder which was spontaneously reduced. Since the fragment was large, it was treated by open reduction and internal fixation.

Figure 181. Postoperative picture following reduction of old unreduced posterior dislocation. At operation the posterior margin of the glenoid was found to be displaced posteriorly.

to cause recurrent dislocation, but repeated injuries may well do so, each one requiring less trauma than the one before. If so, appropriate measures for the recurrent dislocation are in order. A reconstruction operation may be the answer if athletics are to be continued.

In this situation, in which manipulation cannot reduce the fracture satisfactorily, open reduction and internal fixation probably should be utilized, because with the loss of whatever degree of convexity there is of the glenoid, the possibility of subsequent recurrent dislocations is very real. So, even in the spontaneously reduced dislocation, if damage to the glenoid margin is considerable, it probably would be better to replace it and hold it with some degree of internal fixation (see Figs. 180 and 181). The follow-up studies on dislocation without glenoid damage show a 70 to 90 per cent rate of recurrence. With glenoid damage, these rates probably would rise to the vicinity of 100 per cent. The exception to this is the fracture of the inferior rim of the glenoid that was not caused by dislocation of the shoulder. In this instance, one may be able to treat the fracture nonsurgically with a reasonable amount of support. It should heal and give no further trouble unless the shoulder is used actively.

In the spontaneously reduced dislocation in which the shoulder is in normal position at the time of the examination, these glenoid marginal fractures will give good insight into the degree of trauma. What may appear to be a simple sprain or contusion may be revealed as a spontaneously reduced dislocation with attendant damage to the capsule.

Another type of avulsion fracture about the glenoid that is peculiar to athletes is avulsion of a piece of bone by the triceps attachment along the inferior rim of the glenoid. Symptomatically there is pain on active stretching of the triceps muscle, and palpable tenderness along the inferior rim of the glenoid will usually be present. The fragment is difficult to visualize on the x-ray and may appear more as an area of calcification than as an avulsed fragment, particularly if the injury is recurrent in type (Fig. 182). Ordinarily, firm fibrous union will bind the fragment of the glenoid, and there will be no residual symptoms. In the occasional case there will be pain on forcible use of the triceps. This is particularly likely in one who has to throw hard or use the arm in violent overhand motion, as in tennis. In this case removal of the fragment of bone and resuture of the tendon to the bed will result in relief of symptoms.

Following the acute injury, a period of rest with application of heat locally followed by active physical therapy will be of help in rehabilitation. It must be remembered that too early resumption of the violent activity that caused the original lesion will cause prompt recurrence. This accounts for the extremely poor results from treating shoulder lesions of

Figure 182. Fragmentation and calcification of the inferior lip of the glenoid following injury. This may have been from incomplete dislocation or from pull of the triceps tendon.

Figure 183. Series showing progress of calcification in the vicinity of the lower lip of the glenoid. This may well have been a partial avulsion of the triceps tendon, with calcification and the resultant hematoma. (Rex Dively, M.D., Baseball Shoulder, JAMA, Nov. 21, 1959.)

this type in a baseball pitcher. Any change in his throwing habits will usually result in loss of effectiveness, and he soon resumes the same type of activity that hurt him in the first place.

Chronic irritation of the triceps attachment in this area may cause a deposition of calcium, which may be quite diffuse. It may be impossible in a chronic case to distinguish between the primary avulsion of a portion of the glenoid and the deposits of calcium within the tendon of the triceps (Fig. 183). Since the treatment is identical, namely, physical therapy, leading up to final surgical excision if it fails, the exact diagnosis probably is not too important.

Fracture by Direct Blow. The same force applied to the lateral side of the shoulder which may break the humeral head may also fracture the glenoid. This is a stellate fracture and in the athlete is usually without displacement. Gross displacement of the glenoid requires violent trauma. No treatment is necessary other than protection of the arm during the acute period by the application of a sling. The glenoid will tolerate a great degree of deformity, with deep fissures in its surface, without material interference with the function of the shoulder, since weight-bearing is not involved.

A fracture of the glenoid may be caused by falling on the flexed elbow. In this case the humeral head may be driven forward or backward in such a way as to knock off a large portion of the anterior or posterior portion of the glenoid. In either case, if there is gross displacement of the anterior lip of more than

1 cm., the best treatment will be surgical replacement of the fragment (see Fig. 180). If the posterior one third of the glenoid is broken off, posterior subluxation or recurrent dislocation is likely to occur (see Fig. 181). This deformity of the glenoid is easily corrected in a fresh fracture but is extremely difficult to correct following recurrent posterior dislocation. In the athlete such a fracture should be treated surgically, using a posterior approach similar to that employed in recurrent posterior dislocation of the shoulder. When the rim of the glenoid is readily visualized extracapsularly, internal fixation may be utilized to restore the buttress. Similarly, in rupture of an anterior fragment that consists of as much as one fourth of the glenoid, surgical repair should be carried out early.

Figure 184. Professional football quarterback whose left arm was struck while coming forcibly forward as he was tackling an interceptor. Severe pain and loss of function in the shoulder. Unable to throw. *A*, X-ray reveals an avulsion of the tip of the coracoid, with some separation of the fragments. At surgery the tendons involved were found to be the coracobrachialis, the biceps and a small portion of the pectoralis minor. *B*, The coracoid fragment was replaced and held with a screw. He had a good and uneventful recovery and was back playing the same season.

SHOULDER SERIES

SUBLUXATIONS – DISLOCATIONS

Figure 185. *Shoulder Series.* The diagrams above depict the series of exercises utilized by West Point cadets following shoulder subluxation, dislocation or surgery. This exercise program is modified as demanded by range of motion of the injured shoulder and is instituted when range of motion in external rotation and abduction is about 75 per cent of normal.

It should be specifically noted that this is a total upper body reconditioning program with all major muscle groups being challenged. A low weight, low repetition work-out is begun, and the cadet is progressed on individual events as tolerated. Some exercises, particularly 3, 7 and 13, will be very difficult for some who suffer from subluxation or dislocation if they have not had surgery.

It is felt that by employing the above program, re-injury of the involved shoulder or new injury to an adjacent part is minimized. The above program will take at least 40 minutes, even if done by the most aggressive athlete. The cadet is returned to full unrestricted activity when upper body performance is approximately symmetrical.

The exercise contained in the diagrams of the West Point shoulder reconditioning program represent the evolution of rehabilitation spanning many years and involving many individuals. The West Point Orthopaedic Service, Physical Therapy Department and Office of Physical Education have all contributed to the program now in use.

Stellate fractures that simply enlarge the glenoid or increase its concavity will usually not cause disability.

Avulsion of the Coracoid Process

An injury that occasionally occurs in the shoulder is an avulsion of a portion of the coracoid process by the conjoined tendon of the biceps and coracobrachialis and to a lesser extent the pectoralis minor (Fig. 184). The outlook for repair of a tendon is more favorable than it is for rupture of the tendon or of the muscle-tendon junction.

Surgical Repair. Technique for exposure of the coracoid is relatively simple. A linear incision should be made along the deltopectoral interval, from the clavicle down over the coracoid process. Dissection is carried out between the pectoralis major and the deltoid muscles. This interval is marked by the cephalic vein, but often the vein is not encountered until deep in the gutter. I recommend ligating the vein at each end and removing it, since retracting the vein will traumatize it so much that it will probably thrombose anyway. The idea of going through the deltoid and leaving a segment of it to protect the vein is not an attractive one, since the muscle left to protect the vein would be without nerve supply. I have never seen any complication as a result of sacrifice of the vein. Circulation is quite adequate around the shoulder.

After separating these two muscles, deep retraction will permit the coracoid process, lying underneath the deltopectoral fascia, to be readily visualized. The deltopectoral fascia may be divided, further exposing the coracoid. In acute injury one is immediately in the area of the fracture. Depending on the level of the fracture, the fragment will be found in the wound, along with the attachments of the coracobrachialis-biceps tendon. If it is relatively distal (approximately 1 cm.), it probably will not have the pectoralis minor attachment on it, although some portion of the pectoralis minor may have gone with the fragment. In any event, adequate retraction will expose the denuded end of the coracoid. Now the coracoid process may be reduced and held, preferably with a couple of Lewin clamps in order to get good apposition, while a drill hole is made through the fragment across the fracture line and the body of the coracoid. It further extends into the intermedullary area. A single screw is adequate for fixation. In closure, simply let the muscles fall together and approximate them loosely with 2-0 cotton. Careful attention is given to closing the skin, since the skin does tend to fall off in a shoulder wound.

A sling is worn on the arm for four weeks, although use of the forearm and hand is allowed before then. The patient should not participate in contact sports for at least eight weeks. One may expect complete recovery from this type of injury following successful fixation.

REHABILITATION

Rehabilitation is of extreme importance in any condition involving the upper extremity; perhaps it is more important than in any other area of the body. The reader is urged to carefully study the section on rehabilitation in Chapter 22. West Point Military Academy has an unusually fine program of rehabilitation, as exemplified by the exercise diagrams shown in Figure 185, which the staff use and hand out to injured cadets. They have kindly consented to their inclusion in this book.

Injuries of the Upper Arm

8

This chapter deals with the area between the shoulder and elbow joints and does not include discussion of either joint. *Anatomically* the arm consists of a single long bone, relatively circular in cross section, which is completely surrounded by muscles along which various vessels and nerves traverse. Injuries to this area are peculiar to this anatomical type and are similar to those of the thigh.

CONTUSION

There is little subcutaneous bone in the upper arm, since in all locations the skin is separated from the bone by an intervening layer or layers of muscle. The single exception is at the distal attachment of the deltoid to the lateral humerus. *Contusion of the skin*, therefore, is likely to be relatively benign and asymptomatic and to require little treatment. The structures lying between the skin and the bone, however, are quite subject to injury by contusion.

Contusion of Muscle

A direct blow over the biceps muscle in the front of the arm may well result in a contusion and hematoma of this muscle. However, this injury is neither frequent nor often disabling because of the thick muscle pad and the relatively smooth bone. Similarly, a direct blow over the triceps at the back of the arm may result in a painful, tender muscle but is not apt to present major complications.

In the presence of a contusion of the muscle, no matter where it is located, our first consideration is to rule out complications such as hemorrhage, nerve damage and fracture of the underlying bone. If there is any suspicion of fracture, an x-ray film should be made. Careful examination of the muscle and tests of its function will usually reveal whether or not there has been a major rupture of the muscle fibers.

In the absence of any major complication, *treatment* will vary depending upon the symptoms. If there is painful dysfunction, I recommend the early application of a cold pack. The arm should be wrapped snugly with sheet wadding, followed by an elastic bandage extending from the fingers to the axilla. The ice packs are applied over this and held on by a second elastic bandage so that they can be changed at regular intervals without disturbing the pressure on the arm from the underlying elastic bandage. This way it is not necessary to stop the cold treatment by changing the dressing as the ice packs warm up. More pressure should be applied in the vicinity of the contused area. The arm is then placed in a sling to put the involved muscle at rest. If the symptoms persist after 48 hours, the cold pack may be replaced by the application of heat locally, using an electric pad, inductive heat or hot packs. Within a few days after the most acute symptoms subside, pain-free activity may be permitted. The whirlpool bath is a useful adjunct at this stage. The patient should be advised to use the arm strictly within the limits of pain. There is no place for massage or passive motion in the early treatment of a muscular contusion. Rehabilitation may progress parallel to the subsidence of symptoms. In this situation, as in so many others in the athlete, too early and too extensive use of the involved muscle will only prolong the disability—a fact that needs repeated emphasis. Should a hematoma develop, it is treated by aspiration, local injection and a pressure bandage.

Contusion of Tendon and Bones
(Blocker's Exostosis)

An injury of unusual significance is a *contusion of the middle third of the arm in the vicinity of, and actually just over, the attachment of the deltoid muscle on the lateral aspect of the humerus*. In this area the bone approximates the skin quite closely, particularly in the sulcus between the anterior distal portion of the deltoid and the belly of the biceps. This coincides with the area most frequently struck by the blocker as he throws his arm up to check the impetus of the charging, opposing player. A direct blow by the hard headgear and, more particularly, repeated blows in this area will result in contusion of the tendon of the deltoid and of the periosteum of the humerus where the deltoid inserts. Adding to the vulnerability of this particular area is the fact that the anterior edge of the shoulder pad usually extends to about this level, and the edge of the pad itself may well contribute to the damage rather than protect the area. The hemorrhage that occurs ordinarily is not extensive and, indeed, is not enough to be palpable as a hematoma. If this condition is recognized early, it can be treated by adequate protection with a simple fiberboard pad, which prevents recurrence of injury. Suitable measures such as local injection into the bruised area and early application of cold followed by heat usually give prompt relief of the early lesion.

If the condition progresses and becomes chronic, a painful *periostitis* and *fibrositis* may develop. These conditions are manifested by extreme tenderness just lateral to the belly of the biceps at the deltoid insertion. Treatment is by protection against further blows and local injection of a long-acting anesthetic and a corticoid preparation. Frequently dramatic improvement will result following such an injection. There is a definite tendency toward recurrence, however, and once this painful condition has developed, the player should be instructed to wear a suitable contact pad. This must be firmly fastened to the arm so that the pad itself does not slip around and cause further irritation.

As a further sequela of this same condition, there is often spur formation along the bone (Fig. 186). This is not a true myositis ossificans but rather an irritative *exostosis* that arises from the bone and has all the characteristics of bone. It is not infiltrated through the muscle as is myositis ossificans. This exostosis extends anterolaterally, usually with a relatively sharp edge. It may become quite disabling owing to the pain of a direct blow. Once it reaches this stage, it is not easily protected by a pad. The treatment of this condition is surgical excision, but it is extremely important that the growth be entirely mature before its removal is considered. The majority of these cases do not advance to this degree, and if they are asymptomatic, no treatment is indicated. The growth actually may appear and regress spontaneously (Fig. 187). If the mass is surgically removed during the formative stage, it will recur. The author recently had a case in which the original lesion seemed quite mature and was surgically removed before examination here. In a very few weeks there was development of a second exostosis above the level of the old lesion (Fig. 188). Although the main mass of bone seemed mature, there was still a portion of it in the formative stage, and the surgery simply triggered the formation of another spur. For a more complete discussion of myositis ossificans and exostosis, see the general discussion in Chapter 4, page 41, and the more specific discussion in Chapter 17, page 434. Whereas in myositis ossificans of the quadriceps, active use appears to be the aggravating factor, in the described condition in the arm, the exciting factor is repeated contusion. The patient can usually use his arm very well if he avoids a direct blow. The muscles themselves are not primarily involved, since the mass usually lies in the plane between the deltoid and the biceps.

Contusion of the Radial Nerve

As the radial nerve leaves the posterior cord and passes down the arm, it moves in a spiral fashion from superomedial to inferolateral along the muscular spiral groove of the humerus. The nerve here is in closer relationship to the bone but is covered by the bellies of the triceps muscle. As it swings laterally just above the lateral epicondylar ridge, it becomes much more subcutaneous and is quite liable to contusion. A direct blow on the posterolateral arm may cause a serious lesion of the nerve. Usually it is accompanied by a shocking, tingling sensation extending to the radial portion of the hand, and the hand is "numbed."

There is no specific early *treatment* for this condition; treatment is the same as that for contusion anywhere, i.e., early application of cold followed by heat and protection. If there

Figure 186. Typical blocker's exostosis of humerus. *A,* Showing the early formation of bone having the appearance of myositis ossificans. Immature nature of the growth is indicated by irregular margins and relatively light deposit. *B,* The mature growth now appears as an exostosis firmly attached to the humerus with mature bone. *C,* Some months after removal. This mass did not recur because it was allowed to mature before it was disturbed surgically.

Figure 187. *A,* Exostosis in front of the humerus two months after injury. The patient was advised that the growth was immature and should not be disturbed. *B,* Five months later the mass has regressed and matured and is asymptomatic.

Figure 188. Exostosis in front of humerus. *A,* The original lesion appeared mature and was removed with no recurrence locally. *B,* Subsequent recurrence at a higher level without intervening injury.

is an actual radial palsy, suitable splinting should be applied to the wrist and hand to overcome the wrist drop and loss of extension of the fingers and thumb. Usually the involvement is not complete. Sensation may be impaired in the radial distribution, but it is almost always present to some extent. Indeed, there may be complete motor loss with complete retention of sensation. Paresthesia is common. In such a case, early surgery is not advisable, but if the condition continues for three or four months without definite signs of improvement in voluntary motion, surgical intervention is indicated.

Usually the condition is one of constriction and edema rather than actual severance of the fibers and may be relieved by appropriate neurolysis. At operation the nerve is carefully exposed and traced through the contused area. If it is bound down to the humerus or is caught in scar, it must be freed by meticulous atraumatic dissection. Any constrictions of the sheath are released. If the constriction is not too mature, the sheath may be expanded by injecting saline into it and forcing the column of saline past the constriction. After the nerve is entirely free, an effort should be made to suture the muscle layers so as to place an intervening muscle layer between the nerve and the bone. This condition is not frequent but is extremely distressing when it does occur.

STRAIN

Acute Strain

The muscles of the arm are subject to acute strain in excessive muscular activity. This strain may vary from a mild (first degree) irritation of the tendon or muscle to a complete (third degree) rupture. The tendinous strains are discussed in conjunction with the adjacent joints. It may be difficult in some instances to distinguish between contusion of the muscle and acute strain or partial rupture. Indeed, frequently, the two may be simultaneous. That is, while the muscle is under a rather severe strain, it may receive a direct blow and the fibers may rupture. Clinically some distinction can be made between acute strain or muscle rupture and contusion, because in strain or muscle rupture, function of the part is likely to be more painful than palpation, whereas in contusion the reverse is usually true. If a strain is suspected, for example, in the biceps, the muscle should be carefully checked throughout its length and the exact area of tenderness to palpation determined. Palpation may also determine whether or not there is a defect in the muscle or some change in its shape. A test of function, particularly against resistance, will usually reveal a localizing point of pain, tenderness or separation.

Proper *treatment* should be instituted according to the findings. In strain it is extremely important that the muscle be protected from overuse or overstretch. It is therefore more vital to protect the arm in a sling or even a splint than it is to treat the condition locally. Optimum treatment includes the use of the cold pack and then heat, compression and protection by splinting. As the acute symptoms subside, a more definitive diagnosis may be made and subsequent treatment determined. That is, if there appears to be a major defect in the muscle (severe), more extensive treatment will be required than if the strain is mild. If it can be determined that there is an actual rupture of the muscle or musculotendinous junction (severe), surgical repair should definitely be recommended. Since surgical repair is most successful if done early, the importance of an early definitive diagnosis is apparent. The muscle most frequently damaged in the upper arm is the biceps, not only because it is more subject to a direct blow but also because the blow frequently occurs while the biceps is in strong contraction.

If the rupture is at the musculotendinous junction, the same symptoms may be present as with rupture of the tendon, except that the tenderness will be in the muscle rather than over the tendon. Tests for configuration of the biceps with the muscle in contraction may give a definite lead as to the completeness of the rupture (see Fig. 140, page 171). If this condition is to be treated nonsurgically or if the rupture is not complete, splinting should be continued for at least three weeks and should be followed by a sling that restricts extension at the elbow. The patient should be cautioned not to contract the biceps against resistance. In the vast majority of cases the rupture will be incomplete. The intact portion of the muscle protects the injured area and holds the torn fibers in relatively good apposition.

Chronic Strain

Chronic strain is much more likely to occur in a tendon and is considered in our discussion of the adjacent joints. There may be a chronic strain of the musculotendinous junction or in the muscle itself, which is evidenced by pain on overuse—either repetitive overuse or a single massive effort. This will differ from acute strain in that there will be no local signs of hemorrhage, swelling or separation of muscle or tendon fibers. Instead, there is a feeling of strain on forced activity, followed by stiffness and spasm of the muscle after a period of rest. The patient may go to sleep at night with only moderate soreness and awake in the morning with muscle spasm, stiffness and pain much more severe than it had been the night before. The situation may develop in the baseball pitcher or the weight lifter or the javelin thrower.

The only real solution to this problem is rest and avoidance of the type of activity that caused the condition in the first place. This is quite disrupting to the young athlete, and he frequently returns to his activity too soon and has prompt recurrence of his trouble. *Treatment,* therefore. should be local injection, application of heat locally and protection against excessive use but not immobilization. Function should be encouraged, but it should remain strictly within the limits of comfort. Since it is not necessary to use the upper extremity for weight-bearing, the requisite inactivity can usually be accomplished without special apparatus. A sling may be required to remind the youth that strenuous activity is interdicted. The patient should be given a clear understanding of the rationale of the treatment. If this is comprehended, a high degree of cooperation can be expected. The physician interested in the treatment of athletes should acquaint himself as to the anatomical characteristics of the muscles involved in the function of the arm and should be prepared to guide the patient in the selection of those activities which he may continue and those which he should abandon. This is particularly pertinent as rehabilitation progresses and it becomes necessary to permit greater activity. If the strain is the result of a particular activity, as for example, baseball pitching, it may be found that the patient can tolerate some other field position before he can return to pitching, since a somewhat different muscle activity is demanded of the pitcher than of the infielder, for example. So also, the pole vaulter might be permitted to participate in the hurdles or the high jump much sooner than he could pole vaulting.

FRACTURE

Fracture of the humerus may occur but is not a common injury in athletic competition. In any injury that seems to be severe, x-ray examination should be made. The radiograph of the shaft of the humerus leaves little doubt as to whether or not there is a fracture. Fracture almost always causes some interference with function. The exception may be the greenstick fracture in the younger individual in which the bone may be broken but the fragments are not disrupted. This can also be readily determined by x-ray visualization.

As with any injury in athletes, the goal of _treatment_ must be complete recovery. One is, therefore, more justified in adopting definitive treatment in the young person than one is in an older person. If a treatment can be utilized that will permit rehabilitation at a relatively early stage, this of course should be considered. Rehabilitation should be instituted as promptly as possible, but participation in sports must not be allowed until the fracture is entirely healed and the muscles restored to normal size and tone. With an injury to the arm, it is usually entirely feasible to continue conditioning the rest of the body and, indeed, many portions of the arm itself during the actual healing period of the injury.

Injuries of the Elbow

9

ANATOMICAL CONSIDERATIONS

The elbow is a complicated joint consisting of three different articulations: that between the ulna and the humerus, that between the radius and the humerus and that between the radius and the ulna. Although functionally it is primarily a hinge joint and so has motion in flexion and extension, it also participates in the rotatory motions of the forearm through the articulations of the radial head with the ulna and with the lower end of the humerus. The olecranon and coronoid processes of the ulna form a deep socket (the olecranon fossa) which encircles the trochlea of the lower end of the humerus and provides a very stable joint. This joint permits only flexion and extension. The ulna does not rotate. On the other hand, the upper end of the radius makes a very unstable connection with the lower end of the humerus, the buttonlike head of the radius having a shallow depression with the same arc of curvature as the transverse arc of the capitellum of the humerus. On flexion and extension, the head of the radius travels from the front to the back of the capitellum by a simple gliding action. On rotation of the forearm, the button of the radial head rotates through the shallow socket on the side of the ulna, while its proximal end simply turns on the capitellum.

The integrity of the relationship between the head of the radius and the ulna and humerus depends entirely upon ligaments (Fig. 189). The radioulnar articulation is stabilized by the annular (orbicular) ligament, which holds the head and the neck of the radius firmly against the radial fossa of the ulna. The stability of the radius and the lower end of the humerus is largely capsular in character, there being no collateral ligament extending from the outer side of the humerus to the head of the radius. A lateral ligament extends from the lateral epicondyle to a very firm connection with the annular ligament. Thus, the lateral integrity of

this joint also depends upon the continuity of the annular ligament of the radius. On the medial side there are very strong ligaments extending from the medial epicondyle down to the medial surface of the coronoid and downward and backward to attach to the whole length of the olecranon from its proximal tip to the base of the coronoid process. The anterior part of this ligament is cordlike, whereas the posterior part is shaped like a fan with the handle attached to the humerus. With the elbow in extension, the anterior portion of the ligament becomes very tight, whereas with the elbow in flexion, the posterior part of the fan is tight. The capsule of the joint is relatively relaxed. There is no check ligament as such. Extension of the elbow is prevented as the olecranon process impinges against the olecranon fossa of the humerus. Flexion is checked by pressure of the muscles of the forearm and arm or by the coronoid process against the humerus. Rotation of the forearm is entirely dependent upon a smooth radial head with its outer circumference intact.

CONTUSION

There are several areas of subcutaneous bone at the elbow. The entire olecranon is subcutaneous, as are the medial and lateral epicondyles and the supracondylar ridges. As might be expected in these circumstances, contusion to the elbow is a common injury. Falling on the flexed elbow crushes the skin against the hard bone of the olecranon and may result in severe contusion and abrasion or even laceration over the point of the elbow. Since this area is relatively insensitive, the injury is not especially painful; indeed, it may be overlooked. The area of the lateral condyle and the radial head, however, is quite sensitive, and a painful bruise here may follow a direct blow to the side of the elbow—the medial side less often because of its protected position. In

221

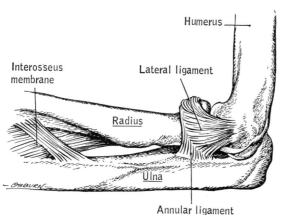

Figure 189. Medial and lateral views of the elbow showing bony and ligamentous structures.

contusion of any of these areas, care should be taken to determine whether there are other lesions. In cases of doubt, x-ray examination is indicated.

In the uncomplicated contusion, *treatment* depends upon the degree of injury. Often none is required. If there is an accompanying hematoma, it should be aspirated, and local injection with hyaluronidase may be carried out. The area is then wrapped in sheet wadding with the elbow at an angle as near to 90 degrees as is comfortable for the patient. A snug elastic bandage is wrapped over the arm from wrist to axilla. In the early stages, cold should be applied using an ice pack. After 48 hours heat may be used if symptoms persist. A sling should be worn if an elastic bandage is used; otherwise, flexion and extension of the elbow against the tight bandage will simply aggravate the contusion.

Periosteal irritation may develop as a result of a direct blow over the subcutaneous bone. In this instance the bone remains tender and is very sensitive to pressure. This condition responds well to local injection of a long-acting anesthetic and protection by adequate pad-

ding. A corticoid may be injected only if the condition is chronic.

Contusion on the back of the arm over the triceps tendon may cause tenosynovitis in the area with resulting pain, particularly on forced passive flexion of the elbow. As a rule tenosynovitis is not severe enough to cause impairment of triceps function. The usual measures prevail. Application of heat, rest and injection usually gives prompt relief.

Contusion of the Ulnar Nerve

Contusion of the ulnar nerve is quite frequent because of its anatomical position at the elbow. As it traverses the inner side of the arm, it passes behind the medial condyle through a tunnel, the floor of which is made up of the ulnar groove of the humerus, the roof being a rather loose fibrous sheath. As the arm flexes and extends, the nerve slides up and down in the ulnar groove. In this region the nerve is subcutaneous and lies directly on the bone. Hence, a direct blow may damage the nerve to a greater or lesser extent, depending upon the strength and direction of the force applied. The so-called crazy bone should have been named the crazy nerve, although certainly the bone does participate in the etiology of the syndrome. A direct blow causes immediate severe pain with a shocking sensation extending down to the ring and little fingers. This paresthesia is usually transient, disappearing after a few minutes or several hours, depending upon the severity of the injury.

Under ordinary circumstances no permanent injury results from ulnar nerve contusion, but occasionally there may be late sequelae. If the injury was sufficient to cause bleeding into the nerve, adhesions may form within the nerve trunk itself, resulting in the development of ulnar palsy. The same effect may occur if the irritation is external to the nerve and there is constriction within the groove. In either event the nerve fibers are constricted, and lose their elasticity, and a progressively increasing ulnar palsy results. A symptom of delayed palsy is gradually increasing numbness along the ulnar distribution of the forearm and hand. This includes the ulnar side of the lower forearm, the little finger, half of the ring finger and the fourth and fifth rays of the hand. The pain is ordinarily much more severe in the hand than at the elbow, although both may be quite painful. As the loss of nerve function continues, there will be marked atrophy of the intrinsic muscles of the hand. It should be recalled that a great majority of the intrinsic muscles of the hand are supplied by the ulnar nerve. One of the early symptoms of ulnar palsy is inability to adduct the little finger so as to place it against the ring finger. The metacarpal shafts will become more prominent because of intrinsic muscle atrophy. Contracture of the fingers will result as the condition progresses, and typical deformity occurs.

Definitive *treatment* in the early stages of ulnar palsy will usually prevent permanent disability. The condition is not amenable to local injection and similar measures. If there is a definite palsy and the nerve appears to be constricted, treatment should be surgical.

Ulnar Nerve Transfer. In an ulnar nerve transfer, a skin incision is made directly over the ulnar groove, extending up on the epicondylar ridge and extending down, for a length of about 10 centimeters, along the medial side of the forearm. The skin flap is reflected, particularly the anterior flap, to expose the flexor pronator muscles in the upper forearm. By careful dissection, the ulnar nerve is identified above the elbow. The roof of the tunnel

is carefully divided along the course of the nerve, and the nerve is freed from the surrounding tissues about 5 centimeters below the elbow and 5 centimeters above. The nerve must be freed proximal to the area where the nerve passes between the muscle bundles. The proximal skin flap must be completely free of the fascia and lifted so that the nerve can be laid beneath it. In the distal dissection, some branches of the nerve extend up into the muscles. Of these branches, only the most proximal one is sacrificed in order to free the nerve enough so that it can slip well forward in front of the medial condyle.

Once the skin has been reflected, the nerve is mobilized and laid anteriorly along the muscle mass. A fairly sharp curve is necessary, and there is a tendency for the nerve to slide back down in front of the epicondyle. However, a few sutures extending from the subcutaneous tissue into the muscle fascia will form a barrier which prevents this from occurring. If there is an hour-glass constriction of the nerve or if the nerve seems to be at all tight, a 25 gauge needle should be used to penetrate the sheath above the elbow and to inject normal saline. Under ordinary circumstances, this will balloon the nerve sheath and smooth any puff or restriction. This method is readily available and is also less hazardous than attempting to release the sheath by sharp dissection. The wound is then closed in the usual fashion and the elbow immobilized at 90 degrees, with the forearm in a position in which the flat of the hand rests against the abdomen. It is not necessary to completely pronate the forearm.

Immobilization of the elbow should continue for about three weeks, and when motion is resumed, it should be with careful avoidance of active stretching. Mobilization of the elbow should be gradual and should be pain-free. The rate of recovery depends on the duration and degree of nerve compression. It may be several months before complete recovery. If this operation has not been delayed too long, very good recovery can be expected.

STRAIN

Muscle-tendon strain about the elbow is quite frequent owing to the extremely forceful action required at the elbow joint in many sports. The powerful triceps muscle attaching to the olecranon is subject to strain anywhere from its attachment on the olecranon to the musculotendinous junction. The symptoms are tenderness over the involved area, pain on forceful extension of the forearm against resistance and pain on complete passive flexion of the elbow. There may well be local heat if the condition is acute enough, although this is not a diagnostic sign. Forceful active extension of the arm, as in throwing, aggravates the condition.

Another common area of strain is in the biceps where it attaches below the neck of the radius. The biceps has a firm tendinous attachment to the radius and through the bicipital aponeurosis (lacertus fibrosus) to the fascia of the forearm. Strain may occur anywhere in this complex and indeed may be severe enough to tear the lacertus or to avulse the biceps from the radius. The signs of tendon rupture may be somewhat obscured, particularly if the radial attachment pulls off and the lacertus remains intact or if the lacertus pulls off and the radial attachment remains intact. Under these circumstances the shortening and bunching of the biceps that are so characteristic may not be present (see Fig. 140, page 171). If there is complete rupture of the radial attachment, it should be replaced surgically. This is true whether the attachment is torn from the muscle, torn in its substance or pulled off the bone. It is not necessary to repair the lacertus in the case of an independent injury. In fact, the lacertus is very infrequently torn, since there is a certain amount of elasticity to its lateral attachment.

There may also be strain about the brachialis near its attachment to the ulna or of the anconeus or indeed of any of the muscles about the elbow. The symptoms are those of disturbance of function of the particular muscle involved.

Another very frequent area of strain is on the medial or lateral epicondyle of the humerus. Overuse, particularly in throwing, may well cause irritation of the muscle fibers at their attachment, with partial rupture of the fibers and hemorrhage. This results in an epicondylitis if not treated promptly. The early symptoms of the condition are tenderness, perhaps local swelling and pain on use of these muscles in forcibly gripping, pronating or supinating the forearm, as the case may be. Gripping causes pain whether the strain is to the medial or to the lateral epicondyle, since in gripping, the extensors and flexors both contract. Treatment of the acute injury is by local injection of a long-acting local anesthetic. Particularly important are immobilization and protection from function. Any painful function should be interdicted. If the third degree sprain

occurs, there may actually be an avulsion of the muscles on either epicondyle (see Avulsion Fracture, page 241).

Tennis Elbow

A type of condition about the elbow that is quite common in athletes, particularly in part-time athletes, is the so-called tennis elbow. Tennis elbow is one of those diagnoses similar to shin splints or belly ache. In this instance the name comes from the location. It has no relation to the type of injury. There are at least four distinct, different conditions that are commonly called tennis elbow. Physical examination will usually distinguish among them. Their histories, however, are very likely to be the same, that is, some unusual exertion involving a grip of the hand, with lateral play of the wrist. The name tennis elbow derives from the fact that it frequently occurs in someone who plays tennis before becoming well conditioned. There is pain in the lateral side of the elbow, sometimes on the medial side of the elbow, aggravated by gripping and rotating. In the days antedating the vacuum sweeper it was also called "rug beater's elbow." There are various other adjectives to describe the condition in relation to the activities that ordinarily involve lateral movement of the wrist, such as tennis playing, beating a rug or using a hammer; even overuse of the elbow, such as in shaking hands at a reception, can bring on the symptoms. This is described in detail in the following section on epicondylitis.

The various conditions on the lateral side which may be labeled tennis elbow are (1) true epicondylitis of the extensor supinator aponeurotic attachment to the lateral epicondyle; (2) radial ulnar synovitis marked by development of a pannus of synovium between the radius and the ulna; (3) strain in the aponeurosis itself, often directly over the radial head; and (4) radial humeral bursitis. It can be seen how the close proximity of the epicondyle, the radial humeral joint and the supinator aponeurosis could result in their being confused. Often, indeed, the different conditions have the same cause, namely, overuse of the mechanism. Ulnar neuritis, which occurs on the medial side of the elbow, is sometimes classified as tennis elbow, although it also is readily distinguishable from medial epicondylitis. I urge that the use of "tennis elbow" to describe any of these conditions be discarded and that more definitive diagnoses be made.

Epicondylitis

A type of involvement that is peculiar to the elbow develops along the medial and lateral epicondyles. The extensor-supinator muscles arise along the lateral epicondyle and the flexor-pronator muscles arise along the medial epicondyle, where they have an aponeurotic attachment. Either by contusion of the area or more commonly by strain, an irritation develops at the attachment of the aponeurosis to the bone that is quite characteristic. There is pain along the epicondyle, which is aggravated by gripping. The pain extends down the corresponding group of muscles, either medially or laterally, sometimes as far as the wrist. In the normal mechanism of clenching the fist, one of the first phases of action is strong contraction of the carpal extensors in order to fix the wrist. If this did not occur, the wrist would go into flexion and an ineffective fist would result. This is exemplified by a hand in which there is radial paralysis. A person is unable to make a fist, not because he cannot flex the fingers but because he cannot stabilize the wrist. So when the hand grasps an object, tension is placed on both the flexors and extensors of the wrist. Hence, gripping will cause pain whether the involvement is medial or lateral. On examination there is tenderness localized to the epicondyle or upward for a short distance along the supracondylar ridge. The tenderness may also extend down over the radial head, but in the true epicondylitis, the acute tenderness is directly on the epicondyle.

This condition may be extremely aggravating, particularly since it is often chronic and is increased by many activities of the forearm and hand. *Treatment* demands rest, and in the severe case, a splint that fixes the wrist in slight dorsiflexion and the elbow at 90 degrees may be needed. Application of heat locally by diathermy, electric pad or whirlpool is useful. Dramatic results are often obtained by local injection, my preference being for a long-acting local anesthetic plus a corticoid preparation. The needle should be inserted directly into the area of involvement, and multiple puncture points should be made. The anesthetic is injected until the tenderness is entirely relieved, after which the corticoid is injected into the same area. Following such an injection, the pain may be much more severe for 12 to 24 hours but then subsides, and the symptoms gradually improve, until by the end of a few days they may be entirely gone. Should the symptoms then recur, a second or even a third or fourth injection may be necessary to obtain permanent relief. Throughout this period the patient must avoid the activities that caused the trouble. This frequently poses a problem, since the activity that caused the condition may be an integral part of the regimen of this particular patient. Thus a pole vaulter may be unable to grasp his pole, a javelin player may be unable to snap his wrist and a baseball pitcher may have trouble gripping the ball or in sharply extending his elbow to throw. Handshaking may be the offending activity, and the resulting disability has been known to interfere with the activities of public figures. If nonsurgical measures fail, the condition can ordinarily be relieved by detaching the muscles from the epicondyle and smoothing the bone, thus eliminating the irritated area and permitting the muscle to heal.

The following technique is used: A curved incision is made in front of the epicondyle and carried across the elbow joint onto the radial head area. There are two peculiarities in this situation. On the medial side, care must be taken to avoid damage to the ulnar nerve. If there is any question about constriction of the nerve, it should be transferred forward (see page 223). On the lateral side, the incision should be carried sufficiently past the radial-ulnar joint to permit the epicondyle to be well visualized.

The skin is reflected, exposing the aponeurotic attachment of the extensor supinator muscle group. By sharp dissection, the muscle tendon is separated from the epicondyle and is stripped from the bone with an osteotome or elevator, thus exposing raw bone, particularly on the anterior surface of the epicondyle. As the epicondylar tissues are stripped from the epicondyle, the radial humeral joint is exposed. This joint should be carefully inspected. If there is synovitis of the joint, it should be trimmed away and carefully coagulated. Care should be taken not to divide the annular ligament around the radial neck.

The bone of the epicondyle is now fully visualized, and any irregularities are smoothed. If there is also involvement along the sharp lateral margin of the epicondyle, exposure is carried posteriorly to free the condyle in this area. The lateral edge is flattened with an osteotome to reduce its sharpness, and all exposed bone is then smoothed with an elevator, rasp or osteotome. As soon as the condyle has been appropriately flattened, the exposed bone is covered with bone wax. At this point, the anterior flaps should contain the flexor supinator group of muscles. The anterior and posterior muscle flaps are pulled back together by direct suture along the posterior part of the linear incision over the epicondylar ridge, without suture to the bone. It is not necessary to drill holes in the bone to reattach the soft tissue because there is always sufficient periosteum and fibrous tissue here to hold it securely in position.

The splint is applied with the forearm in supination if the lateral epicondyle has been repaired, and with the forearm in pronation if the medial epicondyle has been repaired. The sutures are removed in two weeks and immobilization of the arm is continued for another two to four weeks, at which time controlled motion is carefully begun. The patient should be advised during the mobilization period not to forcibly grip with the fingers. The rehabilitative period is relatively slow, but use of the hand is quickly restored. Forceful manipulation to straighten the elbow is not necessary or desirable.

Although epicondylitis may follow a relatively acute strain, it more often results from a chronic degenerative change by attrition of the aponeurotic fibers at the elbow. This occurs in certain types of athletics, such as baseball pitching, but it is not common in ordinary athletic pursuits, acute sprain being the more likely cause. If there is degenerative change, there may be calcification or even spur formation over the epicondyle. The patient presents complaining of an aching pain on the outer or inner side of the elbow which is made more severe by active use of the forearm and hand.

This type of epicondylitis may seriously interfere with athletic competition, not so much because of pain at the elbow but because of restriction of use of the hand. The tender point should be protected by a contact pad. The patient should be warned to avoid gripping. Since this is extremely difficult to avoid in most sports, it may be necessary to forbid participation for a period of several weeks. Another measure to prevent recurrence of this distressing condition is rehabilitation of the muscles involved. Most agree that tennis elbow is a result of overstress from overuse, and it is axiomatic that overuse is very much more likely to occur in the ill-conditioned muscle. Rehabilitative exercises for the wrist and hand (see page 687) are extremely productive in preventing recurrence of the condition and increasing endurance of the forearm and hand.

So, the term tennis elbow is not entirely restricted to epicondylitis. Other conditions grouped under this category are radial head capsulitis and radiohumeral bursitis, each of which is discussed in the following sections.

Sprain

Since the elbow is a stable joint, ligament injury here is relatively uncommon. It is virtually impossible to sprain the elbow by excess flexion. In excessive extension, on the other hand, as the olecranon impinges against the back of the humerus, the continuing force pulls the coronoid away from the trochlea of the humerus. This results in injury to the anterior portion of the collateral ligaments, particularly on the medial side. This injury may vary from a partial tear of little significance (first degree) to complete rupture (third degree) of the ligaments and capsule. As the force stops short of complete rupture, the elbow flexes, the tension is relaxed and there is no feeling of instability at the elbow joint because of its inherent bony stability and because it does not require the degree of stability for weight-bearing that is necessary at the knee.

The patient with such an injury presents with a history of hyperextension of the elbow and severe pain on the medial and sometimes the lateral side of the elbow, which is relieved by flexion, so that he ordinarily will have his hand tucked into his shirt or his thumb hooked over his belt to prevent elbow extension. The symptoms at the time of the examination vary directly according to the severity of injury. Pain is not ordinarily a prominent factor. There is localized tenderness at the site of the tear, either along the ulna on the medial side or along the epicondyle. There may also be pain along the lateral collateral ligaments at the site of the tear. Any attempt to extend the arm causes pain, and complete extension is prevented by muscle spasm. I have never seen a case in an athlete in which I could demonstrate excess motion indicating a complete tear without there being complete dislocation.

The collateral ligaments may also be sprained by lateral motion. Forced abduction of the extended arm will damage the medial ligaments. Forced adduction will damage the lateral. Here again, instability is extremely infrequent, and I find it very difficult to determine whether or not the rupture is complete unless there has been a complete dislocation of the elbow. A "sprain fracture" due to avulsion of the ligament with a fragment of bone may be revealed by x-ray examination.

Symptoms of lateral stresses are localized to the one side, with the same findings as those for hyperextension, that is, tenderness along the site of the tear, local swelling and pain on attempt to reproduce the causative force.

Treatment of such a sprain is relatively simple. In the acute stage, the use of cold followed by heat and a protective sling is adequate. Use of the extremity should be restricted for the first few days, but unless the injury is quite symptomatic, a splint is not necessary. As the acute symptoms subside, more motion may be permitted but always within the limits of pain for at least four weeks. At this time active, unprotected function should be encouraged.

Occasionally there is a complete rupture, particularly of the medial collateral ligament, with instability of the elbow as the stress pushes the forearm laterally. This can be very disabling to the athlete, and considerable time usually elapses before it is identified as a permanent disability. The reconstruction of the joint, although rare, has been done quite successfully by utilization of tendons for grafts to pass along the course of the medial ligament, running from the epicondyle down to the side of the coronary process of the ulna and similarly running down from the epicondyle into the medial side of the olecranon process. Here they are fixed by appropriate drill holes looped back and forth. A complete rupture is unusual, but when it occurs, reconstruction can be successfully carried out.

DISLOCATION

As the hyperextension force at the elbow continues, the olecranon remains fixed in the olecranon fossa, extension of the arm levers the coronoid completely around the trochlea, and the lower end of the humerus slides forward and downward to lodge against the anterior ulnar shaft distal to the coronoid (Fig. 190). At the same time the capitellum, by virtue of rupture of the lateral collateral or annular ligaments, slides forward and downward, so that it rests on the radial neck. There may be a lateral component of this dislocation, so that the coronoid of the ulna may lie behind the capitellum rather than behind the trochlea (Fig. 191), in which instance the radial head is displaced laterally and does not appose the humerus.

Dislocation of the elbow cannot occur without rupture of the collateral ligaments. In many instances the force is relieved before this dislocation becomes complete, and the elbow components slip back into their normal relationship. This subluxation, or spontaneously reduced dislocation, presumably has occurred whenever complete rupture of both collateral ligaments is diagnosed. The dislocated elbow has a rather typical deformity, with the olecranon prominent posteriorly and with the forearm extended beyond a right angle. If the dislocation remains unreduced, immediate, extensive swelling occurs, rapidly obliterating the bony landmarks about the elbow.

Figure 190. Lateral x-ray of a dislocated elbow, showing the lower end of the humerus resting on the ulna in front of the coronoid. Note fragmentation of the coronoid.

Figure 191. A fracture-dislocation of the elbow in a child. *A*, Anteroposterior view before reduction. Note lateral displacement of the forearm in relation to the arm. The medial epicondylar epiphysis is displaced with the ulna. *B*, Anteroposterior view after reduction. Note epicondylar epiphysis caught in joint. Also note the lateral displacement. *C*, Lateral view after reduction. Note epicondyle in joint. This must be surgically removed from the joint and fixed to the medial condyle.

The most pressing requirement on examination of such a patient is to determine the circulatory capacity to the hand, since circulatory changes rapidly become irreversible. One should carefully determine the presence or absence of the radial pulse. Careful attention should be given to the capillary circulation of the nail beds. A second requirement is investigation of nerve function. The median is the nerve most likely to be involved, as it is caught on the end of the humerus as the bone slides forward. Interference with the nerve supply should be carefully determined. It is extremely important to record any neurological change *before* an attempt at reduction is made or else one may never know whether the nerve damage was immediate and was caused by the dislocation or if it was caused by the trauma of reduction or developed later because of swelling and edema.

Treatment. A dislocated elbow is a surgical emergency. The result obtained from treatment of such an injury depends to a great extent upon the length of time the dislocation has been unreduced. If the arm is seen immediately after the injury (for instance on the playing field), one should take the time to investigate the circulation of the hand and to make a rough evaluation of the nerve supply. At this time, while the arm is numb and swelling has not taken place, it may be possible to reduce the deformity at once and without anesthesia. This must be done by the gentlest

means, since forceful manipulation not only will increase the muscle spasm and prevent reduction but also may cause severe damage to the nerve or blood supply, which may have been spared at the time of injury. If the forearm is displaced laterally, usually to the radial side, the upper arm should be steadied by the doctor with one hand while he grasps the forearm just below the elbow with the other. By gentle manipulation, the lateral deformity is usually easily corrected. Once this is accomplished, the right arm of the operator must be shifted to grasp the wrist, and steady, even traction must be applied along the long axis of the forearm as the elbow gradually moves toward extension. If this causes pain and spasm, the attempt should be discontinued. If the patient can relax his muscles, the elbow may slip easily into position. This may be facilitated by slight hyperextension of the forearm, which permits the coronoid to slide under the trochlea, whereupon the dislocation will be reduced as the forearm is gently flexed. If the emergency reduction is not successful or if the patient is not seen immediately, he should be moved to the nearest place where there are proper facilities for x-ray examination and anesthesia administration. X-ray examination before the reduction is highly desirable. This not only provides some idea as to the exact location of the bones but also demonstrates any accompanying fractures (see Figs. 191 to 193).

Figure 192. The white arrows indicate the displaced epicondylar epiphysis in both the anteroposterior and lateral views. Note the fracture of the radial head without displacement (black arrow); it does not require treatment.

Fractures frequently accompany dislocation of the elbow, the most common being those of the epicondyles, the coronoid and the radial head. The fractures are of either the avulsion or leverage type and may greatly complicate the treatment of the dislocated elbow. The coronoid may be injured as it passes under the humerus by combination of muscle pull and direct impingement, the significance being that there may be avulsion of the anterior capsular ligaments and also of a portion of the brachialis attachment. Similarly the epicondyle may be avulsed by the pull of the flexors or extensors. The medial epicondylar epiphysis is most frequently pulled off, since it is the last epiphysis at the elbow to close. It may well be avulsed and the small button epiphysis may be overlooked in its displaced position (see Fig. 191). Many of these fractures require open reduction. If for any reason open reduction of the fracture must be delayed beyond an hour, the dislocation should be reduced at once—under

Figure 193. Dislocated elbow with fracture of medial epicondyle. *A,* Dislocation with displacement of condyle into the joint (arrow) is shown. *B and C,* Reduction with poor position of the epicondyle (arrows) is shown.

Figure 194. The anterior and posterior splints. *A*, Plaster splints carefully molded to the arm over sheet wadding. *B*, The dressing is completed by application of gauze bandage.

anesthesia if necessary. It is extremely important that the dislocation be reduced at the earliest possible moment even if a second anesthetic will be required for later surgical replacement of a fragment. Prompt reduction of the dislocation will prevent excessive swelling in the soft tissues, excessive and long-continued stretching of the nerves or blood vessels and other serious complications. Following reduction, radiographs of the elbow should be made *before application of a splint* (see Fig. 191). I wish to emphasize this point, since it is very difficult to visualize a small displaced fragment about the elbow through a plaster splint using radiography. If there is any doubt at all as to the positions of the epicondyles, coronoid and radial head, similar x-ray films should be made on the normal elbow in a similar position and the two films carefully compared.

Following reduction of the dislocation, one should again painstakingly assess the circulation of the hand. If possible the elbow should be splinted at 90 degrees (Fig. 194). The circulation should again be evaluated in this position both before and after the application of the splint. Similarly, a check of nerve function should be carried out, although this must await the patient's recovery from the anesthetic. It should be done at the earliest possible moment, since it is extremely important to know at what stage nerve symptoms develop. The decision as to the method of management of the nerve injury may depend wholly upon this knowledge. If there is sudden complete loss of function of the nerve at the time of the accident, early repair is indicated, whereas if the

onset is gradual, a more conservative attitude should be adopted. If the circulation is not intact with the elbow at 90 degrees, the elbow should be extended to that position at which the circulation is satisfactory.

If there is evidence of arterial spasm, with a white hand and absent radial pulse, an emergency situation exists that calls for immediate measures to restore the arterial circulation. A stellate ganglion block should be accomplished. Vasodilator drugs should be given. Cold may be applied to the opposite hand. If such measures do not restore the arterial pulsation, the arm should be opened in the antecubital area and the artery identified and examined. Appropriate measures to restore circulation, such as stripping the artery if it is in spasm, and repairing, grafting or ligating it if it is lacerated, are then carried out. These measures must not be delayed until irreversible changes take place in the hand. The hand is extremely vulnerable to circulatory disturbance. Simple loss of radial pulse does not mean arterial insufficiency. Loss of the pulse must be accompanied by signs of actual ischemia of the hand in order to justify exploration of the artery.

The duration of immobilization depends somewhat upon the degree of reaction in the elbow. Immobilization should be by anterior and posterior plaster splints and not by a solid cast (see Fig. 194). There must be no constriction in the antecubital space. By the use of anterior and posterior splints, the degree of tension in the forearm tissues can be assessed readily by palpation along the sides of the splints. The splints may be loosened if necessary and tightened as the swelling subsides. No attempt should be made to mobilize the arm until the swelling is well under control. If the patient has been seen early and reduction has been carried out promptly, there probably will not be excessive post-reduction swelling. In such a case the arm should be immobilized in double splints for two weeks. At the end of two weeks if no pain and swelling are present in the elbow, the anterior splint is removed and the posterior one continued. The posterior splint permits a few degrees of flexion and extension and is worn for one more week, a total of three weeks. The arm is then placed in a sling, which is to be worn another week. At the end of this time (four weeks), unrestricted active use of the arm can be permitted. Passive stretching has little place in the rehabilitation of the elbow. There will be marked stiffness of the elbow following dislocation, but motion should be complete after several months if meddlesome passive stretching is avoided.

Rehabilitation commences immediately and consists of using the fingers and thumb and setting the muscles of the forearm and upper arm, all within the limits of pain. As the course of treatment progresses to the use of the posterior splint alone, active flexion and extension of the elbow are permissible, since this splint "hinges" at the elbow. When the splint comes off, active use is encouraged, again within the limits of pain. Strenuous motions should be avoided for six weeks. Any attempt to forcibly extend the elbow by passive stretching tends to delay the healing, to increase the inflammatory reaction around the elbow and to encourage bony deposits. These deposits are not in the muscle, as in the case of a myositis ossificans, but are infiltrated throughout the capsule and ligaments of the joint (Fig. 195). Gravity is of great benefit in restoring extension, and it may be acceptable to add to the effect of gravity by a lead wristlet (a pound or two). Little is gained by carrying a heavy weight, at least in the first six to eight weeks. A dislocated elbow is a serious injury and therefore requires prolonged aftercare. It should result in little or no permanent disability in the young athlete.

Ossification of the capsule of the elbow occurs not only with frank dislocation but also with many lesser injuries of the ligament and capsule, since this area is particularly prone to ossification. This often results in serious restriction of motion of the joint. The most vulnerable areas are around the coronoid process of the ulna in the anterior capsule, and the

Figure 195. Ossification in the elbow capsule following dislocation.

olecranon process of the ulna in the posterior capsule. Any ossification of either of these areas seriously restricts motion of the elbow. Ossification may also occur as a plaque of bone along the collateral ligaments, where it not only restricts motion but also may be quite painful on function. Occasionally, following dislocation or fracture-dislocation about the elbow, ossification will surround the joint completely, causing serious disability. This tendency toward ossification should be recognized. Prompt care and rigorous management tend to minimize the deposit. Adequate immobilization during the acute stage directly after the injury encourages absorption of the extravasated blood and minimizes ossification. Repeated manipulation at intervals of several days, with resultant irritation, tends to increase the ossification. Later in the rehabilitation, any attempt at forceful motion of the elbow will stimulate ossification in the capsule (Fig. 196). These osseous deposits are not myositis ossificans, since they do not occur in the muscle. *Once the condition begins, treatment consists of immobilization and protection rather than manipulation.* Nothing is gained by trying to prevent stiffness by manipulation once ossifi-

Figure 196. Excessive ossification following dislocation of elbow treated by early active use.

cation is present. The temptation to remove the bone surgically should be resisted for many months. It may ultimately be advisable to attempt excision of some ossific plaques, but any attempt to do this before the deposit is entirely mature and completely stable will only result in increased ossification. Indeed, it may recur in any event.

As noted previously, early ossification around the joint is only increased by manipulative treatment. There has been some recent work, most of it in relation to ossification around the hip, using radiation as a preventive measure. I think this approach has promise. It appears that radiation treatment must be done very early, within 4 or 5 days of the injury, to be effective. By that time it might be virtually impossible to tell whether there has been any ossification or whether it is likely to occur. In the growing child, whose epiphyses are open, care should be taken not to damage the epiphyseal plate by the radiation. As of 1982, this method of treatment was in the early testing stage and was not applicable to elbow dislocation.

FRACTURE-DISLOCATION

As has been noted previously, fractures frequently accompany elbow dislocations. This is particularly true of dislocations in those whose epiphyses have not entirely closed. It is very common for the medial epicondylar epiphysis to be pulled off.

Epicondyles

The epicondyles serve as the attachment not only of the collateral ligaments of the elbow but also of the strong muscle. All these attachments are put under great stress during dislocation of the humerus, whether this dislocation is straightforward or has a lateral component. The bones carrying attachments of muscles are likely to be grossly displaced if the fracture is complete (see Fig. 192). Reduction of the elbow may catch the fragment within the joint (Fig. 191), and this may actually prevent complete reduction. X-ray examination as soon as possible after reduction of the dislocated elbow is imperative, whether or not films were obtained before the reduction (Fig. 193). An avulsed condyle should be replaced surgically, even when the avulsion is simply of a muscle attachment with a small splinter of bone (Figs. 197 and 198), since firm fixation of this attachment will permit much more rapid motion and complete rehabilitation. The detached epicondyle tends to rotate because of the pull on its periphery, so that it frequently presents its cortical surface toward the humerus and its fractured surface toward the skin (Fig. 199). Nonunion is quite common and growth dis-

Figure 197. *A*, Avulsion of medial epicondyle. *B*, Replacement of condyle, held with nail. *C*, Late x-ray shows firm union.

Figure 198. This 13 year old female injured her elbow while doing a handspring. *A*, Original x-ray showed no fracture, although there was much tenderness around the medial epicondyle. *B*, Two weeks later there was separation of the epicondyle with some downward slipping.

Figure 199. *A*, Avulsion fracture of medial epicondyle, with 90 degree rotation of the fragment. *B*, The fragment was reduced and held with multiple Kirschner wires.

turbance inevitable when this occurs and is untreated (Fig. 200).

At operation the muscle or ligament attachment is carefully replaced with or without the fragment of bone. If the fragment is small, it is better removed and the aponeurotic ligament fastened to the raw bone of the humerus. A larger fragment may be held in place by nail or screw or other suitable internal fixation (see Figs. 197 and 199). Once internal fixation is secure, rehabilitative measures can proceed at

about the same rate as if there had been no fracture. Any internal fixation should be removed after four to six weeks, particularly if it crosses the epiphyseal cartilage.

Ulnar Nerve Injury

The ulnar nerve is usually not injured in a posterior dislocation of the elbow. However, in a fracture involving the medial epicondyle,

Figure 200. *A*, Fracture of lateral condyle with growth retardation, causing marked cubitus valgus. *B*, Correction by osteotomy.

ulnar nerve injury occurs with some frequency. This emphasizes the importance of careful evaluation of nerve function prior to any manipulation or surgery. If there is evidence of ulnar nerve damage, the nerve should be carefully examined at the time of the operation on the medial epicondyle. If there appears to be a possibility of its future involvement in scar, it should be transposed forward. On the other hand, if there is no sign of ulnar damage, it may be quite possible to replace the epicondyle without disturbing the nerve. The surgeon must always be conscious of the nerve so that it is not inadvertently damaged by either the instruments or the internal fixation. Hence, it is desirable to locate the nerve early and to be sure of its integrity at the termination of the operation before the wound is closed.

Following the operation, the function of the nerve should be determined at the earliest possible moment. If this is not done and an ulnar palsy is discovered several days later, one may be unable to determine whether it was caused by a gradual constriction of later scar formation or by actual injury at operation. This may have a great deal of prognostic importance. If the involvement is evident immediately after surgery and was not apparent preoperatively, one should seriously consider reopening the wound for examination of the nerve. This is particularly true if the loss of function is complete. On the other hand, if the onset is gradual after a day or two, immediate attention must be given to relieve any possible pressure. If the splint is tight, release it. If the pressure is from internal tension, the splint should be removed and the elbow gently extended to whatever degree is necessary to relieve the tension. Late paresthesia or anesthesia is another problem, and a great deal of judgment is required in determining the proper measures and the proper timing. If the condition is progressive, one must decide whether surgical treatment is necessary. If the nerve is to be transposed, it must be done before permanent changes occur in the nerve.

Coronoid Process

The coronoid may be broken off at the time of dislocation of the elbow (Figs. 201 to 203). If the fragment is small but somewhat displaced, it is best removed. If it comprises the major portion of the coronoid, its replacement may be necessary. This is a difficult procedure and should be postponed until the swelling of the elbow has subsided.

Radial Head

At the time of dislocation of the elbow, the radial head is forcibly driven against the lower

Figure 201. Fracture-dislocation of the elbow. A, Fracture of radial head and fracture of the ulnar coronoid, with displacement. B, Resection of the radial head, replacement of the ulnar coronoid and fixation by screw. Good stable elbow with no restriction of flexion extension resulted.

Figure 202. Case similar to Figure 201. Fracture-dislocation of the elbow with fracture of the radial head and the coronoid. X-rays made 15 months postoperatively, at which time the radial head was removed. Failure to replace the coronoid resulted in complete block in flexion at 115 degrees and in extension at 35 degrees. Patient has traumatic arthritis of the elbow which increases his disability.

Figure 203. A and B, Anteroposterior and lateral views of severe fracture-dislocation of the elbow and fracture of radial head and ulnar coronoid. C, Radial head removed. Remaining coronoid caused extensive ossification in the capsule. This ossification may also be the result of damaged periosteum around the radial neck. D, Same as C; elbow in extension, showing range of motion.

end of the humerus and is frequently damaged. Indeed, many complete fractures of the radial head have probably been accompanied by dislocation of the ulna that has reduced spontaneously. Treatment of a complete fracture of the radial head is almost always surgical, since it is necessary that the head be undistorted if normal rotation of the forearm is to be expected. Therefore, following a dislocation, the head should be carefully examined using radiography (see Fig. 201). A fragment that involves less than one fourth of the entire circumference of the radial head, particularly if it is on the lateral aspect of the head, may be removed and the remaining intact head left in situ. One often discovers, however, that there is also a comminuted fracture of the remaining portion of the head as well as the small segment. These fractures are not avulsion fractures, since there is nothing attached to the rim of the radial head. They are caused by direct force; hence, there may be extensive chondral damage which does not show on the film. There also may be damage to the cartilage of the capitellum of the humerus (Fig. 204). These factors present another argument for early surgery in fracture of the radial head in order that the nature of the lesion can be determined and proper measures undertaken.

If there is a complete fracture of the radial head, particularly if it is comminuted in type, the head should be removed and the annular ligament carefully repaired if it has been disrupted (Fig. 205). Most fractures through the radial neck in adults should also be treated by

excision of the radial head. Fractures occurring in children before the upper radial epiphysis has closed should never be treated by excision of the head because of the disability following growth disturbances and radial shortening. In these cases the head should carefully be replaced by open reduction if manipulation fails, if there is angulation over 30 degrees or if there is any lateral displacement.

Olecranon

Almost all dislocations of the elbow are posterior. That is, the forearm moves posteriorly in relationship to the arm (see Fig. 190 and 193). This frequently has the lateral component indicated previously. A true anterior dislocation of the elbow is virtually impossible without fracture of either the olecranon or the lower humerus. Anterior fracture-dislocation is a very serious injury, usually resulting from force applied directly on the back of the flexed elbow (Figs. 206 and 207). The olecranon breaks, the triceps attachment holds the proximal fragments posteriorly, the lateral ligament gives way and the humerus moves backward and downward into the fracture line. The same force may cause a fracture of the trochlea of the humerus or indeed of the entire distal end of the humerus. As the olecranon is driven into the distal end of the humerus, it may act as a wedge and cause a condylar or T fracture. The radial head is not usually fractured in either of these instances, since the forces applied do not put stress on it.

Figure 204. *A*, Fracture of capitellum with separation of the fragments. This is the same force that might break the radial head. *B*, Following open reduction with removal of small fragments and replacement of major fragments. Excellent function.

Figure 205. Fracture of the radial head. A, The comminution. B, Treatment by resection of the head.

Figure 206. Fracture-dislocation of elbow. A, The dislocation was reduced and the radial fragments allowed to remain. B, Subsequent picture shows good healing of the radial head but with deformity and restriction of rotation, ossification of the medial capsule with restriction of flexion and extension, and pain. Radial head resection would have permitted earlier motion and better rehabilitation. The radial head should now be removed, but the ultimate result will not compare with that of early surgery.

Figure 207. *A,* Fractured olecranon at its base. This will require a long intramedullary screw or pin for firm fixation. Treatment refused. Result—traumatic arthritis of the elbow, with restriction of motion and pain. Fibrous union of the fragment. *B,* Case similar to *A.* A fractured olecranon but with fractured coronoid. Note oblique screw transfixing olecranon and coronoid, with longitudinal screw extending into the shaft. It is probably better to use a longer screw in the shaft, but in a young individual, good purchase can often be obtained without using an intramedullary nail or screw.

This injury must be treated surgically in order to obtain accurate replacement and firm internal fixation of the fragments. The exact type of fixation depends upon the pathological conditions. If the fragment is a single large block, it may be held very well with a long intramedullary screw or pin. If the fragments are more comminuted, a small plate may be needed. Some of the fragments or, indeed, all of the fragments may be removed with suture of the triceps tendon to the remaining olecranon (Fig. 208). One may remove a surprising amount of the olecranon process and not materially impair function of the elbow if the triceps is carefully repaired, since the triceps

sling gives sufficient stability. The elbow tolerates considerably more roughness of the olecranon than the knee does of the patella because weight-bearing is not involved. Open reduction following these injuries permits careful inspection of the cartilage, not only of the olecranon fossa but also of the humerus. The chondral fragments can be removed and the cartilage smoothed with gratifying results.

The following steps are imperative in the treatment of complete dislocation of the elbow:

1. One must first evaluate the circulation of the hand.

2. The nerve function of the hand must be determined before manipulation.

Figure 208. Fracture of olecranon after excision of broken tip and repair of tendon to olecranon. Excellent functional result.

3. Reduction must be completely atraumatic.

4. Careful x-ray study should be made after reduction *before* the splint is applied.

5. Appropriate treatment must be instituted for accompanying fractures about the elbow.

6. The elbow must be immobilized by plaster splints. It is not sufficient to simply use a sling.

7. Early forceful passive stretching of the elbow must *not* be carried out.

8. Patient, active rehabilitation will usually result in normal function.

FRACTURE

A complete discussion of fracture of the elbow, which is a large subject indeed, is not necessary here, the reader being referred to the many excellent standard texts on treatment of fractures. However, there are certain peculiarities in the management of athletes with fracture about the elbow that should be emphasized.

A fracture of the elbow in a growing child is an extremely serious injury. The anatomical structure of the elbow is such that in a child a supracondylar fracture, like a dislocation, may cause irreparable damage to the blood vessels, which may catch over the end of the bone, with resulting impairment of the circulation. The fascia of the forearm is relatively inelastic and subject to intense pressure by swelling, which may result in irreparable damage to the forearm and hand (Fig. 209). Anyone who has seen or treated a case of Volkmann's contracture (Fig. 210) knows what a catastrophe it is. Of particular significance is the acute ischemia resulting from arterial spasm. This is contrasted sharply with the swelling of the hand resulting from venous congestion. The hand is cold and white and feels numb. There is no capillary pulse. This is an extreme emergency and much more serious than ordinary congestion and swelling. It probably will not be relieved by ordinary measures such as straightening the elbow. It is obvious that any gross displacement at the fracture site should be completely reduced, particularly if there is anterior displacement. However, this condition may not be relieved by simple release of the pressure.

This syndrome demands immediate stellate ganglion block and immersion of the opposite hand alternately into ice and hot water. If such measures do not result in prompt restoration of circulation, the artery should be explored by incision in the antecubital fossa. The artery must be inspected and, if caught on a bony fragment, must be released. Often the artery is free but in spasm. Stripping of this artery often relieves the spasm and restores circulation. If the artery is lacerated or severed, it must be repaired, replaced or ligated. Simple ligation often relieves spasm and permits the collateral circulation to supply the distal area, but repair is better.

I know of no injury that requires more skill in management than the fractured elbow in a

Figure 209. Gangrene of the arm following a neglected fracture of the elbow. Amputation just below the shoulder was necessary.

Figure 210. Volkmann's contracture—final result. This is an essentially useless arm and hand despite yeoman efforts at rehabilitation, including extensive surgery.

child. I make it an invariable rule to obtain x-ray films of both elbows and try to ignore any preconceived notions of what normal should be. By actually comparing one side with the other, one can usually determine whether or not there is any displacement of fragments or disturbance of the normal relationships at the elbow.

Avulsion Fracture

In a previous section I discussed fracture of the epicondyle in relation to dislocation. This same fracture may occur as an avulsion fracture as a result of muscle violence without dislocation of the elbow. Not infrequently the medial epicondyle is pulled off by massive flexor pronator muscle contraction, together with abduction stress on the forearm, without dislocation of the elbow. This avulsion will be of the muscle and lateral ligament attachments at the elbow (Fig. 211). An identical force may completely avulse all or a portion of the flexor pronator muscle group at the elbow. I have seen this happen most often in football players who use maximum exertion and terrific force in order to "throw the bomb." In this effort, the whole aponeurosis may be pulled off without any bone, or a single strip of it may be pulled off, such as the flexor carpi ulnaris and the flexors to the ring and little fingers. This acute injury is manifested by severe pain, early swelling, tenderness and particularly pain during the pronation-flexion function. The symptoms are more severe with avulsion of the muscle and aponeurosis than with avulsion of the epicondyle itself. Avulsion of the epicondyle occurs before the epiphysis is united in the young patient, whereas a muscle avulsion occurs after the epiphysis is closed in an older person. Treatment for this condition is ob-

viously replacement of the aponeurosis by direct suture. This should be done as early as possible, since, as pointed out elsewhere, contracture of the muscle soon makes it difficult to replace the aponeurosis. However, if it comes off in a single mass, it may well be replaced with the elbow flexed and the forearm supinated. The treatment for delayed avulsion is a reconstructive problem, which may require some muscle substitutions.

Perhaps of even more concern, since it is so readily overlooked, is the circumstance of violent muscle contraction (as in throwing) which separates the apophysis from the major bone but does not grossly displace it. X-ray pictures often appear to be negative. However, if they are carefully compared with those of the opposite side, the epiphyseal line of the injured arm will appear slightly wider than that of the normal arm (Fig. 212). In these instances the injury does not seem to be too severe, but the recovery is very slow and often the symptoms increase rather than improve with the passage of time. The young athlete suffers distressing recurrence of elbow pain and ineffectiveness in the use of his arm, usually with restriction of extension. This condition should be treated by immobilization for a relatively short time, four to six weeks, until the major bone and the apophysis have reunited. Immobilization should be with the forearm supinated if the lateral epicondyle is involved and pronated if the medial condyle is involved. The apophysis ordinarily will continue to grow without any further symptoms. Anytime a young pitcher or quarterback complains of pain on the inner side of the elbow and x-ray film findings appear to be negative, the physician's index of suspicion should be quite high. In some instances, as indicated in Figure 211, the incomplete displacement will become complete, at which time it is difficult to obtain a normal elbow.

It is possible for the olecranon to be avulsed by violent contraction of the triceps as the forearm is forcibly flexed, but this is unusual. If there is a complete fracture of the olecranon by such a force, the triceps attachement is, of course, disrupted. This should be repaired surgically, regardless of the size of the fragment. If there is simply a "skin" of bone pulled off, it should be treated exactly as tendon avulsion—namely, removal of the fragment and suture of the tendon to bone. If the fragment is larger, it should be attached to the olecranon by internal fixation. The olecranon process fits into the trochlear fossa of the humerus, and perfect positioning of the frag-

Figure 211. *A,* Normal elbow. *B,* Anteroposterior view showing an old epicondylar fracture with displacement of the fragment downward. At the time of operation it was impossible to replace this greatly enlarged epiphysis. It was removed and the aponeurosis sutured to the epicondylar ridge.

ment is necessary to assure normal function. This cannot be obtained in the usual case by immobilization of the elbow in complete extension. Then, too, accurate and firm internal fixation permits rapid rehabilitation, whereas immobilization of the elbow in extension for a period long enough to permit the olecranon to unite will give rise to a great deal of difficulty in obtaining normal flexion later.

Direct contusion of the olecranon with the elbow flexed may result in fracture of the olecranon process. This may be comminuted and accompanied by anterior dislocation of the forearm on the humerus. This dislocation is usually spontaneously reduced before the patient is examined. Careful manipulation may determine whether or not there is instability of the ligaments in this direction. If this dislocation has been present, it greatly complicates the recovery. If the olecranon is broken, it may be replaced and held by internal fixation. It may be necessary to remove some of the comminuted fragments in order to prevent overgrowth of callus. If the fragments are small and at the proximal tip, they may be removed and the triceps sutured to the remaining olecranon.

BURSITIS

The olecranon bursa lying between the tip of the olecranon and the skin is the bursa most commonly involved in bursitis at the elbow (Fig. 213).

Acute Bursitis

Acute contusion to the point of the elbow usually results in hemorrhage into the olecranon bursa. The bursa distends with blood and there is synovial irritation. If this injury is seen early, the blood may be aspirated and a pressure dressing applied. This will ordinarily relieve the conditions, although it may be necessary to aspirate more than once. More frequently, the condition does not receive early care, since the symptoms and disability may not seem severe. The synovial irritation continues and a chronic bursitis ensues.

Occasionally following an injury or indeed without injury, an infection occurs within the bursa and an acute suppurative bursitis ensues. The area is hot, inflamed and red, and the patient presents the ordinary signs of infection

Figure 212. This 11 year old male when pitching four weeks ago threw very forcibly off balance to first base and had right elbow pain. He tried to continue to pitch but had to quit. The elbow swelled. On examination everything appeared to be negative. He gradually improved until he tried to pitch again. Every time he tried to throw his condition worsened. On examination his complaint was all around the medial epicondyle. There was thickening but not gross swelling. There was pain particularly in gripping and pronating the forearm against resistance. *A,* X-ray shows the right elbow with what might be interpreted as a normal epiphyseal plate until compared with that of the opposite elbow (*B*). You will notice that the epiphyseal plate is narrower and smaller. Even in four weeks' time the epiphysis had enlarged in size and traversed downward a few millimeters. Ultimately this may well have regressed to the point of that in Figure 211. The patient was treated by immobilization for another four weeks, with uneventful recovery except for some enlargement of the epicondyle.

with malaise and fever and pain, restriction of motion, tenderness and swelling of the elbow. If upon examination the bursa is found to be full of fluid, it should be aspirated and a culture made of the specimen. In the meantime the

Figure 213. Olecranon bursitis.

arm is immobilized in a sling and treated with the continuous application of hot packs. An appropriate broad-spectrum antibiotic should be given in the hope that the acute inflammation will subside without the necessity for drainage. If the symptoms persist and aspiration does not relieve the effusion, the bursa should be drained surgically. Usually following acute inflammation and drainage, the bursal walls become adherent, and this automatically cures the bursitis. For the duration of the acute inflammation, it is important that the arm be immobilized to avoid constant movement of the elbow. This is particularly true if an incision has been necessary. We advise an incision at either side of the bursa and the use of a through-and-through tissue drain, which should be removed in a few days as the inflammation subsides. Occasionally the infection will progress to spontaneous rupture of the bursa, since the skin over the back of the elbow is rather thin. The rupture usually occurs at the point of the olecranon and may leave a painful, adherent scar.

Much more frequently the bursitis is not suppurative. Because of synovial irritation, the bursa simply fills up with fluid, causing tension within the sac. This should be treated by aspiration, followed by injection of a corticoid into the bursa and use of a pressure dressing. Repeated aspiration may be necessary, but with proper treatment, the acute bursitis will usually subside without apparent residual.

Chronic Bursitis

Since acute bursitis is frequently overlooked, minimized or undertreated, chronic bursitis of the olecranon bursa is quite common. In this case the sac gradually enlarges, at times becoming quite tense with fluid. At other times the bursa is simply boggy and thick. Through the course of many weeks and months, some of these bursae attain amazing size. The author has seen some as large as 7 inches long and 4 inches wide—a veritable bag of water dangling from the point of the elbow. When seen in the early stages, bursitis can often be relieved by aspiration, injection of a corticoid and application of a pressure dressing, with the aspiration repeated at suitable intervals to prevent tension within the sac. Once the chronic bursitis is well established, surgical excision is usually the only means of obtaining permanent relief. Cartilaginous, or occasionally calcific, nodules may develop in the floor of the bursa which are readily palpable beneath the skin. They may become quite tender to pressure, giving rise to severe discomfort, particularly when one rests his weight on the elbow. Surgical excision is simple, since easy access to this area can be obtained. It is important to remove all of the bursa. Tacking the redundant skin to the underlying tissue may serve to prevent reaccumulation of fluid in the space and hence recurrence of the bursitis. Immobilization is imperative and must be continued until the wound is healed (three weeks).

Radiohumeral Bursitis

Radiohumeral bursitis is frequently called tennis elbow and is frequently confused with epicondylitis. The radiohumeral bursa lies directly under the flexor pronator aponeurosis, and it permits the aponeurosis to slide freely over the humeral condyle and the radial capsule. Gripping causes pressure on this area, with resultant pain, simply by tensing the aponeurosis over the bursa, if the latter is inflamed. There usually is not sufficient bursal fluid to cause fluctuation. On examination the tenderness is localized over the radial head rather than over the epicondyle.

This condition responds well to local treatment with injection of a long-acting local anesthetic and a corticoid, followed by elimination of the movements that cause pain. Indeed, it responds very well to the same therapy that relieves an epicondylitis.

Figure 214. X-ray of right (A) and left (B) elbows of professional football player who had gradually increasing disability culminating in sharp restriction of motion of the right elbow after he fell on his elbow. This is a chronic traumatic arthritis which markedly improved by surgical removal of the foreign bodies and spurs. No other joints were involved.

OSTEOCHONDROSES

Osteochondritis dissecans of the elbow is not common except in people who engage in certain activities. The baseball pitcher, for example, is very prone to injury of the articular cartilage with resulting "joint mice," pitting of the cartilage and chondromalacia. X-ray diagnosis of osteochondritis dissecans in articular cartilage at the elbow is difficult. Usually it is not seen until the fragment becomes detached. Indeed, it appears that the deposits may be largely in the nature of concretions formed within the joint as the result of chrondral tags and synovial irritation. Although these occasionally reach an amazing size, they are usually very small and give trouble simply by being impinged between the olecranon and the back

Figure 215. This 14 year old male was wrestling and fell on his left elbow several weeks before I saw him. His complaints were gradually increasing pain on motion, pain as he raised the arm, popping in the elbow when he rotated it and severe pain on snapping the elbow straight. He was comfortable in his sling. On examination there was tenderness on the lateral condyle at the joint line. Neither the radial head nor the epicondyle was tender. Surgical incision revealed a large foreign body consisting of a major portion of the lateral condyle, lying completely free in the joint. This left a gross defect that had been tentatively diagnosed as a cyst. The bed was relatively fresh bleeding bone. Treatment was removal of the fragment and drilling of the bed. A, X-ray shows the radiolucent area adjacent to the subchondral bone on the lateral condyle that could be interpreted as being a cyst, chondroblastoma or chondral fracture. Arrow points to the defect, B. C, Surgical photograph of the lateral condyle with the fragment in situ held in Kelly forceps. D, The defect and the fragment removed from the joint. Note the relatively fresh bed indicating recent injury.

of the humerus. Surgical removal is quite successful, although repetition of the same activity that caused them to form may cause recurrence (Fig. 214). At the time of removal the joint should be carefully explored and any suspicious areas of loose cartilage carefully trimmed away. The joint should be thoroughly lavaged to wash out small rice bodies. If the foreign bodies appear to be the result of chronic synovitis, the elbow can be treated by the usual measures of injection, application of heat locally and protection. In chronic synovitis, extensive effusion in the elbow is not common. The capsule is not redundant and is not prone to distend as it does in other joints during acute inflammation. Complete avoidance of the forceful action that caused the condition may be necessary to prevent prompt recurrence.

Osteochondral Fracture of the Capitellum

One type of osteochondral fracture or osteochondritis dissecans is frequently overlooked and misdiagnosed. The complaint is of pain in the lateral side of the joint, not in the radial head or on the epicondyle of the humerus but on the condyle itself, right at the joint line down to the articular margin. Knowledge of a history of a previous fall on an outstretched hand or some similar trauma may be helpful, since this type of injury would force the radial head directly into the arc of the capitellar articular cartilage. The injury may have been seriously symptomatic at the time, very similar to osteochondritis dissecans at the knee. The complaint is of aching pain and especially of pain on forced snap extension of the elbow, as in throwing a baseball. X-ray examination may be negative, but often the x-ray film reveals a cystic-appearing radiolucency within the capitellum extending down toward the articular cartilage. This may be diagnosed as a chondroblastoma. This location is typical for this tumor insofar as the articular cartilage is concerned, although the elbow is not as common a location for this lesion as is the knee—or it may be called a bone cyst. Although it does not have a trabeculation one might expect to find in a multilocular cyst, it has the appearance of a unicameral bone cyst (Fig. 215). At surgery the true pathological condition is revealed, namely, a large osteochondral fragment including the articular cartilage. The fragment leaves a gross defect in the articular portion of the capitellum. If the fragment is large and fairly fresh, it may be replaced and pinned in situ. Usually it has become chronic, and the best treatment is to remove the fragment and curette the bed down to bleeding bone. If the bed is sclerotic it should be treated by curetting out the fibrous tissue and then by drilling multiple small holes, using a Kirschner wire, into the bed. Since the elbow is non–weight-bearing, the results are predictably good. Whether the defect fills with fibrocartilage or hyalincartilage, it seems to function well. Repeat operation is rare, fortunately, so that we can only speculate on the anatomical result. Functionally the result is very satisfactory, especially in the young person (under 18 years of age) in whom osteochondral fracture of the capitellum frequently occurs.

10
Injuries of the Forearm

ANATOMICAL CONSIDERATIONS

Although to a large extent injuries to the forearm concern function of the wrist and hand, there are certain anatomical considerations in the forearm proper that merit review (Fig. 216). Whereas in the upper arm there is a single bone surrounded by a mass of muscle, the forearm contains two bones with the rather complex interrelated movements that were described in the chapter on the elbow. The ulna, being large at the elbow and small at the wrist, provides good stability between the humerus and the forearm. This humeroulnar articulation permits motion in only one plane, flexion and extension. The ulna is fixed to the humerus and does not rotate, so that the position to the entire shaft of the ulna is constant in relation to the upper arm. At the lower forearm the radius is the larger bone, and it alone articulates with the carpus. The radiocarpal joint is of the ball and socket type, which permits motion in any direction. The range of motion permitted is attributable to ligamentous limi-

tations rather than to any bony block. The axial relationship of the radius to the carpus and hand is constant in the sense that there is little rotary motion between the carpus and the radius. Pronation-supination of the hand occurs by the rolling of the radius and carpus as a unit around the axis of the fixed ulna.

While the two bones of the forearm are essentially parallel to each other, the radius arches enough to allow considerable space between it and the ulna in the middle third, but they are in contact at the proximal and the distal radioulnar joints. The integrity of these two joints is entirely ligamentous. Each joint consists of a small saucerlike bed for the radial head at the upper end of the ulna and a small fossa for the ulna on the lower radius. The two bones are firmly bound together by the interosseous membrane. The fibers of this membrane are interdigitated and decussated so as to permit rotation of the radius over the ulna while maintaining constant tension of some of their fibers. The upper end of the radius is firmly fastened to the ulna by the

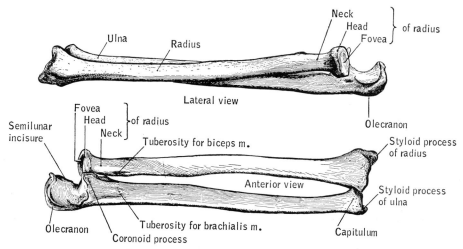

Figure 216. The bony anatomy of the forearm.

orbicular ligament. At the distal end the ulna is bound to the radius by a similar arrangement, so that these ligaments give considerable inherent stability to the two joints. On either side of the interosseous membrane lie the blood vessels and nerves. An extremely intricate complex of muscles attaches along the shafts of the two bones. The synergistic action of these muscles carries out all the complicated motions of the wrist and hand, each of the muscles having a somewhat different function, depending upon the relative position of the hand and the forearm and the arm.

This is not the place for a more detailed discussion of the anatomy of the forearm. The reader is urged to consult a good atlas of anatomy, and he is bound to be amazed by the ingenuity with which the function of the hand is assured. The entire dorsal surface of the ulna is subcutaneous, so that from the tip of the olecranon to the ulnar styloid the bone can readily be palpated beneath the skin. The only subcutaneous areas on the radius are at its proximal and distal extremities.

CONTUSION

The forearm is very subject to contusion because of the substantial area of subcutaneous bone. This is doubly true because the forearm is toward the distal extremity of the most active member of the body and often comes in violent contact with an opposing player or an obstacle. Hence, a contusion may result from a fall on the olecranon process with the elbow flexed or from a direct blow against the subcutaneous shaft of the ulna.

Contusion of the Skin

In either cause of contusion, the result is damage to the skin with typical excoriation, pain, local swelling and hematoma. The most frequent complications that may arise are olecranon bursitis at the elbow and a periostitis along the ulna. Ordinarily, contusion of the skin leads to minimal disability and *treatment* should be largely of a local nature: aspiration of the hematoma, injection of long-acting anesthetic and application of a pressure dressing followed by application of cold in the early stages, to be subsequently changed to heat. The area can be adequately protected by a pressure pad and usually the injury need not interfere with athletic participation. Chronic periostitis, if it results, may require more com-

prehensive treatment, with injection of a corticoid and more extensive physical therapeutic measures.

Contusion Involving the Musculotendinous Structures

Of more consequence than contusion of the skin is contusion involving the musculotendinous structures. This is particularly pertinent in the lower forearm, where the tendons become subcutaneous as they converge toward the carpal tunnel on the volar side and toward the extensor aponeurosis on the dorsum of the wrist. In these circumstances if a tendon and its sheath are caught between the striking object and the underlying bone, a serious and disabling *traumatic tenosynovitis* may result. In this condition there is a history of a direct blow followed by discomfort of a moderate degree. After 12 to 36 hours the pain increases and is particularly aggravated by motion of the part involved. For example, if the extensor carpi ulnaris tendon is involved, there will be pain on dorsiflexion of the wrist against resistance, pain on passive palmar flexion of the wrist and pain on gripping. All these activities are essential to athletic competition. If the tendon happens to be the long supinator, the pain will be on function of this muscle, and so on. A careful analysis of the symptoms involved must be made to determine which tendon is involved. Usually the pain is well localized over the area of the contusion.

Treatment of a traumatic tenosynovitis demands rest of the involved tendon. It is completely futile to try to "work it out," or to use extensive physical therapy and at the same time encourage use. The part must be put at functional rest and the best criterion of the adequacy of immobilization is relief of pain. *Painful motion should be eliminated.* This may mean restriction of motion of the wrist in either rotation or flexion and extension and also interdiction of gripping. If a little time is taken to explain to the athlete the purpose of not exercising the involved part to the extent of causing pain, he can usually be permitted to exercise just short of the pain-producing movement and so continue his rehabilitation to some extent. Local treatment is of value, and injection of the involved tendon sheath with local anesthetic and one of the corticoid preparations is worthwhile. Care should be taken not to inject into the tendon, which not only is ineffective but also may cause degenerative changes in the avascular tendon. Use of a local anesthetic and of corticoids is, however, more successful in the chronic than in the acute stage. In the acute stage rest, local heat and protection will usually result in good recovery. Recovery is likely to be more complete following a tenosynovitis caused by contusion than one caused by strain. Very frequently a chronic tenosynovitis results from strain. This will be discussed later on.

Another complication of contusion is *fracture*. If the condition appears to be severe, the bone tenderness is acute, and function is painful, careful x-ray study should be done to rule out fracture.

Contusion higher in the forearm involving the belly of the muscle is similar in nature to muscular contusion anywhere else and requires the same treatment, namely, aspiration of the hematoma, local injection of an anesthetic, compression, application of cold followed by heat and protection against motion. However, contusion of the muscles of the forearm presents an additional problem in that the motions of these muscles are extremely complex and so may cause considerably more disability for a given degree of contusion than elsewhere in the body. Very early rehabilitative use of the fingers can nevertheless be permitted, always short of pain. Protection may consist simply of prevention of competition and careful instruction. For certain sports it is possible to support the wrist and wrap the forearm so that the injured muscle can be protected. This extensive wrapping should be carefully removed once competition is over to permit resumption of pain-free function.

STRAIN

Strain is a common problem in the forearm, where many tendons glide together in the same sheath or separately. Any one of these musculotendinous units may be subject to strain from overexertion caused by a single active contraction of the muscle against too much resistance, from overstretching of the musculotendinous unit or from chronic overuse of the unit. The unit may be damaged by the actual disruption of some of its fibers by stretching, by a single violent contraction of the muscle beyond its capacity or by repeated contractions of the muscle beyond its fatigue quotient.

Acute Strain

In acute strain the symptoms are pain along the area of strain, usually at the musculoten-

dinous junction or at the attachment of the tendon to the bone. At this stage, overstretching or active contraction of the unit will cause pain at the area of strain. As the condition continues, a tenosynovitis develops with irritation between the tendon and its sheath or mesotendon. This results in hyperemia, local swelling, inflammation and exudation of fluid. As the tendon continues to slide within the irritated sheath, sticky adhesions result and the so-called "snowball crepitation" is elicited; i.e., with the finger over the tendon, soft crepitation can be felt as the tendon slides up and down the sheath. This motion is painful and becomes increasingly so as use is continued. If the condition progresses, the tenosynovitis may become adhesive, in which state the tendon fails to slide and dense adhesions form between the tendon and sheath. In other circumstances the tendon itself thickens and becomes constricted by its sheath.

If the strain is in the muscle belly, the pain will be muscular and more diffuse. This results from either congestion within the muscle, or rupture of some of the muscle fibers, or both. In extreme cases the strain may be so severe that continued use may cause a rupture somewhere in the unit. This may be of the fibers of the muscle itself or at the origin of the muscle or the attachment of the tendon. Very careful analysis of the condition will permit one to determine the exact location and nature of injury and so suggest the treatment. Only by careful examination can one properly regulate the treatment of acute strain, since it will vary from no specific treatment to surgical repair of the lacerated unit.

Treatment of the acute strain depends upon the severity of the condition and the exact unit involved. The principles of treatment are rest, use of heat locally and protection of the injured area. In the very early stage an ice pack and compression bandage may be used, particularly if hemorrhage within the muscle is suspected. Within a few hours, cold should give way to local heat. Until the severity of the condition is determined, it is wise to immobilize the forearm in a position that will relax the involved unit. If the muscles to the fingers are involved, immobilization should include the hand. A word of caution should be sounded against prolonged immobilization of the fingers. In the first place, the fingers do not tolerate immobilization well and the joints tend to stiffen very rapidly. In the second place, active unresisted motion of the fingers will put very little strain on the injured area, the exception being a case of acute tenosynovitis involving the tendons to the fingers themselves.

The strain and, indeed, the resulting tenosynovitis much more commonly involve the muscles to the wrist, so that immobilization is adequate if it terminates at the distal palmar crease with the wrist placed in the slight cock-up position. Careful inspection of the forearm should be carried out at frequent intervals to determine the progress of the condition. As soon as unresisted movement of the wrist is pain-free, complete immobilization may be discontinued and protection substituted. In a strain of moderate severity, pain-free movement will usually be possible in a week or ten days. If the condition has gone on to tenosynovitis, the treatment must be more prolonged and more intensive, with absolute immobilization of the affected tendon and the administration of some sort of inductive heat that can be given through the splint. Once crepitation is detected, any further testing should not be carried out for at least a week, since repeated irritation only encourages adhesions, and complete rest will permit resolution of the lesion. There is no place for local injection in the treatment of acute tenosynovitis. Only occasionally will there be sufficient fluid in the tendon sheath to justify aspiration.

Chronic Strain

Management of chronic strain can be extremely difficult for the physician and disheartening to the athlete. In the usual case the strain is caused by the very activity that the athlete wants to carry out and resumption will cause its recurrence. The condition should be managed by rest and application of heat to the injury. Careful analysis of the cause of the strain may reveal some unusual habit or posture that can be altered to place less strain on the involved muscle. As in so many conditions, it is important that use of the muscle be held within the limits of discomfort and pain and that overuse be carefully avoided. In the management of chronic tenosynovitis the same general dicta apply. In this circumstance, however, local treatment is of considerable value, and injection of a corticoid into the involved tendon sheath may speed up the recovery markedly. There are no areas in the forearm proper in which constricting tenosynovitis is a problem. (See de Quervain's disease, page 259, and Carpal Tunnel syndrome, page 261.)

FRACTURE

The forearm is a common location for a fracture in the young individual, usually caused by a fall on the outstretched arm. Hence, in any instance following a fall in which there is pain with swelling and disability, fracture should be suspected. X-ray examination of the forearm is easy and should be carried out in case of any doubt. One common error in x-ray examination is to obtain anteroposterior and lateral views by simply rotating the hand on the film. This does not rotate the ulna, however, and while it results in anteroposterior and lateral views of the radius, the ulna is shown in the same plane. Radiographic study of the forearm illustrates very well the rule that the adjacent joints should be visualized on x-ray. In making an x-ray of the forearm, the elbow and the wrist should be included. If there is any suspicion of epiphyseal separation or of some abnormality of the forearm, films of the opposite extremity should be taken for comparison.

A detailed discussion of the *treatment* of fractures of the forearm will not be given here, since it is available in many good textbooks on fractures. A few points pertinent to the athlete should be mentioned, however.

Since the radius rotates around the ulna in pronation-supination of the forearm, one should be particularly careful to immobilize the elbow in case of fracture of the radius, even at its distal end. An undisplaced fracture of the radius may become displaced by rotation of the forearm.

The so-called *greenstick fracture*, in which the forearm is bent and one cortex of the radius or ulna is broken and the other is intact, may trap the unwary clinician. It is extremely easy to simply straighten the bone out and apply a splint or indeed a circular cast. Often as the fracture heals, however, the deformity recurs, and on removing the splint, marked bowing of the forearm bones is found (Fig. 217). This is particularly likely to happen if a solid cast is used, since the cast becomes loose as the muscles atrophy and the swelling subsides. As a general rule, the greenstick fracture should be completely broken, and this will usually require anesthesia. An exception is in the youngster in whom the dorsal cortex at the lower end of the forearm is buckled by a fracture equivalent to a Colles' fracture in the adult. The angulation can sometimes be straightened by a quick snap without anes-

Figure 217. *A*, Greenstick fracture of lower radius. *B*, Reduced and in splint without breaking the dorsal cortex. *C*, Recurrence of deformity in splint. This deformity may correct spontaneously, since the child was only seven years old and modeling was already beginning. Surgery is not indicated.

thesia. Following fracture of the forearm, the young athlete should wear some protection on this arm for several weeks.

Typical *Colles' fracture* is quite unusual in the athlete, since ordinarily there will be a distal radial epiphyseal dislocation or fracture slightly higher in the forearm.

Subluxation of the distal radial epiphysis has considerable significance and requires careful handling in order to minimize the danger of growth disturbance. If the pain of the so-called strained wrist is actually at the lower end of the radius, x-ray examination is mandatory. If the x-ray shows any abnormality in the epiphyseal plate, films of the opposite wrist should be made for careful comparison. Many times the so-called sprained wrist will actually be a slipping off of the epiphysis (Fig. 218). In this instance the subluxation either was incomplete or was spontaneously reduced. In spite of normal-appearing x-rays, there will be persistent pain along the distal radial epiphyseal plate. Even if there is no displacement, the wrist should be immobilized until this tenderness disappears. If the epiphysis is displaced (Fig. 219), it should be reduced promptly and completely with as little trauma as possible. In any case of real or suspected damage to the epiphysis, the parents should be warned of the possibility of growth disturbance with consequent radial shortening (Fig. 220). This does not occur often but may be quite deforming

when it does. This same type of injury may result in a dislocation extending partially through the plate, with a fracture extending up the radial shaft (Fig. 221). This also requires very careful reduction. Growth disturbance here may lead not only to overall shortening but also to angulation, which is even more distressing than shortening. The patient's condition should be very carefully followed, and if angulation begins, the viable part of the epiphysis should be closed to prevent increasing deformity.

Complete fractures of both bones of the forearm in the adolescent or adult are extremely difficult to reduce properly and hold in position by external means. One must bear in mind that in this category of patients, correction of the deformity by growth modeling will not take place. The beneficent effects of further growth, which are so notable in the child, will not be seen. Forearm fractures with displacement illustrate well the aphorism that fractures do not spontaneously improve in the splint. If the reduction looks bad before the splint is applied, it will look worse when the splint is removed. There is no place for unguarded optimism in the management of a fracture in the athlete. Every effort must be made to restore the bones to their normal position. This is particularly true in the forearm, where the interrelationships with the wrist and hand are extremely intricate.

Figure 218. "Sprain" of the wrist. Note the buckling of the dorsal cortex which indicates that this is the same injury as shown in Figure 219, which either was spontaneously reduced or was incomplete to start with. No reduction necessary. Splints should be applied. Note that the displacement is actually through the distal radial epiphysis.

Figure 219. A, Epiphyseal dislocation of lower radius. Note the fragmentation of the dorsal cortex, indicating that a part of the epiphysis is probably intact. Should premature closure occur in one portion of this epiphysis and not in another, deformity may occur. B, Atraumatic but complete reduction gives some insurance against premature closure.

Figure 220. Radial shortening from epiphyseal disturbance some years following epiphyseal fracture of the lower radius. Note complete dislocation of the distal radioulnar joint, the ulna being distal to and behind the carpus. This was extremely disabling. Correction was carried out by the shortening of the ulna and osteotomy of the radius.

Figure 221. *A,* Fracture-dislocation of lower epiphysis of the radius. Note the epiphyseal dislocation on the palmar two thirds of the plate, with fracture of the shaft dorsally. *B,* Early accurate repositioning minimizes the chances of epiphyseal disturbance and growth deformity.

Figure 222. This 19 year old male was playing football and fell on the outstretched left hand, after which another player fell across his arm. He heard a cracking and had severe pain in the forearm with obvious instability. An air splint was applied and he was sent to the hospital. *A,* X-ray shows the fracture with the forearm in the air splint. Complete overriding of both bones. Closed reduction was impossible. *B,* Open reduction was readily carried out with a plate on the radius and intramedullary pin in the ulna. *C,* The ulna failed to unite. The pin was removed and bone graft applied, with excellent union. Note proper spacing between radius and ulna with slight bowing of the radius away from the ulna. This is extremely important in the function of the forearm. He missed one season of football.

One must pay particular attention to the alignment of the two parallel bones in the forearm (Fig. 222). In the child, some correction of malalignment may be expected with growth, particularly in the axis of flexion of the adjacent joint. Hence, some posterior or anterior bowing may be acceptable in the adolescent. However, lateral angulation with relative shortening or lengthening of one bone does not correct with growth or with modeling. The bone itself may appear to be straight, but the length will not increase. Therefore an angulation at the wrist is inevitable. This deviation, usually radial, not only will be disfiguring but also will be disabling to some extent. Therefore, in the adolescent or young adult, accurate realignment and correction of short-ening are imperative, even if this should require open reduction and internal fixation.

Fractures of both bones of the forearm in this age group are major injuries requiring excellent care and are fraught with the dangers of disfigurement and disability. Definitive treatment initiated early will be extremely gratifying. One must not shrink from open reduction if this is required to obtain perfect function. The adolescent is not a "child" and must not be treated as one. In treatment of fractures of both bones of the forearm, we should use that method which has the best chance of restoring normal function of the extremity. (See page 268 for distal radial-ulnar dislocation.)

11

Injuries of the Wrist

ANATOMICAL CONSIDERATIONS

The wrist covers the area from the distal end of the radius and ulna to the proximal end of the metacarpals (Figs. 223 and 224). This includes the eight carpal bones, the proximal articular surfaces of the metacarpals, the distal articular surface of the radius and the fibrocartilage at the distal end of the ulna. There is no articulation between the ulna and the carpus, the two being separated by the triangular fibrocartilaginous disc, which also separates the wrist joint proper from the distal radioulnar joint (Fig. 225). The shallow concavity of the distal end of the radius is extended ulnarward by the articular disc, which thus serves to broaden the carpal articulation. At the radiocarpal joint the proximal row of carpal bones together form a smooth convex surface that articulates with the concavity at the lower end of the radius.

The amazing complexities of the articulations of the carpal bones will not be discussed in detail here. It is important to recognize the relationships of these bones to one another and to the forearm and hand. The greater part of the motion at the wrist takes place between the carpals as a unit and the radius. However, there is a definite amount of motion in each of the intercarpal joints. The navicular bone, the most radial of the proximal row, is long and boat-shaped and extends distally to bridge the proximal and distal carpal rows. It is the only carpal bone that is in both rows, and therefore it is much more subject to injury. In a transection through the wrist the capitate and, to a lesser extent the hamate, extend proximally into a concavity formed by the navicular, lunate and triquetrum bones. The two multangular bones are relatively short. Thus, the navicular extends across the two rows of the carpals, its distal portion actually

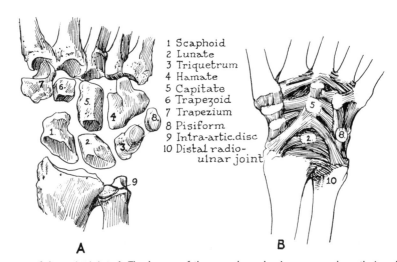

1 Scaphoid
2 Lunate
3 Triquetrum
4 Hamate
5 Capitate
6 Trapezoid
7 Trapezium
8 Pisiform
9 Intra-artic.disc
10 Distal radio-
      ulnar joint

A

B

Figure 223. Structure of the wrist joint. *A,* The bones of the carpal mechanism, opened on their volar surfaces, are irregular in size and shape but fit perfectly like the pieces of a jigsaw puzzle (after Grant). *B,* Many strong ligaments hold the carpal bones firmly in place, connecting their volar surfaces to the radius, the metacarpals and to each other.

The intra-articular disc separates the wrist joint from the distal radioulnar joint and acts as a soft-part hinge upon which the radius swings around the ulnar head in supination and pronation. (From McLaughlin, Trauma.)

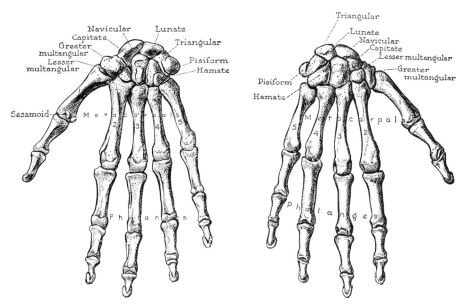

Figure 224. Palmar and dorsal aspects of bones of the right wrist and hand. (From Anson, Atlas of Human Anatomy.)

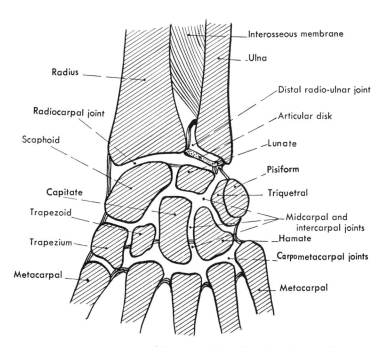

Figure 225. The bones and the joint cavities of the wrist. Note that the radiocarpal and inferior radio-ulnar joint cavities are separate and distinct; that the midcarpal joint is continuous with the intercarpal joints between both the proximal and the distal rows of the carpals; and that the carpometacarpal joints, except for that of the thumb, are continuous with the intermetacarpal joints and with the distal parts of the intercarpal joints, but have no communication with the midcarpal joint. (From Hollinshead, Functional Anatomy.)

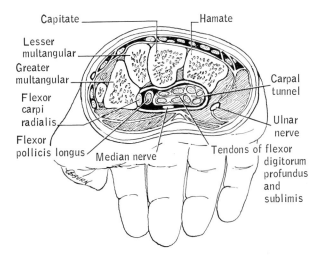

Figure 226. The carpal tunnel.

extending more than halfway down the length of the capitate, which makes it particularly vulnerable to injury on forceful motion through the midcarpal joint.

The entire lower end of the forearm and the metacarpals and carpals are firmly bound together by the volar carpal ligaments, which make a dense impenetrable ligamentous mass on the palmar surface of the wrist. Dorsally, the ligaments are much weaker. These volar ligaments, and particularly the radial and the ulnar collateral ligaments, have various main components. The pisiform bone actually lies within the tendon of the flexor carpi ulnaris, so that in effect this muscle attaches to the pisiform and in turn to the rest of the carpus through the strong ligaments extending from the pisiform bone to the metacarpals and to the hamate bone. Injury to the pisiform, therefore, is in a somewhat different category than injury to the other carpal bones.

In addition to the strong ligaments that bind these bones together, there is a heavy band, the volar carpal ligament, which extends from the greater multangular bone across to the hook of the hamate. By virtue of this ligamentous strap the volar carpal tunnel is formed, three sides of which are made up by the carpal bones themselves and the roof by the ligament (Fig. 226). Through this tunnel pass the flexor tendons to the fingers, together with the median nerve. This sets the stage for the carpal tunnel syndrome. On the medial aspect of the wrist, the ulnar artery and nerve enter the hand by passing through Guyon's canal, which is formed by the pisiform bone medially and by the volar carpal ligament anteriorly. Although the carpal bones are not subcutaneous

in a true sense, they are covered only by ligaments, tendons, blood vessels and nerves, there being no muscular pad in the vicinity of the wrist.

CONTUSION

Contusion of the wrist is a frequent occurrence in athletes. It is not usually caused by a fall but rather by a direct blow by a knee or headgear or foot when the player's outstretched hand is lying on the ground. Owing to the multiplicity of tendons in the wrist, the resulting injury is much more likely to involve them than the skin or bone. Hence, at the time of such an injury the wrist should be carefully examined for associated injury to the underlying structures. If the contusion seems severe, x-rays should be taken of the wrist not only in the anteroposterior and lateral but also in the right and left oblique planes. The carpal bones are not frequently fractured by a direct blow, unless there is an especially severe crushing injury. Tendon injury is quite common from contusion, and if overlooked or minimized, it may progress to a chronic tenosynovitis with all its attendant disability.

Treatment. Contusion of the wrist is treated by the usual measures, according to its severity. If there is any doubt as to underlying injury to either tendon or bone, a splint should be applied. If there is no involvement of the radioulnar joint, the splint may be limited to the forearm. A good test for the adequacy of the splint is to rotate the forearm through a complete arc of pronation-supination. If this causes pain, the splint should be placed above the elbow. In the early stage the splint may be incorporated into the compression bandage and an ice pack used. Ordinarily the contusion is not too severe and an elastic bandage wrapped over a protective pad will be adequate, more extensive treatment being reserved for any complications.

Laceration also is found fairly commonly in contusion of the wrist, although not as frequently as in the hand. This will be discussed in some detail in the section on the hand.

STRAIN

The general treatment of strain in this area was discussed in the section on the forearm. Since there are no muscles in the wrist proper, muscular strain does not occur here. However, this area is particularly vulnerable to tenosynovitis. The tenosynovitis may be the result of contusion of the tendon sheath if the tendon has been caught between a blunt object and the hard bone, or it may be caused by a single violent muscular contraction against resistance or by violent passive motion. The most common cause of tenosynovitis in the wrist, however, is chronic overuse. With the multiplicity of tendons in this area, tenosynovitis may become a highly complicated problem. It will require the usual type of treatment, namely, local injection, rest, heat and protection, as indicated earlier.

Tendon Rupture

Each of the many tendon attachments in the region of the wrist is subject to strain. Those particularly vulnerable are the flexors and extensors of the wrist. The same forces that cause tenosynovitis may rupture some of the tendon fibers at their attachment (second degree strain). Usually the force is a violent passive motion rather than an active contraction of the muscle. The history is of a fall with resultant pain at the site of the attachment of the tendon. The injury may easily be confused with contusion of the wrist or sprain or carpal fracture, the significant finding being pain on active contraction of the muscle involved. Thus, if the extensor carpi radialis is avulsed from its carpal attachment, active dorsiflexion of the wrist against resistance will cause pain. This is not ordinarily the case in a sprain or a fracture. If possible it is important to determine the degree of injury. The detachment is usually not complete.

Treatment. To relieve pain the wrist should be immobilized in the position in which the involved tendon is relaxed. If this tendon is an extensor, the wrist is put in the cock-up position. If it is a flexor, the wrist is placed in flexion. This immobilization, which is most readily accomplished by plaster splints, must continue until the healing is complete, after which the wrist is carefully protected for the remainder of the playing season against the particular motion that caused the injury.

If the condition becomes chronic and there is persistent tenderness at the site of the tendon attachment and discomfort on active use of the muscle, local treatment is of some value. In these instances we advise injection of the area with a long-acting local anesthetic, followed by injection of a corticoid preparation. Steroid injections should not be made directly into the tendon but into the peritendinous area. Necrosis of the tendon may occur if the injection is into its substance. A test of the effectiveness of the injection is that the pain and tenderness should be completely relieved following the anesthetic injection. This indicates that the condition has been correctly located. It should be remembered that many of these tendons have extensive insertions, particularly into the ligaments at the wrist and at the bases of the metacarpals. Following complete relief of pain and tenderness by anesthetic injection, a corticoid is injected into the same area. In the chronic condition it may not be necessary to immobilize the wrist completely, but the patient should be warned against any activity that causes discomfort. Some sort of wrist wrapping or strapping is advisable. Since the wrist flexors and extensors are tight whenever the fingers are made into a tight fist, forceful gripping should be discontinued during the treatment period, particularly if it causes discomfort. X-ray study should be carried out in any such condition involving the wrist. Occasionally the injury can be localized by visualization on the x-ray of a small flake of bone caused by avulsion of the tendon fibers.

If the detachment is complete (third degree strain), it should be repaired surgically.

Certain peculiar characteristics of the wrist predispose to the pathological entities discussed in the following sections.

deQuervain's Disease (Constrictive Tenosynovitis)

As the tendons to the thumb cross over the lower end of the radius on its radial aspect, they pass through tunnels made up of grooves on the lower end of the radius and a fibrous retinaculum forming the roof. In particular, the long abductor and short extensor of the thumb pass directly over the styloid process of the radius, and multiple tendons of the abductor may pass through the same sheath. This sheath is subcutaneous. Tenosynovitis in this area is quite common, usually as a result of overuse of the wrist and thumb. These tendons slide through the tunnel not only in movements of the thumb but also in movements of the wrist with the thumb fixed. As the condition progresses, the tendon tends to swell and the sheath to thicken, and a situation arises analogous to "trigger finger": While one tendon slides through the groove, another one hangs and doubles up. In the early stages it may then slip through the constriction with a palpable click (Fig. 227).

During the early stage of this condition, use of the wrist is increasingly painful. An actual swelling appears over the styloid of the radius, which on palpation is very firm and tender. At this stage the tendons will slide through the tunnel, although with discomfort. A good test for this condition is to grasp the flexed thumb with the fingers, thus fixing the thumb in flexion. Then adduct the wrist. This will cause severe pain in the area of the constriction, since by this maneuver all the tendons are forced through the tunnel at the same time. The condition may progress until no motion of these tendons through the tunnel is possible.

Treatment. If the condition is diagnosed in the early stage, treatment consists of immobilization of the wrist, including the thumb if motion of the thumb is painful. Injection of the tender area with a long-acting local anesthetic and a corticoid may have some value. Care should be taken not to perforate the

Figure 227. Stenosis of the two tendons in one osseo-fibrous canal. (K. L. Loomis, Journal of Bone and Joint Surgery, Vol. 33–A, 1951.)

tendons themselves with the needle, since this may increase the swelling or cause later necrosis. Application of heat locally is a useful adjunct, and if treatment is carried out promptly the condition should subside. Once it is established, constrictive tenosynovitis is very prone to recur.

Fortunately, surgical treatment is extremely effective. The skin incision is made transversely, directly across the radial styloid. Care should be taken not to penetrate deeper than the skin. The skin edges are carefully divided, revealing the cutaneous nerve, which passes directly over the styloid process. This should be protected. Careful dissection and retraction of the skin margins reveals the multicompartmental areas along the radial styloid, where there may be a single tendon through a single compartment, or there may be several tendons passing through one compartment, as indicated in Figure 228. At this point, a linear incision is made directly over the thickened roof of the involved tunnel. Since there are multiple compartments, it may be necessary to divide multiple areas linearly. Some of them will carry a single tendon and some multiple tendons. In addition to splitting the roof, it is advisable to cut out a definite section of it, approximately 2 to 3 mm. wide, so the two· parts cannot reunite and again become adherent. There are all sorts of variations in attachments (see Fig. 228). It is probably best to resect most of the roof of the tendon.

In a recent case in which there was actual snapping of the tendon from one tunnel to the other on lateral deviation of the wrist and particularly on flexion and extension of the thumb, the whole area was explored, and ridges were revealed between the various grooves. A prominent ridge between two of the grooves was shaved down and flattened off so that although the tendons might slide back and forth, they would not pop over an intervening ridge of bone. This is not a common finding, although it is often present in a case with relatively long continued popping. In this particular patient, there was already attrition in the extensor tendon, particularly in the abductor pollicus longus as it popped back and forth in and out of its groove.

In this major type of procedure, it is necessary to splint the arm for at least two weeks, and then to get the skin sutures out. The arm should then be protected again for another week or two, depending somewhat on the degree of reaction, before normal active motion is undertaken.

Figure 228. Variations in the insertion of the abductor pollicis longus tendon, associated with stenosing tenosynovitis. (T. Lacey II, H. L. Goldstein and C. E. Tobin, Journal of Bone and Joint Surgery, Vol. 33–A.)

Carpal Tunnel Syndrome

The carpal tunnel syndrome develops from unusual anatomical relationships on the volar aspect of the wrist. The eight flexor tendons of the fingers, the flexor pollicis longus and the flexor carpi radialis pass through the constricted confines of the carpal tunnel (see Fig. 226). The median nerve also passes through this canal. This vulnerable and compressible nerve lying in this confined space with the incompressible tendons is the innocent bystander that bears the brunt of early compression. The syndrome may be initiated by direct trauma, such as a fall on the outstretched hand, which causes swelling and thickening of the volar carpal ligament. It may be initiated by tenosynovitis of the flexor tendons. It is not an infrequent complication of an injury such as a Colles' fracture or indeed a fracture of any of the carpal bones. Occasionally, the injury is caused by an actual mass intruding into the tunnel. This may be a ganglion, an exostosis, a solid tumor, a fragment of one of the carpal bones, a dislocation of the carpal bones or an adventitious bursa. We recently had a case in which the typical findings were caused by a calcific mass, apparently a calcified bursa, within the tunnel itself (Fig. 229).

The essential ingredients of the carpal tunnel syndrome are swelling of the structures within the tunnel, or constriction of the tunnel, or both. Under these circumstances pressure on the median nerve is evidenced first by tingling in the distribution of the median nerve at the tips of the index and long fingers. The unwary

Fig. 229. Patient is a 20 year old female. Spontaneous onset of carpal tunnel syndrome, with typical gradual increase in pain and numbness of index and long fingers. X-rays show calcified mass in the carpal tunnel. *A*, Tunnel view showing mass. *B*, The opposite wrist for comparison (for x-ray positioning, see Fig. 230). *C*, Anteroposterior and lateral views of same patient.

physician may be deluded into believing that the involvement is in the fingers or in the nerve higher up in the arm. The characteristic distribution in the long and index fingers should lead one to suspect this condition. Careful examination then will elicit tenderness in response to deep pressure on the volar ligament, which may increase the pain and paresthesia in the median distribution. Atrophy of the thenar muscles is a late manifestation. The condition should be diagnosed long before this occurs.

X-rays. A careful radiographic study may be very valuable and should always be done.

Anteroposterior, lateral and right and left oblique views may reveal spurring, osteoarthritis or actual fracture. The carpal tunnel view is extremely important (Fig. 230). Comparative views of the opposite wrist must be done in all projections. The carpal tunnel view may show unusual configuration or, as in the case of the Fig. 229, invasion of the foreign substance.

Treatment. If the syndrome is diagnosed early, immobilization of the wrist may give relief, since it accomplishes two things. In the first place, it puts the swollen parts at rest and thus permits subsidence of the inflammation.

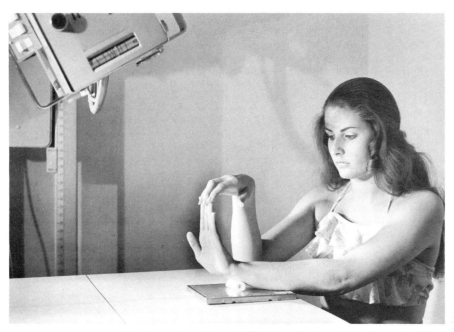

Figure 230. Radiographic position for view of carpal canal. With the patient seated at the end of the table, extend the forearm parallel with the long axis of the table. Center the radial styloid to the center of the cassette. Place a 2 cm. thickness roll of gauze or plastic foam under the wrist. Hyperextend the wrist until the hand is in a vertical position, slightly rotated radially to prevent superimposition of the hamate and pisiform bones. Let the patient hold this position with the opposite hand. With the tube angulated 25 to 30 degrees to the long axis of the hand, direct the central ray approximately 3 cm. above the base of the fourth metacarpal.

In the second place, it prevents the tendons from sliding up and down over the nerve. If the condition does not respond promptly to conservative treatment or if it shows signs of progression, it should be treated surgically. Surgical treatment is highly successful, but in this area it is not for the uninitiated.

Surgical Technique. A proper tourniquet is essential. After preparation of the skin, the hand is placed supine on a suitable table. There are several landmarks for the incision, which begins above the wrist directly over and parallel to the palmaris longus tendon as it passes down to its insertion into the palmar fascia. The incision is just to the ulnar side of the flexor carpi radialis tendon. It begins about 5 cm. above the distal carpal crease and extends down to this crease. At this point the cut passes laterally along this crease until the most proximal end of the thenar crease is reached. It then extends distally into the palm along the thenar crease to a point where the thenar muscle mass terminates (Fig. 231). The skin flap is reflected, including the attachment of the palmaris longus, which is left in the flap.

The palmar carpal ligament is readily defined as a broad transverse band extending from the thenar to the hypothenar eminence. Its proximal and distal margins are defined.

An instrument is passed under the ligament and along the flexor tendons. The entire breadth of the ligament is carefully divided, the incision being protected by an underlying instrument (a grooved director or hemostat). The tunnel is now carefully explored by dis-

Figure 231. Carpal tunnel syndrome, classic. Constriction of the palmar carpal ligament. Note the palmar carpal ligament has been resected and reflected with the retractor.

placing the tendons out of the groove to permit careful inspection. The median nerve is readily visible, together with the many tendons. If there is extensive synovial thickening, it should be removed very carefully to expose the underlying structures. If there is definite constriction of the median nerve, a saline neurolysis, accomplished by inserting a small needle into the nerve sheath above the constriction and forcing saline within the sheath to dilate it at the constricted area, is advisable. This is probably less traumatic than mechanical neurolysis, which entails splitting the sheath by sharp dissection. If irreversible changes of the nerve have not occurred, recovery will be complete. Great care must be taken not to damage the recurrent thenar branches of the median nerve, which usually come off the main trunk of the median nerve just proximal to the distal edge of the ligament. The cut edges of the ligament should be trimmed back to leave at least a 1 cm. defect as an assurance against reunion of the palmar carpal ligament. A forearm splint is applied for protection for two or three weeks, depending on how well the wound heals and on the extent of the pathological condition found. The fingers should be left free after the first 48 hours.

Ulnar Nerve Entrapment

Very similar to the carpal tunnel syndrome is the entrapment of the ulnar nerve branches to the fourth and fifth fingers and to the intrinsic muscles of the hand. As the ulnar nerve winds around the hook of the hamate, it may get caught between this bone and the overlying ligament. The etiology of this condition is more often chronic overuse of the wrist than acute injury. The symptoms pertain to the ulnar nerve and include pain along the hypothenar eminence and in the fourth and fifth fingers. The entrapment may cause aching through the palm and cramping of the intrinsic muscles. Paresthesias of the skin are frequent. This condition is long-lasting. It may eventuate in atrophy of the intrinsic muscles of the hand, since this deep branch of the ulnar nerve does supply almost all of the intrinsic muscles of the hand. Because of the relatively less vulnerable superficial branch of the ulnar nerve, there may be no sensory involvement. This makes the condition even more puzzling. Surgical treatment is indicated if this condition does not respond promptly to immobilization. The nerve or ligament should not be injected with any local anesthetic, since this can only increase the pressure. Surgical release of the ligament and fascial tissue overlying the nerve will usually permit complete recovery if the condition has not persisted for too long.

Strain or Fracture of the Pisiform Bone

Anatomically the pisiform bone does not actually make up a part of the carpal joints. Basically, it lies within the tendon of the flexor carpi ulnaris, but it has a small articulation with the hamate and this attachment, continuing down to the carpus through the ligament, connects the pisiform to the carpus. Forcible strain on the flexor carpi ulnaris tendon may cause injury here quite similar to that of injury around the patella. The tendon may avulse the pisiform (Fig. 232). The pisiform may be pulled loose from its attachments or the bone may actually break (Fig. 233). The injury commonly occurs from a fall on the outstretched hand when the wrist is in dorsiflexion and the tendon is stretched tight. Tenderness along the palmar aspect of the hand, often sharply localized over the pisiform bone, should lead one to suspect pisiform damage. On careful examination the flexor carpi ulnaris tendon can be palpated to its attachment in the bone and determination made of the exact location of the lesion. Both dorsiflexion of the wrist

Figure 232. Avulsion of the pisiform by the flexor carpi ulnaris tendon. Bone removed and tendon repaired to the carpus.

Figure 233. Fifteen year old male noticed numbness of the ring and little fingers, extending into the wrist, while playing football six months earlier. Did not recall the injury but did remember that hand was numb for several hours after the game. Had persistent pain in the wrist since. X-ray film (illustrated) shows avulsion fracture of pisiform bone by the attachment of the flexor carpi ulnaris tendon. At surgery the fragment was removed and the tendon repaired to the pisiform. Six months later he was having no trouble and was back playing sports.

with radial deviation and active contraction of the flexor carpi ulnaris will cause pain. X-ray examination may or may not reveal involvement of the bone.

Treatment. The condition is treated as a strain. Acute dislocation of the pisiform may occur and should be recognized by comparing x-rays of the normal and the injured wrist (Fig. 234). A carpal tunnel view is unusually valuable here. It is not possible to reduce and hold this bone by closed methods because of the distracting effect of the tone of the flexor carpi ulnaris muscle. Early open reduction with threaded K-wire fixation of the bone to the carpus and repair of the ligaments may be effective. Much more often the bone should be removed and the tendinous attachment of the flexor carpi ulnaris secured to the adjacent carpal capsular ligaments (Fig. 235).

If rupture is complete and the pisiform is dislocated, it should be removed and the tendon repaired. If the condition is treated as a contusion, the progress of recovery will be disappointing, since constant reinjury by use of the involved muscle may prolong and even prevent recovery. In a chronic injury in this region, calcification within the tendon is quite prone to occur, the result of a chronic tendinitis with degenerative change or of calcific deposit within the hematoma.

Injury of the Triangular Cartilage

The fibrocartilaginous extension of the radiocarpal joint lying between the ulna and the carpus is subject to injury in sprains or fractures about the lower end of the forearm. The symptoms are tenderness and pain not on the ulnar styloid but in the sulcus between the ulna and carpus. These symptoms are particularly elicited by lateral motion of the wrist, either by impingement as the wrist is pulled into adduction or by distraction as it is pulled into radial flexion. Rupture of the fibers of this ligamentous and cartilaginous structure may result in hemorrhage and degeneration. Calcification is a late manifestation of this same condition.

Treatment. During the acute phase this condition will ordinarily respond well to immobilization, although it is quite prone to recur. In the chronic stage, local injection of an anesthetic plus a corticoid into the area may give considerable relief. If relief cannot be obtained, the cartilage may be excised, including the calcified area. Care should be taken not to damage the ulnar collateral ligament. If the ulnar collateral ligament is damaged it should be adequately repaired, since a large part of the stability of the wrist depends upon the integrity of this structure.

Dislocation of the Extensor Carpi Ulnaris Tendon

This tendon lies in a groove along the medial side of the distal ulna. Dislocation is manifested by a feeling of slipping as the wrist is rotated and by pain in the area. Attempts to hold the extensor in the groove often are not successful. The condition will usually become symptom-free, except for the slipping, and requires no particular treatment.

Figure 234. Acute injury to the wrist. Original x-ray film findings interpreted as negative. Comparable multiple views of each wrist show the dislocated pisiform. *A* and *B*, Anteroposterior and oblique views showing dislocation. *C* and *D*, The normal wrist for comparison.

GANGLION

Ganglion, which has been previously discussed (page 69), has a predilection for the dorsum of the wrist, where it often causes disability, particularly on forceful use. There is lively controversy as to the exact cause of the mass, many believing it to be a degenerative change and others considering it to be a synovial herniation, either from the carpal joints or from one of the tendon sheaths. It probably arises from a variety of causes. In the wrist it usually presents itself as a soft, fluctuant, nontender mass distal to the dorsal carpal ligament. It may protrude between any of the various tendons of the back of the hand but seems to be most common directly over the capitate. Ganglion seems to follow chronic strain or sprain of the wrist, but in many instances there is no history of trauma. It must be differentiated from an effusion within the tendon sheath and from other types of soft tissue tumor. Sometimes amazingly firm, it may feel like a cartilaginous or bony mass under the skin. The mass is usually movable but not freely so, since it has a firm underlying attachment. Effusion in a tendon sheath on the back of the wrist is infrequent, and it is ordinarily not as firm as a ganglion and is more linear. In the case of the firm tumor, x-ray examination should be done to rule out possible bone involvement.

Treatment. A ganglion may spontaneously regress and disappear altogether, or it may

Figure 235. *A,* Patient "sprained his wrist" six months before and experienced constant pain, with impairment of grip. Note subluxation of pisiform; symptoms relieved by excision of the pisiform and reattachment of the tendon to the carpal ligaments. *B,* Carpal tunnel view; note the narrowing of the joint between the pisiform and the triquetrum, demonstrating some displacement as compared with the opposite side, *C.* (For x-ray positioning, See Fig. 230.)

disappear and then reappear. The time-honored methods of breaking the sac and of aspiration usually fail. I have not had satisfactory results from the injection of corticoid, as has been reported by others. If the mass is troublesome, causes pain or is too unsightly, it should be removed surgically. The success of surgical removal depends upon adequate repair of whatever defect is found. Sometimes the tumor can be dissected out intact. In other instances it will be diffuse, so that the presenting part is comparable to the top of an iceberg in that the mass covers a good deal of the posterior carpus beneath the tendons. If the ligaments are split or if there is a defect in the capsule of the wrist, careful suture is necessary after removal of the ganglion. If there is a pedicle communicating to the tendon or carpal joints, as is often the case, it should be carefully closed. After removal of a ganglion, the hand is immobilized in a cock-up wrist splint for at least three weeks. This may result in some restriction of motion of the wrist, but in my experience recurrence is much less likely if the wrist is protected during the healing period.

Ganglion may occur on the palmar aspect of the wrist or on the flexor tendons to the fingers. Treatment is the same wherever the location.

SPRAIN-SUBLUXATION-FRACTURE-DISLOCATION

Since by our definition *sprain* is a ligament injury, it is relatively uncommon in the wrist. Most of the so-called sprains—and the diagnosis is a frequent one—are not sprains at all but are strains of the tendon attachments or injuries to the bone. The ligaments of the wrist permit a large amount of motion in the radiocarpal joint but very little motion in the intercarpal joints. The massive ligaments on the volar aspect of the wrist are so strong that in hyperextension the injury is more likely to be a fracture of the carpal bones which may be incomplete, or a contusion of the articular surfaces, or possibly a chondral fracture rather than a tearing of the ligaments. It is felt by some that in hyperextension there may be actual slipping of one row of carpals on the other, which permits damage to the dorsal carpal ligaments, although this is rather difficult to demonstrate. Suffice it to say that in the very common dorsiflexion injury of the wrist, the damage is usually on the dorsal aspect. One should therefore be very wary of the diagnosis of sprain of the wrist, i.e., ligament damage, in the common dorsiflexion injury. On dorsiflexion of the wrist, pain is more frequent over the back of the wrist and forearm than over the front, although the greatest stress on the ligament would appear to be on the volar side. If there is tenderness over the carpus, careful x-ray study should be done and the carpal bones closely studied as to both their position and condition.

If the findings of the x-ray study are negative, as they usually are, and a diagnosis of "sprain" is made, the *treatment* is immobilization, with the wrist in slight dorsiflexion for two or three weeks, and physical therapy, unless the symptoms completely subside before this time. If facilities permit, the splints may be removed for daily treatment, always within the limits of pain-free motion. When athletic participation is permitted, the wrist should be carefully strapped to prevent re-injury, since these conditions tend to be quite chronic. At the end of the period of immobilization further x-ray study should be carried out, since linear fractures through the carpal bones that did not show on the first film may be revealed on the second. The common carpal fracture is through the navicular bone at its midpoint, since the navicular takes a good deal of stress of the wrist, whether it is in dorsiflexion or palmar flexion, because of its position bridging the two rows of carpals.

Subluxation and *dislocation* may accompany ligament injury and in the wrist they have some peculiar characteristics. Dislocation of the radiocarpal joint is extremely uncommon, although it has happened as a result of violent action (Fig. 236). A complete carpal dislocation is also uncommon and is obviously a serious injury (Fig. 237). In both of these conditions obvious deformity and disability are present, and therefore they are readily diagnosed and ordinarily receive good treatment. The diagnosis of the exact dislocation through the carpus presents great difficulty, but careful x-ray study of the normal as well as the injured wrist in several positions will cut down the margin of error. It is particularly important that these conditions be diagnosed early because, as with most dislocations, the longer the dislocation remains unreduced the greater will be the likelihood of recurrence and of permanent residual disability. So in the presence of major swelling, pain and particularly deformity of the wrist, prompt definitive treatment must be sought if there is any question as to the extent of injury or the perfection of reduction.

Dislocation of the Distal Radioulnar Joint

Dislocation of the distal end of the ulna is not a very frequent injury but it is quite distressing when it occurs, interfering sharply with the patient's grip, particularly when he is gripping and rotating simultaneously (Fig. 238). The distal radioulnar ligaments provide the main support, holding the distal end of the ulna against the distal end of the radius, where there is limited articulation. The round, cartilaginous ulna rotates against the articulation, which is formed by the distal end of the radius, with the radius of the curve being the same in the two bones. Anterior stability here is helped by the flexor retinaculum, which actually forms the anterior ligament between the radius and ulna, thus having clear articulation with the rest of the carpal bones. The flexor retinaculum forms the attachment for the flexor carpi ulnaris, which also attaches to the proximal base of the fifth metacarpal. The flexor carpi ulnaris tendon inserts directly into the base of the fifth metacarpal but has an ancillary attachment to the pisiform bone, which in turn is fastened to the other metacarpals by the carpal-intercarpal ligaments.

The exact pathology in dislocation of the

Figure 236   Figure 237

Figure 236. Radiocarpal dislocation. Result of a serious injury to the wrist. There was a fracture of the radial styloid which was reduced and held by a transfixion screw. The dislocation of the entire carpus on the lower end of the radius was not held reduced. Wrist fusion was the only solution to this painful wrist.

Figure 237. Fracture of hamate caused by forcible dorsiflexion and ulnar deviation of the wrist. At operation for removal of these fragments, very extensive ligament damage to the carpus was found, indicating that the patient had had a carpometacarpal dislocation which had spontaneously reduced.

Figure 238. This 18 year old male was playing football. There was no specific injury. Six months earlier he noticed snapping and popping in the distal forearm when he tried to lift something of 500 lb. *A*, The separation between the radius and the ulna is shown. *B*, Radiograph shows forearm after reconstruction of the ligaments and reduction of the dislocation. The pin was removed eight weeks postoperatively. The four months postoperative x-ray film shows no displacement. Dismissed for full activity. He had no complaints and there was no further slipping.

distal end of the ulna and distal radius is difficult to evaluate. The massive ligaments connecting the carpal bones and, thence, attaching to the metacarpal ligaments do serve to bind the distal ulna firmly to the radius. Actually, the dislocation should rather be of the radius on the ulna, since the ulna is the stable bone at the wrist, with the radius rotating around it. During the acute phase of this condition, treatment may be somewhat of a challenge.

The flexor retinaculum acts as the transverse carpal ligament (triangular ligament) anteriorly and unites the carpal bones, including the pisiform, firmly to the carpus. In the *acute injury* this ligament can ordinarily be identified and directly repaired. The dorsolateral approach to the distal radius is used, which sacrifices some of the circulation but no vital nerve supply. The imbrication may continue by bringing the portion of the ligaments binding the ulna and radius together for a direct overlapping-type repair after transverse section of the ligament. In the acute dislocation one would anticipate a satisfactory functional result following meticulous repair of all injury found.

The *old injury* presents considerably more challenge, because the structures cannot be defined as well and it is very difficult to identify

the exact segment you are dealing with. The carpal synovial sheaths that form a common sheath between the carpal bones and the distal ulna can often be utilized to form a strong, fibrous band from the ulna to the radius. In reconstruction of this joint, various procedures have been recommended. The most feasible ones probably utilize the short extensor tendon from the dorsum of the hand, weaving the tendon through the radius and then through the ulna to stabilize the radial ulnar joint. It is difficult to get firm fixation by tendon transference using the short extensor tendons from the fingers, since prevention of posterior slipping is desired, and this requires firmer fixation than prevention of separation between the two bones. More support can be obtained from imbrication of the ligaments that are locally present. Transfixion of the radius and ulna is secured by a pin to hold the union while healing takes place. I usually leave the pin in place for six to eight weeks. This method permits a stable wrist insofar as the distal radial ulnar articulation is concerned.

Probably the most accessible incision for these conditions is one made along the medial edge of the distal ulna and medial border of the hand. The so-called articular discs can be easily located in this incision for direct imbrication.

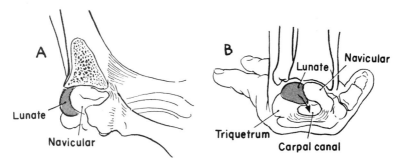

Figure 239. Drawing showing dislocated lunate. (From McLaughlin, Trauma.)

Dislocation of the Lunate (Seminlunar) Bone

The most common dislocation in the wrist is of the lunate bone (Fig. 239). The shape of this bone lying between the massive capitate and the lower end of the radius makes it particularly prone to volar dislocation, since it is narrow in its dorsal portion and quite wide at its volar margin. Forceful compression of the lunate against the capitate by dorsiflexion of the wrist slips this bone forward much like an apple seed pinched between the fingers (Fig. 239B). The dorsal carpal ligament, which is attached to the lunate, gives way and the lunate slips forward, its convex proximal sur-

face lodging along the undersurface of the capitate. If the dislocation is more pronounced, the bone may be completely extruded from the space and may locate almost anywhere on the volar surface of the carpus. If the disrupting force is relatively mild, the subluxation or dislocation may reduce spontaneously but the damage to the dorsal carpal ligament will remain. Indeed, this may be the mechanism of sprains of the wrist in which the force is dorsiflexion but the ligament injured is actually on the side that is not overstretched.

It is extremely easy to overlook a dislocation of the lunate (Figs. 240 and 241). Clinically, the wrist will be painful. It will be tender on the dorsum just distal to the lower end of the

Figure 240. Dislocated carpal lunate. The patient fell forcibly on the outstretched arm and another player fell over him. Note (A) the complete forward displacement of the lunate in relation to the carpus. B, Anteroposterior view shows the fracture of the styloid of the radius and styloid of ulna. The carpal dislocation was overlooked in treating the radius and ulna. It was recognized later, and the lunate was removed with consequent disability.

Figure 241. Fracture dislocation of the wrist. Note that in this case the navicular fractured and the lunate dislocated. Compare with Figure 240, in which the navicular remained intact and the radial styloid fractured as the lunate dislocated.

radius. Brawny swelling will usually prevent palpation of the space where the lunate should be. On the palmar aspect of the wrist, particularly if it is examined early, there is a palpable thickened area under the flexor tendons, quite unlike the corresponding area on the opposite wrist. Motion may not be acutely painful if the lunate is not locked under the volar ligaments; if the lunate is locked, motion may be completely prevented. In such a case careful x-ray study will reveal the deformity, particularly if the film is compared with a similar one of the opposite wrist.

Occasionally the displacement will be accompanied by neurological symptoms, since the extruded lunate tends to compress the carpal tunnel. Frequently there will be paresthesia and pain in the median distribution of the hand, i.e., the first and second fingers, but in the acute injury these are easily overlooked because of the pain. It has been aptly said that the sprained wrist accompanied by symptoms of involvement of the median nerve in the

hand is an indication of lunate dislocation (Fig. 239B).

Treatment. Treatment of these cases is often casual until late complications call attention to the diagnosis. By that time succcessful treatment will be virtually impossible. If the diagnosis can be made early, manipulative treatment is highly successful. Under complete anesthesia, straight traction combined with moderate dorsiflexion of the wrist opens up the space from which the lunate was displaced, and direct pressure against the lunate on the volar surface of the wrist will slip it into position. Once the bone is reduced the wrist should be moderately flexed. This tends to close the space again and maintain the proper position. Following reduction, the wrist is protected by splinting in semiflexion for three weeks. It should then be moved into a neutral position for the fourth week. After this it is protected against dorsiflexion for several more weeks, particularly if athletic competition is to be permitted. It should be emphasized that closed reduction should be prompt if it is to be successful. If the bone is going to reduce at all, it will reduce by gentle manipulation. Force is neither necessary nor advisable. If closed reduction fails, open reduction should be carried out.

In far too many cases the diagnosis is not made early and the patients present several days or several weeks after the injury. Closed reduction should not be attempted after the lapse of more than a week, since by then it is virtually impossible to open the space and reduce the bone. Even if the dislocation is reduced, it is with so much attendant trauma that necrosis is inevitable. Open operation is relatively successful if carried out within the first few weeks. After this period removal of the bone is probably more desirable than an attempt to force the lunate into its normal position. As is true in other dislocations, the longer the lunate remains dislocated, the greater is the likelihood of circulatory changes. For this reason, many surgeons advise removal of the bone if it has remained dislocated for more than two or three weeks. However, this does not produce a normal wrist, and I believe that in the athlete one should attempt reduction of the bone even if this means it later must be removed because of avascular necrosis. As might be expected, a dorsal incision is much preferred, for two pertinent reasons. In the first place, considerable damage may be done to the remaining blood supply if the bone is dissected out from the front, since the only remaining attachment to the lunate is the volar ligament. Second, it is necessary to traverse very vital structures on the volar aspect of the wrist in order to reach the dislocated bone. Dorsal exposure, while it may present some difficulties in actually reaching the bone, will be much less traumatic from both standpoints. In the very late case in which a firm decision has been made to remove the bone, a volar incision should be made. I cannot emphasize too strongly that the principal peril in these wrist injuries is that the true diagnosis will be overlooked and hence the ideal opportunity for definitive treatment will be lost. Any of the other carpal bones may be dislocated, although this is quite uncommon.

Perilunar Dislocation

In dislocation of the lunate this bone dislocates in relation to both the radius and the carpus, so that there is a true dislocation of the lunate alone. In the so-called perilunar dislocation (Fig. 242) the lunate remains with the radius, and the carpus dislocates on the lunate and radius. This is almost never a pure dislocation. Usually either the navicular bone dislocates and the whole bone remains with the radius and the lunate or, more commonly,

Figure 242. Perilunar dislocation. Note that the lunate has remained with the radius, whereas the rest of the carpus is dislocated dorsally. This case is unusual in that the navicular is intact. Frequently the proximal half of the navicular remains with the lunate, the remainder of the bone dislocating with the rest of the carpus. The "1" on the dome of the greater multangular in *B* should appose "2" on the concavity of the lunate, as in view *C*.

the navicular fractures at its vulnerable waist and its proximal fragment remains with the lunate and the radius. There are many possible combinations; for example, the entire proximal row of carpal bones may remain with the radius and the dislocation may be intercarpal, or any combination of these bones may remain with the radius.

Treatment. This is an extremely serious type of fracture-dislocation and bodes ill for normal function of the wrist. For this reason it should be handled by a specialist. It is extremely important not only to get a perfect reduction but also to maintain it. This dislocation is notably unstable because of the extensive damage to the carpal ligaments. Each of the carpal bones must fit exactly against the other if function is to be normal. Even if reduction of the displacement is obtained, one still must deal with the fracture, so that the overall problem becomes very complicated. Time is of the essence, since the dislocation rapidly becomes irreducible because of the occurrence of massive fibrosis through the wrist. Should this occur, wrist fusion is practically the only procedure offering some salvage of function of the wrist.

Chronic arthritic changes are common in these fracture-dislocations even under the most favorable circumstances. One must be precisely analytical in studies of these obviously serious injuries to the wrist. X-ray diagnosis of a fracture-dislocation through the carpus is difficult and only by very careful examination, with x-ray comparison of the injured wrist and the normal one, can one have a reasonable hope of success. One should be particularly suspicious of the sprain that is slow to recover or of the wrist that feels thick from front to back. For this reason no wrist injury should be treated for a long period of time without repeated careful observation, since the deformity, which may be obscured by swelling, may become quite evident once the swelling has been reduced.

Dislocation of the Navicular Bone

A rather unusual injury of the carpus is dislocation of the navicular. This injury is much more readily determined by x-ray study, since the radial-carpal relationship is more obviously disturbed than in the lunate dislocation. It is unusual for this dislocation to occur as an isolated injury; it is frequently the residual of an incompletely reduced perilunar or intercarpal dislocation.

Treatment. If the dislocation is seen and recognized early, it may be reduced by manipulation. The wrist is placed in complete ulnar flexion to open up the space between the styloid of the radius and carpus, after which the navicular may be rotated in position by direct pressure of the fingers. It must be obvious that this can be much more readily accomplished early than late in the course of the injury. As with most dislocations, the longer the navicular remains displaced, the more likelihood there is of an aseptic necrosis of the bone. If the dislocation is recognized after several weeks, an attempt at open reduction may be carried out. If to obtain open reduction the navicular will have to be forced into position or held in position by forcible radial flexion of the wrist, it may be advisable instead to remove it. However, if there seems to be some possibility of restoration of the circulation to the bone, reduction can be tried and fusion of the wrist or excision of the navicular done at a later operation if the first procedure fails.

Sprain-Fracture

Avulsion of the ligament from the bone results in a sprain-fracture. Careful x-ray study made in various positions may reveal the flake of bone lifted up from one of the carpals or from the lower radius or the ulnar styloid. As a general rule, sprain-fractures require a longer period of time for union than does a simple sprain. In some instances painful nonunion may develop between the flake of bone and the parent bone. In such a case it may be necessary to remove the fragment surgically and suture the tendon to its original bed.

Avulsion of the Ulnar Styloid

The styloid process of the ulna may be pulled off by the ulnar collateral ligament. This is in reality an injury to the ulnar collateral ligament and should be treated as such. It usually will heal with fibrous union without instability. If instability does occur, or if the area is painful on function, the styloid should be removed and the ligament sutured to the lower end of the ulna.

Avulsion of the Radial Styloid

The styloid process of the radius is not as vulnerable as is the styloid of the ulna, nor are

Figure 243. *A,* Fracture of the styloid of the radius; presumably the fragment was pulled off by the lateral ligament. *B,* Note perfect union one month following screw fixation.

its ligament attachments as strong. Usually a force that will break the styloid of the radius will either tear the radiocarpal ligament or break the lower end of the radius. A sharp ulnar flexion of the wrist with little or no dorsal component may cause avulsion of the radial styloid (Fig. 243). In such a case the symptoms will be those of a sprain. There will be pain on ulnar deviation of the wrist but little pain on flexion and extension. The tenderness will be at the tip of the styloid, just at the base of the thumb. Careful examination will distinguish between tenderness over the navicular or over the base of the metacarpal of the thumb and that over the radial styloid. These areas are all subcutaneous and can be readily palpated. In palpating the dorsal surface of the radius one may be misled into believing that the condition is a sprain, since the tenderness will be lateral rather than dorsal. Any injury of this severity requires x-ray films taken in anteroposterior, lateral and oblique planes. Careful study of the films will be necessary to reveal the precise nature of the lesion. A very small fragment, hardly recognizable on the x-ray, should be treated as a carpal sprain. On the other hand, a significant amount of the styloid may be pulled away (Fig. 243). Poorly planned x-ray films may fail to reveal the displacement.

Treatment. Since this fracture involves the articular surface of the radiocarpal joint, it is subject to the same requirements of treatment as articular fractures elsewhere. The fragment

must be perfectly reduced and firmly held until union is secure, or it must be removed and the ligament sutured to the radius. If the fragment is as substantial as the one in Figure 243, where it involves roughly two fifths of the articular surface, it should be replaced. The main problem is recognition of the nature of the injury. It will be futile to try to replace the fragment and maintain fixation by any bizarre position of the wrist. Internal fixation is an absolute necessity.

FRACTURE

Fracture of the Navicular Bone

For reasons previously mentioned, the most common carpal fracture is of the navicular. Contributing factors are that the navicular bridges the intercarpal joint, that it is directly impinged upon by the lower radius on dorsiflexion and radial deviation of the wrist, and that it has a rather narrow waist (Figs. 244 and 245). The force is usually hyperextension—as in a fall on the outstretched hand—a force similar to that causing lunate dislocation or Colles' fracture. Following such an injury there will be pain through the wrist, not at the lower end of the radius but just distal to it. Findings of careful x-ray study often are negative. The diagnosis of sprain of the wrist is acceptable here if one is prepared to treat the sprain

Figure 244. Acute fracture through the waist of the carpal navicular (*A*). Treated by plaster cast, with solid union four months later (*B*).

Figure 245. *A*, Avulsion fracture of the carpal navicular by traction on the radiocarpal ligament. *B*, Solid union four months later following cast immobilization.

adequately, that is, by immobilization of the wrist for two to three weeks. At the end of two weeks the wrist should be re-x-rayed, care being taken to get oblique views (Fig. 246). Frequently a fracture line will be revealed in this second x-ray (Fig. 247). If this later x-ray still does not reveal a fracture and symptoms persist after four or five weeks, films should be made again with the wrist in various positions, since it must be assumed that there is a fracture of the navicular until this diagnosis can definitely be ruled out.

Undisplaced Fracture

The treatment of an undisplaced fracture of the navicular is immobilization for a period long enough to permit the fracture to heal completely. This will be many weeks or months. The progress of union should be checked by radiographs. The original dressing should be anterior and posterior splints extending from the proximal interphalangeal joints to below the elbow, with the wrist in slight dorsiflexion. The proximal phalanx of the thumb is included. This type of fixation is continued for a variable time, depending upon the amount of swelling. If there is little reaction in the hand and no danger of constriction, a solid cast may be applied at the first visit. In the presence of considerable swelling, however, plaster splints with some compression are used instead, the use of the cast being postponed until the size of the wrist has somewhat stabilized. In any event, immobilization should be early and complete, with the hand held in the grasping position. A bizarre position of the wrist is neither necessary nor desirable. Since complete immobilization is important (Fig. 248), the gauntlet cast should be changed if it becomes loose, as it usually does. This may require a change of cast every two or three weeks, at which time the x-ray check of the progress of union should be made. When union appears to be secure across the fracture line, as revealed in a good oblique x-ray picture, the gauntlet may be supplanted by a leather wristlet or adhesive strapping. If athletic competition is to be permitted, dorsiflexion of the wrist must be prevented by an adequate support. In the fracture without displacement, it may not be necessary to immobilize the thumb. My own practice is to include the base of the thumb to the metacarpophalangeal joint and thus to permit phalangeal but not metacarpal motion.

Complete Fracture

In a complete fracture and particularly in a fracture with displacement or instability, the type of immobilization described will not be adequate. The management of such a fracture requires the utmost in skill and judgment. If there is displacement an attempt may be made by manipulation to reduce the fragments. The hand is checked in radial deviation or in ulnar deviation, flexion or extension to determine what position makes the fragments the most stable. It is my own opinion that such a fracture should be treated by operation to obtain perfect reduction and held with transfixion screws or pins. By this method immobilization can be assured at the fracture site, although at the expense of some further sacrifice of circulation to the fragments. If the fracture line is actually unstable so that in various positions the fragments can be shown to move on each other, it is extremely unlikely that simple immobilization of the wrist will prevent motion. Indeed, immobilization of the wrist does not prevent rotation of the forearm, and in rotation of the forearm there is inevitably some torsion at the radiocarpal joint.

Following operation, the same treatment should be carried out as for a fracture without displacement. The aftercare of such a fracture requires sound judgment. There seems little justification for continuing immobilization for many months if union does not appear to be progressing or if the fragment has become sclerotic or cystic. True enough, prolonged immobilization has in some cases finally resulted in bony union, but in my experience these are few and far between. The displaced fracture that has gone unrecognized and is discovered after several weeks is also probably doomed to nonunion. As the union or nonunion is seen on x-ray study, a decision must be made in each case whether to continue immobilization or to recommend some other type of treatment. If union is not at least proceeding satisfactorily after three or four months, I would advise removal of the external fixation to allow function of the wrist.

Many of these ununited fractures are entirely pain-free and allow remarkably good wrist function (Fig. 249). If this is the case surgery is not advisable, since any type of open reduction and grafting for delayed union or nonunion has a high percentage of failure. If symptoms persist and are disabling (Fig. 250), then one must consider the various possibilities for treatment of nonunion. I know of no treat-

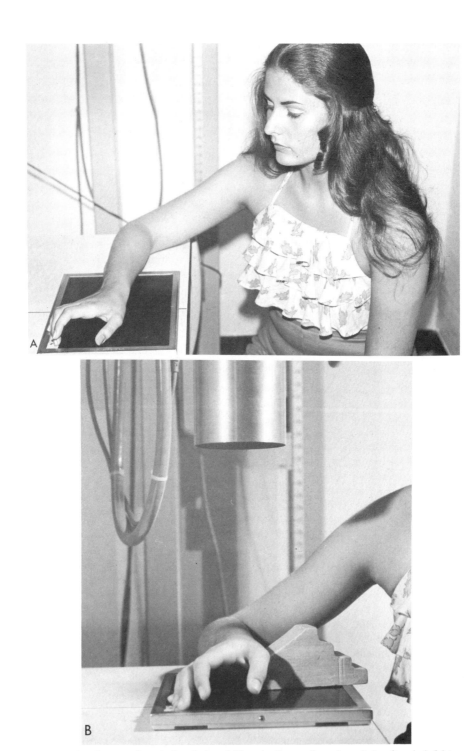

Figure 246. Positioning for carpal navicular. *A*, In addition to the routine views it is often helpful to position the patient's wrist in a routine anteroposterior view but with as much lateral deviation as possible. *B*, The oblique view is best obtained by supporting the palm of the hand on a nonopaque object such as a 35 degree angle balsa wood block. The wrist should be abducted as much as the patient can tolerate.

Figure 247. *A,* Acute sprain of the wrist. Note normal-appearing navicular on the day of injury. *B,* Two weeks later showing some separation. *C,* Following several months of immobilization. Note the union.

Figure 248. Classic fracture through the waist of the navicular, showing fibrous healing with spur formation following inadequate immobilization.

Figure 249. Long-standing nonunion of the carpal navicular fracture, which occurred in football. Patient is now 60 and has advanced degenerative arthritis of the radiocarpal joint and sclerosis of the adjacent margins of the fragments.

Figure 250. Untreated fractured navicular with resultant cystic changes and considerable disability. This type of case is not amenable to bone grafting. The salvage procedure here would probably be radial styloidectomy, although this would not completely relieve the symptoms.

ment that can guarantee a normal wrist, and the choice is a very difficult one. One must depend to a large extent upon the nature and condition of the navicular bone. If there is carpal arthritis and particularly arthritis of the radiocarpal joint, solid union of the navicular will not relieve the symptoms (Fig. 251). If the fracture is central and the bone fragments are relatively viable, bone grafting should be attempted and is frequently successful. Since following this procedure there often will be chondral damage around the fracture site, it is advisable to remove the styloid of the radius (Figs 251 and 252) so that the fracture line does not articulate across the lower end of the radius. Indeed, if the arthritis is localized to this area, a radial styloidectomy may be the treatment of choice either with or without grafting of the navicular. If, on the other hand, one fragment is small or there is comminution of one or the other fragment, these fragments should be removed (Fig. 253). Indeed, this probably should be done as a primary procedure in such a case. Because of the very poor prognosis in nonunion, it is extremely important that these fractures be diagnosed early, since treatment of the acute fracture is highly successful, while treatment of nonunion is very unsatisfactory. Currently electrical stimulation has been utilized in nonunion. I have not seen any series on navicular fracture nor have I utilized this procedure for this conditon.

Should one be allowed to participate in sports following a fracture of the navicular bone? Most teams will not allow a member to play while wearing a plaster cast; therefore,

the athlete should not be allowed to participate during the period in which union may still be expected. If the injury occurred during spring practice and several months have elapsed and union is not expected, should the patient be allowed to participate? I have permitted this when it seemed that nonunion was inevitable and there was no justification for further immobilization. I recall one player who "sprained" his wrist in spring practice. The navicular fracture was revealed after several weeks, and he was treated by immobilization throughout the summer; union did not occur, and he was permitted to play the following season wearing a suitable leather gauntlet. At the end of the season, bone grafting was carried out (Fig. 254). Whether or not this is justifiable I think depends upon the drive of the particular patient and the importance to him of his participation.

Compression Fracture

Since the carpus is made up entirely of cancellous bone and since it is subject to compression forces such as a fall on the clenched fist or on the outstretched hand, it would seem that compression fractures of the carpal bones would occur frequently. The fact that they are so rarely diagnosed does not necessarily mean they rarely occur. I am sure that many of the so-called sprains of the wrist which improve with that tardiness which is so aggravating to the athlete may well be compression fractures of the carpals. Diagnosis is

Figure 251. *A*, Unrecognized fracture through the waist of the carpal navicular which has gone on to union but with marked narrowing of the joint space and radiocarpal arthritis. This house painter was unable to work. *B*, His symptoms were ameliorated by radial styloidectomy.

Figure 252. *A*, Fracture of middle third of navicular, with nonunion and bone spurring on the navicular and the radial styloid. *B*, Treated by excision of the radial styloid and bone graft with navicular pegs. Solid union. Good clinical result.

Figure 253. *A,* Compression fracture of the body of the navicular caused by sharp radial flexion of the wrist, so that the bone is impinged between the radial styloid and the triquetrum. *B,* This painful injury was relieved by removal of the fragment. Athletics resumed. If recognized early, this condition should be treated by immobilization with the wrist in ulnar flexion so that the carpal capsule will tend to pull the fragment back into position.

Figure 254. *A,* Fractured navicular through the waist as an acute injury. This was immobilized in plaster for four months *(B)* with no bony union. The patient was allowed to play football with the arm carefully protected in a brace, and at the end of the season, radial styloidectomy with peg grafts of the navicular was carried out with solid union *(C).* Arrow indicates well-preserved radial navicular joint space.

virtually impossible by early x-ray. Later x-rays which might be expected to show some atrophy or condensation of bone are extremely difficult to interpret because many of the bones are superimposed. Clinically the diagnosis of compression fracture is also difficult, since the ordinary findings of this fracture are quite confusing in the wrist. Local tenderness is present whether the injury is a sprain or a fracture. Pain on forced motion is also likely in either. The unusual fact that many of the "sprains" of the dorsum of the wrist are caused by dorsiflexion forces may give a clue. It is possible that many of these dorsal flexion "sprains" may actually be compression or chondral fractures of one or the other of the carpal bones. Sprain of the dorsal ligaments of the wrist is caused by palmar flexion, which puts stress on these ligaments. Dorsal flexion is the usual force in the so-called sprain of the wrist, but this puts no stress on the dorsal ligaments. On the contrary, dorsal flexion puts all the stress on the palmar side. Hence, pain on the dorsum of the wrist following falling on the outstretched hand is more likely from osteochondral damage to the dorsal part of the carpus than from sprain of the ligaments on the dorsal side. For this reason a second set of x-rays should be taken after two or three weeks, particularly if pain persists on the dorsum. There may be fragmentation of the edges of the bones. Even though early x-ray findings are negative, a period of immobilization is imperative so that any chips of cartilage that

may have been fissured or cracked will have a chance to heal. This particular injury to the wrist should be treated with the wrist in a neutral position or possibly with a little palmar flexion, whereas if the ligament is injured ("sprain"), the wrist should be treated in dorsal flexion. This is not difficult to determine if one has a high index of suspicion. The two conditions, i.e., palmar sprain and dorsal impaction, are easily distinguishable, if one takes the trouble to make a definitive diagnosis.

No specific *treatment* is required for the acute condition other than rest and protection. Since this is also the treatment for a sprain, one does not err in applying protective support to any wrist injury provided one is first assured that no condition is present that requires more definitive treatment. A compression fracture will heal much more slowly than the ordinary sprain. If the symptoms persist over a long period of time, one may be unable to decide whether the lesion is a compression fracture, a synovitis or some type of chondral damage. Since all will require basically the same treatment, namely, protection against the motion that causes the pain, a definitive diagnosis may be academic, except that the prognosis may be somewhat more grave in one condition than in the others. The wrist should be protected against painful motion progressively by splint, by a leather wristlet, by adhesive strapping and finally by elastic wrapping. Only thus may we minimize the tendency for occurrence of chronic arthritis, which can be extremely seri-

A   B

Figure 255. *A,* Classic Kienböck's disease (osteochondritis of the lunate), old, in which the bone involuted incompletely, leaving a sclerosed, deformed bone, causing painful carpal function. *B,* The symptoms were relieved somewhat by removal of the carpal lunate. Early recognition of this osteochondritis and immobilization would have prevented this poor result.

ous in the carpus, where there are so many interrelated joints. In the final analysis, the treatment for persistent chronic arthritis is fusion of the wrist. The intervening treatment should be physical therapy, local injection and other measures ordinarily employed for chronic traumatic arthritis elsewhere.

Kienböck's "Disease"

Kienböck's disease (Fig. 255), which is a late involvement of the lunate, may well be the result of compression fracture of this bone. The condition is variously called osteitis, osteochondritis or malacia of the lunate and is most common in the adolescent. In this condition there is definite involvement of the lunate with bony changes, the bone going through various stages, i.e., atrophy followed by sclerosis and later decalcification, often with fragmentation resulting in marked change in shape of the bone. The deformity may be prevented by early recognition and protection. Should a youth with an osteochondritis of the lunate be permitted to participate in sports? Certainly he should not during the early stage. He should never play unless there is adequate protection in the form of a gauntlet cast or a reinforced wrist and forearm splint. The period of resolution of this bone may be a couple of years. The same condition may involve the other carpal bones and requires the same treatment.

Chondral Fracture

Almost the same can be said about chondral or osteochondral fracture (see Chapter 4) as has been said previously about compression fracture. It seems inevitable that there will be serious damage to the cartilage of the carpus in many injuries of the wrist. These cannot be visualized on x-ray in the early stages. The late changes to be expected are those so often associated with chronic arthritis, namely, irregularity of the joint cartilage, narrowing of the joint space, painful motion and tenderness upon pressure. If actual fragments of cartilage loose in the carpal joints could be recognized early, surgical excision would be the treatment of choice. They are, however, almost impossible to diagnose unless the fracture includes a small portion of bone. Many wrists that show small "flakes" of bone on x-ray are very likely to have a rather large chondral fragment. I feel sure that if one would analyze the injury carefully and come to this conclusion, the final result would be markedly improved by early removal of this fragment. The mild chondral injury goes on to a good recovery. The moderate ones leave aching pain and pain on forced motion. The severe ones terminate in intercarpal arthritis.

SUMMARY

From the foregoing the conclusion is inevitable that successful treatment of the carpal injury can be expected only when one takes the time to analyze the injury carefully. Diligent evaluation of the forces applied will be extremely rewarding. Precise clinical study involving location of tender points with the rubber end of a pencil may enable one to pinpoint the lesion. A painstaking study of the effect of the various directions of motion will give invaluable aid. In short, the treatment must depend upon a very careful and exact analysis of the condition one is treating. Only by such methods can one avoid the embarrassment and humiliation of realizing that he is dependent upon Father Time for his diagnosis, often to the extreme detriment of the patient. Once the lesion has been identified and a reasonable degree of recovery has occurred, rehabilitative exercises can be a major factor in preventing recurrence of the condition (see p. 687).

Injuries of the Hand

12

with GAEL FRANK

ANATOMICAL CONSIDERATIONS

The hand is a highly complicated, intricate, mechanical device and sensory organ. Most functions of the upper extremity are directed at positioning the hand in the best manner to perform the intended task. Before undertaking any treatment of this complex organ, one should be thoroughly familiar with its functional as well as its gross anatomy and aware of the principles of treatment which have been developed over the past half century. Those not familiar with the treatment of hand injuries can do far more damage than that occurring in the original injury by an oversight as simple as splinting the hand in a nonfunctional position.

Position of Function

The key to proper functioning of the hand is the overall configuration which the hand assumes in the resting position. This is known as the position of function, and it is the position which the hand assumes when the wrist is dorsiflexed approximately 45 degrees and the thumb is placed parallel to the forearm in a position of opposition to the fingers. The fingers are flexed 45 degrees at the metacarpophalangeal and interphalangeal joints. The importance of the position of function cannot be overemphasized. A hand which is stiff in a flat position is useful only as a paddle, whereas a hand which is stiff in the functional position is able to utilize even a small amount of motion to perform useful operations. In this position the intrinsic and extrinsic muscles are balanced and can perform with optimum efficiency (Fig. 256).

When the hand is in the functional position, its form assumes two arches. One is formed in a sagittal plane, with metacarpals and pha-

langes forming the elements of the arch. The other arch is in the transverse plane and is seen best in the curve formed by the metacarpal heads. The transverse arch motif is carried proximally to the wrist, where the bony elements of the wrist form the carpal tunnel. The thumb represents a mobile post against which the fingers can function in pinch and grasp.

Joints and Ligaments

The bony elements of the hand are formed by the metacarpals and phalanges (Fig. 257). The metacarpal of the thumb articulates with the greater multangular in a saddle-type of joint. The capsule is thickened laterally and dorsally to form ligaments. This gives the joint a wide range of motion combined with good stability. The ulnar and radial lips of this metacarpal provide bony stability. This stability is lost when either lip, but most commonly the ulnar lip, becomes fractured. The four finger metacarpals articulate with the distal row of the carpal bones and with each other. These articulations form arthrodial, or gliding-type, joints. The metacarpals articulate with the proximal phalanges by means of a condyloid joint, a joint which allows motion in all planes except axial rotation. The interphalangeal articulations are of the ginglymus type, allowing motion in only one plane.

At the finger carpometacarpal joints very little motion is possible, and there are no specifically named ligaments. The capsule is thickened on the dorsal and the palmar sides to form capsular ligaments. The capsules of the metacarpophalangeal and interphalangeal joints are thickened on the sides to form collateral ligaments and on the volar surface to form a volar plate. These joints articulate with a camlike action. The heads of these bones are shaped like a cam, and the collateral ligaments

286

Figure 256. Drawing shows the hand in the position of function. Notice in particular that a very small amount of motion in the thumb and fingers is useful motion in that it can be utilized to pinch and grasp. Notice the close relationship of the tendons to bone. The flexor tendons are held close to bone by a pulleylike thickening of the flexor sheath, as represented schematically. With the hand in this position, intrinsic and extrinsic musculatures are in balance, and all muscles are acting within their physiological resting length. The key to abbreviations is as follows:

EDC, Extensor digitorum communis
EPL, Extensor pollicis longus
FDP, Flexor digitorum profundus
FDS, Flexor digitorum sublimis
FPL, Flexor pollicis longus
EPB, Extensor pollicis brevis
APL, Abductor pollicis longus

i, Interossei
tm, Transverse metacarpal ligament
l, lumbrical
ad, Adductor pollicis brevis
ab, Abductor pollicis brevis

are tightest in flexion and most relaxed in extension. Therefore, these joints should always be splinted in some degree of flexion when stiffness is anticipated, because from this position the fingers can eventually be straightened. This is possible because with straightening the ligaments become more relaxed. With the joint splinted in extension, flexion is extremely difficult, since it involves stretching the collateral ligaments, which are quite refractory to this type of stretching.

Binding the finger metacarpal heads and necks together are the very important transverse metacarpal ligaments. The lumbrical tendons pass anterior, and the interosseous tendons posterior, to these ligaments.

Skin and Fascia

The skin covering the hand not only provides cover but also contains the sensory end organs. These give the hand its highly specialized sen-

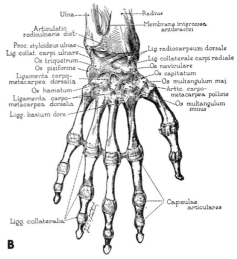

Figure 257. Bones and joints of the distal forearm, wrist and hand. *A*, Palmar (ventral) aspect. *B*, Dorsal aspect. (From Anson, Atlas of Human Anatomy.)

sory function and enable it to distinguish various sensations and to identify objects in a highly discriminatory manner. The skin covering the palmar surface of the hand and fingers is more firmly fixed to the underlying soft palmar tissues than that on the dorsum of the hand. Beneath this palmar skin there is a cushioning pad of fat separated into multiple compartments by fascial septa. This enables the hand to grasp objects with a tremendous amount of pressure and with a surface which does not slip beneath the grasp. On the dorsum of the hand the skin is highly mobile. This is necessary because the wrist and fingers have a wide range of flexion and extension. In flexion the skin is stretched tightly across the convex surface, and its mobility is necessary to accommodate to the shape of the hand. The subcutaneous layer beneath this dorsal skin is primarily areolar tissue, which makes possible gliding motion.

The fascia on the palmar side of the hand is primarily a deep layer, there being no superficial fascia in the palm. This deep fascia is divided into bands and septa termed *palmar fascia,* which separate the palmar structures and divide the subcutaneous tissue into compartments.

Blood Supply

The blood supply to the palmar surface of the hand is provided by two palmar arches formed by the terminal branches of the radial and ulnar arteries. The superficial palmar arch gives rise to the common volar digital arteries, except those to the thumb and the radial side of the index finger. These latter arise from the deep palmar arch. The deep arch gives origin to the metacarpal arteries, the first one forming a proper volar digital artery to the thumb and another to the radial side of the index finger. Through this complicated network of arches and anastomoses, the hand is assured of a good collateral circulation and a very adequate blood supply. On the dorsum of the hand, the dorsocarpal arterial arch is formed by a branch of the radial artery and a branch of the dorsal branch of the ulnar artery. This arterial arch gives origin to the dorsal metacarpal arteries, which terminate in the dorsal digital arteries. This dorsal anastomosis is not as important as the volar network in supplying the fingers and does not extend beyond the proximal interphalangeal joints of the fingers.

Nerves

The motor nerves to the intrinsic muscles of the hand arise from the ulnar and median nerves. The median nerve supplies most of the intrinsic muscles of the thumb and the two most radial lumbrical muscles. The ulnar nerve supplies the remaining intrinsic musculature of the hand and extends across the palm to supply the transverse head of the adductor brevis muscle of the thumb. Motor function of the hand results from a balanced action between intrinsic and extrinsic musculature.

Tendons and Associated Structures

An important consideration in regard to the flexor tendons of the fingers is that they are

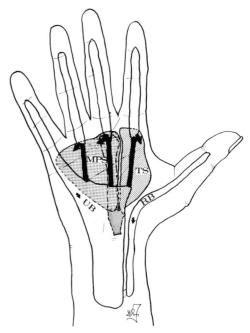

Figure 258. A schematic representation of the flexor tendon sheaths and the fascial spaces of the palm. To avoid confusion, it is important to remember that the tendon sheaths are termed bursae and the potential spaces deep to these bursae and their tendons are termed spaces. Notice that whereas the flexor tendon sheaths of the little finger and thumb communicate proximally with their bursae, the index, center and ring bursae end at the metacarpophalangeal joints. Flexor tendon sheath infections starting in the thumb and little finger can therefore migrate proximally into the wrist, whereas infections in the index, center and ring fingers are limited proximally to the metacarpophalangeal joints. Should the infection from these three fingers point and drain at this proximal termination of the flexor sheath, they will drain into the potential spaces, as indicated by the arrows. RB, Radial bursa, UB, Ulnar bursa. TS, Thenar space. MPS, Midpalmar space.

enclosed in a flexor sheath throughout most of their excursion through the palm and fingers. These flexor sheaths provide a gliding mechanism through which the tendons slide. Also, since the tendons must glide around two or three completely flexed joints, the flexor sheaths act as pulleys to keep the tendons from bowstringing across the interval. As one might suspect, the more joints crossed, the more important the pulley action of the flexor sheath becomes. In the fingers, where there are two flexor tendons and three joints to cross, the flexor tendon sheaths are quite restricted. The communications between these flexor sheaths are important in hand infections. The flexor sheaths to the index, center and ring fingers are interrupted in the palm, and infections originating in the flexor sheath of these fingers do not migrate past the metacarpophalangeal joints when carried along the flexor tendon sheath (Fig. 258).

With the extensor tendons of the thumb and fingers there is no need for pulleys, so there is no extensor sheath for the thumb or fingers

distal to the wrist. The intrinsic musculature of the hand is divided into the muscles of the thenar eminence, the muscles of the hypothenar eminence, the interosseous muscles arising from the metacarpals and the lumbrical muscles arising from the flexor digitorum profundus tendons (Figs. 259 to 261). The primary function of the muscles of the thenar eminence is to bring the thumb into opposition. The muscles of the hypothenar eminence control the little finger and help cup the hand. The lumbrical muscles flex the metacarpophalangeal joints of the fingers and, through their insertion into the dorsal hood mechanism, extend the distal interphalangeal joints. The prime function of the dorsal interossei is abduction of the fingers away from the center finger, that of the volar interossei is adduction toward the center finger.

Deep to the flexor tendons and their associated structures lie two potential spaces which become important only in the presence of infection (see Fig. 258). The dividing line between these two spaces is formed by a septum

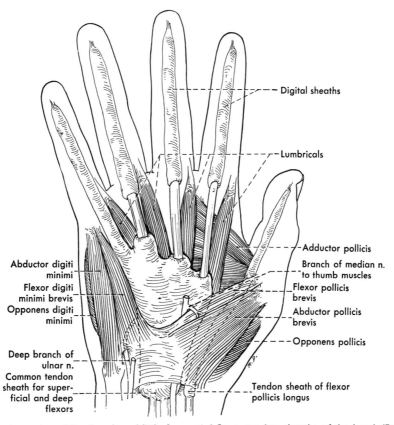

Figure 259. Short muscles of the thumb and little finger and flexor tendon sheaths of the hand. (From Hollinshead, Functional Anatomy.)

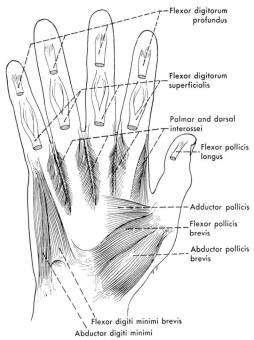

Figure 260. The flexors of the interphalangeal and metacarpophalangeal joints. Note that each joint has its own special flexor or flexors. (From Hollinshead, Functional Anatomy.)

running from the shaft of the center metacarpal along the palm toward the thumb and associated with the attachment of the transverse head of the adductor brevis of the thumb. The potential space lateral to the center metacarpal and superficial to the adductor pollicis muscle is known as the *thenar space*. That space which lies to the ulnar (medial) side of the septum is called the *midpalmar space*. As previously indicated, this space becomes important only in the presence of infection and will be discussed later.

GENERAL CONSIDERATIONS IN THE MANAGEMENT OF HAND INJURIES

In addition to a detailed patient history and careful physical examination of the injured area, appropriate x-ray studies are of paramount importance. The physician must insist on radiographs taken to show the injured area to best advantage. Specific films of the individual fingers or thumb in the desired projections should be ordered, avoiding such vague orders as "x-ray of the hand." If one suspects a specific injury, detailed and localized x-rays of that area should be ordered, whether it is an

interphalangeal joint or the hook of the hamate.

Be sure that the athlete understands the reason for the proposed treatment program. Make it abundantly clear that he must accept responsibility for unauthorized departures from the treatment program. It is inexcusable for an athlete to remove a protective device during an athletic contest and then attempt to replace a loss of natural ability with a subsidy from the physician's malpractice insurance.

In today's medicolegal climate, it is important to document advice given to the injured athlete. In many instances, hand injuries tend to be regarded as insignificant by the patient. The physician who treats today's athlete owes it to himself to provide adequate protection in the form of entries in permanent office records.

CONTUSIONS AND ABRASIONS

The hand's location at the end of the extremity and its function expose it to a wide variety of traumatic episodes. Many of its functions automatically increase the possibility of contusion. The athlete does not ordinarily receive severe crushing injuries such as those seen in industry. The most common contusions of the

Figure 261. The flexor tendons on a finger—anterior and lateral views. (From Hollinshead, Functional Anatomy.)

hand in the athlete occur as a result of direct impact, such as from a foot stepping on the outstretched hand with the fingers extended or from a blow of the fist with the fingers closed against an opposing blunt object. Very often these will result in a combination of an abrasion and a contusion or a contusion and a laceration.

Although the hand, and particularly the back of the hand, is prone to rapid swelling, hematomas are not common. The blood on the back of the hand is much more likely to infiltrate up and down under the loose skin than it is to collect in a localized pool. On the palmar surface of the hand there is no room for excessive hematoma formation because of the very nature of the tightly closed spaces. The bleeding is usually in the form of extravasation through the tissues rather than collection into a pool. If a hematoma can be demonstrated, it should be treated by aspiration and a pressure bandage under strict surgical asepsis. When a large hematoma is seen on the dorsum of the hand, one should suspect a defect in the clotting mechanism such as is found in hemophilia (Fig. 262).

The Dorsum of the Hand

The skin over the back of the hand is so loose that it swells rapidly, but it is not subject to hematoma formation between the skin and underlying fascia. Certain complications do occur from contusion which should be thought of, particularly if the contusion appears to be serious. Nerve damage is not likely from direct contusion because the major nerves lie on the volar aspect and are well protected. The tendons, however, lie subcutaneously and may be caught between the underlying bone and the contusing object. So, too, if the fist is clenched and the knuckle forcibly driven against a hard object, there may be chondral damage to the end of the metacarpal, damage to the extensor tendon as it passes over the metacarpal head or a fracture or infraction of the head.

These areas, mainly subcutaneous, are readily available for careful physical examination. One can frequently determine whether there is a fracture of the underlying bone by simple palpation and careful manipulation. Active and passive motion of the fingers should be carefully checked to determine whether there is any loss of tendon function. Nerve function should also be noted. This can be done quickly and may save many headaches later. If the contusion seems severe with local tenderness, pain and swelling, an x-ray should be made and carefully studied.

Treatment. *Early treatment* of the contusion should be initiated by very careful cleansing of the skin with soap and water. The athlete is likely to be in an area where there is dirt, dust or various other contaminants, and these may be ground into open cuts or abraded areas. The cleansing should be done at once. Copious amounts of running water and bland soap are much better than alcohol or various antiseptics. There is no necessity for painting the part with an antiseptic. Following such cleansing,

Figure 262. A large collection of blood on the dorsum of the hand should immediately alert the examiner to the possibility of a defect in the clotting mechanism. Before one injudiciously sets about to drain such a hematoma by aspiration or incision, a careful check should be made of any history of bleeding tendencies. This particular individual has hemophilia.

the area can be protected by a water soluble unguent, a thin strip being appropriate. Some may prefer an antibiotic ointment, and I see no objection to this if inquiry is made as to any possible sensitivity. Once the skin has been carefully cleaned, attention must be given to the underlying condition. It is best treated by a compression dressing with mechanic's waste or similar soft material placed over the contused area and snugly wrapped in place with an elastic bandage. An ice pack is then applied. Careful inspection of the hand is carried out after 12 hours, and if the swelling is under control, the ice may be discontinued. It is inadvisable to use heat therapy for the first 36 hours.

Subsequent treatment will depend upon the extent of the contusion. If the area remains swollen, edematous and painful, and particularly if there is pain on active extension of the fingers, one should protect the hand much longer because of the possibility of tenosynovitis, which may be quite crippling and last for many weeks. If function of the fingers remains pain-free, a rigid protective dressing may be applied over the back of the hand and snugly held in place by an elastic bandage. Participation in sports may be continued, always provided that function of the fingers is pain-free. Careful re-examination from time to time will detect any possible late complication such as involvement of the intrinsic muscles of the hand, localized phlebitis, lymphangitis, delayed tendon rupture and so forth.

The Palm

A particularly distressing injury to the hand is a contusion of the palm in which there is damage to the intrinsic muscles. This occurs most commonly at the base of the hand in the thenar and hypothenar eminences where the intrinsic muscles to the thumb and to the little finger are involved. This injury is of the "stone bruise" type and may require considerable time to subside. The palmar portion of the hand is a relatively closed space and any localized swelling here can be distressing. Contusion directly over the transverse ligament may give rise to the carpal tunnel syndrome (see p. 261). Contusion of the distal part of the palm may cause severe tenderness over the metacarpal heads, so that gripping a hard object such as a golf club or a tennis racket may be painful. This condition may be very disabling; if it persists, later treatment may be necessary, consisting of local injection of a long-acting anesthetic and a corticoid prepa-

ration. Physical therapy, particularly with the heat modalities, is appropriate.

FINGERTIP INJURIES

Injuries to the athlete's fingertip usually involve the nail and the pulp, sometimes in combination with fractures of the distal tuft. These most commonly result from direct trauma to the fingertip.

Injuries to the Nail

The nail is very closely apposed to the bone, being separated only by the nail bed. Contusion here is likely to cause hemorrhage into the closed spaces under the fingernail or in the tip of the phalanx. As the hematoma develops, it causes pressure symptoms and throbbing pain that are very distressing. The immediate treatment is application of cold, the hand being held in direct contact with crushed ice or in ice water. If swelling subsides early enough, the severe symptoms may be prevented. Should blood accumulate under the nail at this early stage, it is advisable to drill the nail to relieve the pressure. This should be done under aseptic technique, since infection in this space has extremely serious consequences. Everyone has his preferred method for drilling the nail. I prefer to drill carefully through with a convex-type knife blade, such as a No. 10 Bard-Parker, which will drill through the nail without pressure. However, there are many other suitable ways to open this space. After the bleeding stops, the treatment with ice or cold water may be discontinued, but heat should not be applied for 48 hours. A protective splint will usually give considerable relief.

Badly lacerated nails can be either repaired with sutures or removed if damage is extensive. Various complications are seen in this condition, making careful examination of the area mandatory. In order to clean the area thoroughly, it is usually necessary to anesthetize the finger by injecting lidocaine (Xylocaine) into either side at its base. Never use a local anesthetic with epinephrine when blocking digital nerves. Once the finger is insensitive and the pain is gone, a more definitive examination can be carried out. The nail should be carefully studied. Frequently the root of the nail has slipped out from under the eponychial fold, and its proximal end is found lying on top of the skin (Fig. 263). In this case enough of the proximal end of the nail should be cut away to permit the nail to fall back into the nail

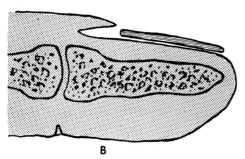

Figure 263. Lateral drawing of tip of the finger, showing (*A*) the nail avulsed from its root and lying on top of the skin on the dorsum of the finger and (*B*) the proximal end of the nail cut off to permit the nail to fall back into the nailbed.

bed. The finger is then dressed carefully with a petrolatum strip, and a splint is applied with moderate pressure. The nail must be carefully protected in the athlete. In many instances the root will not adhere to the nail bed, and protection will be needed until the new nail grows out from under the injured part. It is well to clip off the old nail just distal to the advancing edge of the new nail.

Avulsion Lacerations of the Fingertip

If the injury is less than 1 cm. in diameter and if the bone is not exposed, treatment consists of simple cleaning of the wound and application of a sterile dressing. The wound epithelializes fairly rapidly and can be healed within two weeks. Wounds greater than 1 cm. in diameter without exposure of bone are treated by the application of a heavy split-thickness skin graft or a full-thickness skin graft taken from the volar surface of the forearm in the male or some less conspicuous spot in the female. If the patient has preserved the avulsed fingertip, after defatting it can be replaced as a full-thickness graft.

All the injuries just mentioned can be asso-

ciated with fracture of the tuft or shaft of the distal phalanx. A fracture with significant displacement should be reduced insofar as possible to prevent the development of a deformed nail.

More severe injuries of the fingertip are not commonly seen in the athlete, but when they do occur they can be repaired by (1) excising enough bone to allow primary closure, (2) covering the defect with a split- or full-thickness graft, (3) creating cross finger flaps, or (4) creating a palmar pedicle flap or an abdominal or axillary pedicle.

One must be extremely penurious in sacrificing the length of the finger simply to effect closure. It is far better to use a primary split graft, deciding later on definitive treatment, including the possibility of amputation. It is not proper to rush a patient with such an injury to the emergency room and clip away the distal tip of the finger until one has analyzed the blood supply very thoroughly. In many instances what may appear to be a hopelessly unsalvageable fingertip may actually be viable when properly replaced (Fig. 264). We have witnessed many instances in which a seemingly lost fingertip was saved by replacement of the avulsed portion as a full-thickness graft. Extreme conservatism must be practiced in sacrificing any tissue in the finger.

Before undertaking a complicated program of pedicle grafting, consider how important the added length may be to the patient, especially if it will be devoid of sensation. Injuries of the fingers are often lightly treated, resulting in various deformities which may be quite painful in the very sensitive area at the end of the finger. We cannot overemphasize the importance of cleanliness in treating all these injuries.

LACERATIONS OF THE HAND

Lacerations of the hand may have extremely serious consequences and should never be minimized. The laceration penetrates the skin with the fingers in various degrees of flexion or extension. When the cut is examined, all too often the finger may be in another position, and superficial examination of the cut may reveal normal structures. It is dangerous to assume that the deep structures are not involved unless the cut is carefully examined with the finger in various positions.

Treatment. The first step in treatment of the lacerated hand is an assessment of the function

Figure 264. This water-skiing accident illustrates a principle of treatment of fingertip injuries. The patient sustained an extensive injury to the tip of the index finger which resulted in avulsion of a portion of the distal phalanx (A). This was repaired as a primary procedure, and the ischemic area was allowed to demarcate, as indicated in B. Once demarcation was complete it was possible to remove the gangrenous tissue and close the finger tip with the viable flap of skin on the radial side of the finger (C). Injudicious amputation as the primary procedure would have resulted in a much shorter phalanx or anesthetic skin coverage on the fingertip.

of the part. This includes all motions of the involved area, both active and passive. One should then carefully check the nerve function, bearing in mind the distribution of the nerve which is likely to be injured. This check may be made without removing the dressing from the hand; in fact, there is no excuse for repeatedly removing the dressing to examine the hand if the laceration appears to be severe. As the player comes off the field, a sterile dressing should be applied immediately and a firm pressure bandage wrapped around the injured part. He should then be taken to the infirmary or hospital in which he is to receive definitive treatment. At that time, and at that time only, should the dressing be removed. After the dressing has been carefully removed and the wound has been thoroughly inspected, determination should be made of the type of anesthesia indicated. If there is disturbance of tendon function, if there is loss of nerve function or if there appears to be any joint involvement, it is advisable to use a general anesthetic, which makes easier the use of a tourniquet to control bleeding. Occasionally a tourniquet placed on the forearm is well tolerated and may be used with local or regional nerve block of the hand; in this case a general anesthetic will not be necessary. An x-ray study should be made to detect any abnormality of the bony structures of the hand.

After preliminary preparations, the patient is taken to the operating room and given the appropriate anesthetic, either nerve block or general. Any definitive treatment is best carried out under tourniquet control. The dressing is removed and the surgeon, wearing sterile gloves, should carefully inspect the hand. This is not the time for a detailed examination of the wound itself. The next step is a thorough cleansing of the hand. If necessary, a detergent is used to remove grease; otherwise, soap and water are employed to cleanse the entire hand, with particular attention being paid to the site of the wound. The wound is thoroughly lavaged with running water.

The hand is now redraped with sterile drapes; the medical team puts on new gowns and gloves. Only then is the wound itself investigated. It is thoroughly lavaged again, all exposed areas being brushed with a sterile sponge. Examination should make it possible to determine the extent of involvement of nerve or tendon. It may be that a tendon has been partially cut. This can be determined only by moving the finger through a full range of motion while inspecting the tendon throughout the area which might have been exposed in this wound. Ordinarily it is not necessary to enlarge the wound simply for diagnostic purposes. If there is nerve damage, and if the wound is relatively clean, the wound should be enlarged enough to expose the nerve ends and permit nerve suture. If there is a combination of nerve and tendon damage, the tougher structures should be sutured first.

Repair of Lacerated Tendons and Nerves.
No attempt is made here to describe in full the repair of lacerated tendons and nerves, but a few principles should be emphasized. As a general rule, it is not advisable to suture lacerated nerves unless the wound is scrupulously clean. Lacerated nerves are best repaired at a later date, after scarring in the perineurium renders them easier to suture. The volar digital nerves can be repaired primarily in most instances. Lacerated extensor tendons can also be repaired primarily, and delayed repairs are not necessary or advisable. With flexor tendons an entirely different situation exists, because they must glide in a very tight fibro-osseous compartment at the level of the fingers, and repair of the flexor tendons within the flexor tendon sheath of the fingers is not advisable. Certain rules have been established for repair of these particular tendons. The profundus tendon cut close to its insertion into the base of the distal phalanx can be advanced and sutured into the base of the phalanx, excising the distal segment of the tendon. Lacerations of both flexor tendons between the area just proximal to the insertion of the profundus tendon and the distal palmar crease are in "no man's land." If both sublimis and profundus tendons are lacerated in this location, it is best to obtain primary closure of the skin and do a flexor graft later. With the advent of modern surgical technique, it is becoming more and more acceptable to perform primary tendon repairs in "no man's land."

If only the sublimis tendon is lacerated, repair is not indicated. If the profundus tendon is cut, and the sublimis remains intact, a tenodesis procedure, fixing the distal interphalangeal joint in flexion, or fusion of the distal interphalangeal joint in flexion, will yield the most consistently satisfactory results.

If it is determined that the laceration is within the sheath and it nevertheless seems advisable to repair the tendon, the sheath should be partially excised. Never repair two tendons within the same sheath. If both the flexor digitorum profundus and sublimis have been severed within the same sheath, the sublimis should be sacrificed and the profundus alone repaired.

Tendon or nerve suture in the hand is a highly specialized procedure, and one should be thoroughly versed in the proper technique before attempting even a simple repair. Therefore, although these injuries are not common in the athlete, when they do occur they are extremely important. I know of one instance in which the classic mistake of suturing a lacerated flexor tendon to the median nerve was accomplished, and needless to say, the function of neither the tendon nor the nerve was restored.

Following repair of the tendon or nerve, the extremity must be placed in the position that most relaxes the area of repair and held there for at least three weeks to permit the early stages of repair to take place. Following the three-week period, if the finger can be securely splinted with a dressing that is acceptable to the athletic authorities, participation in sports might be permitted.

Many of these injuries are locker room accidents, such as from thrusting the hand through a glass door, and may indeed involve multiple tendons. One of our patients was a young athlete who was in the hospital to have his knee cartilage removed. He attempted to close the transom window over his bed by driving the heel of his hand against the glass. The glass broke and the jagged edges sectioned all the flexor tendons and the median nerve at the level of the wrist. The only good thing about this accident was that he was in the proper locale to get early treatment. This could hardly be called an athletic injury, although it certainly was an injury to an athlete. In this instance we were able to repair the tendons and the nerve, since the tendons at this level are not within a sheath.

PUNCTURE WOUNDS OF THE HAND

Puncture wounds of the hand are infrequent in athletes, although they are common enough in others. A wound in the hand made by a sharp cleat is almost always a laceration, because the skin in the dorsum of the hand tears as the cleat hits it and skids. Puncture wounds may be caused by contaminants on the playing field or by sharp projecting points on the players' equipment. After a puncture wound, particularly on the palmar side, the hand should be carefully checked for disturbance of nerve or tendon function. If this function remains intact, the wound should be treated expectantly; that is, the surrounding area should be thoroughly cleansed, a sterile dressing applied and the wound regularly observed. If any sign of deep-seated infection appears, adequate drainage must be provided immediately, since infection within the closed spaces of the hand can be very severe and may lead to a crippling disability. The player should be instructed that if he experiences fever or malaise, or if he has aching or throbbing in the hand, he should report at once for a careful examination to determine the severity of the involvement. In the early stage there may be considerable deep soreness. This should not be confused with infection, since infection is unlikely to develop for several days.

Here once more is illustrated the great value of careful primary examination. If the initial examination elicits no particular soreness anywhere in the hand, any soreness that develops after several days is much more significant. When treating the hand, one must be particularly careful to prevent an iatrogenic lesion. An unclean or incautiously used scalpel or scissors may readily spread infection into the tendon sheath or palmar space or may actually sever a nerve or a vessel. It is axiomatic that any puncture wound requires administration of tetanus toxoid. A broad-spectrum antibiotic may be required.

In any penetrating wound one must always suspect the presence of foreign material, particularly glass. Clothing or similar material is not frequently carried into the tissues of the hand.

Human Bite

A wound in the athlete that has a particularly grave connotation is the "knuckle" wound caused by striking the human tooth. It is a contaminated wound and should be treated as such by meticulous cleansing of the part. Again, the extensor tendon, which is part of the capsule of the metacarpophalangeal joint, may be cut while the finger is flexed. When it is examined with the finger in extension, the laceration of the tendon has now traveled considerably proximal to the cut in the skin and the defect may be completely overlooked.

Treatment. To treat such a wound as a casual "barked" knuckle is to court disaster. In the first place, infection from a human bite is one of the most difficult to treat. In the second place, there will remain not only a defect in the capsule but also irregularity of the metacarpophalangeal joint. In this instance, the proper treatment is to retract the wound edges carefully, to lavage the wound thoroughly, and to clip away any obviously necrotic tissue but to be very wary about sacrificing tissue. Then examine the tendon carefully by flexing the finger. If necessary, the wound may be enlarged to permit careful suture of the tendon. When the skin is ready to be closed, the contused, devitalized edge may be trimmed away very sparingly. It is impor-

tant to effect well-demarcated skin edges. The wound may be closed without drainage but must be watched very carefully. The patient should be observed for signs of any developing infection. One should give a prophylactic broad-spectrum antibiotic in any case. If infection is imminent or actually present, the skin edges should not be closed. They should be opened if the wound was closed primarily and infection has supervened.

INFECTIONS OF THE HAND

There is no place on a team for a player with an infected hand. His dressing should not be changed in the dressing room or training room, since the spread of infection to other members of the team may be disastrous. This applies as well to any infection elsewhere. If a player has an abrasion that is contaminated and draining pus, he should be barred from the dressing room until the purulent stage has passed. The hand should be treated with warm saline dressings. After the suppuration has cleared, the abraded area should be carefully protected with unguent and a suitable dressing. Even at this stage the player should be warned not to peel off his dressing and throw it on the floor or in the shower or any other place where it could contaminate the room.

Infection About the Fingernail

Although not strictly in the category of an athletic injury, this subject should be considered here since it frequently involves the athlete. Indeed, it may often follow relatively minor injuries about the nail with impingement of the paronychial fold against the side of the nail.

Simple contusion of the nail or along the side of the nail may cause some abrasion or laceration of the skin. An inflammatory reaction about the nail produces the familiar picture of a red, inflamed, swollen nail fold. This may be an extremely distressing condition and may materially handicap the athlete, particularly if it is on the thumb or first or second finger. In the early stage it is best treated by heat applied locally. It should be carefully explained to the player that adequate care in the early stage may well prevent considerable disability later. Soaking the area several times a day or continuous warm soaks and the use of a heat lamp may prevent suppuration.

If an abscess develops, it should be drained. If the involvement is close to the nail, an instrument can be passed between the nail and the paronychial fold and the nail lifted gently, permitting the pus to exude through this defect. This route of drainage has the advantage of not requiring a cut on the skin. It has the disadvantage that the nail fold tends to close down readily over the nail and the abscess does not drain. If this occurs, or if the infection seems to be away from the nail, a straight linear incision parallel to the nail edge will usually suffice for drainage. The incision is carried down to the abscess. Ethyl chloride applied locally will suffice for anesthesia. This incision will tend to gape open rather than to seal, and drainage will be adequate. Hot soaks should be continued, and the dressings applied should be sufficiently protective to prevent contamination of the finger from extrinsic infection and to prevent the finger from being the source of contamination to the patient or to others.

An infection of the base of the nail may have more serious consequences, because it tends to burrow under the proximal edge of the nail at the root and so to form a subungual abscess. Prompt, adequate drainage must be carried out or else the nail bed may be destroyed and permanent damage will result. If the pus has actually elevated the proximal section of the nail, this portion should be removed to permit exposure of the nail bed at its root, thereby preventing further undermining. As much of the nail should be removed at the proximal end as is undermined by the infection; otherwise the detached nail lying over the nail bed will serve to form a pocket of infection. Following complete drainage by resection of the base of the nail, the area must be carefully protected to prevent external contamination of the wound and the spread of infection to other parts of the body. If the drainage has been carried out promptly, there is every reason to expect regrowth of the nail. If drainage is delayed, destruction of the nail root and bed will lead to gross and often painful deformities of the nail.

Felons

A felon is an abscess located within the fat pad of the fingertip. The important consideration here is that pus creates pressure in the closed septal spaces, which exist primarily to provide a cushioning effect from the fat on the palmar side of the finger. When these spaces become infected, abscess pressure builds up, because it is not easily decompressed by expansion of the skin. The abscess continues to

Figure 265. *A*, Illustration shows the importance of an adequate incision and drainage of a felon. The pus is contained in compartments, and all compartments must be decompressed to prevent erosion of bone and osteomyelitis. The line of incision is outlined extending through all compartments. *B*, An unfortunate result of an inadequately treated felon which led to osteomyelitis. Most of the bone of the distal phalanx was destroyed. Treatment of an abscess, even in this day of modern miracle drugs and antibiotics, is still drainage through an adequate incision.

invade tissue adjacent to it, gradually enlarging until the whole fingertip may become involved. This can lead to osteomyelitis of the phalanx if the abscess if not adequately drained (Fig. 265*A*).

Treatment. Treatment consists of incision and drainage, by making an adequate incision along either the medial or lateral border of the phalanx. Combining both in a fish-mouth type of incision is usually not necessary or desirable. It is important to decompress all involved compartments (Fig. 265*B*). The wound should be held open with petrolatum gauze or a through and through rubber drain. It should be allowed to close in two to three days when the inflammatory reaction has subsided. The tragic complication of osteomyelitis of the phalanx should never be permitted to develop.

Flexor Tendon Sheath Infections

Infections in the fingers which enter the flexor tendon sheaths will present symptoms of swelling and pain along the flexor sheath, limited painful extension and flexion contracture. Infections entering the little finger or thumb flexor sheath will travel proximally to the wrist and palm and may join to form a horseshoe abscess. Infections in the index, center and ring finger sheaths will stop at the metacarpophalangeal joints. Infections from the index finger which escape the sheath at the metacarpophalangeal joint will enter the thenar space; infections in the ring and long fingers will enter the midpalmar space when they escape the confines of the flexor tendon sheath (see Fig. 258).

Treatment. Treatment of all these infections requires proper drainage of the abscess from the space or bursa involved. This drainage should be preceded and followed by continuous hot sterile soaks until the infection subsides.

The collar button abscess is one in which the primary abscess cavity is located deep to the palmar fascia and only a small portion of the abscess is seen superficial to the palmar fascia. This creates two abscess cavities which are separated by a small neck, giving the appearance of a collar button. It is important to recognize that the most superficial portion of the abscess does not represent the entire abscess. A similar situation exists with a felon in which there can be a small collection of pus immediately beneath the dermis overlying the more important felon beneath.

Traumatic Inflammation of the Flexor Tendon Sheath

Repeated trauma to the flexor tendon sheath can result in an inflammatory reaction with swelling that restricts the normal gliding of the flexor tendons within their sheath. This is especially true of the already thickened portion of the sheath that forms the pulley at the level of the distal metacarpal. A small nodule already present in the flexor tendon can become impinged on either the proximal or distal side of the pulley, creating either a snapping sensation or completely locking the finger in either the flexed or the extended position.

This is the so-called *trigger finger*. It can be treated initially by rest and anti-inflammatory agents such as phenylbutazone given systemically or cortisone injected into the sheath.

Frequently surgery is necessary to correct the problem. Surgical treatment is directed toward removing the thickened pulley at this level. It should be performed under general anesthesia or adequate regional block. A tour-

niquet is a must, as is adequate visualization of the involved portion of the flexor tendon sheath. Adequate excision of the pulley and a portion of the adjacent sheath will prevent a distressing recurrence of the problem.

STRAIN (MUSCULOTENDINOUS INJURIES) IN THE HAND

With the vast complex of muscle-tendon units in the hand, it is obvious that strain will occur frequently.

There are two basic categories of these muscle-tendon units: the long flexors and the long extensors, which are entirely tendinous in the hand; and the intrinsic muscles, in which the entire musculotendinous unit is contained within the hand itself.

Strain in the hand has two primary causes. One is excessive overuse against resistance, and the second is overstretching of the unit beyond its normal extensile range. In the intrinsic muscles of the hand the former cause is by far the more common and usually results from repeated use beyond the total capacity of the unit rather than from a single excessive contraction. This is not a common injury in athletic competition but may occur in sports such as gymnastics or those requiring constant gripping, such as rowing, tennis or golf. The initial symptoms are cramping and fatigue of the muscles involved with pain on function against resistance. If the activity is discontinued at this stage, recovery is prompt and without residual. Continuation of overuse may result in persistent muscle spasm or even contracture. Tenosynovitis is not common in the intrinsic muscles of the hand, since the tendons do not have a synovial sheath.

Strain in the long musculotendinous units may be manifested in the forearm near the musculotendinous junction. This has been discussed previously (see the section on the Forearm). There may also be a tenosynovitis in the palm or more distally in the fingers. There may be irritation at the attachment of the tendon to the phalanx. Irritation or strain of the attachment of the wrist flexors and extensors as they reach the base of the metacarpals may cause symptoms in this area. Those conditions which result from overuse must be treated primarily by rest. Rest is the essential ingredient for recovery. Other modes of treatment that may accelerate recovery are the use of heat applied locally, particularly the penetrating modalities, and the local injection of an anesthetic and a corticoid. These are of considerable value if the irritation is specifically within the sheath or tendinous attachment or even at the musculotendinous junction. Injection is much more successful if the condition is local. A local spot of discomfort over the dorsum of the base of the second metacarpal, with tenderness on pressure and pain on dorsiflexion of the wrist against resistance, may be interpreted as strain of the attachment of the extensor carpi radialis. Local injection in this area will give prompt and often permanent relief, provided that the etiological factor is eliminated. To avoid further strain, the hand and wrist should be supported by a forearm splint with the wrist in dorsiflexion. When competition is resumed, the wrist should be taped. Keeping in mind that the cause is overuse rather than overstretch, one must be careful to avoid active use of the muscle. Hence, a serious involvement of the carpal flexors or extensors will prohibit participation in athletics.

Whereas strain of the short flexors is most often within the muscle and is due primarily to overuse, long flexor involvement may well be in the tendon and is frequently due to overstretch, particularly against resistance. For example, a wrist that is forcibly dorsiflexed with the wrist flexors contracted may suffer strain of the flexors. This strain may be anything from a slight separation of some of the fibers in the musculotendinous junction or at the attachment of the tendon in the hand (mild) to a complete avulsion (severe). Symptomatically, there will be pain at the site of involvement, pain on active contraction of the muscle and pain on passive stretching of the muscle. If the rupture is complete, there will be loss of function of the muscle. In this case there may be bunching up of the muscle as it contracts with the distal end of the tendon pulling free, so that the muscle may actually shorten while the wrist does not flex.

If the tendon is avulsed, surgical treatment is indicated and the tendon should be sutured to its attachment. Much more frequently the strain is partial (mild to moderate). The treatment in this instance will be protection, first against overstretch, second against overuse. This protection must be continued for a sufficient time to permit the strength of the tendon to be restored. With only slight involvement (mild) little or no immobilization will be needed, whereas if there is extensive tearing (moderate), protection must be provided for several weeks. One can usually assess the degree of involvement by the rate of subsidence of symptoms and so regulate the extent

of immobilization of these long flexors. If there is irritation within the tendon sheath, the part must be immobilized. Injection of a steroid into the tendon sheath, together with physical therapy, is of considerable value. Corticoids must not be injected into the tendon itself. Rupture may result as a direct consequence of their adverse effect on collagen formation. Function should be resumed very slowly here or there will be prompt recurrence of symptoms. Although it is difficult to elicit in the hand, snowball crepitation can sometimes be felt along the tendon sheath. If present, it is diagnostic.

Avulsion of the Flexor Digitorum Profundus Tendon

This lesion is seen very infrequently but can occur. The tendon is usually avulsed from the attachment to the base of the distal phalanx. The earlier the lesion is recognized, the better the chances of obtaining a satisfactory result from surgical repair. Inability to actively flex the distal interphalangeal joint and problems with the flexor tendon sheath strongly suggest an avulsed tendon. This, together with a high index of suspicion, will lead to the correct diagnosis in those rare instances of tendon avulsion without x-ray evidence of avulsed bone.

SPRAIN-SUBLUXATION-DISLOCATION

It should be emphasized again that injuries to the components of the hand are extremely serious from the functional point of view. One must always bear in mind that almost the whole function of the upper extremity rests in the capability of the fingers and thumb. Despite this fact, injuries to the hand proper are often considered minor injuries and all too frequently the treatment they receive can be classified as minor, too. The treating physician does not recognize the magnitude of the maximum deformity occurring at the peak of injury unless an accurate history is taken or unless stress films can be obtained. Much damage to ligaments will have occurred before the joint is returned to normal. Since there is a considerable difference functionally and anatomically between the thumb and the remaining fingers, or more accurately between the first ray and the remaining rays of the hand, they will be discussed under separate headings.

Thumb Ray

Carpometacarpal Joint

Since the thumb is the opposing member of the group, of necessity it must have more mobility. The carpometacarpal joint is extremely mobile, its action in effect being that of a universal joint so that it moves in all directions—flexion and extension, adduction and abduction, circumduction and rotation. For this to occur the stability of the joint to extremes of motion must be maintained almost entirely by ligaments and other soft tissues, since there is no bony restriction to any particular motion. Forced motion in any direction beyond the strength of the ligamentous support will cause a sprain, which may be mild (first degree), moderate (second degree) or severe (third degree). If the force is continued, a subluxation or dislocation will occur. For example, forceful wide abduction of the thumb produces hyperextension of the carpometacarpal joint, which throws a strain on the anterior portion of the capsule. If the force is arrested, the injury may be mild or moderate and a sprain results. If it continues, the injury will be severe, and the base may dislocate as it passes out through a rent in the capsule. The thumb in this case is actually bent backward over the wrist owing to complete disruption of the anterior structures of the joint. Similarly, the dorsal capsule may be injured by hyperflexion. The foolish habit of grasping the thumb within the fingers and then striking a blow with the clenched fist tends to rotate the base of the metacarpal dorsally and to rupture the dorsal ligaments. Subluxation is more likely to occur here than dislocation, although disruption of the capsule may be complete. There may be sprain of the lateral and less frequently of the medial components.

Treatment. Treatment will vary according to the severity of injury. Mild sprain of the carpometacarpal joint is extremely common and causes pain around the joint, tenderness to pressure over the area and pain on reproduction of the motion that caused the injury. Within a few hours the area of the base of the thumb will be swollen and edematous and almost any motion will cause pain. Treatment should be directed toward reduction of any residual subluxation and protection of the joint against stress until the healing is complete (Fig. 266). If the injury is mild, simple adhesive strapping will suffice to prevent overstretch (Fig. 267). If the injury is moderate to severe, the joint should be immobilized by plaster fixation in a position which would be assumed

Figure 266. This patient sustained subluxation of a carpometacarpal joint in a bowling injury. Notice the lateral subluxation of the base of the first metacarpal (arrow). Although the injury appeared to be quite minimal on x-ray, the patient was in severe pain until the subluxation was reduced by traction and pressure at the base of the thumb.

by grasping a 3 in. ball (see Fig. 256). It is not necessary to immobilize the fingers, but the splint should include the hand and wrist and the thumb as far as the middle of the proximal

Figure 267. Basket-weave strapping of thumb. (Courtesy of Rawlinson, Modern Athletic Training. © 1961 by Prentice Hall, Inc.)

phalanx. The duration of the immobilization will vary with the severity of the injury. As a general rule, the cast should be left on about three weeks and the thumb should be protected against strain by adequate taping for the next three weeks. Later the thumb should be protected during contact sports if the ligament rupture was complete.

If there is subluxation or instability of this joint, great care must be taken to immobilize the joint in its normal relationship. If the subluxation cannot be reduced and held by simple plaster fixation, traction should be applied. In these cases immobilization will be considerably longer, since at least six weeks is needed for the ligament and capsule to unite firmly, even under the most favorable circumstances.

Simple dislocation of this joint is not a frequent injury. If the force is sufficient to disrupt the joint, a fracture-dislocation will occur (Fig. 268*A*). The so-called Bennett fracture leaves a small portion of the lip of the metacarpal fixed to the anterior capsular ligaments, whereas the remaining portion dislocates. This is discussed in the section on fractures.

It may be that when a frank dislocation does occur it is reduced spontaneously, and by the time it is seen by the physician there is no deformity. If dislocation persists, it should be reduced by traction along the long axis of the thumb and by gradual abduction, while local pressure is placed on the dorsal aspect of the proximal end of the phalanx to force the metacarpal back into its normal carpal relationship. If it is unstable in this position, some form of internal fixation, such as percutaneous insertion of a K-wire, is advisable, since it is extremely difficult to hold it by plaster alone. While the thumb is held manually, a transfixation pin may be drilled through the base of the metacarpal and into the adjacent carpal or into the adjacent second metacarpal (Figs. 268*B* and 269). Ideally it probably would be better at this time to open the dorsal aspect of the joint and repair the ligaments. The fact that one so often sees a hypermobile, painful and even subluxating joint following this injury would suggest that some improvement in treatment is indicated. The usual error is that of inadequate immobilization rather than incomplete reduction. After dislocation of the thumb, the athlete should wear supportive strapping for the rest of the season (see Fig. 267).

Treatment of the chronic sprain is difficult, since continued participation in sports causes frequent reinjury. The first requirement is an adequate support that is tolerable to the patient and yet protects the joint. Adhesive strapping is not dependable, since someone is required to reapply it and frequently it is not done properly. An injury may occur while the strapping is off. A little slip-on protector that fits around the wrist can be devised by the bracemaker and is quite effective. At the time

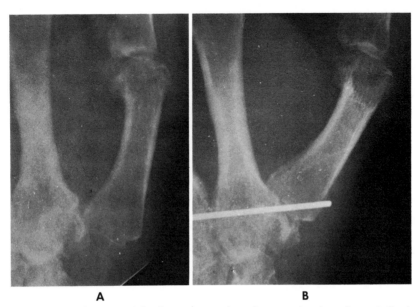

A   **B**

Figure 268. *A*, A fracture-dislocation of the first metacarpal on the trapezium by a force similar to that causing a Bennett fracture. *B*, The same case as *A*. Excellent postoperative fixation was obtained by transfixation through the metacarpal base into the base of the adjacent metacarpal. (For positioning for x-ray, see Fig. 269.)

Figure 269. For the visualization of the carpometacarpal joint of the thumb, the most comfortable position for the injured patient should be assumed. *A*, Posteroanterior view. Place the hand in a lateral position with the thumb abducted and supported on a nonopaque pad. Direct the central ray to the base of the thumb. *B*, Lateral view. Pronate the forearm. Support the slightly elevated palm enough to place the lateral aspect of the thumb, slightly abducted and flexed, on the cassette. Direct the central ray to the base of the thumb. These same views show the Bennett fracture.

of acute recurrence of chronic sprain, local injection of a corticoid into the joint is effective, and the usual physical therapeutic measures also help.

Metacarpophalangeal Joint

The metacarpophalangeal joint of the thumb (Fig. 270A) permits motion primarily in flexion and extension. However, there is an element of adduction and abduction permitted by the convex-concave lateral curvature of the head of the metacarpal and base of the phalanx. The collateral ligaments definitely restrict adduction and abduction. This joint is extremely vulnerable to sprain, because as the thumb is abducted the metacarpal becomes fixed, and the force applied to the end of the thumb is directed against the metacarpophalangeal joint. When the lateral stress is toward either adduction or abduction, the sprain is to the collateral ligaments. When the force is in straight extension, the strain is to the anterior

capsule. If the force is limited, the resultant injury is low-grade and no instability results. If the force continues, subluxation occurs as the result of tearing of the stressed ligament (see Fig. 270B). Thus, if the force is abduction, the medial collateral ligament will be avulsed (Fig. 271) or torn (Fig. 272), the phalanx and metacarpal will separate and the joint will open on the medial side. As soon as the force is released, the thumb falls back into its normal position and reveals no obvious abnormality. The pain will be along the medial side of the joint and, as with sprains elsewhere, in the final analysis the determination of the degree of lateral instability is of utmost importance. If the force involved is hyperextension, the metacarpal head thrusts forward through the anterior capsule (Fig. 273). Here again, if the force is relieved, the joint may slip back into position and be spontaneously reduced.

A sprain to the area of the metacarpophalangeal joint may cause chronic disability for months or years or even permanently. Inade-

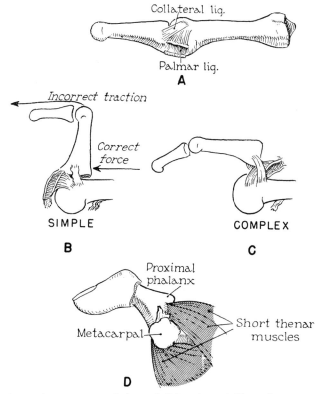

Figure 270. Simple and complex metacarpophalangeal dislocations. *A,* The volar aspect of a metacarpophalangeal joint capsule is reinforced with a palmar ligament or fibrocartilage. *B,* In a simple dislocation the phalanx is hyperextended, and the palmar ligament hangs like a curtain over the metacarpal head. Traction may pivot the phalanx on the intact collateral ligaments and interpose the palmar ligament between the bones. The phalanx should be pushed into place. *C,* In a complex dislocation the finger is hyperextended so that it is more parallel to, but not on, the metacarpal. The volar joint capsule and palmar ligament are interposed, which usually prevents reduction by manipulation. *D,* In the metacarpophalangeal joint of the thumb, the short thenar muscles augment the pivot force, thereby predisposing the joint to complex dislocation. (From McLaughlin, Trauma.)

Figure 271. Lateral ligament injury of the metacarpophalangeal joint of the thumb, avulsing the corner of the proximal end of the phalanx. This is really a ligament injury and requires repair by either pinning the fragment or removing the fragment and repairing the ligament.

Figure 272. Demonstrations of a lateral deviation injury at the metacarpophalangeal joint of the left thumb, with a complete tear of the collateral ligament of the ulnar side. A, Stress film showing the extent of dislocation possible. B, An operative photograph of the torn ligament held in the forceps. Here the orientation is the same as on the x-ray, looking into the dorsomedial aspect of the metacarpophalangeal joint through the first web space. The dorsal creases of the interphalangeal joint are marked with i–p.

Figure 273. Complete dislocation of the metacarpophalangeal joint of the thumb. This could be reduced only by open reduction, since the flexor tendons were looped around the metacarpal head.

quate treatment of an initial injury is mainly responsible, since it permits the ligament and capsule to heal with redundancy. Thus recurrent subluxation is easily produced. Many baseball players, particularly catchers, have such an involvement, and the least hyperextension of the thumb or flexion of the thumb across the palm will cause recurrence of the painful, swollen joint. The thumb should be immobilized for at least three weeks if the injury seems severe. It should then be protected for several more weeks by very comprehensive strapping that permits only a minimum of motion in the metacarpophalangeal joint but leaves the distal phalanx relatively free. The degree of immobilization and duration of protection will depend upon the response to treatment. As long as the interphalangeal joints are given motion relatively early (within three weeks), one need not fear immobilization. I have yet to see an instance of restriction of motion in the metacarpophalangeal joint that could be attributed to overlong immobilization. Protection of the joint in the young patient is particularly important. One has only to experience a recurrent or chronic sprain of this joint to appreciate the seriousness of the resulting handicap to the budding athlete.

With a *complete dislocation* (see Fig. 273), the very fact that the dislocation reaches the physician unreduced is a warning signal. Under ordinary circumstances this dislocation will reduce spontaneously. If it does not do so at once, or if it does not do so spontaneously, the injured person himself almost certainly will have grabbed the thumb and pulled it into position, often with the eager help of one of his teammates. Hence, if the dislocation can

be reduced by simple traction and manual manipulation, it will already be reduced before the doctor sees it. If this dislocation is seen almost immediately after injury, one is justified in attempting an atraumatic manipulation without anesthesia. The traction should be in the long axis of the deformed phalanx, whatever its position. Direct distal pressure of the operator's thumb against the base of the phalanx will slide it into position as the phalanx is flexed. This dislocation cannot be reduced by traction along the long axis of the metacarpal, since this simply locks the dislocation in position.

If a complete dislocation does not reduce readily by such methods, one should proceed to open reduction on the assumption that the metacarpal head is caught in the rent in the capsule or between the long flexor tendon and one of the intrinsic tendons. The hand should be prepared for surgery, the anesthetic given and a second attempt made to reduce the dislocation under anesthesia. If it does not reduce promptly with minimal stress, manipulation should not be pursued, since it only damages the periarticular structures. Open operation should be carried out at once. It should be emphasized here, as in all dislocations, that time is of the essence and one must not wait days or even hours before final reduction is carried out.

Lateral stress injuries are treated using the same principles as for hyperextension injuries, with the exception that surgery is performed to repair ligaments rather than to effect reduction. If complete instability is demonstrable following acute injury, repair of the involved ligament is indicated (see Fig. 272). If x-ray shows an avulsion fracture with separation, the ligament should be opened and repaired (see Fig. 271).

Postoperative Care. If the injury is moderate or if deformity is spontaneously reduced, or if open reduction has been done, the thumb should be treated by immobilization of the joint, plaster splints being my preference. The splints in this instance go out beyond the interphalangeal joint extending back to the wrist and down onto the thenar eminence. It is not absolutely essential to immobilize the wrist. After the splint is applied, motion of the thumb itself should not increase the discomfort. If it does, the wrist should be included until the muscle spasm has subsided, possibly a week. After approximately a week in splints, a thumb spica cast may be used to complete three weeks of immobilization. Since the ligaments are not securely healed at this stage, the thumb should be carefully taped to prevent the motion that puts stress on the involved ligament. This should continue for at least three additional weeks. After this the thumb must be taped during athletic participation until all tenderness is gone.

A sprain of the medial collateral ligament of the metacarpophalangeal joint of the thumb may be extremely distressing to the athlete, particularly if he has to handle a football. Actually the pinch of the thumb opposing the fingers when the ball is grabbed for throwing or passing back, such as by the center, depends upon the stability of this joint. Because this joint is unstable, when the pinch occurs it simply opens up. When the index finger presses the ball toward the thumb, it opens up this inner side of the joint and results in serious disability. Recently we had two patients with sprain at essentially the same time. One was a center and one was a quarterback on the same team (Fig. 274). Both obtained excellent results from reconstruction by advancement of the cuff of the capsule without any additional reinforcement. It requires considerable study of the anatomy of this portion of the hand in order to recognize the various components. It is a much more favorable injury if the ligament is actually torn off the metacarpal head, which was true in each of these cases, and reconstructive repair was carried out by simply detaching the ligament from the scar which had formed, advancing it down on the shaft and securely suturing it with drill holes through the metacarpal shaft.

Interphalangeal Joint

Sprain of the interphalangeal joint is not nearly as frequent as sprain of the other two joints of the thumb. The leverage factor is such that more strain is applied to the other joints than to the interphalangeal joint. Lateral motion of the distal phalanx may tear the opposing collateral ligament, and the pain will be on the same side of the thumb as the applied force. Since the interphalangeal joint is a hinge joint, there is no appreciable lateral motion

Figure 274. Two months ago this 22 year old football player caught his thumb in the equipment of another player when he was blocking and threw the thumb into wide abduction. He continued to play with a tape splint but now has complete instability of the ulnar side of the metacarpophalangeal joint of the thumb. He is unable to grasp the football in order to throw it. *A,* Neutral position is shown. The small fragment is pulled off the ulnar side of the base of the proximal phalanx of the thumb. *B,* Stress, toward the radial side. *C,* Stress, toward the ulnar side. Note the phalanx actually subluxes off the metacarpal head.

and the joint should be carefully checked for lateral instability. If instability is evident or if a small fragment of bone is revealed on the x-ray, one must assume that the collateral ligament has been avulsed or torn, and the protection should be correspondingly protracted. If one can diagnose with certainty a complete tear of the collateral ligament, primary repair of the ligament is the treatment of choice. All too frequently the instability is not recognized until several weeks following the initial trauma, when swelling, pain and disability persist and one notices the phalanx is deviating to the opposite side. At this time one may belatedly discover instability of the collateral ligament. Reconstruction rather than repair is then necessary, and it is correspondingly difficult and less successful. If injury to the interphalangeal joint is relatively severe, immobilization is indicated for at least three weeks, followed by protective strapping for three more weeks.

Finger Rays

Metacarpal Area

Sprain may occur at the carpometacarpal, the metacarpophalangeal and the intermetacarpal head area.

Sprain at the *base of the metacarpal* is not common. This entire area is firmly bound together by the dorsal and palmar ligaments of the wrist and hand so that they are firmly adherent not only to each other but also to the carpus. There is little lateral motion in these joints, and lateral stresses are not readily applied. The sprain is much more likely to involve the wrist than the carpometacarpal joint, since the same force puts stress on both areas and the wrist is much more vulnerable than the carpometacarpal joint.

At the *distal end of the metacarpals* the joints are in effect universal, permitting flexion and extension, adduction, abduction and circumduction, but not axial rotation. Extremes of these motions may cause a sprain of the capsular ligaments. The digits most likely to be injured in collateral sprains are the index and little fingers, since either one may be forcibly abducted away from the hand, whereas it is much more difficult to abduct the other two fingers to the extent required to damage the capsular ligaments.

The most common injury is damage to the transverse metacarpal ligaments. The same force that pulls the fingers apart may tear the ligament binding the metacarpal heads together, and this may occur at any space. That is, the long and ring fingers may be forcibly separated and tear the ligament between the third and fourth metacarpals. This is much more likely than a tear of the capsular ligament of the metacarpophalangeal joint. This injury is readily overlooked. It is usually minimized but may cause weeks or months of disability of the hand and, indeed, may lead to chronic sprain with repeated reinjury and resultant disability. The injury is readily recognized if the hand is examined with this condition in mind, since simple separation of the two involved fingers will cause severe pain. The areas most commonly affected are between the fourth and fifth metacarpals and between the second and third. Treatment is relatively simple. If the hand is dressed in a manner that will hold the fingers together, free motion can be permitted to the phalanges, and athletic competition can actually be continued if fixation is firm enough to prevent separation of the metacarpal heads. Protection should be continued for another three weeks. This injury is not particularly disabling, and essentially free function of the hand can be maintained so long as the patient wears the protective dressing.

The force most likely to cause a sprain of the metacarpophalangeal joint is hyperextension. In this instance the anterior capsule becomes tight. As the force continues the capsule may tear. The injury may be mild or moderate or it may be a complete avulsion (severe), leading to dislocation. It may involve a single finger or more than one.

Symptomatically, any sprain involving the metacarpals will manifest tenderness at the area of the tear, and pain will be caused by reproduction of the motion that caused the injury.

Sprain of the metacarpophalangeal joint may be severe enough to cause actual dislocation. This is infrequent and is readily recognized as a very serious injury which demands definitive care by an experienced physician. Dorsal dislocation of the base of the phalanx at the metacarpophalangeal joint occurs as a result of the same hyperextension that causes sprain of the anterior capsule. As the force continues, the proximal phalanx moves backward over the metacarpal. The anterior capsule tears and the soft tissues are pulled dorsally, being displaced posterior to the metacarpal head. The phalanx dislocates onto the back of the metacarpal, where it stands at a 90 degree angle to the metacarpal. As men-

Figure 275. *A*, Drawing showing the normal position of the thickened portion of the capsule, which is termed the volar plate. Notice that it attaches well proximal to the head of the proximal bone. *B*, Illustration of the first effect of hyperextension, which is either sprain of the ligament or avulsion of its attachment to the bone (arrows). *C*, The end point of complete hyperextension, with a torn capsule and dislocation of the involved phalanx. The arrows indicate the direction of the forces which should be used in reduction. If the phalanx is merely straightened, the situation in *D* will possibly prevail, with the head of the proximal bone protruding through a rent in the capsule.

tioned previously, it is quite unlikely that this dislocation is seen in its original position; inevitably someone has attempted to straighten the finger. If an attempt has been made by simply flexing the phalanx, it will usually result in sliding the phalanx back along the dorsum of the metacarpal and impinging a flap of capsule between the phalanx and metacarpal head. Such manipulation is to be discouraged and should be avoided by the physician who attempts reduction (Fig. 275).

If the deformity is of the right angle variety, reduction can frequently be accomplished by applying pressure distally along the base of the phalanx in the direction of the long axis of the metacarpal while the finger is maintained in hyperextension. This permits the base of the phalanx to slide over the metacarpal head, and as it resumes its normal position in relation to the metacarpal head, flexion of the finger will

reduce the dislocation. An attempt may be made to carry out this manipulation without anesthesia provided that the dislocation is seen very early and that there has been no traumatic attempt to carry out reduction earlier.

If the finger and metacarpal are parallel to the phalanx resting on the back of the metacarpal neck, it is unlikely that the dislocation can be reduced without anesthesia. In such an instance it is well to be prepared to perform a surgical procedure at the time the anesthetic is given, since it may be impossible to reduce the dislocation even under anesthesia. Under anesthesia, traction may be placed on the phalanx along the axis of the metacarpal. This maneuver often will successfully reduce the dislocation. If it does not, the phalanx may be very carefully hyperextended to an angle of 90 degrees to the metacarpal, placing it back in the position it occupied at the time of the

Figure 276. *A* and *B,* The anteroposterior and lateral views of a dislocated metacarpophalangeal joint of the index finger. Avulsion of the attachment of one of the collateral ligaments to the first metacarpal has taken a small piece of bone with it. Dislocation of this joint should be opened through an incision in the palm because the metacarpal head becomes caught between the lumbrical tendon laterally, the long flexor tendons medially, the capsule distally and transverse fibers of the palmar fascia proximally. In this instance the avulsed ligament was repaired through a separate dorsal incision (*C*).

dislocation. This may remove the interposed tissue and permit classic reduction. If such a reduction cannot be done without undue force, the attempt should not be continued, and one should proceed to an open reduction in order to disengage the interposed tissue and permit the metacarpal head to move backward under the phalanx (Fig. 276). Since the structures blocking reduction are located anteriorly, the incision is most logically placed in the palm. The head of the metacarpal becomes caught between the flexor tendons medially, the lumbrical laterally, the volar plate distally and the transverse elements of the palmar fascia proximally. A transverse incision over the metacarpophalangeal joint gives excellent access to these structures. Identify and protect the digital vessels and nerves. A midlateral incision will result in a three-hour bungling attempt at the same thing. Some surgeons prefer a dorsal incision dividing the extensor tendon. Following reduction, immobilization should be carried out for about two weeks, but it is not necessary to immobilize the interphalangeal joints. Thus, rehabilitation can start at once.

Finger Area

Sprain of the interphalangeal joints may be caused by hyperextension of the joint, which causes the anterior capsule to be torn (see Figs. 275A and B), or by excess lateral motion of this hinge joint (Fig. 277). The interphalangeal joints have definite collateral ligaments which are tight in flexion and relatively loose in extension. Lateral angulation of the phalanx will cause damage to the collateral ligament. This usually occurs with the involved joint in extension. A torn collateral ligament may be a very painful injury and may result in disability if left untreated. On the other hand, if it is immobilized, disability may result from stiffness. Careful examination of the finger will permit one to determine whether or not there is instability. If there is instability the joint should be immobilized in extension with appropriate lateral deviation to close the joint on the involved side. This should be maintained for about two weeks. After that, some motion may be permitted, but flexion beyond 90 degrees should not be permitted for at least four weeks.

Figure 277. A neglected injury to a collateral ligament of the proximal interphalangeal joint results in a finger which is unstable in lateral deviation. *A,* The joint remains chronically swollen. *B,* A stress x-ray shows correction of the deformity.

Sprain of the anterior capsule can be demonstrated by pain when an attempt is made to completely extend this joint. If the injury is severe, it may actually be possible to hyperextend the joint. In such an instance the joint should be immobilized in moderate flexion for two or three weeks. If there is no instability but only pain, it should suffice to protect the finger for a week or 10 days and then permit motion, warning the patient that he should not completely extend it. If athletic competition is permitted, either game or practice, the finger splint should be replaced during actual play for at least four weeks, since relatively minor repetition of the original injury may cause recurrence.

Dislocation of the interphalangeal joints is ordinarily caused by the same forces that cause sprain of the anterior capsule (Fig. 278). As the hyperextension continues, the anterior capsule tears, and the head of the more proximal phalanx thrusts through the palmar surface of the joint; it may, indeed, pierce the skin. Such an injury should be regarded as very serious (Fig. 279). It is frequently spontaneously reduced, particularly if incomplete. Even if the dislocation is complete, it will usually be reduced by the time one sees it if it is readily reducible.

In the dislocations that do not reduce, the head of the phalanx is usually caught either in the capsule or in the flexor tendon. If this is seen immediately after the injury, it may be reduced by manipulation. The first step is to reproduce the hyperextension to unlock the base of the dislocated phalanx and then, by traction along the line of the dislocated phalanx, the base of the bone can be readily pushed down into contact with the head of the more proximal phalanx. If it does not reduce readily, lidocaine block may provide adequate anesthesia, since muscle relaxation is not necessary. If the dislocation is open, the wound is given a very thorough cleansing using copious amounts of soap and water. The head is then reduced. If it is a recent injury, the skin edges are sutured as a primary procedure.

Following any of these dislocations, the finger should be immobilized with the joint in some flexion. The finger should not be flexed as much as 90 degrees, even though this may seem to hold the dislocation more firmly. In this position the collateral ligaments are under undue tension, and healing occurs with the ligament too long.

The dislocation may occur without actually tearing either collateral ligament. After the finger is reduced, particularly if the procedure is performed under anesthesia, careful check should be made to determine whether or not

Figure 278. *A,* The anteroposterior and lateral views of a dislocated proximal interphalangeal joint. Usually this can readily be reduced by hyperextending the dislocated joint and applying distal pressure to the base of the middle phalanx. When the overriding has been corrected, the joint is flexed. *B,* A similar situation is shown in the distal interphalangeal joint, which is reduced in much the same manner. *C,* The taping for a sprained or dislocated finger. Flex the injured joints slightly. Using ½ inch adhesive tape, apply a basket weave over the injured joint. Place ⅛ inch thickness of soft sponge, felt or cotton between the fingers to prevent maceration. Using ½ inch tape, strap the finger to an adjoining finger, which will act as a splint, leaving the index finger free if possible. (Courtesy of Rawlinson, Modern Athletic Training, © 1961 by Prentice Hall, Inc.)

Figure 279. *A,* and *B,* Dislocation of the proximal interphalangeal joint of the little finger. This dislocation usually entails severe injury to the collateral ligaments and is likely to heal with a swollen, stiff joint or instability, or both. The ligament should be repaired as the primary procedure.

there is instability. If instability is present, one should repair the collateral ligament. In many of these conditions there is redundancy of this ligament with migration of the more distal phalanx toward the opposite side, and a painful, unstable, nonfunctional joint may result.

The same components are present in dislocation of the interphalangeal joint as in dislocation of the knee. It is a serious injury and may well result in permanent disability, particularly if treatment is too casual. One should study the x-ray carefully, particularly after reduction, since it may provide evidence of an avulsion of the ligament or possibly a fracture of one of the margins of the phalangeal base. Our belief is that severe and complete tears of the collateral interphalangeal ligaments should be treated by surgical repair. It is very difficult to obtain reliable figures relating to the rate of permanent instability in these cases. Many patients are treated quite casually and never see the doctor. The ones who do have severe dislocations which will not reduce or old ones which have already healed but which have instability. Certainly it is very difficult to repair an old tear. Reconstruction is not always satisfactory. Hence, we recommend surgical repair early if there is gross instability in the involved joint. Remember that the most stable position in the interphalangeal joint is at 90 degrees of flexion rather than at complete extension. In complete extension most interphalangeal joints do have some lateral motion.

Chronic Sprain of the Interphalangeal Joints

A joint that has sustained repeated sprains or several inadequately treated sprains, or even the joint that has been treated properly, will occasionally become swollen and stiff and defy all efforts at rehabilitation. Local steroids or systemic phenylbutazone is helpful, and avoiding repeated trauma provides the best complete cure of the painful swollen joint that is compatible with satisfactory hand function.

Fracture-Dislocations

When the dislocation is associated with a fracture, the fracture will frequently appear to be the primary injury; however, attention should still be directed toward reducing the residual subluxation of the joint. Frequently when the subluxation is reduced, the fracture fragments will mold themselves into proper position. If the deformity of the phalanx is a volar subluxation, this should be corrected and held with a K-wire inserted percutaneously across the joint. Similarly if the subluxation is dorsal, it can be reduced and held in position with K-wire. Molding of the fracture fragments will sometimes offer surprisingly good results (Fig. 280). If a medial or lateral subluxation fractures one of the condyles of the phalanx, it can be similarly returned to its normal position by reducing the subluxation and holding the condyle in place by a K-wire inserted percutaneously without opening the fracture site. Occasionally, however, it must be opened.

If a small fragment of bone attached to the capsule at the base of the phalanx is pushed distally at the time of the dislocation, it can be returned to its normal relationship by hyperextending the joint (Fig. 281). If the small chip is merely avulsed and returns to its normal position with flexion, the finger can be immobilized in moderate flexion for two to three weeks (Fig. 282).

FRACTURES OF THE HAND

In dealing with fractures of the individual bones of the hand, it is important to remember that each presents unique problems, but none of the problems associated with the healing of the fracture should overshadow the importance of obtaining satisfactory hand function. The necessity of obtaining a good reduction should be weighed against the possibility of producing joint stiffness and tendon adherence. On the other hand, malposition of a fracture cannot be tolerated if it interferes with the balance between intrinsic and extrinsic function, which is achieved with the hand in the position of function. Frequently immobilization of the hand in this position will help with the reduction of the fracture. It is important to remember that the tendons glide in close proximity

Figure 280. *A,* A volar fracture-subluxation of the proximal interphalangeal joint. *D,* A dorsal fracture-subluxation. *B* and *E,* Each injury was treated by reducing the subluxation and holding the joint in the reduced position using a K-wire strategically positioned so as not to cause separation of the fracture fragments. *C,* Although a perfect x-ray result was not acquired, notice the complete range of motion obtained. There was no swelling about the joint. *F,* A much better reduction with an equally good functional result. This same situation exists at the base of the proximal phalanx at the metacarpophalangeal joint.

Figure 281. *A,* Snubbing fracture of the anterior flange of the proximal end of the middle phalanx. *B,* Note reduction of the fragment by extension of the finger.

to the bones in the hand, and careless treatment of fractures will result in adhesions of tendon to bone.

Fractures are caused by indirect violence or by direct violence with a direct blow to the bone involved. Indirect violence coupled with hyperextension or medial or lateral angulation of the hand produces damage to any one of three elements: The first element is composed of the ligaments and their bony attachments,

Figure 282. Avulsion injuries of the volar plate, pulling small fragments of bone from the base of the phalanx. *A,* A very small flake of bone. *B,* A larger chip of bone. Frequently, careful questioning regarding the mechanism of the injury and oblique x-rays in several planes will reveal the presence of these fragments when they might otherwise be overlooked.

the second element is the epiphyseal plate and the third is bone. Treatment of the ligamentous injuries, including their bony attachments, has been discussed previously and will be found in the section on sprains. Epiphyseal fractures and fractures through bone present essentially the same problems of treatment and will be discussed together. In fractures of the epiphyses and in fractures close to the joints the reduction should be as nearly anatomical as possible. Again, since the thumb and fingers present unique problems, they will be discussed separately.

Thumb Ray

Metacarpal Area

The same forces that produce dislocation of the thumb may also cause fracture. A fracture peculiar to the thumb is the *Bennett fracture,* which is in reality a fracture-dislocation of the carpometacarpal joint with fracture of some portion of the medial proximal margin of the base of the metacarpal (Fig. 283*A*). The same force that causes dislocation by direct force down the shaft of the metacarpal, such as a

blow with the fist, drives the base of the metacarpal proximally and dorsally. Instead of the anterior capsule tearing, the bone breaks. The injury causes not only fracture-dislocation of the metacarpal but also tearing of the dorsal ligaments and capsule of the metacarpophalangeal joint. On examination the thumb appears foreshortened. It is thick at its base, with prominence of the base of the shaft of the metacarpal. Traction-abduction readily reduces the dislocation and one may not suspect the fracture unless x-rays are made (see Fig. 269). On relaxing the traction, the deformity promptly recurs (Figs. 284 and 285).

Theoretically traction and abduction with pressure against the base of the phalanx should adequately hold this fracture. However, this method is unnecessarily cumbersome and ineffective. If traction is elected, skeletal traction should be used through either the distal end of the metacarpal or the shaft of the proximal phalanx. The wrist must be flexed to the ulnar side, and the thumb widely abducted with traction along its long axis. The cast is applied in this position, care being taken to place a felt pad at the pressure area on the base of the metacarpal. Elastic traction is then applied by an outrigger (Figs. 286 and 287). The pull is

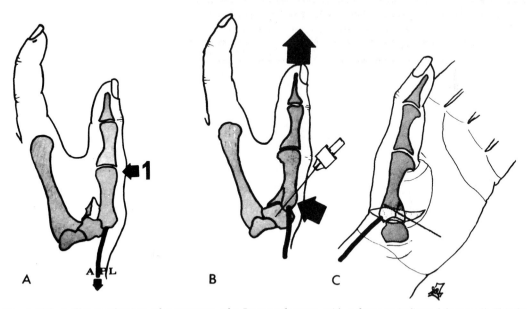

Figure 283. *A,* The mechanism of occurrence of a Bennett fracture, with a force as indicated (arrow 1). This force drives the thumb into the palm and results in a fracture of the ulnar lip of the base of the metacarpal, which holds the base on its saddlelike articulation. The abductor pollicis longus (APL) contributes a deforming force by pulling the base of the thumb from its saddle. *B,* The principle of reduction with closed percutaneous pinning. Longitudinal traction is placed on the thumb, and pressure is applied at the base of the thumb, in order to reposition the metacarpal on the greater multangular so that the fracture is reduced in the same manner that fracture-dislocations of the fingers are reduced (see Fig. 280). Notice how an intact periosteum helps mold the fracture. The K-wire must not enter the fracture site, since this will merely cause distraction of the fracture fragments. *C,* The principle of open reduction of this fracture. The fracture is visualized through an incision at the base of the thumb and held in the reduced position with one or two small threaded K-wires inserted across the fracture site. These are best inserted with a motor drill.

Figure 284. *A*, A Bennett fracture. This fracture is completely unstable. *B*, Reduction is best maintained by internal fixation. The wire shown is not well placed but did hold. (For x-ray positioning, see Fig. 269.)

Figure 285. This 19 year old male had pain and disability of the thumb because of a football injury. *A*, X-ray shows the dislocation of the base of the metacarpal, with the triangular fragment of bone remaining adherent to the ligaments. *B*, This was treated by closed reduction and transfixion pin across the base of the metacarpal of the thumb and into the base of the metacarpal of the index finger rather than into the carpus. This gave very adequate fixation. *C*, Complete healing is shown. (For x-ray positioning, see Fig. 269.)

Figure 286. *A*, Transverse fracture of the base of the thumb with displacement. *B*, Fixation in wide abduction maintained by plaster cast.

Figure 287. Transverse comminuted fracture of the base of the thumb, treated by traction. Note distraction of the metacarpophalangeal joint.

along the long axis of the metacarpal. This position must be maintained for several weeks until union is fairly firm. The traction can then be removed, but the cast must be replaced holding the thumb in abduction. It is notably difficult to hold this position, and recurrence of deformity is frequent (Fig. 288). An alternative method of holding the reduction in-

Figure 288. The result of an inadequate reduction of a Bennett fracture. There is nonunion of the fracture (arrow) and osteoarthritic spurring about the carpometacarpal joint.

volves insertion of a K-wire to hold the base of the metacarpal on its saddle (see Figs. 283 to 285).

Since an inadequate reduction will lead to osteoarthritis later, the best result is obtained by a nearly perfect reduction. Our preference is to try to reduce the fracture under anesthesia by manipulation and traction. If reduction is good, percutaneous threaded K-wire fixation across the base of the metacarpal through the fragment and into the carpus is attempted. If this is successful and if it holds firmly, a gauntlet thumb spica is applied. If it fails to reduce or if the fixation fails to hold, primary open reduction should be carried out and completed by properly placed internal fixation of the shaft to the fragment without involving the carpus if possible. This will permit motion of the thumb before the fixation is removed, which may be a quite important factor.

With *fractures of the shaft* and of the neck of the metacarpal of the thumb, it is important to obtain and maintain good position. The fracture of the middle of the shaft of the metacarpal will usually angulate dorsally and may be reduced by abduction of the thumb and pressure over the fracture site. It may be held in this position by an appropriate plaster cast. If the position is not secure or does not hold, open reduction with internal fixation or percutaneous insertion of K-wires is the treatment of choice.

Figure 289. *A*, An example of a fracture at the base of the thumb metacarpal produced by essentially the same force as that causing a Bennett fracture. However, this is an impacted fracture of the base and is corrected by simply abducting the thumb, thus straightening the angulation (*B*).

Fractures of the proximal phalanx of the thumb are not nearly as common as those of the fingers (Fig. 289). If a fracture is complete, it is much more difficult to hold because of the extreme mobility of the normal thumb. Fixation should be with the thumb in flexion, at both the metacarpophalangeal and the interphalangeal joints. This may be maintained by a suitable plaster splint until swelling is stabilized. Then a plaster cast is applied. It is imperative to secure good position in order to preserve the function of the thumb. One must be particularly careful that there is no rotation of this phalanx. When the thumb is flexed into the palm, it should cross toward the base of the fifth metacarpal head, not toward the second. This permits opposition of the thumb to the various fingers. The so-called mallet finger, or baseball finger, is unusual in the thumb and treatment is the same as in the fingers. The same is true in fractures involving the interphalangeal joint and in crushing injuries of the tip of the distal phalanx.

Finger Rays

The subject of fracture of the metacarpals and phalanges is a voluminous one. The reader is referred to standard works on fractures or treatment of injuries to the hand for adequate detail. Some of the details particularly pertinent to the athlete will be reviewed.

Metacarpals

Fracture of the *base of the metacarpal* (Fig. 290) occurs from a direct blow against the end of the metacarpal, which transmits the force down the shaft, as exemplified by a blow with the clenched fist. It may also be caused by a direct crushing force over the back of the hand as it rests on a solid surface. The metacarpal bases are so closely bound together that the fracture is not displaced. Diagnosis may be made by history of the character of the injury and by the local findings. Tenderness will be extreme at the site of the break (Fig. 291). Direct pressure over the injured area is painful. Pain is elicited by tapping the end of the bone, the force being transmitted down the shaft of the metacarpal to the fracture site.

Careful x-ray study is important, since in many instances the fragments are impacted. This, combined with the fact that the bones normally overlap, may make x-ray interpretation difficult. One may be amazed to see, after several weeks, fractures that did not appear at

Figure 290. An oblique fracture at the base of the metacarpal; notice the shortening. This can be corrected by traction with a Z-wire of fishhook type inserted into the neck of the metacarpal.

all on the original x-ray. A particular effort should be made to assess any possible dislocation. Since the palmar ligament is so much stronger than the dorsal, the force may drive the shaft backward, break off the anterior margin of the metacarpal and permit the shaft of the metacarpal and dorsal part of the proximal end to displace dorsally (see Fig. 290). This can be readily palpated immediately after the injury but is later concealed by swelling, edema and infiltration of blood. Very careful lateral x-ray views in several planes may be necessary to actually demonstrate this dislocation.

One may be chagrined after treating what appears to be contusion or sprain of the hand to find gross deformity of one of the bases, particularly of the second and third metacarpals. On the other hand, if the injury is recognized early it may be reduced by traction. It may be difficult to maintain reduction by cast fixation only. Internal fixation is relatively simple because the bone may be transfixed by percutaneous insertion of K-wire after reduction without actually opening the fracture site. After reduction, transfixion wires may be placed through the metacarpal into the undisplaced proximal fragment. A little ingenuity will be well rewarded provided that the diagnostic acuity has been sufficient to reveal this lesion. If the fracture is incomplete or without displacement, simple immobilization of the wrist and hand is adequate. It is not necessary to immobilize either the metacarpophalangeal or the interphalangeal joints. Protection should continue as long as the symptoms persist. The inherent stability here is such that in many circumstances immobilization may be discontinued within two weeks.

As the location of the injury moves distally

Figure 291. Fracture of base of the fifth metacarpal resulting from a blow with a clenched fist against the opponent's head. This comminuted type of fracture requires traction—in this instance straight traction—for reduction and fixation.

to involve the *metacarpal shaft,* management becomes more complicated. Many fractures of the third or fourth metacarpal, being surrounded on two sides by intact bone, may be without displacement and so require little treatment. Angulation of the shaft of the third or fourth metacarpal is not common. If it occurs, it should be reduced by traction on the fingers, direct pressure over the metacarpal adjacent to the fracture site and then transfixion of the shafts by K-wire drilled across and through the two adjacent and intact metacarpals above and below the fracture site (Fig. 292). These can be cut off beneath the skin, and virtually no external immobilization is required after the first few days. This internal fixation is more likely to be necessary in the oblique than in the transverse fracture (Fig. 293). The long spiral fracture ordinarily will maintain adequate position and a few millimeters' shortening of the bone will be of little consequence. When the fracture involves more than one metacarpal, or when it involves the second or fifth, stability is much less secure. It has been our experience in the athlete with a fracture and displacement in the shaft of either of these metacarpals that some sort of internal fixation is advisable. This is particularly true because fixation by plaster is cumbersome and very often fails.

If plaster fixation is elected, the wrist should

Figure 292. Oblique, comminuted fracture of the shaft of the fourth metacarpal, treated by manual traction and K-wire transfixing two intact metacarpals. This is an excellent method.

be dorsiflexed. Direct pressure is applied over the metacarpal adjacent to the angulated fracture site while traction is placed on the involved finger. If the fracture is unstable, skeletal traction may be necessary using any of the

Figure 293. Spiral oblique fracture of the middle of the shaft of the fourth metacarpal. Note that in the anteroposterior view the fracture line is not visible, although the bone does look somewhat shorter. Because of the shortening, traction is indicated even though the fracture should heal well without treatment.

various methods, such as a Z-hook K-wire through the dorsal cortex of the distal fragment or transfixation traction through the proximal phalanx laterally. After traction is applied and the fracture is reduced, a palmar splint should be applied with the wrist dorsiflexed, the metacarpophalangeal joint semiflexed and the proximal interphalangeal joint rather sharply flexed (90 degrees). This should be supported by a posterior splint plus a felt pressure pad adjacent to the fracture site, permitting direct downward pressure against the angulated fracture fragment. This pressure must never be exerted directly over the fracture site, since it may force the extensor tendon into the fracture

site and lead to adhesions (Fig. 294). This position is maintained by manual traction until the splint is hardened. Sometimes additional felt pads can be inserted after the splints harden. After the plaster sets, some sort of outrigger must be applied to maintain traction on the involved finger. Bear in mind that this cannot be done with the fingers in extension but must be done with the fingers flexed.

It is much more difficult to treat a metacarpal fracture by skeletal traction than it is by some form of internal fixation. Consequently, if the fracture is not adequately supported by the cast alone without traction, I would abandon further efforts to hold it and would use

Figure 294. *A*, A typical deformity produced by fracture of the midshaft of the metacarpal. Note that once the intrinsic-extrinsic balance of the finger is upset, a series of deformities are produced, each one contributing to another deformity. In this example, the angulation of the metacarpal produces tension on the extensor digitorum communis (EDC), which in turn hyperextends the metacarpophalangeal joint. This places tension on the lumbrical (1), which helps produce more bowing at the fracture site, and also places tension on the flexor digitorum sublimis tendon (FDS). The first principle to observe in treating fractures of this type is to place the hand in a position of function which will correct the deforming forces. *B*, An x-ray of this type of fracture. *C*, A very satisfactory reduction obtained by splinting the hand in the position of function. If additional pressure padding is needed to help maintain the reduction, felt is used. It is never placed over the fracture site but adjacent to it; this avoids pushing the tendons into the fracture site (arrows).

Figure 295. Fractured metacarpals resulting from athletic injury. Reduction is maintained by K-wires. These wires transfix the metacarpal head and should be removed as soon as the union is solid enough. The fingers should be immobilized until the wires are removed.

internal fixation. Internal fixation is carried out with wire loops or a small plate or by K-wire transfixion of the fractured metacarpals to the intact ones. Another method is to use an intramedullary pin inserted into the distal end of the bone with the metacarpophalangeal joint in complete flexion (Fig. 295). It should not be left in place for more than three or four weeks.

It must be emphasized again that fractures of the metacarpals are serious injuries. If one intends to treat them, he should properly prepare himself by adequate study of the various factors involved both in causing the deformity and in preventing its recurrence.

Fractures of the *neck of the metacarpal* are very common, the most frequent being of the fifth. They are often caused by the impact of the knuckle of the clenched fist against someone's skull as he ducks a blow to the face. The result is almost always a flexion deformity with the head rotated over the neck, so that the head presents itself in the palm. Examination of the metacarpal bone will show why forward rotation of the head causes such prominence in the palm of the hand. The head normally hooks forward to be much more prominent on the palmar than on the dorsal surface. Forward angulation causes this normal prominence to be exaggereated. On examination, this abnormality is readily palpable. This fracture is usually impacted but should not be left unre-

duced. It should be noted that there is usually more trouble with the third and fourth heads than with the others because they are less mobile, and any gross displacement of the head into the palm will cause disability not only by the impingement of the head but also by pressure on the nerve and restriction of motion of the joint.

In addition to the preceding factors, some angular deformity can be accepted in index and little finger metacarpal neck fractures. Angular deformity without a rotary element merely increases the transverse metacarpal arch. If the function does not appear to be compromised by the impacted fracture and the cosmetic deformity is acceptable to the patient, the hazards and risks of breaking up the impaction occasionally outweigh the potential benefits. Each case should be individualized and reasons for proceeding in the manner chosen discussed with the patient. As a general rule, function should not be sacrificed for cosmesis, but occasionally the patient has strong feelings to the contrary.

These fractures are usually readily reduced. Anesthesia is required. Under anesthesia it may be possible to manipulate the head by pressure of the surgeon's fingers over the shaft dorsally and pressure backward with his thumb against the head. However, the fracture may be impacted so much that this simple manipulation is ineffective. In such a case the proximal phalanx can be utilized to push the head dorsally on the metacarpal shaft after flexing the metacarpophalangeal joint to 90 degrees. One should not be deluded into believing he can flex the proximal phalanx into the palm, apply a pressure dressing and so reduce the fracture. The fracture must be disimpacted and reduced before any dressing is applied. Very frequently, it may be held in a simple splint, maintaining the fingers in semiflexion (see Fig. 294).

If the fracture seems unstable, it has been advocated that greater stability can be obtained by flexing the proximal phalanx to 90 degrees and splinting the finger in this position on the theory that pressure upward on the phalanx and downward on the back of the hand will hold the position. My experience with this method is not favorable. It is my belief that if the fracture will hold in this position it will probably also be held securely by a splint in the functional position. It is impossible to keep constant pressure on the back of the hand and on the distal end of the proximal phalanx in an active individual.

If the fracture is unstable, my preference is to transfix it with a K-wire (Figs. 295 and 296). With the uncomplicated case one can go through the end of the knuckle and down the shaft of the metacarpal. This wire can be removed at the end of three weeks, since the fracture stabilizes itself rapidly. The more se-

rious injuries of the hand involving multiple metacarpals with fractures and dislocations will require a high degree of skill, and no effort should be spared to restore the function of the hand to normal.

Phalanges

Proximal Phalanx. The *proximal phalanx* is more commonly fractured than the other two phalanges. This is primarily due to the fact that the entire leverage of the fingers is brought to bear on the proximal phalanx, whereas in the middle one there is a much shorter lever arm. Any of the phalanges may be fractured by a direct blow. This may be caused by a football cleat as the hand is stretched out on the hard ground or by catching the finger between two hard opposing objects such as the football helmet and the ground or the fiber pad on the pants against a helmet or a shoe. This type of fracture from a crushing injury is ordinarily stellate and without displacement. Whichever phalanx is involved, it may be treated by simple immobilization of the bone, including the joint above and the one below, provided there is no rotational deformity.

The finger is not often broken by direct impact, as in boxing, since the flexed position tends to protect it from this force. The more serious fractures usually result from leverage

Figure 296. *A,* An unstable type of impacted fracture of the neck of the metacarpal. Once the impaction was corrected, the metacarpal would not maintain its normal length because the head kept slipping into maximum deformity (*B*). *C,* K-wires were inserted to maintain the reduction. Each K-wire obtained purchase on the head and also into the neck. These wires were inserted percutaneously without opening the fracture site.

action. In the proximal phalanx this action is usually hyperextension of the fingers, the same force that causes dislocation of the proximal interphalangeal joint or the metacarpophalangeal joint.

At the *base of the proximal phalanx* the injury may actually be a fracture-dislocation. As the phalanx slides backward over the metacarpal head, the dorsal margin is broken off by direct impingement against the metacarpal or the palmar margin is pulled off by traction of the capsule. The dislocation in this instance is usually spontaneously reduced, since the base does not tend to lock out of position. The result is that the player presents with a painful, swollen, very tender metacarpophalangeal joint without obvious displacement. However, if the fractured fragment is large enough, instability results and the joint will subluxate (see Fig. 280). The tenderness will be at the base of the phalanx rather than over the metacarpal head. Careful x-ray examination will reveal the triangular-shaped shadow of the fragmented bone. If the fragment is the posterior cortex, the metacarpophalangeal joint must be placed in extension in order to obtain apposition. If it is the palmar border, the finger should be placed in flexion (Figs. 282 and 297C). Following the repositioning of the finger, careful x-ray study should

be made to determine the exact alignment of this fragment (see Fig. 297B). If it is not correctly positioned and held, the fracture should be treated by open reduction and pinning with a small threaded K-wire. Since the joint surface is involved, the aphorism "the nearer the joint, the more perfect the reduction must be" is pertinent.

This same type of fracture may occur on the lateral margins of the index or little fingers as a result of forced abduction of the finger away from the midline (see Fig. 271). These injuries are in effect capsule or ligament injuries and should be treated as such (Fig. 298).

The *shaft of the proximal phalanx* may be fractured at any level by the same hyperextension force; the break occurs most commonly through the middle third (Fig. 299). The fracture is transverse or oblique and the distal fragment will angulate dorsally (Fig. 297A and C). It may or may not be completely displaced. If the fracture is a stable fracture or can be made one, it may be supported in complete flexion of the finger by simple splint fixation. This applies particularly to the transverse fracture and more so to the transverse fracture in which the fragment is angulated but not displaced. Careful manipulation will reduce the angulation, and the fracture will be quite stable because the finger is held with all the inter-

Deformity of proximal phalanx

Tape

Reduction and immobilization

Sheet wadding

C

Figure 297. Fracture of the base of the proximal phalanx. *A*, Lateral view. Note the classic deformity. *B*, The finger is best held in the flexed position as illustrated. Traction is not necessary. *C*, Drawing of the strapping as described in the text. (Modified from Ochsner and DeBakey, Christopher's Minor Surgery.)

Figure 298. *A*, Transverse fracture and epiphyseal dislocation of the proximal phalanx of the fifth finger, treated by manipulation and splint. *B*, Solid union. No growth interference.

phalangeal joints and the metacarpophalangeal joint in complete flexion (Fig. 297). It can be held in this position for about three weeks by a well-padded dorsal splint and then gently mobilized. In the young individual the resulting stiffness is not permanent.

We have not found it necessary in these cases of transverse fractures to use traction in the flexed position. Instead, we prefer the following dressing (Fig. 297*C*): The involved finger is joined to its immediate neighbor, i.e., if the ring finger is the one involved, include the little finger; with the index finger, include the long finger; with the long finger, include the ring finger. This serves two purposes. It permits the fingers to be held in this position without strain and provides some stability from the adjacent finger not only for angular but also for rotary position. After the finger is flexed, a piece of adhesive tape is started over

the metacarpal head, passed over the finger, down into the palm and up along the palmar surface of the hand and wrist. It is advisable to place a strip of sheet wadding between the two fingers and through the flexor creases of the fingers. This position, when held by the tape, will be quite secure. A strip of 1 in. tape is then passed from the back of the hand, through the palm just proximal to the tip of the flexed fingers and back onto the dorsum of the hand. This serves to anchor the palmar strips. The whole is then included in a firm wrapping of gauze bandage. The fingers need not be flexed beyond the point of comfort, and if the hand is uncomfortable after the dressing is applied, the dressing should be loosened sufficiently so that there is no feeling that the joints are overflexed. If the hand swells or the fingers feel numb, the tips should be carefully checked for circulation. If desired, this dress-

Figure 299. Fractures of the proximal phalanx. *A*, All the muscle forces acting upon a fracture of the proximal phalanx collaborate to produce an angular deformity, apex forward. *B*, Proximal phalanx fractures must be immobilized by well-fitting splints, with the finger flexed. Unstable fractures may require supplemental traction. (From McLaughlin, Trauma.)

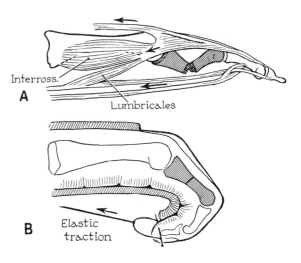

ing may be buttressed by a plaster or plastic-type splint about 2 in. wide, beginning at the tips of the fingers and extending over the dorsum of the hand. This will protect the hand against a direct blow on the injured area.

If the fracture is unstable, as will be the case in a comminuted, oblique or spiral fracture, traction may be required to maintain the reduction. There are many ways in which this traction can be applied. The finger should be in flexion, since it is unwise to apply traction with the metacarpophalangeal joint extended. On the other hand, there is no particular objection to extension of the proximal interphalangeal joint. We prefer a plaster cast which includes the wrist and hand and goes down to the proximal interphalangeal joint on the palmar surface and to the metacarpal heads on the dorsal surface. The plaster should be molded so that the proximal joint can be flexed at least 45 degrees. An outrigger, such as a bent piece of coat-hanger wire, can be incorporated into the back of the cast behind the fingers and flexed to the same angle as the proximal phalanges. Traction can then be applied to the fractured finger distal to the proximal interphalangeal joint. This can be done by a small K-wire passed through the base of the distal phalanx or a fish-hook type wire drilled into the dorsum of the middle phalanx. Traction can be exerted by rubber bands. It is undesirable to include more than one finger in the traction, but the splint should include an adjacent finger.

Open reduction of the fracture of the proximal phalanx is usually not necessary. It is neither desirable nor easy, since internal fixation is very difficult to apply to this phalanx. It is not for the uninitiated. Intramedullary fixation can be carried out by passing the wire through the distal end of the proximal phalanx with the middle phalanx flexed at 90 degrees (Fig. 300). The finger must be supported with the joint flexed until the wire is removed, since the wire will interfere with and cause irritation from motion. The wire may damage the proximal articular surface of the middle phalanx unless movement is prevented. There is not room in the finger for plate fixation without interference with tendon function. Any internal fixation that is used should be removed as promptly as stability will permit.

Fracture of the *distal end of the proximal phalanx* usually is a flexion fracture quite similar to fracture through the neck of the metacarpal. The distal end of the phalanx is snubbed downward toward the palm, with palmar angulation of the distal fragment. This is usually a *transverse type* of fracture, often impacted. It can be readily reduced by hyperextension of the middle phalanx with pressure against the shaft of the proximal phalanx. The fragments will frequently move into position and be quite stable. In this instance the finger must be immobilized in complete extension in order to prevent recurrence of deformity. The pull on the anterior capsule of the joint by the extended middle phalanx will hold the head of the proximal phalanx in the proper position. The finger should not be maintained in this position more than two weeks, since undue stiffness will result. At the end of two weeks,

Figure 300. *A,* Fracture of the proximal phalanx treated by K-wire fixation. The middle third is treated by a wire through the proximal end of the phalanx. *B* and *C,* Similar type of fracture with the wire through the distal end. This is the more acceptable of the two procedures.

| A | B | C |

Figure 301. The effect of rotation upon a fractured finger is shown. In this case most of the deformity is due to rotation. The injury was produced when the finger was caught and the hand rotated. *A,* The fracture. *B,* Anteroposterior and lateral views show that the reduction is obtained by simply correcting the rotation. This type of fracture should be splinted with the adjacent one or two fingers in flexion to be sure that proper rotation is maintained, or the final result may resemble *C,* which shows marked rotation. Note flexed finger rests on its neighbor, a nonfunctional position.

the finger should be slightly flexed and the splint continued.

Our preference for a splint for the transverse type of fracture is carefully molded plaster, applied as follows: A small splint about 1 in. wide and six layers thick is begun at the base of the finger on the palmar surface, passed over the end of the finger and back to the metacarpophalangeal joint. This is placed over the single layer of compacted sheet wadding. The splint should actually be applied with the finger in the position in which it is to be held, so that the splint will not cause undue pressure such as might occur if it is applied before the finger is positioned. After the splint has set, a few circular turns of 1 in. gauze bandage may safely be applied from the base of the finger to the distal interphalangeal joint, leaving a gap at the tip of the finger, covered only by gauze. This will permit the finger to be inspected for adequate circulation. If this dressing is uncomfortable, it must be changed. Pressure necrosis can almost always be avoided by careful follow-up care, because the finger should not be painful once the fragments are reduced.

"T" fracture of the distal end of the proximal phalanx poses a more severe problem, since it is quite unstable. Frequently the "T" fracture can be stabilized by careful reduction and transfixation across the condyles with a threaded K-wire. It may then be treated as a stable fracture. The interphalangeal joint will not tolerate gross irregularity of the articular surface, and open reduction should be resorted to if it is needed to secure good apposition.

Rotation of the distal fragment is of extreme importance in fractures of the proximal phalanx (Fig. 301). Rotation causes a concealed deformity which results in the finger flexing in the direction of the long axis of the forearm rather than toward the tubercle of the navicular. Normally, as the fingers are flexed together into the palm, only the long finger flexes directly downward toward the tubercle of the navicular. However, if flexed individually, all fingers converge toward the base of the thumb, so if a line is drawn down the axis of each flexed middle phalanx, these lines will converge to the navicular tubercle at the wrist. Hence, any fixation of the finger should be in this axis rather than along the axis of its metacarpal. This is particularly true in the unstable fractures. The traction must be directed along this line. It is distressing to have a healed fracture in which the fingers overlap as they flex because the physician failed to recognize the converging long axis of the flexed fingers.

Middle Phalanx. Fractures of the middle phalanx present many of the same problems as those of the proximal phalanx. The fractures of the base of the phalanx should be treated in the same way. In any fracture without

Figure 302. *A,* Avulsion fracture of the palmar lip of the proximal end of the middle phalanx as a result of hyperextension of the finger. This mild displacement requires no treatment other than fixation of the finger in a splint. *B,* Note the old baseball finger deformity in the distal phalanx (arrow) and the healed fracture of the middle phalanx.

displacement a simple finger splint, preferably of aluminum, will be adequate to maintain all the joints of the finger in a semiflexed position (Fig. 302). It should be emphasized that the phalanges do not require a long period of immobilization. To do so invites adhesions of the closely overlying tendons.

In complete fractures of the middle phalanx that are unstable, the deformity will vary considerably according to the location of the fracture because of the tendon attachments to this finger (Fig. 303). The extensor tendon has an attachment to the base of the phalanx, whereas the flexor sublimis attaches to the middle of the palmar surface of the phalanx. If the fracture lies between these two tendon attachments, the distal fragment will move forward with the sublimis tendon and the proximal fragment will be pulled backward by the extensor retinaculum. If the fracture is transverse, it may be stable after reduction. The finger may be splinted in extension (not hy-

Figure 303. The type of deformity seen in fractures of the shaft of the middle phalanx. Here the lumbrical is relaxed, and the deformity is maintained by the pull of the flexor digitorum sublimis attaching to the distal end of the proximal fragment, very close to the fracture site (*A* and *B*). *C,* The final result is obtained by splinting the finger in the position of function, with a little extra padding placed over the distal interphalangeal joint. There should be no padding placed on the volar side of the fracture to push the flexor tendon into the fracture site. If something is placed in the palm, it should be a soft roll of felt, never a hard roll of gauze.

perextension) by simple plaster or aluminum splint. It should be noted that the splint must be rigid and so applied and maintained that it will hold a constant position without direct pressure over the fracture site.

In a fracture distal to the sublimis attachment (see Fig. 303), the angulation of the proximal fragment is forward in the same manner as in the proximal phalanx and the same treatment will be necessary; that is, the maintenance of flexion of the fingers in all joints. This may be accomplished by the same apparatus as indicated for the proximal phalanx. If the fracture is comminuted or spiral and unstable, it should be treated by traction, in this instance with the splint extended slightly beyond the proximal interphalangeal joint and traction applied to the distal phalanx along the long axis of the middle phalanx, which will ordinarily be at about 45 degrees of flexion from the extended position. This traction may be by K-wire through the base of the distal phalanx or by pulp traction at the tip of the phalanx. Our preference is K-wire through the distal phalanx. Once the fracture is fixed, careful x-ray study should be done to determine that the alignment is correct. The importance of rotation in fractures of either the proximal or the distal phalanx should be emphasized. Rotation in the long axis of the finger will change the relationship of the interphalangeal joints with each other and present an obvious deformity after healing occurs.

Avulsion of the Central Extensor Tendon Slip at the Proximal Interphalangeal Joint (Boutonnière Deformity). A tendon avulsion problem which gives a classic deformity is usually less well recognized than the baseball finger deformity discussed later. The lesion is avulsion of the central slip of the extensor mechanism at the proximal interphalangeal joint. Unfortunately, the resulting boutonnière deformity with inability to actively extend the proximal interphalangeal joint does not always lead to the correct diagnosis, and the injury is then seen after a flexion contracture of the joint takes place. The correct diagnosis might be made earlier if it shows on x-ray. When seen late, the flexion contracture must be corrected before surgical repair will be successful. This contracture can be corrected with the application of a dynamic splint. A simple splint is the so-called clothespin splint or a reverse finger knuckle bender, available in prefabricated forms from several of the surgical supply houses. This same splint can also be used to prevent deformity while healing takes place in the incompletely avulsed tendon for which

surgical repair is not elected. As noted earlier, the diagnosis is the key to correct treatment and would be made in more cases if x-ray evidence of avulsion with a bone fragment were present, but it is not.

An untreated boutonnière deformity will require reconstructive surgery.

Distal Phalanx. Fractures of the distal phalanx are almost always *crushing injuries,* except for the avulsion fracture of the flexor or extensor tendons. The injury may involve the tuft at the tip of the finger, in which case the fracture itself is of much less significance than the crushing injury (Fig. 304). It may involve the shaft or indeed extend back to involve the base and articular surface. Usually these fractures require no treatment other than attention to the soft tissue injury. However, the two more distal phalanges of the finger should be immobilized by a metal splint in order to protect against a direct blow and to prevent later deformity. In the occasional case in which there is a transverse fracture through the shaft with displacement and instability, the fracture may be reduced and readily stabilized by an intramedullary K-wire drilled through the distal end of the finger and down to the distal interphalangeal joint. Angular deformity of the distal phalanx should not be ignored, since it may cause distressing disability (Fig. 305).

If the fracture is directly across the base of the finger and seems unstable, the wire may be passed across the joint and down into the middle phalanx. In this instance the finger should be immobilized in the position in which the fracture is most stable, preferably in a few degrees of flexion. The threaded wire should be removed as soon as healing has accomplished stabilization, which will occur at two or at the most three weeks. If the fracture involves the articular surface in the nature of a "T" fracture or a fracture across one angle of the base, it may be transfixed by drilling the wire laterally across the finger after reduction of the fracture. If reduction cannot be obtained otherwise, open reduction should be done using a transverse incision distal to the fracture. Great care should be taken not to involve the nail root lest deformity of the nail result.

Tendon Avulsion Injuries With or Without a Bone Fragment. Fractures of the base of the phalanx involving the dorsal or palmar surface are almost always *avulsion fractures,* in which the flexor or extensor tendon pulls off a segment of bone as the distal phalanx is hyperflexed or extended. Unfortunately, a fragment of bone is not always avulsed with the tendon, and the physician looking for the "classic" case

Figure 304. Tuft fracture, lateral (*A*) and anteroposterior (*B*) views. Note swelling of the tip of the finger.

Figure 305. *A,* Compound crushing injury of the distal phalanx. This was treated by simple dressing. The wound healed, but the finger remained so painful that the patient was unable to work for four months. *B,* X-ray revealed malposition and nonunion. Treated by resection of the fragment, with good recovery.

Figure 306. The deformity caused by a finger in which the extensor tendon is avulsed from the base of the distal phalanx is shown. Any attempt to extend the distal phalanx results in an imbalance between the intrinsic lumbrical tendon and the extrinsic long extensor tendon. The metacarpophalangeal joint is slightly flexed. The proximal interphalangeal joint is hyperextended, and the distal interphalangeal joint is flexed. Tension on the fracture fragment can be alleviated by flexing the proximal interphalangeal joint and hyperextending the distal interphalangeal joint. The finger can be maintained in this position by casts or a K-wire, but maintaining it with a splint is very difficult. In an old fracture in which there has been nonunion, the intrinsic-extrinsic imbalance can be relieved by sectioning the attachment of the long extensor to the base of the middle phalanx.

overlooks the injury. This is doubly unfortunate because pure tendon injuries require surgical repair more often and earlier than those involving avulsion of a chip of bone. In injuries of the dorsal surface involving the tendon, which give rise to the so-called *baseball finger* (Figs. 306 to 308), it may be possible to immobilize the finger by flexion of the proximal and extension of the distal interphalangeal joints. The plaster can be applied dry to the finger over a tube gauze covering. The finger is then dipped into water and held until the plaster hardens. This method of applying the cast avoids much fumbling and loss of position during setting of the plaster.

We have been unable to hold this fracture satisfactorily by simple splint fixation and have not been particularly pleased with the method of passing an intramedullary K-wire down the distal phalanx and across the extended distal interphalangeal joint and then out through the palmar cortex of the middle phalanx to transfix the proximal phalanx. We have had better success in passing the K-wire across the extended distal joint and down into the middle phalanx, stopping short of the proximal joint. One must supplement this by splinting, holding the middle phalanx flexed.

Some of these fractures should be treated by open reduction and internal fixation. If the fragment is large enough, it may be reduced and held by a transfixion pin through the fragment and into the distal phalanx. If the fragment is too small for this, it may be held by wire suture passed through the fragment from the fracture line back through the tendon and looped back to emerge into the fracture line again. It then passes through holes drilled in the distal phalanx to emerge on the palmar surface of the finger. It is then tied over a button. A pull-out wire will permit its easy removal after healing. Great care must be taken not to cause pressure necrosis on the skin of the palmar surface of the finger by the button or the splint.

Avulsion fracture of the flexor tendon at-

Figure 307. Baseball finger. *A*, Note fragment is not reduced by extension of the phalanx, (*B*) nor does it widely separate by flexion. However, the patient lacked complete extension. Treated by open fixation.

Figure 308. Baseball finger showing (*A*) the deformity, (*B*) poor position by hyperextension of the finger and (*C*) poor result, with dislocation of the phalanx, because of improper immobilization. It should be noted that this fracture involves over one half of the articular surface.

tachment may be fixed in similar manner with the finger in flexion. Again, the preference is open reduction, obtaining fixation either with a small pin through the fragment and distal phalanx or by wire fixation utilizing a pull-out wire. In this instance the wire may be passed directly through the nail bed over a button on the fingernail. In either instance surgical repair should be supplemented by appropriate splinting, in the dorsal fracture with the distal phalanx extended and in the palmar fracture with the distal phalanx flexed.

Open Fractures

Open fractures occur in the finger due to the fact that the bone is so close to the skin, particularly on the dorsal surface. They should be treated as open fractures are elsewhere. If the injury is seen early enough, very careful and thorough lavage of the tissue may permit primary closure. If seen later, the wound should be left open and appropriate drainage used. It must be closed as soon as possible, since long-standing chronic infection of the finger will result in stiffness of the interphalangeal joints. It is impossible to clean a finger adequately without administering anesthesia, either local block or general. Great care should be taken not to sacrifice any skin. Even if there is some question as to the vitality of the skin, it should be saved, and a decision made later as the line of demarcation is formed.

Arterial Injuries

Following direct trauma to the palm of the hand, an occasional case of thrombosis of the palmar arterial arch and its tributaries occurs. It is most prevalent in older people but happens occasionally in young athletes following direct trauma to the ulnar border of the hand. The symptoms are point tenderness and swelling over the hand, most commonly on the ulnar border of the hand. The fingers may be pale and cool compared with those of the opposite hand. The symptoms are most pronounced in cold weather.

Physical examination discloses tenderness, swelling and evidence of decreased circulation. Allen's test should be performed in cases in which thrombosis of the palmar arterial arch is suspected. The test is performed by obliterating both the radial and ulnar arteries at the wrist by pressure from the examiner's fingers. The patient is then asked to open and close his hand repeatedly until blanching occurs. Pressure over the ulnar artery is then released and the pressure on the radial artery is maintained. If the ulnar artery is patent, an almost immediate erythema develops throughout the palm and fingers. If the ulnar arch is obliterated in the palm, this erythema will not occur.

In the presence of the findings just mentioned, an arteriogram should be performed, and surgery consisiting of thrombectomy, carried out through multiple arteriotomies, or other appropriate procedures, are indicated.

Injuries of the Chest

13

RIBS

Anatomical Considerations

In discussing functional anatomy it is very difficult to separate the trunk from the extremities and the various parts of the trunk from each other since, by the very nature of their function, the extremities depend to a large extent upon the trunk not only for stability but also for mobility (Figs. 309 and 310). So, in the chapters on the upper extremities we have included a good deal about the chest. The discussion in this section will be largely confined to injuries of the chest proper, excluding the spine but including the sternum.

The thorax is the most rigid part of the human trunk. Not only are the vertebrae much

Figure 309. Upper skeleton, viewed from the front. (From Anson, Atlas of Human Anatomy.)

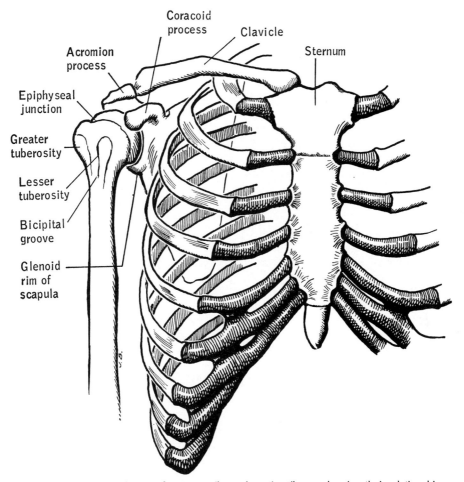

Figure 310. Anatomical view of sternum, ribs and costicartilages, showing their relationships.

more firmly integrated in the dorsal spine than in other areas but the formation of a rough oval by the spine, ribs and sternum serves to stabilize the whole structure. Each rib articulates with its appropriate vertebra and is firmly attached by strong ligaments both to this vertebra and to the one above and to its fellow ribs above and below. The end of the rib abuts directly against the articular process on the body of the dorsal vertebra on the lateral surface of the pedicle, and the articular tubercle of the rib articulates on the anterolateral tip of the transverse process of the same vertebra. The capsular ligaments hold the rib firmly against the body of the vertebra and against the transverse process. There also are dense ligaments extending vertically from the transverse process above to the upper surface of the rib below, so that the ribs are held firmly against the vertebrae and are bound to each other and to the adjacent transverse processes.

These attachments are so firm that they are rarely damaged.

The oval of the chest is much smaller at the top (see Fig. 310). The first ribs, together with the first thoracic vertebra and first piece of the sternum, form a much smaller and more circular ring than those below. The ribs down to the 7th are progressively longer. The upper seven ribs are attached directly to the sternum by the costicartilage. The costicartilage is short in the upper three or four ribs, becoming progressively longer in the lower ribs. Whereas the costicartilage on the first rib may be no more than a fingerbreadth in length, the lower ones extend for several inches. The ribs are relatively horizontal at the top, running more and more obliquely downward until the 12th ribs may actually be more vertical than horizontal. The 8th, 9th and 10 ribs do not attach to the sternum, but each of their costicartilages attaches to the costicartilage of the rib above.

The distal tips of the 11th and 12th ribs are ordinarily free of any bony or cartilaginous attachment to the thoracic cage. The general alignment of the ribs is oblique from above, downward and forward.

The muscles which elevate the ribs, consisting of the intercostals and many other accessory muscles, serve to pull the ribs upward and forward so that the anteroposterior diameter of the lower chest is increased by elevation of the ribs. Correspondingly, the anteroposterior diameter of the chest is diminished by depressing or compressing the rib cage. The ribs are quite elastic in a child and become increasingly brittle with age. In the young athlete there still remains an amazing degree of rib elasticity. Some of this results from the shape of the chest itself and some of it is in the costicartilages, but there is a good deal of "spring" in the structure of the rib cage proper.

The ribs are largely subcutaneous in the anterior half of the chest, but in the posterior half the lumbar muscle mass covers the thorax. The intercostal muscles have a shingling effect, since each intercostal arises from the anterior margin of the inferior surface of the rib above to course downward and forward to attach to the posterior margin of the superior surface of the rib below. The intercostal vessels and nerves pass forward from the spine, nestling in a groove on the undersurface of the rib. The intercostal muscle protects this bundle from an external blow, but the nerves and vessels are easily damaged by an injury to the rib above. The constant position of the neurovascular bundle makes it readily available for local injection. The abdominal muscles attach to the lower ribs in front to give fixation from the bony thorax to the pelvis below.

The ribs are further secured to each other by the intercostal membrane. The anterior intercostal membrane is an extension of fascia over the external intercostal muscle. This muscle extends from the articular process of the vertebra around to cover about four fifths of the rib; the remaining one fifth is covered by the intercostal membrane, which extends forward to attach to the sternum. Similarly, they are held together posteriorly by the posterior extension of this membrane, the posterior intercostal membrane. The internal intercostal muscle is in two layers, the more superficial layer extending from the sternum two thirds of the way backward to be continued in the spine as the posterior intercostal membrane, so that the ribs are held together by this membrane both posteriorly and anteriorly.

The sternum is in three pieces (see Fig. 310): the manubrium, the body and the xiphoid. The first rib articulates on the manubrium, the second on the junction of the manubrium and body, the third, fourth, fifth and sixth on the body, and the seventh on the junction of the xiphoid and body. These costicartilages are firmly adherent to the sternum and to each other by interdigitating ligaments, the so-called sternal intercostal ligaments.

Contusion

Contusion of the chest is frequent, the resultant injury depending upon the location of the trauma. Contusion of the anterior half of the chest is likely to be either to the skin or to the bone itself, whereas posteriorly the muscles of the back cushion the blow to the ribs and the injury will be to these muscles. The history is that of a direct blow with resultant pain. If the blow is severe enough, the "breath is knocked out" and subsequent muscle spasm may make breathing quite difficult for a short period. As soon as these preliminary symptoms are over, the patient becomes aware of a localized area of the chest that is tender to palpation. This does not interfere with breathing unless extremely deep breaths are taken. Examination at this time will reveal an area of localized tenderness, either directly over a rib or in the skin. If the periosteum is involved there will be considerable tenderness on the rib itself, whereas if the skin is involved the tenderness will be more superficial. This distinction can be made by sliding the skin upward or downward over the rib. If the tenderness remains constant in the skin, one can assume that the contusion is of the skin and subcutaneous tissues. If the tenderness remains on the bone, regardless of what area of skin is over the bone, one can assume the damage is to the bone.

Contusion of the chest wall often does not require extensive *treatment*. If there is a complicating hematoma, it may be aspirated. There is much more likely to be infiltration of blood, and this may be injected with hyaluronidase early and a corticoid preparation several days later if symptoms persist.

Another complication is fracture of the ribs. If several ribs have been fractured, the diagnosis can be made quite readily on the basis of severe pain on breathing and crepitation, ecchymosis and edema along the chest wall. If, as so frequently happens in athletes, a single rib is broken, the adjacent ribs with the intercostal muscles splint it well and the major findings will be tenderness over the rib and pain on forced inspiration. However, if compression of the chest is carried out by placing one hand over the back of the chest and the other over the front of the chest, pressing from front to back, there will be pain along the point of contusion if the rib is broken or cracked. Rarely, lateral compression will cause pain. This sign is not significant, however, if pressure is applied directly over the bruised area.

If there is no complication accompanying the contusion, no splinting is required. If the player is to continue in competition, particularly in a contact sport, an adequate protective pad should be placed over the contusion to prevent re-injury.

In the muscular areas of the chest, particularly on the posterior one third, there may be painful contusion as the muscle is caught between the ribs and the striking force. This is treated as a muscular contusion anywhere, including the complication of hematoma. Myositis ossificans is not common in the muscles in the back of the chest. In the front of the chest, the lower portion is almost entirely subcutaneous. The superior anterolateral portion of the upper chest is covered with the pectoral muscle, which fans out over all of the upper ribs as it extends out to its attachment on the humerus. This muscle is subject to all the injuries inherent in the muscular system and may receive a painful contusion with hematoma formation. Some of the fibers may be avulsed from the attachments to the ribs. This becomes essentially an injury to the shoulder rather than the chest, however, since the disability is primarily in use of the arm.

Overlying the pectoral muscle is the breast. The breast of most males is a recessive structure, but it may receive a painful contusion. This may result in inflammation locally centered around the nipple and areola with redness, tenderness and local heat. The breast may become quite prominent. On examination there is a palpable hard ring surrounding the nipple which is tender to touch. Serous fluid may exude from the nipple. This is really an inflammatory condition resulting from contusion and should be treated as such with application of local heat and protection of the area. The acute symptoms may subside, leaving a firm, palpable area around the nipple which may be moderately tender and should be protected by contact pads. Occasionally a painful fibrous nodule remains which may require excision.

With more participation in athletics by girls, something should be said about the female breast. The adolescent with immature breasts needs no particular protection, but any injury to the breast should be treated promptly and adequately and athletic competition eliminated until inflammation has subsided. Early application of cold followed by heat and protection and support by a binder or brassiere should be maintained as long as there is swelling or inflammation. The more mature breast should be protected by an adequate brassiere during strenuous athletic competition. This not only will protect the breast from direct blows but also will prevent overexuberant motion of the breast during strenuous activity. Any contusion of the breast that does not respond promptly to local treatment will require consultation with a physician experienced in the management of breast conditions. The adolescent girl often will not mention a breast injury. Coaches and advisors should advise young women to report any discomfort in this area promptly.

Be very wary of any persistent localized nodule in the female breast. Of equal importance are the symptoms of generalized chronic mastitis with aching pain, deep tenderness, and a tendency for "caking" of the gland.

Strain

Since a multitude of muscles attach to the chest, almost any manifestation of strain may occur. Strain may be caused by violent exertion or by overstretching of the muscles. The symptoms will depend entirely upon the area involved. In the long muscles of the back of the thorax, this condition may be indistinguishable from, or may be part of, a lumbar strain. In the front of the chest the strain may involve the muscles of the abdominal wall where they attach to the lower ribs. Strain may also involve the intercostal muscles, although this is not frequent since they are well protected by other muscle structures and these muscles do not often act forcibly enough to rupture their fibers. A strain is much more likely to involve an area connecting to the chest than the chest itself. This is particularly true of the scapular muscles, e.g., strain of the rhomboids will occur either at the scapular attachment or along the spine much more frequently than at the costal attachment. Similarly, the serrati may more likely be injured in their substance or at their attachments to the shoulder than in their costal origins. Careful analysis of the active motion that causes the pain will usually determine the proper muscle group, although it may be quite difficult to relate it to a specific muscle.

Strain of a muscle at its attachment to the rib is likely to be more painful than it is disabling. There may, however, be considerable attendant muscle spasm, which will tend to splint the chest and interfere with deep breathing. It actually may prevent certain types of activity. A strain of the abdominal recti attached to the lower ribs may interdict a sport such as rowing or wrestling, where forcible use of the abdominal muscles is required. Similarly, spasm of the shoulder muscles may interdict throwing.

Treatment. Since most of the attachments to the chest are diffuse muscular ones, they do not lend themselves well to local injection. After one has determined what muscular activity causes pain, this activity should be restricted, either by appropriate splinting or simply by reducing the activity of the individual. If the muscles attaching to the scapula are involved, the arm should be put in a sling. If there is serious involvement of the abdominal muscle attachments, the patient should be put to bed with the head rest and knee support elevated in order to flex his spine and relax the abdomen.

Treatment will depend entirely on the muscles involved. Local treatment may be of some value. In the early stages application of ice will minimize the inflammation and blood infiltration. Later, local heat will give considerable comfort and promote improved circulation. Many of these injuries will be relieved by wearing a snugly fitting binder on the lower ribs. Any webbing band such as a rib belt (Fig. 311) or Elastoplast strapping or, indeed, simply wrapping the lower chest with an elastic bandage may relieve the symptoms considerably. As with many muscular strains complete recovery may be very lengthy. At just about the time the player begins to get rid of his muscle spasm and have some expectation of recovery, he is likely to step up his activities to the point where he reactivates the process. The classic measures of rest, heat and gradual rehabilitation are quite pertinent here.

If after the first week or ten days there remains an area of persistent tenderness, local injection of this area with a long-acting local anesthetic may dramatically relieve the symp-

Figure 311. Drawing of rib belt on a patient.

toms. Infiltration of several levels along the origin of the muscles to the ribs may be necessary. Our method usually has been to outline the areas of tenderness to palpation and check against active contraction and passive stretching of the involved muscle. If these measures cause pain in the area where there is palpable tenderness, one may assume there is local inflammation at this spot. These areas are carefully infiltrated with a local long-acting anesthetic. Proof of the effectiveness of the procedure will be complete elimination of pain on palpation, active contraction and passive stretching. If the pain is not relieved, at least while the anesthetic is effective, the involved area has not been adequately infiltrated. If the pain is relieved, this same area should be infiltrated with a corticoid and the patient should be encouraged to continue his activities but to avoid excess of either active or passive motion.

An example of the condition just described is found in the serratus posterior, which rises from the lower ribs and passes over to the lumbar aponeurosis in the midline. There may be an area of tenderness extending from the inferior angle of the scapula directly down over the ribs which corresponds to the attachment of this muscle. Complete expansion of the chest or leaning toward the opposite side will cause discomfort here. Actively pulling toward the involved side will also cause discomfort in the same area. If these feelings of discomfort can be eliminated by injection of a local anesthetic, one may assume that the area of the trouble has been reached. This local treatment should be supplemented by the use of inductive heat. In many cases, support by appropriate strapping will be of value.

Muscle ruptures are unusual about the

thorax. They are very difficult to diagnose unless they involve the small attachment of a single large muscle such as that of the latissimus dorsi to the upper extremity. This does not directly involve the chest, since the chest component of this muscle is an extremely extensive attachment to many ribs and is not susceptible to strain.

Floating Ribs

Some mention should be made of the characteristics of the 11th and 12th ribs—the so-called floating ribs. The tip of the 12th and often the 11th rib do not reach the sternal attachment and have no costicartilage as such. These ribs articulate with the spine with a single articular facet that has no tubercle and no head, so that there is much less stability and comparatively free motion at the spine. They are invested in the abdominal musculature and completely surrounded by muscle attachments. These ribs do not actually participate in respiration to any major extent and are more likely to be involved in injury of the spine than of the chest. They will be discussed in relation to injury of the spine.

Sprain-Subluxation-Dislocation

The areas subject to ligament injury in the chest are primarily at the vertebral and the sternal attachments of the ribs.

Vertebral Attachment

As has been mentioned previously, the ribs are bound firmly at their vertebral attachments. The degree of motion in this area is necessarily quite restricted and the forces which cause tension against these ligaments are primarily compression forces against the chest or rotation forces. The excursion of movement is relatively small so that there is no forcible lateral bending at a costal vertebral joint, such as might occur at the knee. A direct blow on the rib itself is more likely to break the rib than to knock it loose at either end. A compression force applied to the whole thorax in the athlete is usually from front to back and the major strain of this force is applied at the angle of the ribs owing to flattening of the oval of the chest by the compressing force. The greatest strain is correspondingly felt at the widest extremes of the oval. There are in-

stances of damage to the vertebral joint. In this case the symptoms will depend upon the degree of involvement. If the sprain is mild, there will be point tenderness over the injured ligament and little discomfort on movement of the chest. In the athlete, this area is well covered by the lumbar muscles, making the diagnosis of a mild sprain virtually impossible.

If the sprain is more severe, there may be some pain on deep inspiration or on forced rotation motions of the chest. Here, also, isolating the injury is extremely difficult, since other conditions may cause essentially the same symptoms. It is difficult to separate forceful motion against the ligament of the joint from overstretching of a neighboring muscle. Active contraction of a muscle may cause pain in the injured joint in the same manner as it would if the muscle itself were injured.

I have never seen a complete dislocation of the proximal end of a rib in an athlete. It is possible that subluxation or spontaneously reduced dislocation may occur and be unrecognized. In any event _treatment_ will be symptomatic: early application of cold followed later by heat and protection against that motion which causes pain. If a localized spot of tenderness can be palpated or if there is constant localized pain caused by pressure on the involved rib, local injection with a long-acting local anesthetic may give prompt relief. And if it does, this is diagnostic of dislocation or subluxation.

If deep inspiration causes discomfort, a rib belt (Fig. 311) may be used to restrict inspiration. If rotation or flexion motions of the chest cause pain, these may be eliminated by adequate strapping of the back. Strapping in this instance should consist of strips extending from the shoulders to the pelvis and parallel to the spine. It is my practice to use 3-in. tape with three or four strips to each side, each overlapping about 50 per cent. These strips can be anchored by circumferential tape extending from the pelvis to include the lower rib cage. Cross-stretch adhesive gives much firmer fixation (Fig. 312).

The strapping will to a considerable degree restrict forward or lateral bending and is equally applicable for ligament and muscle sprains of the back. Physical therapy, particularly with inductive heat, will expedite the recovery. Active participation in sports may be impossible for several days while the condition is acute, but after a lapse of a week or ten days, particularly with adequate strapping, participation ordinarily may be resumed.

Figure 312. Back strapping to prevent rotation and flexion motions of the chest. Included also is a rib belt. The two are not usually used together. The rib belt does not add to the back support.

Recent studies have indicated that occasionally a subluxation remains unreduced or there may be an actual dislocation of the rib, in which case the symptoms are those of a second degree sprain but more severe; that is, local tenderness, local muscle spasm and painful motion. In addition, there may be the symptoms of irritation of the neurovascular bundle which passes very close to this articulation. There may be symptoms of intercostal nerve involvement, either hyperesthesia indicating some neuritis or hypesthesia indicating pressure. Manipulation has been advocated as treatment for this condition. Hyperextension of the spine in this local area, allowing the shoulders and arms to fall backward with backward pressure against the anterior portion of the chest, may be effective. Successful manipulation results in complete relief, with only residual soreness remaining. If a dislocation goes unreduced, chronic symptoms develop such as spurring or degenerative arthritis of the costovertebral joints. It has been suggested that open operation with resection of the proximal end of the rib, including its articulations, will give substantial relief. I have never had occasion to carry out this procedure.

Anterior Attachment

Ligament injuries at the anterior end of the rib are considerably more frequent than those of the posterior end. Possibly it should be said that they are more often recognized. Although the ribs are firmly bound to the sternum, these ligaments are more subject to sprain than the posterior ones by virtue of the forward thrust which occurs with lateral compression of the chest or by direct force applied to the sternum, which drives the sternum backward while the ribs swing forward (see Fig. 310). A sprain of the chondrosternal joint should be distinguished from injury to the costochondral junction, which will be discussed under fractures.

The player complains of tenderness in the chest localized over the area of injury. This area is readily palpable since it is subcutaneous. Often, the symptoms may be confined to a single chondrosternal articulation. Pressure directly over the joint or pressure over the adjacent sternum will usually cause discomfort. The symptoms vary with the degree of injury. If the sprain is a mild one, there will be local tenderness and possibly a little local swelling—and that is all. If the injury is severe but still short of avulsion of the ligament, the local symptoms will be more intense. There will be no displacement. The tenderness will be more diffuse and will be accompanied by local swelling. There may be infiltration of blood or even hematoma formation directly over the joint. Deep inspiration will cause pain definitely localized at the involved joint. If there has been an actual subluxation or spontaneously reduced dislocation of the joint, the symptoms will be even more severe. The subluxation may recur on deep inspiration or on lateral compression of the chest. Some degree of subluxation may persist, apparently caused by dehiscence of the anterior ligament while the posterior ligament remains intact, so that the rib will slide forward in relationship to the sternum. There may be a palpable prominence. In the early stage this may be reduced by direct pressure. This movement may cause an audible snap and will certainly cause pain.

Treatment. Treatment of these injuries is quite unsatisfactory if they are severe. The mild (first degree) injury may be handled without support but with local injection of an anesthetic plus hyaluronidase and application of heat locally. In the more severe injury where there is pain on motion of the chest, the chest should be strapped with adhesive or a suitable rib binder to prevent further stress on the injured ligament. The binder should not be put on tightly enough to increase the pain but should be used primarily to prevent wide expansion of the chest. If there is a chronic subluxation, it will be virtually impossible to hold the involved rib down in its normal position.

An acute subluxation, as with dislocation, may require open exposure for fixation. A threaded fixation pin passing through the rib and into the sternum will hold the rib in place. If the separation is at the costochondral junction, the pin can be threaded through the rib and into the cartilage, preferably far enough to reach the sternum. This gives temporary fixation; ultimate recovery must be by plication and repair of the capsular ligaments, reinforcing them with periosteum and with the soft tissue at hand. This procedure is not successful unless it is done within the first two weeks, since scar formation is not compatible with successful reconstruction. Since the subluxation is usually diagnosed after it is a chronic condition, surgery for this situation is rarely indicated (see Chronic Subluxation, page 345). One must be satisfied to immobilize the chest to eliminate pain and accept the minimal deformity caused by undue prominence at the tip of the rib. The injury may be extremely tedious to the player because of its chronicity, and there will be many disheartening episodes of recurrence of pain following forceful activity.

The technique of injection of the chondrosternal area is quite simple. Repeated infiltrations should be used until all pain and tenderness are eliminated. Because of the interdigitation of the ligaments, the injury may be more widespread than first suspected. It may be advisable to infiltrate into more than one area. I do not find it necessary to infiltrate the joint itself as frequently as I do the surrounding ligament. Once the pain and tenderness are eliminated, these same general areas should be carefully infiltrated in the early case with hyaluronidase and in the more chronic case with a corticoid.

In the chronic case, as mentioned, player participation in sports is often not permissible. If the rib binder is applied snugly enough to prevent deep breathing, it may seriously interfere with the player's ability, since it will be necessary for him to breathe deeply in the course of his participation. One must carefully evaluate the source of the discomfort. If it is from direct pressure or direct contact, the discomfort may be prevented by a suitably placed protective pad. If the pain is actually caused by compression of the chest, I know of no appliance that will completely eliminate it. However, a snugly fitted rib belt or corset will tend to hold the chest in a more circular

position and so may well eliminate the stress at this particular point. If on the other hand the pain is caused by deep inspiration, it can be checked by a suitable binder. In most conditions I do not approve of local injection to permit participation, but in this particular condition, and especially if it is restricted to one or two ribs, it is difficult to believe that injection to eliminate the pain would increase the hazard of further injury. One may give the player substantial relief by local infiltration. The question of surgical treatment of these conditions does not often arise. If the pain seems to be from a chronic traumatic arthritis of the joint or from calcification in the anterior fissure of the joint, one may resect a portion of the costicartilage adjacent to the sternum. I have never had occasion to do this to treat an athletic injury or in order to permit participation.

A frank dislocation of the rib that persists should be reduced at the earliest possible moment. Dislocation of an isolated rib is rarely seen but it may be more frequent than is apparent because so often the dislocation reduces spontaneously. If seen, the deformity should be promptly reduced. For reduction, either local or general anesthesia is usually required since, if the dislocation could be reduced easily it probably would have been reduced before it reached the doctor. After injection of a local anesthetic, the rib may be snapped back into position by pressure over the chest and direct pressure with the thumb over the rib end. If it cannot be reduced by manipulation, it may be reduced by making a small incision across the chondrosternal joint paralleling the rib. The rib can be gently levered into place with an elevator. Following open reduction, an attempt should be made to repair the ligaments. If the rib tends to slip back out of position, it may be fixed by a suitable transfixion pin through the end of the rib and into the body of the sternum. Such treatment is rarely necessary. Following open reduction, a rib belt should be applied with a felt pad directly over the dislocated rib.

Fracture

Fractures of the ribs are relatively common in athletes. They usually are caused either by a direct blow from a blunt object—in which instance there is likely to be a fracture of a single or at the most two ribs—or by forceful compression of the chest in one of its diameters—in which case there may be single or multiple fractures. In the first instance, the player will give a history of a blow on the chest which may be forceful enough to "knock out his wind" and cause severe localized pain. As he gets his breath and tries to breathe deeply, there is severe pain. Muscle spasm tends to splint the chest and to prevent deep breathing. The result is rapid, shallow respiration due to the combination of air hunger plus pain on inspiration. In the second instance the player may give a history of being crushed in a pile-up or of falling forcibly on his side with the ball or a helmet between him and the ground. Here again he will have difficult breathing accompanied by severe pain. Careful examination at the time of injury will elicit tenderness localized directly over the rib or ribs. There is pain in this same area on deep breathing. Compression of the chest, even though direct pressure on the involved rib is avoided, will cause pain. For example, if the 6th rib is broken at the anterior axillary line, pressure made directly backward on the sternum will cause pain in the area of the fracture and deep inspiration will be painful. Any attempt at coughing or sneezing is disastrous. The player grabs his chest and attempts to restrict its motion manually. There may be a palpable defect in the rib if the fracture is complete, and it may be possible to elicit crepitation, but the ribs should not be manipulated.

Fracture can be differentiated from a simple contusion by the fact that a contusion does not usually cause pain on motion of the rib. X-ray examination must be carried out but is often unsatisfactory in the early stages. Negative x-ray findings do not rule out fractured ribs. The obliquity of the rib, the depth of the thorax, the intervening soft tissues, together with the oblique nature of the fracture line and the frequent lack of displacement, make the fracture very difficult to recognize. An exception is the unusual complete fracture in which the ends are separated.

Treatment

Complicated Fracture. The vast majority of fractured ribs are uncomplicated by any more serious condition. In the occasional case, however, the complications may be more critical than the injury itself. Fortunately, the bones of the young athlete are elastic enough so that they do not usually splinter into sharp-pointed fragments. When splintering does occur in the fractured rib, the sharp fragment may damage the internal mammary artery, or penetrate the lung and cause pneumothorax, or even pene-

trate the pericardium. A more frequent injury is damage to the intercostal vessels and nerves, which will result in rather marked local swelling and formation of a hematoma.

Following an injury to the chest, if the patient does not promptly recover from the initial period of difficult breathing, one should carefully investigate the possibility of internal injury. The patient may remain short of breath, may become somewhat cyanotic or may complain of increased difficulty in getting enough air. All these things suggest decreased lung capacity. If these conditions come on rapidly, a critical situation may arise in which immediate decompression of the chest is necessary. In such a case the patient should obviously be taken to the hospital at once. After careful x-ray study to determine the degree of collapse of the lung or shift of the mediastinum, a decision is made about aspirating the air or blood (Fig. 313). If the hemothorax is small, it is probably better left alone. If the hemopneumothorax only partially collapses the lung, closed drainage of the pleural cavity will be the likely course. The vast majority of these cases fortunately are not emergent in character and ample time may be taken to complete the diagnosis. When the diagnosis is in doubt, consultation should be obtained from one who is well versed in the treatment of such conditions in the chest.

There will occasionally be subcutaneous emphysema from fracture of the ribs, with leakage of air into the soft tissues causing diffuse swelling, which extends along under the skin and produces characteristic crepitation. This condition may reach alarming proportions, even to the extent of a swelling of the neck that extends to the level of the angle of the jaw. It rarely requires any very radical or specific treatment. If there is any likelihood of internal injury, the patient should be hospitalized until all doubt concerning the presence of a serious complication has been resolved. Needless to say, x-ray study should be repeated, since there may be very rapid changes in the chest which may alter the indications for treatment.

Uncomplicated Fracture. In the absence of any complication, local treatment may afford the player considerable relief. If there is marked pain and muscle spasm, local anesthetic may be infiltrated into the intercostal nerve, at least a hand's breadth proximal to the fracture (that is, toward the spine). The needle is inserted directly under the margin of the rib, the plunger carefully withdrawn to be

Figure 313. X-ray (retouched) showing collapse of right lung following trauma. Note absence of lung markings in periphery of lung.

sure there is no blood, and 4 to 5 ml. of the agent are injected. The injection into a single rib may be quite effective, but it is usually necessary to inject two or three or even four ribs before relief is complete. If a long-acting anesthetic is used the relief may be quasi-permanent, since a good deal of the pain is caused by the muscle spasm pulling at the fracture site. While the spasm will be relieved by injection, the recurrence of pain can be prevented only by support of the chest.

Once the pain is relieved, the chest should be properly immobilized to prevent motion of the rib. In any injury below the upper two or three ribs, the support should be circumferential and to the lower chest. It is not necessary to strap directly over the fractured 5th rib, for example. The purpose of the dressing is to splint the chest and prevent expansion of the thorax and elevation of the ribs. This can be done by pressure around the lower ribs and never needs to be any higher than the top of the xiphoid. There is little to be gained by strapping half of the chest, since this certainly does not restrict expansion to any marked degree. I do not like adhesive tape because of the inevitable irritation of the skin due to the constant sliding during respiration. A commercial or homemade rib belt, which need not be more than 4 to 6 in. wide, can be pulled snugly around the chest and may be adjusted by the patient. His discomfort index is a very good

criterion for the proper tightness of the dressing. He may loosen it at night when he is breathing easily and may want to tighten it during the day when his activities are more extensive.

Another advantage of the rib belt is its usefulness in strapping the female chest. Nothing is more futile than trying to strap adhesive over the breast. In the first place it cannot be placed tightly enough to give any real restriction, and in the second place there is such insecure foundation that it has little effect on the underlying structures. In addition, it is extremely uncomfortable. If the lower chest only is constricted, the problem of the pressure on the breasts is eliminated.

The support should be continued as long as the discomfort in the rib is greater than that from wearing the restraint. This will vary considerably in different individuals. For at least six weeks a binder should be worn during any contact sport. A local rigid pad should be incorporated into the binder to prevent a direct blow on the area. The rib may remain quite tender for many weeks. I do not believe that one is justified in injecting local anesthetic into the intercostal nerves in order to permit participation of the player with *recently* fractured ribs.

In the case of injury to the upper two or three ribs, the pain may be more closely related to motion of the shoulder and neck than it is to expansion of the chest. This can be readily checked by appropriate test movements. If chest expansion does not hurt, there is no advantage in using a rib binder. There may be some value in strapping directly over the shoulder, the straps beginning in the back and crossing across the base of the neck, over the clavicle and down over the front of the chest. This strap tends to minimize elevation of the shoulder girdle when the arm is thrown up in the air. Considerable comfort may be obtained by carrying the arm in a sling. The support of the sling is not as important as the fact that the sling limits the use of the arm to routine movements with the arm at the side and, hence, forcible activity of the shoulder girdle is restricted.

Nonunion is not a common complication of fractured ribs. Malunion is of little importance. If there is troublesome pain and discomfort from a malformed rib that rubs against its fellow, this segment of the rib may be removed without noticeable disability. Before this is undertaken, diagnostic check should be made by intercostal nerve block to make sure that the pain can be relieved.

Fracture of the Ribs Below the Diaphragm

As has been mentioned previously, the lower ribs, particularly the 11th and 12th, have no firm fixation anteriorly and participate more in the abdominal muscle mechanism than in the chest. It should be emphasized here, however, that blows over the lower chest involving injury to the ribs below the diaphragm are potentially abdominal injuries and should be treated as such. The danger of complication is much more real than is the danger of the injury to the rib itself, since the underlying structures of the spleen on the left and the liver on the right might well be injured. This will be discussed in detail under injuries of the abdomen.

Costochondral Injury

The rather unusual anatomical situation in which the anterior end of the rib attaches directly to the corresponding end of the costicartilage sets the stage for an annoying and sometimes quite disabling injury to the chest.

Acute Injury

Following trauma, instead of rib fracture there may be an actual dislocation at the junction of the cartilage and the rib. Occasionally the same general circumstances will arise in fracture through the costicartilage itself. The symptoms vary, depending upon the level of involvement. If the injury occurs in any of the upper seven ribs where there is direct attachment to the sternum, it can usually be diagnosed quite readily (see Fig. 310). The dislocation may be incomplete and without displacement and will be manifested only by tenderness at the costochondral junction, with pain on forceful expansion of the chest or on direct pressure. Such a condition will usually subside without the necessity for treatment.

If the dislocation is complete, there may be an actual offset and overriding so that the tip of the rib rests in front of the costicartilage. In many cases I am sure that the dislocation was originally complete and was spontaneously reduced. The patient will present for examination complaining of pain in the anterior chest, which is particularly notable on coughing or sneezing. Since the area is readily palpable, he will have determined that he has a spot of localized tenderness and swelling one or two fingerbreadths lateral to the sternum. Careful examination will reveal the localized character of the lesion, with pain on direct pressure, pain on pressure against the corresponding rib in the axillary line and pain on pressure downward on the sternum. There may or may not be a palpable deformity and it may be possible to elicit a click as alternating pressure is applied on the sternum and on the involved rib or costicartilage. The subluxation may be minimal and be very difficult to determine, or the rib may completely dislocate. X-ray study is of little value in this condition. The costicartilages are not visualized by x-ray. The rib deformity is not sufficient to be revealed by even the stereoscopic film.

Treatment. If there has been no demonstrable displacement or if there is no palpable click, one may assume that at least a major portion of the ligamentous investiture is intact and treatment can be directed toward preventing further injury and relieving the discomfort. The latter is accomplished by local injection of a long-acting anesthetic agent. The lower half of the chest should then be firmly bound with either a rib belt, Elastoplast or similar strapping. The purpose of strapping is to prevent wide excursion of the ribs. If there is any possibility of recurrence of the subluxation, a direct pressure pad may be incorporated in the strapping with a piece of felt 1½ by 2¾ inches placed over the inner end of the rib but not overlapping onto the cartilage. In the male this can be strapped firmly in place with adhesive strips. This part of the dressing may be quite uncomfortable. Straps over the shoulder should be used only if the lesion is high and insecurity is apparent at this level. If adequately protected, this lesion may heal within six to eight weeks. Costicartilage union is very slow, as is separation between the rib end and the costicartilage.

Chronic Subluxation

Far too often the player does not present himself until the condition already has become chronic, and one is then faced with a different problem. Here again, *treatment* will vary according to the amount of instability in the area. If there is no instability and the major complaint is pain, the condition may respond well to injection of a local anesthetic and a steroid in the usual fashion; that is, the anesthetic agent is injected until the area is symptom-free, after which the same area is infiltrated with a corticoid preparation. The patient should be warned that he may have increased pain beginning in several hours and continuing for several more. He may then expect improvement. If none is seen after three days, the chances are that this treatment will fail. If there is improvement but after a week or ten days the symptoms recur, the area should be reinjected. It may be necessary to repeat the injection three to four times, and one expects to obtain longer and longer periods of remission of symptoms after succeeding injections until finally but little residual remains. In the occasional case a single injection may be effective permanently. There is no necessity for repeating the injection if the symptoms do not recur or if the first injection does not give relief.

In the case with or without displacement in which the symptoms persist and are severe enough to be disabling, one has to consider surgical intervention. The symptoms in such a circumstance are due to a pseudoarthrosis with, in effect, a chronic traumatic arthritis in a false joint. This may be remedied by means similar to those used at the acromioclavicular joint, namely, resection of enough of the apposing surfaces so that they do not actually rub together. One must be careful, however, that in so separating the bone and cartilage the end result is not instability and a snapping joint. After ½ to ¾ inch of the cartilage is resected, the chest should be put in various positions and subjected to various pressures to make sure that the ribs and the cartilage do not interfere on chest movement. Fusion of the rib to the cartilage surgically is extremely difficult, and I can think of no justification for internal fixation in an effort to obtain union in an old condition.

If the chronic condition includes subluxation or dislocation, instability is already present and treatment must be based on different principles. Whereas in the case without subluxation the symptoms are presumably due to chronic irritation with minimal amount of motion, the case with subluxation contains a built-in aggravator because every time the rib slips over the cartilage the irritation is increased. It should be emphasized that the mere fact that it is slipping is not sufficient justification for surgical treatment. In an occasional case the slipping makes the patient so nervous that there may be sufficient justification, but the justification is then the nervous tension and not the slipping itself. If the slipping is symptomatic and it causes pain or spasm or local swelling, there is little hope of a cure short of surgical intervention. Local measures such as injection and heat may be palliative but chances are they will fail. There is no justification for strapping in the chronic case. The relief given will be purely temporary, and indeed the strapping may be more of an aggravation than a relief. If the symptoms justify it, treatment is surgical removal of a section of the costicartilage or of the end of the rib so that the two do not impinge. The fact that the end of the rib remains somewhat unstable will usually not be a problem. This rib is firmly bound to the one above and below and does not have wide excursion. In fact, it may actually slip less after resection, since there is no lever action to slide it up over the costal cartilage and catch it in this position.

Costicartilage injury is usually not severe enough to require stopping athletics. In the acute case, however, the dislocation should be reduced and held by strapping. Following the reduction, contact sports should not be permitted during the eight weeks required for union to become secure. Fortunately, this condition is not a common athletic injury.

STERNUM

Anatomical Considerations

The most anterior portion of the chest is the sternum, which in the newborn is in many segments corresponding to the ribs. These segments later fuse to form three separate bones.

The upper one, the manubrium, carries the attachment of the first rib and the upper portion of the second; the middle segment, the body, contains the attachment of the lower one half of the 2nd rib and the whole attachment of the 3rd, 4th, 5th, 6th and sometimes the 7th ribs; and the lower segment, the xiphoid, hangs from the distal end of the body, its upper portion sometimes giving attachment of the 7th costicartilage. The 7th costicartilage usually attaches along the junction of the body and the xiphoid. The sternum is subcutaneous throughout anteriorly and is readily palpable. Posteriorly, it protects the vital structures of the upper mediastinum.

Since in athletic injury we are usually dealing with young individuals, it is of some importance to recognize the considerable variations in the time of fusion of the segments which make up the body. In the child under 6 years of age, the sternum will usually present six different segments much as the sacrum does (see Fig. 321). As growth progresses, the third and fourth segments are fused around the seventh year to form the body. Hence, an x-ray of a 10 or 12 year old youngster will show definite segmental lines between the first, second and third pieces of the body. The second and third segments will fuse around the fourteenth year, and the first and second are not fused until age 21. Any one of these segments may delay in fusion, particularly the first and second. Contrariwise, there may ultimately be a fusion between the body and manubrium and indeed between the body and xiphoid, so that in an elderly person the sternum may appear as a single, solid bone. Hence developmental facts are important from the standpoint of injuries, since one must be wary not to interpret a persistent fusion line as a fracture.

The superolateral angles of the manubrium carry the articular facets for the clavicles. Just below this is the facet for the first costicartilage. The second costicartilage, on the other hand, fits into the notch formed by the manubrium and the body. The manubrium is a heavy, thick bone. It is prominent and bulges forward at the lower end so that the most prominent portion of the sternum is the junction of the manubrium and the body. The body is somewhat thinner and elongated, roughly rectangular in shape and tends to slope slightly forward so that the lower ribs are more prominent than the upper ones at the costochondral junction. The xiphoid process may actually be recessed behind the body and its proximal end may be somewhat posterior to the distal end of the body. The tip of the xiphoid hangs free

in the infrasternal notch and carries the attachments for the lineae albae and abdominal muscle aponeurosis, particularly those of the recti. There is usually free motion at the xiphisternal junction. There is normally no demonstrable motion between the manubrium and the body.

There are many aberrations in rib attachments which are not particularly significant clinically as long as one keeps in mind that the ribs do not necessarily attach in a consistent pattern. For example, the 2nd rib may be horizontally attached to the manubrium and the 3rd may attach at the manubrial-body junction. Whereas usually the 7th rib is the last rib to attach directly to the sternum, it may carry attachments also to the 6th rib and the 6th rib may attach directly to the 5th.

Contusion

Since the sternum is directly subcutaneous it is readily subject to contusion. The periosteum or skin is damaged by a blow from a hard object. If the blow is a severe one, there may be considerable shock reaction so that the player breathes with difficulty and will believe he has had a serious injury. However, the shock is well cushioned by the bony thorax and the intrinsic organs are well protected so that the effect is transient. After this transient period the patient will note tenderness along the sternum, usually localized in a particular area. There may be local swelling, infiltration of blood and symptoms similar to those of contusion of any subcutaneous bone. If the condition is uncomplicated, deep breathing or compression of the chest will not increase the tenderness.

Treatment is usually not necessary. Local treatment, if used, is by local injection and cold followed by heat. There is no need to strap the chest, but a protective pad should be worn unless the athletic equipment includes such protection. In football the shoulder pads protect the sternum very well, the injury frequently occurring when the players are without pads. One may expect uncomplicated and complete recovery.

Sprain-Subluxation-Dislocation

The same forces causing contusion of the sternum may cause sprain. We have discussed elsewhere sprain of the costochondral junction (see page 340). Sprain of the ligaments connecting the manubrium and body is possible but quite unusual, since there is seldom enough motion at this joint to permit ligament damage. Sprain will frequently occur by actual subluxation; that is, the body will be displaced rather than angulated backward on the sternum. The same force that would break the bone may separate the connection between the two, causing a ligament injury; hence the lesion is really subluxation. The general contour of the chest causes the subluxation to be spontaneously reduced.

The patient presents with pain directly at the manubrium–body junction. Examination at this time will reveal tenderness here. Rarely, pain may be elicited by alternate pressure on the manubrium and body. Ordinary breathing does not cause discomfort but there is sharp recurrence of the pain on ballottement with the heel of the hand against either the body or the manubrium.

Treatment. If the condition is acute, participation in contact sports should not be permitted for the first week or ten days. Subsequently a tailored plastic pad, hollowed out to protect the sternal angle and diffuse the force over the entire anterior thorax, may be placed over the sternum, particularly out over the adjacent ribs. This will usually be adequate to prevent recurrence of the trauma. If the condition is more chronic, injection of a local anesthetic plus a corticoid with the usual physical therapeutic measures may be effective.

If the dislocation is complete and persistent (Fig. 314), with the one bone caught over the other, it can readily be reduced under anesthesia by appropriate measures, first to separate the bones and then to slip one over the

Figure 315. Method of reduction of fractured sternum. If necessary an assistant may apply traction by grasping patient's arm at the axilla and pulling cephalad. Insert shows detail of the forces applied in reduction. (Redrawn from DePalma, The Management of Fractures and Dislocations.)

other (Fig. 315). Usually the bones will maintain themselves in a stable normal position unless the injury has been a major one—and this is not likely in athletes. It may be possible to reduce the dislocation without use of an anesthetic. The supine patient is positioned with a sandbag transversely under his shoulders slightly below the spine of the scapula. The arms are raised above the head and allowed to drop backward, thus overextending the dorsal spine (see Fig. 315). As the head drops backward the dislocation will frequently reduce. The dislocation is almost always of the manubrium over the body so that, if it does not go into position, manual pressure against the dislocated edge of the bone and directed toward the head will usually effect reduction. Frequently closed reduction is accomplished but the dislocation promptly recurs. In this case internal fixation is required. It should be done under direct observation by surgical exposure.

If the dislocation cannot be reduced by manipulation even under anesthesia, open reduction is required. A transverse incision is made directly across the sternal angle. This will permit one to lever the fragment gently back into position. Following open reduction the junction, if it seems unstable, should be fixed by three or four wire loops which extend only through the anterior cortex of the sternum.

Since only a major force will dislocate the sternum, one should be alert to the possibility of a visceral injury. Even if the immediate shock reaction with difficulty in respiration and a tendency toward collapse is only brief, the patient should be placed in bed for careful

Figure 314. Fracture through upper portion of body of sternum, with distal fragment overriding proximal one. Similarly the body and manubrium may overlap. (Redrawn from DePalma, The Management of Fractures and Dislocations.)

observation. X-rays of the chest should be made to determine the possibility of an injury to the structures beneath the sternum, and a careful check for hemoptysis is indicated. If it is acute, the dislocation may cause difficulty in respiration.

Sprain at the xiphisternal junction is not common, since the anterior-posterior motion at this junction is quite free in the young individual. A blow in the substernal notch may seem quite severe but usually the resultant disability is small. There is little likelihood of any dislocation at this joint.

Fracture

The same forces that cause dislocation of various segments of the sternum may also cause fracture. The manubrium, a large bone almost cuboid in shape, will successfully resist almost any force tending to break it transversely. The fracture is usually through the upper portion of the body of the sternum and is caused by the identical forces operating in manubrial-body dislocation. The body is driven forcibly backward while the manubrium is held forward by the rigid first and second ribs, so that the upper portion of the body tends to override the lower. This fracture may be complete or incomplete, with or without displacement (Figs. 316 to 318). The complete fracture has undoubtedly had displacement at one time. Since there is a strong tendency for the chest to resume its normal contour, the displacement corrects itself.

The history will be of a severe blow to the sternum with immediate loss of breath. There

A B

Figure 316. This 20 year old football quarterback was involved in an automobile accident. When seen one week post-injury, examination revealed extreme tenderness over the body of the sternum, with definite, palpable offset between the first and the second segments. *A*, X-ray confirms this position, with the proximal end of the body overriding the distal end of the manubrium. Note there is complete fusion between the manubrium and the xiphoid, which indicates this is actually a fracture rather than a dislocation. Under anesthetic this could be readily reduced by manipulation, but there was no position in which the reduction could be maintained. *B*, Open reduction and internal fixation with wire loops passing through the anterior half of the bone secured good fixation. Six months later he returned to playing football as a quarterback. Patient asymptomatic.

Figure 317. *A*, Another instance of a fracture through the body of the sternum. In this instance a stable fracture which went on to uneventful union (*B*).

Figure 318. During an automobile accident this 16 year old female struck her chest on the steering wheel. Her immediate symptoms were inability to breathe freely followed by persistent pain in her chest and severe pain on sneezing or hiccupping. X-ray reveals the snubbing fracture of the proximal end of the body of the sternum on the ventral aspect. This was treated symptomatically by a rib belt.

Figure 319. Fracture across body of the sternum. Note fracture line across the body, not through the line of fusion.

is a relatively prompt recovery from the general symptoms, but pain persists in the sternum. If the fracture is complete there will be pain on even ordinary respiration so that respiration will be shallow. If the fracture is incomplete, normal respiration will not cause pain but deep inspiration will. Examination will reveal tenderness in the immediate area of the fracture site, with local swelling. Any deformity, if present, will be readily palpable in the early stages. Radiographs of the area should be taken promptly. Adequate x-ray visualization of the sternum is difficult, but by positioning the patient in a few degrees of rotation with the sternum toward the cassette, one can shift the sternum to the side of the spine and get a satisfactory anteroposterior view (Fig. 319). The lateral view may be instructive if there is displacement (Fig. 320). X-rays may be quite deceptive, however, since the various symphyses of the body of the sternum may be interpreted as fracture lines (Fig. 321). A spontaneously reduced fracture is usually not unstable, but alternate pressure above and below will often cause pain at the fracture site.

Treatment. Treatment is local and includes application of cold, followed by heat and compression of the chest by a rib binder or by circumferential adhesive tape. The test of effectiveness of the dressing is relief of the discomfort on normal breathing or ordinary activity.

A displaced fracture in which the fragments are caught or locked on one another should be reduced (see Fig. 315). If the fracture line is oblique, the displacement will tend to be minimal and is not important. The degree of disability will depend almost entirely on the stability, with or without strapping. Participation in contact sports should not be permitted for the first few weeks, unless the patient is completely pain-free on deep breathing and on direct compression of the chest. The sternum can be protected from a direct blow with padding, as indicated earlier, the heavy plastic pad resting on the anterior ribs and protecting the sternum from direct contact. However, this

Figure 320. Patient fell directly on top of his head, receiving injuries to his neck and chest. An x-ray at the hospital revealed fractures of the spinous processes of C-5 and C-6, with displacement. Ambulatory treatment was instituted. Patient developed emphysema accompanied by difficulty in breathing and was re-examined six days later. A recheck x-ray of the cervical spine showed the fractured spinous processes and also revealed a fracture of the manubrium of the sternum, with gross forward and upward displacement. Management by cervical traction cleared up the chest symptoms and materially reduced the deformity. *A* and *B,* The recheck films six days after injury. *C,* Six weeks later. Solid union. Patient asymptomatic.

Figure 321. *A*, Lateral view of sternum in a child showing unfused separate segments. *B*, Note the closing spaces between the segments of 2, 3 and 4, which will fuse to become the body, and the much wider space between 1 and 2, which will persist. *B* is of a child older than the one in *A*.

dressing will not eliminate chest expansion, so it must be supplemented by adequate strapping.

Complications. One must be constantly aware that acute fracture is a major injury and may be accompanied by damage to the underlying structures, with hemorrhage into the pleura, pneumothorax or subcutaneous emphysema. These conditions may develop insidiously over several hours. For this reason the patient with a sternal fracture should be kept recumbent in a hospital and carefully observed for signs of intrathoracic injury such as increasing difficulty in breathing, impending shock or acceleration of the pulse, so that definitive treatment may be carried out if needed.

PENETRATING WOUNDS OF THE CHEST

A penetrating wound of the chest is not an athletic injury but may occur in the athlete. Any suspicion of penetration of the chest by a sharp instrument demands immediate hospitalization for careful clinical and x-ray study and prompt attention by a surgeon competent to handle conditions of the heart and lungs. There is no time for vacillation in treatment of penetrating chest injuries. One should assume that the worst has happened until it can be proved otherwise.

Injuries in the Area of the Abdomen

14

ANATOMICAL CONSIDERATIONS

The area under discussion is that from the top of the diaphragm to the bottom of the pelvis (Figs. 322 and 323). The abdominal area has two functions. One is as a cavity to support and protect the abdominal contents. The other is as a continuation of the trunk to support the body weight and to transmit musculoskeletal forces from the lower extremities to the body. Posteriorly, the lumbar spine gives the necessary skeletal support. In this area the massive

bones, completely surrounded by heavy muscle, form a solid buttress which has some degree of mobility but provides a sturdy trunk to support the chest, upper extremities and head. The lumbar spine also serves to protect the abdominal contents from damage. Before the erect position was assumed, the great majority of insults to the abdominal area were posterior ones, which the back is well constructed to withstand.

Extending from behind and moving forward are the abdominal muscles which traverse in

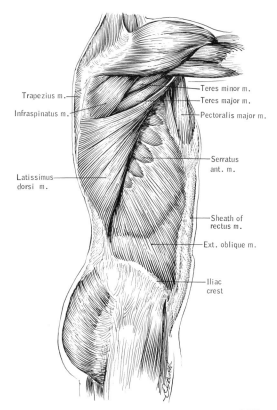

Figure 322. Laterial view of abdominal area, showing the interdigitation of the abdominal muscles with the muscles of the back, shoulder and chest at the top and with the attachment to the iliac crest below. Note the external oblique attachments along the many ribs. The anterior attachment is to the fascia extending in front of the recti to converge at the linea alba in the midline in front.

Trapezius m.
Infraspinatus m.
Latissimus dorsi m.
Teres minor m.
Teres major m.
Pectoralis major m.
Serratus ant. m.
Sheath of rectus m.
Ext. oblique m.
Iliac crest

Figure 323. Drawing showing the intimate relationship between the muscles of the chest and the muscles of the abdomen. Note the ingenious attachment at the pubis in the insert. Also note the tendines contained within the recti, which may be subject to strain. Observe the layers attaching to the iliac crest, with the transversalis coming well forward on the crest, whereas the obliques come only partway forward.

several criss-crossing layers to converge into the fascia in front; this in turn splits to include the vertical recti muscles and then converges at the linea alba in the midline. Superiorly, the lower ribs protect the upper part of the abdominal cavity and overlie the major portion of the liver, pancreas and spleen. Inferiorly, the abdominal cavity terminates in the pelvic cavity, which has a strong, bony structure for protection of the urogenital tract. Anteriorly, the two recti muscles passing from the lower ribs to the pubis serve to help support the trunk by acting as a dynamic support in the maintenance of the erect position. They also serve to assist the anterior spinal muscles in forward flexion of the spine. Thus, we have a massive group of muscles posteriorly, a relatively thin layer of muscle anteriorly and several overlapping layers extending peripherally from posterior to anterior. The whole makes an extremely synergistic muscle mass that permits motion in any direction—forward, backward, lateral, rotatory, or any combination of these—on the relatively flexible trunk of the lumbar spine.

Hence, it can be seen that abdominal injuries to athletes will fall into two very distinct categories, although they may occur together: first, injury to the abdominal wall; second, injury to the abdominal contents.

INJURY TO THE ABDOMINAL WALL

The abdominal walls are subject to those injuries peculiar to the musculoskeletal structure. We will later discuss injuries to the posterior portion of the abdomen, namely, the lumbar spine (page 391). We have also elaborated upon thoracic injuries (page 383), but some further word is warranted on the subject of injuries to the lower ribs.

Contusion

Contusion of the abdominal wall is frequent, but with the exception of certain specific areas, the damage to the wall itself is not usually serious. The muscles of the anterior and lateral abdomen are resilient. They overlie the soft abdominal content and hence are not severely injured by a direct blow. Occasionally a contusion against the tightly contracted rectus, as when a pitcher is struck by a batted ball, may cause a painful injury that may even cause some bleeding into the recti muscles. Under these circumstances the treatment must be directed toward the muscular injury, namely, the application of cold locally followed by the use of heat and protection of the muscles until such time as the tenderness has disappeared. The physical condition of the athlete is such that he is not likely to have a severe contusion of the abdominal wall.

Contusion over the iliac crest at the attachment of the abdominal muscles may be extremely distressing. This will be discussed elsewhere (see Iliac Crest, page 408).

Contusion of the upper abdomen may cause injury to the ribs. The 12th, the 11th and, to a lesser extent, the 10th ribs are much more mobile than the ribs above. Since the proximal end is relatively free and the distal end does not have a bony attachment, an isolated fracture of these ribs is not common. The rib simply moves away from the blow. The contusion may cause periosteal reaction with a subperiosteal hematoma, which may require local injection and some protection. It is extremely unusual to see any displacement of the fragments of a fractured rib in this area, since in this instance the rib is well enclosed by the muscle mass and the stresses are such that there is no overpull on one fragment as compared with the other, such as may be found in the clavicle.

The one fact of overriding importance in contusion of the abdomen is injury not to the wall but to the abdominal contents.

Strain

Since under our definition strain involves the musculotendinous unit and since the abdominal wall is essentially muscular, strain is a frequent occurrence. The symptoms will vary according to the location of injury. Thus, a strain may involve the recti muscles, with pain at or near the upper attachments, or at the pubic attachments below or at the horizontal fibrous bands within the muscle itself. The strain may be from a sudden, violent effort which may actually cause rupture of the muscle fibers or some of the tendon attachments, or it may be from continued overuse. In the first

instance the onset will be acute, with pain, muscle spasm, some rigidity and dysfunction. This may be readily distinguished from injury to the abdominal contents, since the rigidity is localized to the muscle involved or at least to the group involved. Pain is aggravated by active contraction or passive stretching of the muscle. There occasionally may be some concern as to whether the painful muscle is due to acute inflammation of an underlying organ (appendix, for example), but with diagnostic acumen there should be no real confusion. Painful muscle spasm on the right side suggests appendicitis. However, the clinical symptoms are quite different, since the patient with a diseased appendix will have signs of inflammation, some degree of peritonitis, positive laboratory findings and fever, none of which will be present in the patient with the acute strain.

In the great majority of cases, strain does not actually tear the muscle fibers and recovery is relatively rapid. In those instances of musculotendinous injury at the ribs, pubis, or iliac crest, the symptoms may be quite prolonged and cause a distressing degree of disability since resumption of athletics inevitably causes recurrence of the symptoms. The pole vaulter or high jumper who has strained his abdominal wall by excessive stress may require many weeks before he can return to active competition. In fact, he may never be able to return as long as he keeps trying to compete. The best treatment for this condition is to rest the muscle until the symptoms have subsided. This is not incompatible with rehabilitation, since activity may be allowed so long as it is kept within the limits of pain. The primary problem, then, in abdominal strain is that of diagnosis, and careful attention to the actual physical findings will usually rule out any intra-abdominal complication.

It is difficult to use any appliance to protect the abdominal wall against strain and still permit competition. A well-fitted corset (see Fig. 361, page 395) will serve to give abdominal support and will restrict motion sufficiently to eliminate passive tension on the injured area. The corset does little, however, in preventing the vigorous muscle contractions responsible for the symptoms.

Actual muscle or tendon rupture in the abdominal wall is an unusual injury, the exception being avulsion of the muscle from the iliac crest. I have never had to repair any other avulsion or ruptured muscle in the abdominal wall except avulsion from the iliac crest. However, any complete rupture should be repaired.

Hernia

There is no necessity to discuss in detail the various hernias involving the abdominal wall. It seems quite unlikely that any of them are caused by athletic injuries. However, it is inescapable that many hernias will become symptomatic by increased abdominal tension, such as the straining of weight-lifting or the violent exercise of rowing. I believe that if a player has a symptomatic hernia and that if the symptoms are made more severe by athletics, either the hernia should be repaired or athletics discontinued. This is not to say that because the patient has a suspected hernia he should lead a sedentary life. I would recommend that this patient see a capable surgeon and be guided by his judgment as to whether or not the hernia should be repaired. Following successful repair, I see no reason for excluding the patient from sports.

INJURY TO THE ABDOMINAL CONTENTS

In the abdominal area, by far the most significant injury is the visceral one. When, following a blow or occasionally from violent exercise, abdominal symptoms arise, it is imperative to determine at the earliest possible moment the exact nature of the injury. *An intra-abdominal injury is an acute surgical emergency.* The team physician who is not a capable abdominal surgeon and who is not prepared to handle the extremely complicated situations which may arise from intra-abdominal injury is unwise to carry out a policy of "watchful waiting" over any prolonged period. If there is *any* doubt in his mind as to whether or not there is injury to a viscus, the patient should be transferred immediately to the care of the physician or hospital who will provide definitive treatment if the need arises. These injuries are extremely infrequent in athletics, but when they occur they may be disastrous and even fatal. This is another instance in which timely diagnosis makes a simple problem out of what may otherwise develop into an extremely complicated one.

The injury may involve a solid viscus, such as the spleen, liver, kidney or pancreas. It may involve any portion of the gut. It may involve the peritoneum or mesentery, the bladder or, in the female, the genitalia. While in the final analysis it is extremely important to determine just what the nature of the injury is, by far the most important consideration is to determine whether or not *any* intra-abdominal injury is present. It is the responsibility of the abdominal surgeon to determine the diagnosis and the definitive treatment, and he must be given this opportunity at the earliest possible time.

Diagnosis

History. History is of vital importance, not only as a guide to what injury to expect but also to ascertain the progress of events up to the time of the examination. A detailed description of the accident is important. Was this a direct blow by a blunt object, and if so what was the object? Was it the helmet, the knee or the heel? What was the position of the body at the time of the blow? What was the location of the injury? Was it over the back, which is well equipped to protect against trauma, or was it in the flank or anterior abdomen? Were the muscles tense and the player alert or was he relaxed and unguarded? The period of time from when the blow was received to the examination and what happened during that time are of vital importance. Did the patient think he had a serious injury? Was he brought immediately to the doctor or did he report late manifestations, having minimized the original injury? Information should be obtained as to whether or not he had recently eaten. Was his bladder full or empty? Did he have a recent bowel movement?

Observation. Observation of this patient is important. It may be that you were fortunate enough to be present at the time of injury and so were able to observe the actual development of the symptoms. The rapidity of their development is significant. The patient who has received a blow on the stomach or the so-called "solar plexus" may immediately present with agonizing symptoms such as air hunger, severe pain and cramping, which may lead to involuntary defecation and urination. If seen at once he may show symptoms of early shock. However, these symptoms subside rapidly, usually before medical attention can be obtained. Such a patient may appear essentially well when examined by the physician. However, the fact that he has survived the acute injury does not rule out the possibility of late manifestations from injury to a solid organ. The left lobe of the liver which lies directly under the xiphoid is particularly vulnerable (Fig. 324). The right lobe of the liver which extends down to the lower ribs is often injured in contusion of the right flank. While such a patient ordinarily presents no real problem, he

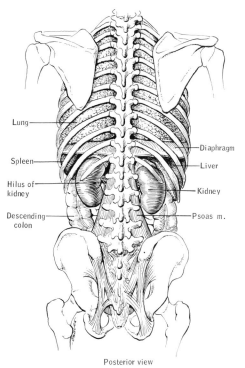

Posterior view

Figure 324. Drawing indicating the position of the spleen on the left side to demonstrate why a blow on the lower rib on the right might damage the liver, and a blow on the left, the spleen. Note the liver on the right side.

should be warned to report any recurrence of his symptoms.

If the patient is in immediate collapse and does not recover rapidly with or without treatment, he has an extremely severe injury that demands emergency care and immediate transportation to a hospital. In the less emergent situation the patient should be observed for pallor and cold, clammy skin; his respiration should be noted; and he should be watched particulary for signs of impending shock, which together with other symptoms will suggest hemorrhage.

Palpation. Careful palpation will be extremely informative in abdominal injury. Rupture of a hollow viscus or indeed bleeding into the abdomen will almost always cause peritoneal irritation and muscle rigidity. This ordinarily will be diffuse. Localized rigidity in a certain area of the abdomen suggests a walled-off lesion with local bleeding or leaking from a viscus. If the abdomen is not tense and not rigid, one may proceed with a more detailed examination, palpating for tenderness around the spleen, liver and kidneys. Loss of peristaltic sounds may be quite significant, since this is a frequent sign of early hemorrhage or other intra-abdominal injury.

Laboratory Findings. The laboratory may be of considerable value. In case of doubt, one should not wait for laboratory reports. Bloody emesis, bloody urine and bloody stool all have significance. Change in the blood count usually will only confirm the diagnosis of abdominal injury, since by the time hemorrhage is manifested by reduced hematocrit or hemoglobin level, the decision should long since have been made that there was injury within the abdominal cavity.

X-ray Studies. X-ray examination is important but only when there are positive findings. Negative x-ray results by no means rule out abdominal injury. Fracture of the lower ribs on the left may suggest damage to the spleen; on the right to the liver (Fig. 324). Fractured lateral processes may suggest kidney damage. Free air in the abdomen demands immediate attention (Fig. 325). Other findings such as obliteration or enlargement of the splenic shadow (Fig. 326), blurring of the psoas margin, change in the level of the diaphragm, generalized dilatation of the bowel (Fig. 327) and dilatation of isolated loops of the bowel all have significance.

Specific Diagnosis

Although at this stage we are not primarily concerned with an exact diagnosis, a few words

Figure 325. Ruptured diaphragm. Anteroposterior view shows air under left diaphragm and scattered throughout abdomen. Severe crushing injury to the chest.

Figure 326. Flat plate of abdomen. Note the enlarged spleen in the upper left quadrant. Following injury, this would suggest intracapsular hemorrhage.

might be said about this problem. As a rule, injury to a solid viscus will be suggested by the history of the blow which makes one suspect the injury, by the location of the abdominal pain over liver, kidney or spleen, or by localization of tenderness and rigidity. The other significant findings are usually related to bleed-

Figure 327. Ileus. Note tremendous dilatation of bowel.

ing and as such are not particularly diagnostic as to the organ involved. They consist of the signs of blood loss, such as rapid pulse with low pulse pressure, dizziness, fainting and finally syncope, and the signs of impending shock. Examination may reveal shifting dullness in the abdomen due to free fluid. Abdominal tap may reveal free blood. It should be recalled that nausea and vomiting frequently accompany any type of abdominal injury and do not necessarily mean injury to the gastrointestinal tract.

Splenic injuries are particularly likely to be insidious because the symptoms here are caused entirely by bleeding. This bleeding may be walled off and may actually stop spontaneously, only to be re-initiated by some other activity at a later time. The physician may be faced with the situation in which his patient is doing very well and then goes into a relatively sudden collapse. Splenic injury should have an extremely low mortality rate, since the spleen can be removed without apparent handicap to the individual if done before dangerous collapse has occurred.

Liver injuries, on the other hand, are much more likely to be rapidly dangerous and carry a high mortality rate. As might be expected, the patients who die do so quickly before they have had a chance to receive supportive treatment. There may be secondary abdominal symptoms from bile leakage as a late sequela to a relatively minor liver injury from which the patient has apparently recovered.

Pancreatic injuries are very uncommon in athletes.

Intestinal tract injuries are extremely uncommon in athletes or at least they are not commonly diagnosed. Contusion of the abdominal wall may well cause some contusion to the underlying stomach or intestines, but these organs are pliable and usually "give" with the blow enough so that they are not caught between the abdominal wall and the spine. This injury also is much less likely because the player's stomach and intestine are usually empty.

The stomach is the most frequently injured organ of the gastrointestinal tract. Following such an injury there may be tarry stools or possibly coffee-ground vomitus, which would make one suspect intrinsic damage to the stomach or bowel. Either of these should put one on the alert but neither is necessarily serious. An injury of sufficient caliber to rupture the bowel will produce immediate, serious symptoms, with abdominal pain, tenderness and spasm, nausea, vomiting, ileus and other signs of peritonitis. Since such symptoms could occur without actual viscus rupture, some confusion may arise as to whether or not these symptoms are from the immediate shock of the blow or from the resultant complications. Here the rapidity of development of the symptoms is extremely important. If the vomiting is simply a process of emptying the stomach and if the symptoms of shock rapidly diminish, one may be permitted more latitude. Persistence of such symptoms and, more particularly, accentuation of these symptoms, constitute an emergency which demands immediate hospitalization with appropriate examination and treatment.

Treatment of Injuries to the Abdominal Contents

It is not our intention here to discuss the detailed care of the patient with intra-abdominal injury. As indicated earlier, there is a diagnostic problem in determining whether or not the patient should be placed under the care of a surgeon. Some generalities about treatment are pertinent, however, since they serve to emphasize the necessity for diagnosis.

Treatment of any intra-abdominal injury is basically surgical. That is not to say that every patient must be operated upon, but in the presence of a real or suspected intra-abdominal injury, surgery must be immediately available if needed. It follows that the responsible surgeon must be in close touch with this patient and ready to carry out whatever procedure is indicated.

In the period prior to reaching a definitive diagnosis, the cardinal points for treatment are bed rest under constant observation and repeated examination by the physician, who notes the local condition of the abdomen and the general condition of the patient. The patient should be covered, but heat should not be applied to either abdomen or extremities. The patient's head should be lower than his feet. If he has abdominal distention, a gastric suction tube should be inserted. If he is unable to void, an indwelling catheter should be used. His apprehension should be quieted, but he should not be heavily sedated. Morphine or any of its modifications or derivatives should be avoided, since they serve to lower the blood pressure still further. Of even greater importance is that opiates may screen vital symptoms. Barbiturates may be used. If the patient is obviously seriously injured and awaiting transportation to the hospital or arrival of the

surgeon, certain other measures should be taken. An intravenous infusion should be started, which not only gives the patient some support but also has the advantage of maintaining a patent vein, which may be hard to obtain if the patient goes into collapse. Blood should be matched for transfusion if possible. Oxygen and suction should be available.

None of these measures is ordinarily necessary in abdominal injury received from a direct blow in the athlete. If they are necessary, a very serious injury is indicated.

INJURY TO THE KIDNEY

It is probable that a mild degree of kidney injury is relatively common in any contact sport. In fact, it has been shown that red blood cells are frequently present in the urine from violent exertion alone. This has nothing to do with trauma to the kidney proper, so that the mere finding of red blood cells in the urine does not necessarily indicate a kidney injury. Certainly not everyone who has pain in the flank has an injury to the kidney. On the other hand, anyone who has this type of injury does deserve examination to rule out the possibility of kidney damage.

Contusion

The most common injury to the kidney is contusion. This may be the result of a blow from a knee or helmet, with the shock penetrating the muscles and transmitted to the kidney. The result of a minor contusion is slight kidney damage (Fig. 328), with local extravasation of blood under the capsule. This causes only mild pain that persists for a few days. Red blood cells may be recovered from the urine. Such an injury is of no serious consequence and need not make the athlete

Figure 328. Anatomical view of kidney showing various types of injury.

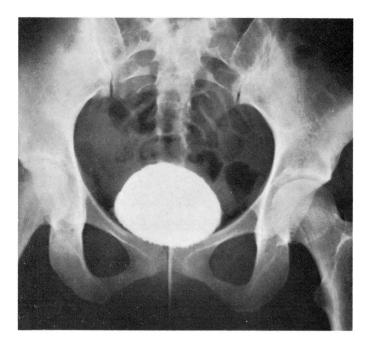

Figure 329. The intact bladder.

overcautious once complete recovery has occurred.

Late manifestations are possible, principally localized infection in the area of the hematoma. This will be indicated by the general symptoms of infection plus local signs of urinary tract infection. In any kidney injury it is advisable to examine the patient and make a urinalysis some two weeks after the injury to determine whether any complication is developing.

A more violent blow may cause serious damage to the kidney (see Fig. 328). The capsule may rupture, with development of perirenal hematoma. There may be subcapsular hemorrhage which progresses to kidney

Figure 330. Severe fracture of pelvis, with extravasation of urine from ruptured bladder.

necrosis. The rupture of the kidney may actually extend into its substance, even to the extent of penetrating the kidney pelvis. The symptoms and signs will be related to the type of injury. In extrinsic hemorrhage, unless this is quite severe, the signs will remain quite localized, with pain and muscle spasm in the flank and lumbar muscles, together with painful function of these muscles. It may be difficult to distinguish this from muscular hematoma or contusion, and the two may well co-exist. It may be impossible to determine the underlying kidney injury unless there are renal symptoms, particularly blood in the urine.

If the kidney substance itself is damaged, extravasation of urine may occur. This is extremely unusual in an athletic injury. In case of doubt, careful study by a urologist is in order. There may occasionally be serious hemorrhage from an injured kidney. It is important to determine not only the severity of injury but also the location, since a major vessel may be damaged. The most outstanding signs here are those of hemorrhage. First these are local: signs of hematoma formation, extravasation of blood along the flank with tenderness and swelling, and possibly positive x-ray findings. If these are accompanied by systemic signs of bleeding, one is dealing with a surgical emergency. An intravenous pyelogram may give useful information. This can readily be taken during the course of examination.

INJURY TO THE BLADDER

Bladder injuries are extremely uncommon in athletics. The nervous tension of the athlete prior to competition is axiomatic. It is almost always manifested in repeated trips to empty the bladder. Since the collapsed bladder is practically never injured, the scene is not set for bladder rupture.

Contusion of the bladder may cause blood cells in the urine but otherwise no symptoms except some indefinite tenderness above the pubis.

Rupture of the bladder (Figs. 329 and 330) is an extremely serious but quite unlikely complication. The patient should be asked to void. If he is unable to void, a catheter should be inserted and left in place. An intravenous cystogram is easily done but may be quite unsatisfactory. The injection of a measured amount of fluid into the bladder, followed by an attempt to recover the same amount, may be informative if radiopaque fluid is used. However, great care must be taken to fill the bladder only by gravity flow. Pressure with a syringe may force extravasation from the ruptured bladder. The intravenous method is far better. Signs of shock with lower abdominal pelvic pain are also danger signals. An accurate visualization of the distended bladder may help. The presence of the dye outside the bladder indicates urine extravasation, and urological consultation must be sought at once.

Injuries of the Spine

15

The spine is readily subdivided into the cervical, dorsal (thoracic) and lumbar sections (Fig. 331). We shall consider these areas separately, since the management of their injuries varies in many particulars.

CERVICAL SPINE

Anatomical Considerations

From the standpoint of the athlete, the cervical spine is by far the most important part of the spinal column. It has two major functions. The first is the musculoskeletal function, which provides support to the head in such a fashion as to permit the person to utilize the various sense organs, such as the eyes, ears and nose, to the best advantage. This requires enough stability to support the weight of the head, yet sufficient flexibility to permit the extreme ranges of motion which are necessary. From the evolutionary standpoint the neck has been one of the most adaptive areas. In various mammals there are wide differences in its structure, from the extreme length and flexibility of the neck of the giraffe, whose small head rests on top of the neck at an amazing distance from the trunk, to the apparent absence of neck in the pig, whose snout seems to extend right back into the body.

The other major function of the neck is to transmit the major nerves from the head to the rest of the body and to give them adequate protection. The requirements for these two functions are to a great extent contradictory. The best protection for the nerves would be a rigid tube with the spinal roots and cord inside. However, the musculoskeletal function demands extreme flexibility. The amazing ingenuity by which both functions are accomplished merits comprehensive study, which cannot be given here.

Free flexibility of the head demands much more vertebral motion than is available anywhere else in the spine. The degree of rotation that can be obtained from the oval vertebrae rotating on each other is strictly limited. Al-

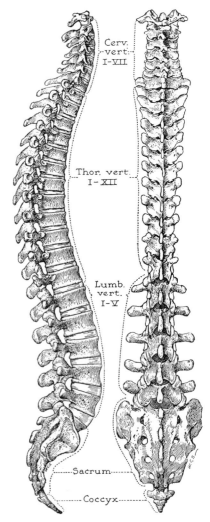

Figure 331. The vertebral column as seen in lateral and posterior views. (From Jones and Shepard, Manual of Surgical Anatomy.)

though this is very much greater in the cervical spine than in other areas by virtue of the relatively flat articular processes, still any major degree of rotation will simply subluxate or dislocate one facet on the other. Similarly, a much more localized range of flexion and extension is necessary to nod the head than can be obtained in any ordinary vertebral joint or series of joints. Hence, the two top cervical vertebrae are entirely different in structure and function from the remaining vertebrae. The first cervical vertebra (atlas) is a large ring bearing the articular facets, on its anterolateral sides, those above articulating with the skull, those below with C–2. The neurocanal in C–1 extends forward to occupy the space which in other vertebrae contains the body. This forward extension is separated from the main neurocanal by a strong fibrous band, thus creating an open ring of three-fourths bone, and one-fourth dense membrane. This space forms a socket to receive the odontoid process of C–2. Developmentally, the odontoid is the body of the first cervical vertebra, which has detached itself from the first vertebra to become a portion of the second. The superior articular facets of C–1 are long and shallow, and on these facets, the head can nod with a hinge motion. There is no rotatory or lateral motion between the cranium and the first cervical vertebra. This wafer of vertebra would readily dislocate were it not for its firm fixation to the odontoid of C–2.

So much for the flexion and extension of the head. The rotatory motion of the head, which in the human is equally, if not more, important, is provided at the atlanto-axial junction. The head and first cervical vertebra rotate as a unit around the pivot of the odontoid process of the second cervical vertebra. The comparatively elongated articular processes permit this sliding motion between the atlas and the axis.

The remaining cervical vertebrae are very similar to the dorsal vertebrae in general structure. There are certain variations characteristic of the function required. The massive cervical spinal cord with its extreme vulnerability to injury requires a ring large enough so that the cord can be suspended in the middle of it without being in direct contact with the surrounding walls. The other and opposing requirement, namely mobility, is obtained by the articular processes, which in the cervical spine are relatively horizontal. The rather flat convex upper surface of the articular process of each vertebra fits into the shallow concavity of the inferior articular surface of the vertebra above

in a much more horizontal plane than in the dorsal area. The angle of these facets is about 45 degrees from the horizontal. The connections between cervical vertebrae are much less secure than those between the vertebrae below the cervical spine, since in the dorsal and lumbar spines these articular facets are vertical. The bodies of the cervical vertebrae are relatively light, since the weight to be carried is only that of the head. The spinous processes are long and extend horizontally backward in the upper portion of the neck but obliquely downward in the lower portion. They are bifid to add further to the area available for the attachments of the multitude of ligaments and muscles that provide good stability and yet free mobility. The seventh cervical spinous process is longer and more prominent than the other cervical vertebrae and, hence, is the most vulnerable to injury. The transverse processes of all the cervical vertebrae are short and light because the massive muscles that attach lower in the spine are not present in the neck. Mobility is more important than strength. The foramina, through which the rather large cervical nerve roots pass, are relatively shallow. The nerves pass almost horizontally through the nerve root canals and so are quite subject to traction injury. The discs between the cervical vertebrae are relatively shallow and much less strong than those between the vertebrae below, since there is less weight to support.

The vertebrae are bound together by the annular ligament. Its dorsal and ventral thickenings hold the bodies snugly but not rigidly together. The ligamentum nuchae extends from the external occipital protuberance to attach along the tips of the cervical vertebrae as far as C–7 and then extends downward as the supraspinous ligament. This ligament is a thin septum, wider posteriorly but narrowing in the anterior direction. It serves to separate the muscles of the posterior portion of the neck at the midline. The interspinous ligaments lie between the spinous processes. The ligamentum flavum secures the laminae. The capsular ligaments bind the vertebrae at the articulations. Together, these ligaments stabilize the vertebrae in their relative positions, each to the one above and the one below. In the neck they are much less stable than anywhere else in the column. This combination of extreme mobility plus the necessity for protection requires an amazingly intricate interdigitation of muscles as well as the support of many ligaments.

The muscles of the vertebral column are extremely massive in the lower back, becoming less massive but with wider excursion as the cervical spine is reached. Since the neck is an isolated column, it requires support in the nature of dynamic guy wires in each direction. The fact that these musculotendinous guy wires can be varied in length permits the neck and head to be moved in any direction while maintaining a constant degree of support. Nowhere is the synergistic use of muscles better demonstrated than in the neck, where the function of each muscle depends altogether upon the position of the head at the time the contraction takes place. It is not advisable here to discuss in detail the individual muscles of the neck, since their number is legion. It suffices to say that the muscles are so arranged as to permit traction to be applied in any position of the head or the spine, so that with appropriate contraction of one group and relaxation of others, synchronous motions occur. As might be expected, the heaviest groups of muscles are posterior. Many of the muscles of the neck pass distally to attach to the muscles in the shoulder girdle as well as to the trunk itself.

In front of the neck lie many vital structures that are poorly protected in the upright position. The veins and arteries on either side, the esophagus behind and the larynx and trachea in front are all quite vulnerable unless the head is held down to permit the chin and thorax to protect the front of the neck.

Emergency Management

Injury to the neck often results in major disability. If there is any question at all as to the severity of a cervical injury, it should be assumed that the most severe injury is present. Under no circumstances should the patient be asked to sit or stand. If he is lying on the ground with a possible serious injury to his neck, he should not be moved until an evaluation of the situation has been made. This may require some time, but delay of the game is of no consequence under such circumstances, and the physician must not be hurried in his evaluation and so permit what may be fatal movement. If the player is conscious, a few words will determine his own feelings in regard to his neck. One should determine whether he has normal function of his hands and feet. This does not require a detailed physical examination but does entail sensible evaluation. The patient should then be moved to a stretcher and adequate help must be present so that this can be done without any motion between the patient's head and trunk. Under ordinary circumstances the athlete will be conscious. He

should be placed on his back with his head carefully supported. On occasion this may dramatize and overemphasize what turns out to be a relatively minor injury. On the other hand, it may save a life or prevent a lifetime of paralysis.

Once the player has been moved to a place for better examination, detailed study should be made, after which the physician should have a definite impression as to the severity of the injury. He should observe such deformity as may be indicative of unilateral or bilateral dislocation. He should attempt to localize the pain. Even if it is decided that the injury is only relatively severe and the patient can be moved to the hospital for evaluation, great care must be taken in his handling. The head may be stabilized by a sandbag on either side or by someone sitting at the patient's side holding his head. It may be stabilized quite well by a simple head halter, which may be made by placing a muslin strip under the occiput and another under the chin that is attached to a weight hanging over the end of the carrier or bed. If it is decided that x-rays should be done, they must be under the same precautions. Under no circumstances should the x-ray examination be carried out with the patient sitting up until one can be sure that there is no instability of the neck. Once a diagnosis is made of a serious injury to the neck, consultation should be sought immediately with the person who is going to carry out the definitive care. This may be the orthopaedic surgeon or neurosurgeon, or both. I cannot emphasize too strongly that the patient must not be asked to sit up. Forceful manipulation of the head to see how well it moves must be avoided. The patient must not be allowed to walk from the field. If he already is sitting or standing, this position may be maintained, again with greatest precautions and support.

In spite of utmost care, symptoms may develop insidiously. The patient receives his injury but may seem quite well, only to succumb to some inadvertent motion later. Any complaint of the neck by a player demands that he be removed from the contest and that a definitive examination be made. This will tend to minimize the tragedies that occur in the locker room or at home following the initial injury.

Contusion

Contusion in the vicinity of the neck has many serious consequences, not in relation to the integument, since the skin is rarely damaged, but in relation to the vital underlying structures. In the back of the neck, the blow may be received on the spinous processes, particularly in the lower cervical area, and since these are long, the leverage exerted at their bases may be quite powerful. If the blow is received with the neck in forward flexion, the combination of tension on the ligament and muscle plus the striking force may break off a spinous process anywhere from its tip to its junction to the body. Such an injury will be painful. There will be local tenderness, particularly on moving the head forward. Palpation will usually be unrewarding in fracture, but careful x-ray study will reveal the lesion. A word of warning: X-ray of the lower cervical area is difficult, and the physician must be sure that he is visualizing the area of involvement. It is worthwhile to insert a hypodermic needle into the tender area at the time the picture is made in order to localize the tender spot on the x-ray.

If a fracture is found, it should be treated appropriately, as is indicated in a following section. Contusion of the bone without fracture is treated according to its severity. Ordinarily no treatment is necessary. Painful bruising of the cervical muscles may cause the usual complications of muscle contusion, with hematoma formation (Fig. 332), muscle spasm, stiffness, pain, etc. In such an instance, local treatment is of value, with application of heat,

pain-free massage and local use of an analgesic balm. Some degree of protection with a cotton collar may speed up the recovery. Muscle spasm can be relieved by antispasmodics, and participation in athletics should be minimized. Ice massage may be useful in relaxing spasm.

Occasionally a blow on the back of the neck will have a direct effect on the spinal cord, and the resultant *shock* may cause transitory paralysis. Much more often there simply is a generalized feeling of numbness, which is extremely transitory and of little significance. In case of persistent neurological symptoms, such as numbness and paresthesia, a more thorough search for interspinal injury should be carried out. Certainly the patient should be kept under observation, and no participation in contact sports be permitted so long as there is any doubt as to the diagnosis. *Concussion* of the cord may be quite alarming, but complete recovery is the rule.

Contusion at the side of the neck, which is less frequent, may cause distressing symptoms by a direct effect on the brachial plexus, with the feeling of shock to the neck and numbness in the arm. These symptoms are usually quite transitory, and the player is able to shake them off. Occasionally there may be permanent damage to some of the components of the brachial plexus. Frequently the contusion may occur with the neck flexed in the opposite direction, so that there may be strain as well as contusion.

In the front of the neck, contusion may be quite severe. The athlete usually learns to protect the neck by carrying his chin low and forward, so that the interval between the chin and sternum is relatively narrow. Given an opportunity, he will protect himself further by dropping his head forward when the blow is impending. The structures most likely to be damaged by a direct blow are the *larynx* and *trachea*. A blow to the throat may cause extreme distress, even to the extent of systemic shock. The player is speechless, with severe dyspnea. He struggles for breath, is completely unable to phonate and, for a period, has the feeling of impending doom. Under ordinary circumstances he recovers quickly, the spasm of the vocal cords subsides and he is able to breathe more easily, although the hoarseness may persist. Immediate treatment should be complete bed rest with a cold pack on the neck. Body activity should be discouraged in order to cut down on the oxygen requirement. Reassurance is vital. Sedation should be given cautiously, particularly if there are signs of systemic shock. Recovery may be complete within a very few minutes, with no damage

Figure 332. Calcification superficial to ligamentum nuchae following neck injury with hematoma. This mass does not move with the spinous process.

done, and the patient may be able to resume play.

In the more severe case, there may be a hematoma, either intrinsic in the larynx or extrinsic from the muscles in the neck. If severe, this can be a dangerous complication. It usually is not. There may actually be *fracture of the thyroid cartilage,* of the *hyoid bone* or of the *trachea,* but this is not common in young athletes, since these structures are quite resilient. If there is persistence of symptoms beyond the day of injury, carefu laryngeal examination should be carried out, particularly if dyspnea persists. In case of doubt as to the diagnosis, the patient should be sent to a hospital, where oxygen, suction and intravenous therapy are available. Laryngoscopy is indicated if there is any question as to intrinsic injury. If signs of increasing intrinsic bleeding appear, the patient should be carefully observed, since the neck will not tolerate much pressure either from the bleeding or from the attempt to arrest this by application of a pressure pack. It is axiomatic that if there is any persistence of these symptoms, the patient should be kept at rest and under careful observation.

It probably is not advisable to attempt to aspirate a hematoma in the neck unless all the facilities of the hospital, together with a trained laryngologist, are available. If the bleeding appears to be increasing, the pressure becomes more severe and ice packs do not control the situation, consultation is mandatory.

Strain

Muscular strain in the cervical area may be extremely complex. The large number of small muscles with multiple attachments are capable of different functions with the head in different positions. It is an area quite subject to strain. It may be very difficult to distinguish between strain and sprain or between sprain and muscle spasm caused by secondary nerve root involvement. Although the athlete is quite subject to strain of the cervical muscles as a result of violent movement of the head, he is also subject to sprain of the joints, with its attendant complications. Indeed, the strain and sprain may well coexist.

Diagnostically, there is some value in the patient's history, even though it may be quite misleading. Although strain may follow overuse of the muscles of the neck, it is even more likely to be the product of an avulsion force against a muscle resisting a violent motion.

Since this same violent motion may cause sprain, subluxation, dislocation or fracture, a muscular strain may well be a secondary consideration. When strain occurs as a separate entity, active function as well as passive stretching of the involved muscle will be painful. The exact diagnosis becomes somewhat academic if the injury is a serious one. In the more minor injuries, diagnosis is not so difficult. The muscle spasm that follows this injury is a universal accompaniment of any injury to the neck and is of little diagnostic significance. Tenderness within the muscle itself or at its attachment may give a clue that the injury is strain.

If the strain seems to be relatively mild, the *treatment* may also be mild. Application of heat locally, rest and reduction of activity are important. All too often, what begins as a minor strain ends up as a rather severe spastic type of wryneck, which may be completely disabling while it lasts. The actual injury seems at the time to be minimal. It is not until 24 to 48 hours later that the constant irritation of the injured muscle causes spasm of all its fellows. This condition requires more definitive treatment. Bed rest with light cervical traction, 4 to 6 lb., is preferable to massive traction in the upright position (Fig. 333). This treatment also has the undoubted value of being good for any injury to the neck, so that if one's diagnostic acumen has been somewhat at fault, at least the treatment is suited to whatever lesion may be present. Bed rest, cervical traction, application of heat locally, use of muscle relaxants and mild sedation will result in prompt relief of symptoms. The danger is recurrence. If the strain is indeed quite mild and recovery is complete within 24 to 36 hours, no protection needs to be applied to the neck. The patient should be advised against participating in forceful activities and told to move his neck as freely as he can but strictly within the limits of pain and not against resistance. If the condition seems to be more severe and traction has been needed for several days, a cervical support, such as a cotton collar (Fig. 334), may be necessary for two to three weeks. As in any strain, careful rehabilitation is needed to prevent prompt recurrence of symptoms. Protection here is not against motion of the neck as in sprain but against overuse of the muscle involved. This requires a cooperative patient who understands his problem. The posterior spinal muscles are the ones most commonly strained—the result of forcible extension of the spine against resistance, as in wrestling. However, any of the muscles may be involved in strain.

Figure 333. Patient in cervical traction. The traction apparatus is placed at the foot of the bed instead of at the head, with the type of halter as shown. Note that the traction apparatus is positioned so that the neck is held in extension.

Sprain-Subluxation-Fracture-Dislocation

Injuries to the spine are difficult to subdivide into specific categories of sprain, subluxation, dislocation and fracture, since one extends indistinguishably into the other and there is often a combination of all four. A much more serviceable classification can be made on the basis of the mechanism causing the injury. Although there is a great deal of overlap and the motion may be much more complex than simple motion in one direction, there is a predominant motion in one direction which is almost always the major cause of the damage. I suppose it is virtually impossible to have pure flexion of the neck without some degree of rotation or vice versa. Nevertheless, the injury characterizes itself by the primary motion.

Whereas the strain discussed earlier is caused by overuse of the muscle, sprain is caused by forcing a joint through an abnormal

Figure 334. Cotton collar. The collar illustrated is a single strip of tapered quilted outing flannel; small end is 3 in. enlarging to 6 in. and 6 ft. long. Same can be made of alternating wraps of sheet wadding and gauze. This should extend far enough to support the occiput and chin.

range of motion, and the ligament designed to prevent this motion is damaged. Sprain of the neck is a very common injury and may be mild (first degree), moderate (second degree) or severe (third degree). The mild injury is of little significance and will require but little treatment. The moderate injury in which there has been some loss of ligament strength will require protection primarily from the forces that caused the injury. Much more complicated is the severe injury in which there is complete loss of integrity of the ligament. As this ligament loses its function, the motion that it is designed to prevent is unrestricted. The forces that ordinarily are controlled by this ligament are then transferred to other areas of the lever. This ligament injury may progress into subluxation, in which the joint partially dislocates; or indeed the capsular ligament may tear completely and the joint completely dislocate. Other ligaments in the spine that are not related directly to the articulations may be involved. The interspinous ligament posteriorly restricts flexion of the neck. The anterior longitudinal ligament anteriorly prevents anterior separation of the bodies of the vertebrae and so hyperextension. There is usually some combination of ligament damage, so that when the one ligament tears, the force is shifted to another ligament and damages this one also. This may continue until there is complete disruption of all the supporting ligaments and complete dislocation of one vertebra on another. So also a fracture may supervene. That is, as the ligament gives way one place, a fracture may occur elsewhere, or as the ligament holds, the edge of the bone comprising the fulcrum or counterlever may give way. Some attempt will be made to describe these injuries under the categories of the forces applied.

Flexion Injury

Interspinous-Supraspinous Ligament Injury (Sprain). The supraspinous and interspinous ligaments, which attach along the spinous processes from the occiput to the dorsal spine, serve as a checkrein to prevent overflexion of the neck. Although they are somewhat elastic, their fibers are not tight when the neck is in extension. They become increasingly tight as the neck flexes forward. The mechanism causing sprain is a forcible hyperflexion of the neck. As this force is applied, the cervical bodies are forced together. The vertebrae rotating on the sagittal axis of the articulations force the spinous processes to separate (Fig. 335) This force is arrested by the combination of the pressing of the intact bodies together and the checking action of the dorsal muscles and the ligamentum nuchae. If the force continues and the bodies maintain their integrity, the ligaments may tear (see Fig. 335A). This sprain may be mild (first degree), moderate (second degree) or severe (third degree).

The mild (first degree) sprain is of little consequence. There will be no particular weakness in the ligament. All the symptoms will be local, with tenderness and pain at the site of injury. Ordinary cervical flexion within normal range will be pain-free. Forcing the neck beyond this range may cause some distress. This injury is not likely to arouse muscle spasm, since the symptoms are mild.

In a moderate (second degree) sprain, which involves some loss of function of the ligament, a portion of the ligament has actually been torn away. This may be within the ligament itself or may be at its attachment to one of the cervical processes. In this instance the symptoms will be more severe. The patient holds his head in extension and resists any attempt to flex it forward because of pain at the site of injury. There is localized tenderness. After the passage of several hours, there is likely to be muscle spasm of the posterior spinal muscles (Fig. 336); and the neck, instead of being pulled to one side or the other, is held in extension. The direction of force applied may indicate the expected location of the injury. If the patient can rotate his atlanto-occipital joint, that is, nod his head without pain, one may assume that the injury is below C-2. A further guide as to the location of the injury is the location of tenderness.

If there is sharply localized tenderness in the spinous processes or ligament, injection of this area with a long-acting local anesthetic if the patient is seen early or a corticoid preparation if he is seen late may provide substantial relief. This injection may need to be repeated several times. In this case, traction is ordinarily not indicated, since holding the head up will relieve the tension. However, this becomes quite tiresome, and tension headache is common, with spasm of the posterior cervical muscles. The patient will be relieved by a cervical collar that holds the chin up (Fig. 337). He may be more comfortable at night in light cervical traction, although usually this is not necessary. Physical therapy is of value here. Great care should be taken that any manipulative treatment is pain-free. This injury may be quite disabling to the athlete, since six to eight weeks will be needed for the ligament to heal, which is enough to seriously disrupt his season. Rehabilitation exercises are extremely important because final stability depends upon strong cervical muscles (see page 682). A well-fitted cotton collar may permit the patient to participate in athletic activity much sooner. The collar must be carefully fitted so that the ligament will not be reinjured by forward flexion of the neck.

Figure 335. Flexion force. *A,* Forcible hyperflexion. The cervical vertebra rotates on the axis of the apophyseal joints (x). The cervical bodies (y) maintain their integrity. The interspinous ligament (z) ruptures. *B,* Same force. The ligament (z) holds. The rotation is around (x), and the adjacent edges of the bodies of the cervical vertebrae buckle. *C,* Same force. The interspinous ligament (z) gives way. The bodies (y) maintain their integrity. The center of rotation (x) advances (to x') as the interarticular ligaments rupture to slide the inferior articular process of the upper vertebra in front of that of the lower, with subluxation or dislocation.

Figure 336. X-ray, lateral view, made with the neck in forward flexion. Note reversal of the curve, caused by muscle spasm of the lower cervical segment, so that this is held in extension while the upper part of the neck flexes forward. This is indicative of muscle spasm such as accompanies strain or sprain.

If the ligament injury is severe (third degree), there is complete separation of the ligament. The ligament may be torn from a single spinous process, and the main body of the ligament may remain intact. This is a much less serious injury than that occurring when the ligament itself is pulled in two. If the ligament is ruptured either in its substance or torn from one of the processes, the symptoms will be quite severe, with sharply localized pain. If palpated early, a defect may be felt in

Figure 337. A, An adjustable cervical brace. B, A plastic cervical collar.

the ligament, particularly if the neck is forced into some degree of flexion. Further flexion will be bitterly resisted. The patient will feel that his head is insecure and will tend to hold his neck quite rigid. Painful spasm soon supervenes, and the head is pulled into hyperextension. At this time it may be quite difficult to determine the exact nature of the injury. Careful x-ray study may reveal an avulsion of a portion of the bone with the ligament (Fig. 338). X-rays made with the head and neck in flexion may reveal unusually wide separation of the spinous processes at some level. This is quite suggestive of ligament injury, particularly if it coincides with the level of local symptoms. There is normally a wide variation in the amount of separation of the spinous processes in the normal neck at different levels.

Treatment for avulsion of the tip of one of the spinous processes is surgical removal of the fragment and repair of the ligament. This treatment seems to be well accepted, especially since the diagnosis can be confirmed by x-ray. The same treatment would be ideal for complete ligament avulsion. Usually, however, this condition is not diagnosed in the early stage and is treated nonsurgically as a moderate sprain. Indeed, if the head is kept in hyperextension, thereby bringing into contact the tips of the spinous processes and with them the ligament ends, the ligament may grow together at near normal length. If this same force breaks the spinous process at the lamina or if it fractures the spinous process without displacement, uneventful healing will occur by simple immobilization of the neck in extension. Avulsion of the tip often results in nonunion, since the separation is usually wide. The treatment of a painful nonunion is excision of the fragment. Athletic competition should not be permitted until union is complete—either union of ligament to bone if the fragment is removed or bony union of the fragment to the vertebra.

Other Flexion Injury

Subluxation Dislocation. In the more severe flexion injuries of the neck, the damage is usually not confined to the interspinous ligament. As the neck is flexed, the cervical discs compress. The bodies are forced together anteriorly and apart posteriorly, and excess of motion occurs at the apophyseal articulations. If the interspinous ligament gives way while the body remains intact, the force is received on the laminal and articular ligaments as well

Figure 338. Avulsion fracture of the tip of the spinous process of C-7 following acute flexion injury. The articular facets and the bodies are spared.

as on the posterior longitudinal ligament, which is relatively weak. As long as the front of the body remains intact, the dislocating force will separate the articulations and rupture the capsular ligaments, and a subluxation of the cervical vertebrae will occur (see Fig. 335C). Indeed, this may happen without actual rupture of the posterior longitudinal ligament. As the flexion is continued, there is a shearing force of the head forward on the trunk that causes the superior articulations to displace forward over the ones below. If some of the ligaments are left intact—either the interspinous, the laminal or possibly the articular ligaments plus the anterior and posterior longitudinal ligaments—a great deal of stability is still present in the spine, and the articular process of the vertebra above slips in front of the superior articular process of the vertebra below. This dislocation locks in the unreduced position. Subluxation followed by spontaneous reduction probably occurs quite frequently in flexion injuries of the neck. This is one of the reasons, already mentioned, why the neck should be carefully protected against a repetition of the flexion shearing force in order that complete dislocation does not occur with a subsequent injury.

In bilateral dislocation (Fig. 339), the head is characteristically held thrust forward but with hyperextension. The spinous process of the vertebra below is prominent, with a corresponding defect above, whereas the proximal portion of the neck will appear to be flexed. The patient is usually extremely apprehensive and will resist any attempt to move his head in any direction. Indeed, he will often hold his

head with his hands. I well remember being called to the hospital one Saturday afternoon to see a man who had ridden in his car to the hospital holding his head in his hands following an episode with a bull. He absolutely refused to take his hands away from his head, making the statement that if he did his head would fall off, nor would he relinquish his grasp to permit examination until he was supine in bed, and even then only reluctantly.

This injury has serious potential for cord and root damage, and a careful examination should be made for the presence of a neurological deficit. This absolutely must be done before any attempt at reduction is made. The injury is obviously a serious one, but fortunately it is extremely infrequent in the athlete. It demands the prompt care of the orthopaedist. In the interim, the patient should be placed supine and the head should be protected by sandbags on either side. Since the exact nature of the injury will not be evident until x-ray studies have been carried out, it is imperative that precautionary traction of a few pounds, using a head halter, be applied as soon as possible. Needless to say, the patient must be transported with extreme caution. Definitive care demands reduction at the earliest possible moment; hence the necessity for early diagnosis (Fig. 340).

The same flexion, forward shearing force that causes the dislocation mentioned previously may continue with the destruction of the remaining ligamentous support at this level, so that one body may slide forward on the other until the back of the neurocanal of one vertebra is at the level of the front of the neurocanal

Figure 339. Fracture dislocation of C-6 on 7 from tackling. *A,* Anteroposterior view. Notice lateral displacement of mass of C-7, with rotation of C-6 forward. *B,* 24 hours in traction reduced the dislocation. *C,* Lateral view in traction shows no displacement, no obvious fracture. *D,* Recent lateral films in flexion and extension showing subluxation, with persistent collapse of disc between C-6 and C-7. This boy developed latent neurological deficit in the long thoracic nerve, which has persisted.

Figure 340. Fracture-subluxation of C-5 on 6 with fracture of the articular process of C-5. The deformity was corrected under traction, recurred in the brace and has persisted. Neurological deficit was persistent, with hypesthesia in the right thumb.

of the vertebra below (Fig. 341). This applies a shearing trauma to the cord and may cause complete quadriplegia. With this injury there is such instability that the neck will frequently fall back into correct apposition, and findings of the local physical and x-ray examinations may be entirely negative. One must not be misled as to the severity of the injury by the negative x-ray findings. The same dislocation

may have been complete and reduced, without cord damage, only to have cord damage occur because the injury was not recognized, and subsequent activity caused a dislocation.

As this dislocation occurs, the posterior portion of the neural arch may break and remain posterior (Fig. 342). This break may take place at the pars interarticularis or further back on the lamina. In any event, this protects the cord

Figure 341. A, Complete dislocation of C-5 on 6 without fracture. The intact arch caused transection of the cord and complete quadriplegia. B, Postoperative picture showing complete reduction with internal fixation from C-4 to 6 plus bone graft. Partial laminectomy at C-5.

Figure 342. Fracture-dislocation of C-2 on C-3. Note that the fracture separated the arch and lamina from the body, which relieved the tension on the cord, and there was no neurological deficit. This picture shows the reduction and plaster fixation. Complete healing. Asymptomatic. Arrow indicates fracture.

to a considerable degree, since the shearing action of the posterior portion of the ring is prevented as the ring itself expands. This accounts for the condition of complete dislocation of the vertebra forward, with no neurological symptoms. Careful x-ray examination will often reveal that the arch has remained posterior. Such cases serve to emphasize the importance of intelligent handling of the cervical injury. The same force that causes bilateral dislocation with forward flexion and shearing may well cause fracture of the articular processes, which may complicate the recovery and result in painful joints.

A unique type of injury that may occur as a result of forward stress is dislocation between the first and the second cervical vertebrae (Fig. 343). It will be recalled that the odontoid is held firmly to the anterior portion of the body of C-1 by the transverse ligament, which keeps the body of C-1 from displacing forward. On a sharp forward thrust of the head, particularly combined with some forward shearing, the odontoid is forced sharply against this ligament. If the ligament tears, the articular ligaments also give way and dislocation occurs, leaving the odontoid within the neurocanal of the first cervical vertebra. The large vulnerable cord of this area is very likely to be damaged, with resulting death. Occasionally there is a congenital shortness of the odontoid, so that it can slip forward under the transverse liga-

Figure 343. Fractured odontoid with forward subluxation of C-1 on 2. Only transient neurological deficit. Treated in traction, cast, and brace, with complete clinical recovery but some persistent subluxation.

Figure 344. Fracture of the ring of the first cervical vertebra, without displacement. No neurological deficit. Treated by plaster immobilization.

ment without actually tearing it. This is the so-called somersault dislocation caused by sharp hyperflexion of the neck. Many of these cases will not have serious nerve involvement. They may actually be in the nature of recurrent dislocation and slip forward and spontaneously reduce. If they do not reduce spontaneously, they can usually be reduced. Owing to the very large brain stem at this level, reduction is better done by mechanical traction with weights than by manipulation. The traction should first be with the neck well flexed and then with it gradually moved toward extension. This dislocation may be very difficult to distinguish from fracture of the odontoid, since the latter, when it accompanies dislocation of the first cervical vertebra, is not readily seen in the anteroposterior x-ray view. Careful study after the deformity is reduced will reveal the character of the lesion (Fig. 344).

A much more frequent injury appears to be the fracture of the odontoid from the body of C-2. In this instance there is much more leeway for the cord, and it is much less likely to be impinged. This fracture may be complete or incomplete. The patient usually realizes that he is seriously hurt. The usual careful management should be carried out. Definitive diagnosis is made by x-ray examination. The severity of this major injury demands early, adequate treatment, which may well be surgical. Of some consequence is the incomplete tear, with damage to the transverse ligament.

The initial relatively minor injury may be followed by a fatal accident at a later time.

Fracture. Aside from the laminal fractures mentioned previously, which are essentially a component of dislocation, there may be fractures of other portions of the vertebrae. It has been mentioned that the spinous process may break rather than the ligamentum nuchae tear. As the flexion force is applied and the spinous processes separate, the cervical bodies are forced together and a fracture of one of them may occur (Fig. 345A). In fact, a fracture of the cervical body is more frequent than a complete tear of the posterior longitudinal ligament. If the fracture is not accompanied by a dislocation, the cervical body may compress as much as 75 per cent. The front part of the body will be down to 25 per cent of its normal height, and the posterior part will maintain its normal height. Since the axis of rotation is at the articulations, which are adjacent to the posterior portion of the body, the force is primarily applied at the extreme front. These injuries are not often accompanied by cord damage, since the neural canal is not impinged upon. The patient will have extreme forward flexion of the neck and severe pain, with the feeling of insecurity that accompanies severe ligament injury or dislocation. The same careful study described previously will reveal the fracture.

The fracture will require definitive treatment by traction to restore the bony contours and prolonged immobilization to permit union.

Roentgenographic study of the neck presents many difficulties, and the team physician would be wise to consult a competent radiologist or orthopaedist before concluding that the x-ray findings of the neck are negative. The potentialities of permanent disability are so great that one can ill afford to "wait and see" in these injuries (see Fig. 345B).

Extension Injury (Dorsiflexion)

Anterior Longitudinal Ligament Injury (Sprain). The anterior longitudinal ligament extends throughout the cervical spine and serves to prevent separation of the anterior margins of the cervical vertebrae by hyperextension of the neck. As the neck moves into extension, the spinous processes tend to impinge on each other and, as the force continues, the lever changes from the first degree, with the fulcrum at the cervical articulations, to the second degree, with the fulcrum at the tip of the spinous processes. Distraction force

Figure 345. *A*, Compression fracture of C-7. This does not require reduction but requires protection so that the body does not collapse. A period of traction until the spasm subsides and then a Minerva cast is adequate treatment. *B*, Inadequately treated cervical fracture-dislocation. This is a flexion film made some months after the injury, showing anterior dislocation of C-6 and compression of C-7. A film made in extension determines gross instability because in extension the dislocation is reduced, indicating nonunion.

is applied to the anterior longitudinal ligament and to a lesser extent to the articular ligaments. This results in some degree of damage to the anterior longitudinal ligament. The anterior ligament may tear or avulse a fragment of the body (Fig. 346). If the ligament maintains its integrity, there may be a fracture of the spinous processes. If the spinous processes hold, the ligament may tear. The tear may be of any degree, and if it is severe enough, it may permit actual dislocation of the cervical spine. If the force is arrested, the neck returns to its normal position and there are relatively few symptoms, since the normal position of the neck puts no strain on the anterior longitudinal ligament. Usually the player knows that he has had a neck injury, and examination will reveal that the pain and tenderness are anterior and that the symptoms are aggravated by extension of the neck.

If the injury is mild (first degree), no particular treatment is indicated, except that as a hedge a cotton collar should be applied. If the injury is moderate (second degree), the same

Figure 346. *A*, Fracture of anterior quadrant of C-2, with anterior rotation of the fragment. No neurological symptoms. *B*, Five months later, solid union. All manipulative efforts to replace the fragment failed. This was undoubtedly an extension injury.

treatment may be used as for the posterior sprain, except that the neck should be placed in some degree of flexion rather than extension, whether using traction or a collar. The motion to be prevented by the brace is extension rather than flexion.

If the injury is severe (third degree) and there has been actual tearing of the anterior longitudinal ligament (Fig. 347), the symptoms will be more extreme and protection must be prolonged. This is the reason for mentioning that in the mild injury it is well to protect the neck until it is pain-free. The ever-present danger is repetition of the force that caused the original injury. Riding in a car, participating in a scrimmage, etc., should be ruled out without protection of the neck to prevent this motion. If muscle spasm supervenes, the head will be pulled forward by the bilaterally tight sternomastoid muscles. This may be extremely painful and to a considerable extent disabling, since the patient has difficulty in raising his head to the erect position. It must be determined by examination that the difficulty is not actually from weakness of the dorsiflexors but from tightness of the forward flexors.

The severe case will require the same careful handling as any potentially serious injury of the neck. The patient should be put at bed rest, with the neck in a position of slight flexion, and light traction (4 lb.) applied. The use of muscle relaxants, sedation and application of heat locally are all important. Attention should be called to the fact that the symptoms are very similar to those resulting from bilateral dislocation of the articular facets, and careful x-ray examination is needed to rule out possible bone or joint damage. Physical examination will help determine the diagnosis, since in this instance, forward flexion very carefully, even gingerly, applied will be pain-free, whereas an attempt to extend the neck will cause increased spasm in the sternomas-

toids. On the other hand, with a dislocation of the neck, the patient is quite willing to dorsiflex his neck. A few hours of traction, with application of heat locally and sedation, will relax the spasm, and a more definitive diagnosis can be made. The patient must be protected for several weeks against dorsiflexion of the neck. This is incompatible with active athletics.

Subluxation-Dislocation. If this same extension force continues, the anterior edges of the bodies are separated, the disc is disrupted (see Fig. 347*B*), the posterior longitudinal ligament tears, the articular ligaments tear and the vertebra may actually be displaced backward over the vertebra below it. This hyperextension type of injury is extremely serious and accounts for many of the cases accompanied by complete paralysis below this level, yet with entirely negative x-ray findings. The cord will tolerate posterior displacement even more poorly than it will anterior. This injury is not frequent in athletics. There is a limiting factor in that the lever of the spinous process is potentially a weak one and it may well give way (see Fig. 347*C*) at any time during the application of this posterior flexion. This buckling of the process may save the cord, since it permits the vertebrae to rotate near the spinal canal rather than to open up on an axis of the posterior tip of the spinous process. The patient with paralysis presents no great problem to the examining physician, since it is obvious he has a major injury. More puzzling is the injury that does not cause primary paralysis. Findings at examination may be relatively negative. X-ray findings are negative. An incautious or unrestricted motion may lead to disaster. One should try to determine whether or not the direction of the force that caused the injury was extension or flexion. The initial traction in bed followed by use of a cervical brace should be designed to prevent extension of the neck. Permission to resume active athletic par-

A   **B**   **C**

Figure 347. Extension injury of the cervical spine. *A*, Hyperextension forces the spinous processes together at (z), dislocates the front of the vertebra at (y). The center of rotation changes from (x) to (x″) as the spinous processes impinge and the vertebrae are torn apart. *B*, Continuation of the same force dislocates the articulations, rupturing the discs and anterior and posterior longitudinal ligaments, and a frank dislocation may occur. *C*, With application of the same forces, the spinous processes break, which relieves the tension, and the vertebrae fall back together without major damage to the cord.

Figure 348. *A,* The older style helmet. Note the hard posterior edge of the helmet is directed at about C-6 and 7. However, it is at least 2 in. away from the spinous process, with the head forcibly extended by pressure on the face bar. *B,* The new style helmet. Note the soft leather roll against the skin with the hard plastic edge 1½ in. away, so that the hard plastic edge is 4 in. from the bone. This is the same player.

ticipation, if ever, will depend upon the individual case.

A present concern in the causation of extension injuries involves the modern headgear. There can be no reasonable doubt that today's headgear is a great improvement over the types previously used, particularly in preventing blows to the head and face. However, there has been an unwelcome result of this improvement that is particularly related to cervical injuries. The plastic headgear is extremely solid and unyielding. Its posterior edge is no exception. In many types of headgear, the posterior edge strikes the upper cervical area, so that with the head in complete extension, the edge of the headgear drives toward the spinous processes. A major improvement in the headgear has been utilization of the face bar, which has markedly diminished facial injuries. However, the long bar projecting well forward, which is preferred by many, presents a convenient handle that the opponent may consciously or inadvertently grasp in his contact with the player. Indeed, he does not need to grasp it. The blocker coming up with the shoulder or elbow may catch the bar and forcibly extend his opponent's neck. The hazard is greatly increased if the bar extends well forward. A severe force is applied to the back of the neck by the combination of the leverage action on the front of the helmet and impingement of the unyielding back of the helmet against the spinous process. This may actually

break off a spinous process, which is not of transcending importance. Much more vital is the fact that the back of the helmet may tend to support the tip of the spinous process, so that it maintains its fulcrum as the front of the bodies of the vertebrae are separated. The force is concentrated at a single point, further encouraging extension injury.

There has been a great deal of study in regard to this problem of spinal injury from headgear in the last few years. Better design of the helmet, with addition of a posterior roll or flap, has been an improvement. The face bars have been better fashioned and do not protrude so far forward. Strict officiating, with immediate, automatic penalty, has sharply discouraged the temptation to use the face bar as a hand hold or as a lever.

Until lately the designers of helmets have concentrated on protecting the head of the wearer. Less thought has been given to the effect of the helmet on other portions of the player's or his opponent's anatomy. A recent modification of the helmet is designed to improve these conditions. The helmet previously used by the University of Oklahoma and the one now used are seen in Figure 348. In Figure 348*A*, the headgear is of solid, unyielding plastic, with a small leather roll over the back edge of the helmet and no padding over the top of it. The new helmet (Fig. 348*B*), has had the plastic back of the neck cut away and replaced with an apron so that it is impossible for the edge of the plastic to impinge against the neck proper. Formerly this same helmet had a strip of plastic foam, about 6 in. wide, beginning at the forehead and extending up over the crown of the helmet, which served as protection for the opposing player. However its use has been discontinued because of the additional weight and heat. The helmet also has plastic pads inside. Although the players complain of its being somewhat hotter, it certainly seems to be more protective. The addition of the external and internal padding accounts for an increase of only 1 oz. in weight. Incidentally, the single face bar for protection has been supplanted in many places by double bars. These do not need to extend as far forward, since they cover more of the facial area and so reduce the leverage somewhat. They are harder to grasp because of the spread between the bars. The blocker is also less likely to get his elbow, shoulder or knee under the bars, since the lower one is considerably closer to the chest. The second bar adds about 10 oz. to the weight of the helmet, but this probably can be reduced in newer models by using lighter weight material. Trying to improve the protective helmet and face bar is certainly much more valid than condemning them and recommending their abandonment.

Rotatory Injury

Sprain. This sprain is usually the result of rotation of the neck in which the head is forcibly turned beyond the tolerance of the vertebra involved. The chin is pulled toward the opposite shoulder, and excess strain is placed upon the ligaments as the neck is not only flexed to the side but rotated the same direction. These capsular ligaments tear to some degree. The force is released. The result is some damage to the ligament fibers, with hemorrhage into the capsule and, indeed, into the joint. In the vast majority of cases, no actual subluxation occurs. As soon as the head resumes its normal position, the spasm subsides, but soreness will persist. In many cases, if the examination is made early, the level of involvement can be determined by palpation directly over the joint. Active function of the cervical muscles will not cause pain, even against resistance. If the sprain is on the left side of the neck, forcibly pulling the head to the left against resistance will not be painful. On the other hand, passive flexion and rotation to the opposite side to reproduce the force that caused the injury will cause pain.

If the sprain is mild (first degree), the symptoms will be few. The player will shrug it off. On the following day he will have soreness and stiffness in the neck but will usually recover completely without either treatment or protection.

If the sprain is moderate (second degree) and some portion of the ligament is actually torn, the symptoms will be much more pronounced. Although the injury may not have appeared to be serious at the time of its occurrence, on the following day muscle spasm will intervene. Spasm of the muscles will have pulled the head toward the involved side and will resist any effort toward reproducing the motion that caused the sprain. The pain may become quite severe, not primarily from the ligament injury but from the resulting muscle spasm. The patient may present several days later with the ear pulled toward the shoulder on the same side and the chin rotated toward the same side, with pain and spasm along the same side (Fig. 349A). The treatment of this condition at any stage will depend upon the severity. If there is painful spasm, the best way to relax it is by bed rest and light cervical traction, accompanied by application of heat locally. Muscle relaxants will give relief. Indeed, the treatment is the same as that indicated for strain previously. Here, too, the extent of the treatment will depend upon the symptoms. It may be that the spasm will subside in a few hours or a day or so, but be assured that it will return if the patient is allowed unprotected activity. This patient must wear a cotton collar or metal or plastic brace to protect the ligament against reproduction of the motion that caused the injury. Athletic competition cannot be permitted for several weeks if the injury was serious. If it appears to be less severe, the player should be protected with a cotton collar during the time of his participation.

Subluxation. If this force continues, subluxation or unilateral dislocation may occur. The spontaneously reduced subluxation has the same symptoms as the sprain mentioned previously. In the cervical spine, the articular process may slide partially off and become locked in this position rather than dislocate entirely forward. This patient will have the same history of injury and the same complaints of pain as one with sprain, but the pain is usually more severe. He will immediately have sharply restricted motion of the neck so that he is unable to rotate his neck at all to the affected side. The chin will have turned

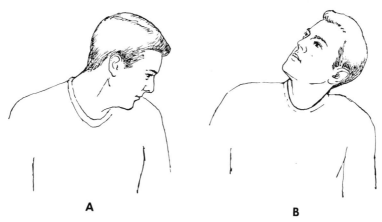

Figure 349. *A*, In sprain the head is tilted and rotated in the same direction. *B*, In wryneck the chin is rotated toward the opposite side, and the head is tilted toward the affected side. The condition of the left side is shown.

toward the opposite side, and the head will be tilted to the opposite side. The sternomastoid muscle on the involved side will be tight. The essential problem here will be muscle spasm due to tightness of the muscles that prevents replacement of the dislocation. Subluxation may occur without actual ligament damage if the ligaments of the neck are somewhat relaxed. In the athlete it ordinarily occurs as an acute injury and with some damage to the ligaments. The reason for separating the two is that in the subluxation without actual ligament damage, the joint is not affected, and once the subluxation is reduced, the patient is essentially asymptomatic, usually with no residual. This injury may be compared with the recurrent dislocation of the shoulder which has become so loose that it slips out without further damage to the ligament, and once the dislocation is reduced, it is pain-free. These recurrent subluxations may well be the result of an untreated sprain in which the ligament was allowed to heal with redundancy.

The condition that is seen as an acute injury, without patient history of subluxation, should be treated as a severe sprain. It is important first to reduce the subluxation. This is accomplished not by massive overhead traction but by bed rest with 4 lb. cervical traction, accompanied by application of heat locally, use of muscle relaxants and sedation. I have yet to see one of these cases of subluxation persist overnight if the patient slept. This is not a complete dislocation, and the articular processes are not locked. Reduction of a subluxation does not heal the ligament injury. As soon as the reduction is accomplished, the condition should be treated as a sprain and the neck protected against recurrence of the injury until

the ligament healing is complete. This will take six to eight weeks.

Dislocation-Fracture. If this same force continues, a complete dislocation of the articular process occurs on one side. In this instance, the articular process slips forward and lodges in front of the superior articulation of the vertebra below, where it is held securely in position. The patient will have had severe pain located at the side of the neck. Muscle spasm will be immediate. At examination the chin is turned away and the head is tilted away from the dislocation. The patient obviously has a serious injury, and it should be handled as such. True enough, if the injury was due to a rotatory force and the major ligaments are intact, the patient is in little danger. One cannot be sure, however, that the injury is not major, and the same care should be assumed in management as in the case of complete bilateral dislocation.

Ill-advised attempts at manipulation should be discouraged. In the first place, manipulation is often unsuccessful, and in the second place, it may cause irreparable damage. Definitive treatment should be carried out by the surgeon skilled in this type of injury. If manual manipulation is to be attempted, with or without the patient under anesthesia, the earlier it is done the more successful it will be. For manipulation without anesthesia, the patient is sedated heavily and the head is tilted forward and rotated in the direction to increase the deformity until the vertebra is unlocked. The cervical spine is slightly flexed, traction is increased and the head is carefully turned and tilted back toward the injured side and into hyperextension. Repeated efforts to do this without anesthesia are unjustified. With the patient under anesthesia,

Figure 350. The Minerva jacket for high cervical fracture-dislocation. The forehead and parietal regions are included to limit rotation and nodding of the head, which take place chiefly in the occipitoatloid and atlantoaxial articulations. In cases of lower cervical injuries, the chin piece may be cut out if the forehead piece is firm.

the same manipulation may be carried out but must be done with utmost precaution, bearing in mind that the safety factor of the patient's muscles has been eliminated.

Many of these dislocations may be reduced by cervical traction, although one is inclined to fear that if reduction is too easy, one or both of the articular processes may be fractured. Following reduction of the deformity, light traction may be continued with the neck in extension, or the patient may be promptly put in a Minerva-type jacket (Fig. 350). The head should be placed so that the neck is slightly hyperextended. The chin should be supported and the cast should extend over the forehead and rest on the iliac crest. Anything short of this cannot immobilize the neck. It should be borne in mind that the dislocation entails a ligament injury, which will require the usual period for healing.

Many of the rotatory injuries are accompanied by lateral stress, so that as the head is twisted to the opposite side, the articular process slides forward on the involved side. A great deal of force is applied to the lateral mass of the vertebra on the opposite side from the inflicting force—that is, on the side toward which the head is turned and flexed. This may cause a fracture of the articular processes on

the opposite side (see Fig. 340) or of any portion of the lateral mass. If this patient is treated as indicated, the fracture will not particularly complicate the picture, since it will have healed by the time the ligament injury has. Casual treatment of the ligament injury combined with failure to diagnose the fracture may court disaster.

Unilateral subluxation and dislocation are extremely difficult to visualize by x-ray examination, particularly if they occur around C-6 and C-7, where the intervening shoulder muscles, particularly in a well-developed individual, interfere with good visualization. In order to determine the nature of the damage, it may be necessary to obtain repeated anteroposterior, lateral, oblique and stereoscopic views or even laminograms or CAT scans.

Many of these rotatory injuries are relieved by simple repositioning of the spine. It may be extremely difficult to convince the eager athlete that he has an injury that demands prolonged treatment. One must exert every effort to prevent him from injudicious exercise in his effort to hasten his rehabilitation, since this only results in prolongation of his recovery and may even result in permanent disability.

Torsion Injuries to Nerve Elements

Brachial Plexus and Nerve Root Injuries. Although flexion and extension of the neck account for the major dislocations, in twisting injuries there may be serious involvement of the nerve roots. As the neck is forcibly rotated in one direction and flexed the same way, undue tension is placed upon the cords of the brachial plexus, particularly if traction is applied at the same time to the outstretched arm. For example, when someone is tackling a player by grabbing him by his right arm and someone else is pulling his head to the left, considerable tension is placed upon the nerve structures. This may result in transitory paralysis of the arm, with the familiar numbing or shocklike feeling, which within a few seconds or minutes completely disappears. It may, however, result in a more serious neurological pathology, even to the extent of tearing the nerve roots from the cord. This is an irreparable injury. Damage to the cords of the brachial plexus also may occur. This latter may well be remediable.

Following such an injury, any evidence of nerve involvement of the extremities that persists more than a few hours demands very careful study, with an attempt to delineate the exact root or trunk involved. Frequently there will be a generalized involvement of the arm, with diffuse numbness and a feeling of heaviness, which gradually disappears. Certain specific neurological defects may be persistent, however, and may easily be overlooked. Damage to the posterior cord affecting the use of the triceps, for example, may be easily overlooked, since the arm will readily fall into extension by the effect of gravity, and several days may pass before the physician realizes that a loss of function of this muscle is actually present. It behooves him to make a careful neurological examination of the extremity after such an injury. The earlier this is done the better, since it provides a base for measuring the progress of the condition by successive examinations. In case of increasing involvement, surgical neurolysis may be indicated. The neurosurgeon should have the opportunity to determine the necessity for this and decide on the best time for the procedure.

Major tears of the nerve roots are extremely rare. When they occur, they are manifested by complete loss of function of the components involved. Unfortunately, they are not amenable to surgical repair. However, one is usually able to distinguish between damage to the more peripheral portions of the brachial plexus and damage to the nerve root. This is of vital importance, since the plexus injury may be reparable.

ASSOCIATED CERVICAL INJURIES

Nerve Root Injury

Any of the previously described forces may cause damage to the nerve roots, ranging from brief irritation with a transient numbing, shocklike feeling in the arm to complete severance of the root. As a rule, the important consideration is to determine if possible the exact nature of injury, in order to know what should be done with the patient. Once he gets well-developed symptoms of nerve root damage, he should be referred to the neurosurgeon or the orthopaedist. There is nothing specifically diagnostic about nerve root pain. It may be caused with equal facility by the pressure of a cervical disc, by fracture of a portion of the nerve root foramen or by pressure on the nerve root from hematoma or hemorrhage within the nerve. Certainly a diagnosis of nerve root syndrome is no more specific than one of bellyache or headache.

The nerve root symptoms that are caused by a sudden twist of the head and that are transient and disappear rapidly are usually of little significance. In exceptional cases, they indicate a subluxation, particularly if the symptoms were the first of their kind to occur in this patient. Some players have repeated episodes of pain in the neck, with nerve root symptoms into the arm which seem to be accompanied by no particular pathological condition in the neck. These must be interpreted as resulting from an impingement of the nerve, either due to hypermobility of a joint or to narrowing of the nerve root canal, so that the nerve is pinched by a motion that ordinarily would leave it amply free. So also may adhesions about the nerve root cause traction on the nerve on an unguarded motion, which ordinarily is prevented by protective muscle tension. Although careful study may be rewarding in eliminating some remediable lesions, one is often in a quandary as to whether or not athletic participation should be permitted. The decision will depend partly on the patient's desire and mostly on the physician's own judgment of the situation.

Scalenus Anticus Syndrome

The scalenus anticus syndrome, like many other syndromes, is much less frequently diagnosed now that it is possible to make more specific diagnoses, for example, of cervical rib, cervical disc and various vascular conditions. The symptoms arise because of occlusion of the artery or vein or pressure of the brachial plexus caused by spasm of the anterior scalene muscle. Certain anatomic characteristics, particularly the presence of a cervical rib, make these symptoms more apt to occur. The pain usually originates at the lower roots of the plexus and continues along the ulnar distribution, particularly whenever the arm is over the head. This is combined with a tendency toward vascular occlusion, resulting in inability to work with the arms higher than the shoulders because of pain and the feeling that the arm "goes to sleep." This is not an athletic injury. It is mentioned because it may at times be confused with cervical injury. A little attention to the patient's history will help in the diagnosis. A classic diagnostic sign is obliteration of the radial pulse as the arm is pulled over the head and the neck is pulled to the opposite side. A well-established syndrome will require surgical treatment.

Cervical Rib Syndrome

This syndrome is mentioned along with the scalenus anticus syndrome because the two are quite similar. The presence of a cervical rib makes injury to this area of the plexus at the base of the neck somewhat more likely. A blow at the base of the neck over a cervical rib may well cause a sharp accentuation of, or may indeed initiate, the neurological and vascular symptoms of cervical rib. Recognition of the possibility of a cervical rib will usually permit adequate diagnosis and treatment (Fig. 351).

Injury to the Long Thoracic Nerve

Injury to the long thoracic nerve frequently occurs in conjunction with sprain or other injury at the base of the neck. This nerve comes directly off the nerve roots and does not participate in the brachial plexus. It passes down and supplies the various serrations of the serratus anterior. Bruising or damage to this nerve may occur and pass unrecognized until distressing winging of the scapula is noted (Fig. 352). The cause of the injury may be a sharp blow at the base of the neck laterally that impinges the nerve against the lower cervical vertebrae. Since this is primarily a motor nerve, there is usually little pain or discomfort to guide the physician. There may be weakness or complete paralysis of the nerve, resulting in loss of fixation of the scapula to the chest wall, so that as the arm is pulled forward, the vertebral border of the scapula swings outward.

The ideal treatment for this condition has not been found. If it is recognized early, recovery would probably be expedited by immobilization of the arm in abduction and external rotation in order to hold the scapula against the chest wall and protect the muscles from undue strain. Since it is usually recognized quite late, there is some question as to the value of immobilization. Surgical treatment is not acceptable, since recovery will usually take place without it. The injury is usually a contusion rather than a separation. Since the involved area is extremely inaccessible, making any sort of repair virtually impossible, neurolysis should probably not be attempted, even if the injury is recognized late. After a period of a few weeks there is no reason to forbid active use; in fact, athletic competition within the patient's capacity should be encouraged.

Injury to the Spinal Accessory Nerve

The spinal accessory nerve, located as it is somewhat superficially near the surface in the

Figure 351. Bilateral cervical rib C-7. This is congenital and not necessarily disabling.

Figure 352. Photograph illustrating winging of scapula.

trapezius muscle, may be injured by a direct blow across the trapezius muscle. This injury may be confused with contusion of the muscle. The player may have difficulty elevating the shoulder toward the ear and will have severe aching pain. The injury requires no specific treatment other than physical therapy. Application of heat and superficial massage will usually relieve the symptoms, and restoration of the motor function of the trapezius muscle is rapid. For a few days there may seem to be serious paralysis.

Snapping Neck

Another and more common condition in the cervical area may give the player and the physician a good deal of uneasiness. This is the presence of an audible and palpable click or snap of the neck on certain rotations. The cause of this popping or snapping is varied. It may be due to irregularity at the articulations. Much more commonly it is due to forcible snapping of a tendon over a bony prominence. As with most conditions of the neck, there is a very considerable apprehension factor which does not seem to be present in joints more distal from the head. The player who can pop his neck on certain rotatory movements is quite certain that he has a gross pathological condi-

tion. He usually holds the neck stiff. He may become amazingly adept at this snapping, since if he learns to hold certain muscles tight, the snapping becomes much more audible. There is undoubtedly a functional component in this condition, and the player has an almost uncontrollable impulse to pop his neck, whereupon he proclaims that he gets great relief.

The treatment for this condition is to avoid the snapping. If the patient is willing to stop demonstrating the snapping, it will usually disappear. A word of warning should be sounded, however. One must make sure that no underlying pathological condition is present that needs to be treated, such as irregularity of the articular facet, tenosynovitis of a tendon or muscle spasm that tends to bow the tendon across the bony prominence. For this reason, a fairly extensive regimen of physical therapy should be instituted. In the true "snapping neck," pain is not an important symptom, whereas apprehension is. A very careful physical examination, together with x-ray study, may be followed by a frank conference with the player in which the situation is thoroughly explained. He is assured that he has no serious condition and that many joints are prone to snap. He should then be urged to avoid, if possible, getting in the position where the phenomenon occurs. Frequently after a suitable period, either the snapping disappears or the player learns to ignore it.

Rehabilitation

Almost any involvement of the neck which is long-standing will require an extensive rehabilitative effort to prevent recurrence. See page 682, where exercises are detailed.

DORSAL SPINE

Anatomical Considerations

The dorsal thoracic spine (see Fig. 331) is the most stable section of the vertebral column. No description of the anatomy need be given here other than to mention a few pertinent points. The 12 dorsal vertebrae, together with the ribs and sternum, combine to form the bony thorax. The whole structure of the thorax is such that it tends to limit motion of the spine. The general contour of the spine is one of dorsal convexity, and extension from this position is resisted by the thoracic cage.

The spine itself has a good deal of intrinsic stability, the vertebrae being very firmly bound together by the various ligaments. The articular processes are vertical and face in such a manner that the inferior processes of the vertebrae above lock behind the superior processes of the vertebrae below to completely prevent any forward displacement of the upper vertebrae on the lower unless there is a fracture of the arch. Sufficient displacement to permit the articular processes to displace upward the full length of the articulation is necessary before the joint can become dislocated. The angle of these processes is such that the inferior processes on the superior vertebrae above fit within the arc of the superior processes of the lower vertebrae, the articular face of the lower vertebrae facing inward almost 45 degrees. The bodies themselves are slightly higher behind than in front, which causes the convexity and again adds to the stability. The ribs, articulating as they do between two vertebrae, tend to reinforce the column at the level of the back of the bodies. The column is also supported by the very immobile articular processes.

The disc spaces are narrow, and the thoracic discs have much less elasticity than either the cervical or lumbar discs. The spinous processes, rather than extending backward as in the cervical and lumbar spines, extend downward, overlapping each other as shingles on a roof. In many instances one actually rests upon its fellow below, so that the leverage of the interspinous ligaments is greatly increased because these spinous processes actually have to separate as the spine flexes forward. These processes immediately impinge on each other as the spine is flexed backward. They are subcutaneous at their tips.

The stable dorsal spine serves for attachment of many of the muscles (Fig. 353) of the trunk, shoulder and arm. The trapezius muscle attaches to the spinous processes from the upper cervical spine well down to lower dorsal spine. In the lower part of the dorsal spine, the trapezius muscle overlaps the long attachment of the latissimus dorsi, which attaches to the spinous processes beginning at middorsal level and extending to the pelvis. These are the most superficial layers of the muscles in the back and serve to enclose the deeper layers. These deeper layers are broad, flat muscles and are not frequently subject to injury. The scapular muscles, including the levator scapulae and the rhomboideus major and minor, underlie the trapezius in the upper portion of the dorsal spine and extend down toward the level of the upper limit of the latissimus dorsi. Still deeper are the muscles running from the spine to the ribs—and deepest are the sacrospinalis group, which is a combination of many muscles whose course essentially parallels the spinal column. The sacrospinalis group fills the

Figure 353. Anatomical drawing of muscles of the back.

sulcus between the spinous processes and the bodies of the vertebrae and the arc of the ribs. They interdigitate in such a manner that each tends to support the other. These muscles make up the so-called lumbar mass of muscle that extends from the occiput to the sacrum just lateral to the spinous processes. They all have multiple actions, depending upon the inter-relationship between them. In one instance they may serve to stabilize the spine in a certain position while another portion moves; in another they may serve to move the spine; and in yet another they may serve to anchor the spine while other muscles move some other portion of the body. The nerve supply is direct from the spinal roots and so is well protected and seldom damaged.

Contusion

Contusion of the spine is relatively common but is not often severe. The subcutaneous spinous process may receive a blow that crushes the skin against the protruding bone beneath or may damage the underlying bone. However, the most common contusion of the spine is of the muscles lateral to the spinous processes. These muscular contusions are similar to contusions elsewhere. One should make an effort to determine whether or not there is some underlying pathological condition. The contusion may cause a hematoma within the muscle that will require the usual treatment with cold pack, local injection and pressure, followed by heat.

The most common complication of contusion of the muscle is residual stiffness, which causes aching pain and restriction of motion for a few days subsequent to the injury. This should be treated by heat, pain-free massage and careful exercise. If the contusion is over the spinous process, there may be some periosteal reaction or reaction in the supraspinous ligament which will result in pain and tenderness that is very sharply localized to the involved area. It may be painful enough to suggest the possibility of a fracture. Indeed, there may be an infraction or crack in the spinous process which cannot be demonstrated by x-ray examination but which may be diagnosed clinically. The resultant painful area can usually be relieved by physical therapy. Local injection of a long-acting anesthetic is of considerable value here and should give rather prompt relief, although more than one injection may be necessary. If athletic participation is to be continued following contusion, a lo-

calized protective pad should be placed over the area.

Strain

The spine is particularly susceptible to muscular strain because of the multiplicity of muscles involved in holding the body erect. Strain of these muscles may be extremely distressing. In the early stages it may be rather difficult to distinguish strain from contusion, since the contusion may cause some hemorrhage within the muscle and may well cause pain on function of the muscle. However, the early history may be a valuable guide in diagnosis. The patient may mention some unusual occurrence. In athletics it is usually a major effort while he is somewhat off balance, such as a shot putter throwing a 16 lb. shot from an imperfect stance. Strain in the athlete does not as a rule result from simple repetition of a motion, as it does in the industrial worker, since the athlete is usually in good enough shape that his muscles will tolerate the degree of strain he puts upon them in athletic use. Basically, the strain is caused by violent contraction beyond the strength of a muscle against a fixed resistance or by overstretching as the muscle attempts to resist this stretch.

On examining the patient with such an injury, it is quite difficult to identify the exact muscle involved. In the shoulder girdle, where one may be able to check a certain specific muscle function, as for example that of the rhomboid or levator scapulae, and find painful function limited to one motion, such identification may be quite simple. In the spine, however, the physician will consider himself fortunate if he can determine which group of muscles is involved and, in some instances, even which side of the back is involved, since there is a great deal of generalized muscle spasm. There will be tenderness over the involved muscle and pain caused by passive stretching or active contraction. If, for example, the spinalis group is involved on the *right side*, one will find tenderness just to the right of the spinous process. Pain is elicited by passive forward flexion, whereas active forward flexion within limits, even against forceful resistance, is pain-free. Passive backward bending will be pain-free, since the involved muscle relaxes in this motion, whereas active backward bending against resistance (as, for example, when the patient is lying prone and raises his chest from the table) will cause pain. Passive flexion to the right is pain-free. Active flexion to the right against resistance will cause pain. To the left side, passive flexion is painful, and limited active motion even against resistance is not. If the condition is fairly severe and well established, there will be tenderness and spasm in the whole group of spinal muscles as they endeavor to restrict the motion of the spine and to reduce the pain. In this instance, the spastic muscles themselves may become painful, even though they were not originally involved. Diffuse pain in the back is the result. The patient presents with a poker spine that will resist motion in any direction.

Treatment is general and local. If there is muscle spasm, muscle relaxants are of considerable value. Preparations are available today that have a minimal sedative effect (e.g., carisoprodol) and these may suffice. Tranquilizers such as meprobamate may be used if there is an element of apprehension or nervous tension in the individual. Local treatment is directed at the local lesion and to relieve muscular tension. If there is an isolated tender area, a so-called trigger point, local injection of an anesthetic agent into this area will tend to break the reflex arc and relax the tension. Similarly, if there is evidence of rupture of the muscle fibers, with hematoma formation, local injection of hyaluronidase may be of value. Physical therapeutic measures are important and should consist of application of heat locally, massage and careful active motion limited to that which is pain-free. The patient may be placed in the prone position and hot packs used in a manner similar to the use of blanket packs in acute anterior poliomyelitis. A body whirlpool, if available, may be used, although I think that application of heat is more effective when the patient is lying down. For this reason I prefer the use of diathermy, infrared rays, electric pad or electric baker.

As soon as the muscle spasm shows signs of subsiding, rehabilitative measures may be commenced but should be carried out strictly within the limits of pain. Far too often in the athlete, the urgency of his participation in athletic activity persuades the doctor or trainer to rehabilitate him too rapidly, with recurrence a discouraging aftermath. It is difficult to protect the upper dorsal spine by a corset. The lower dorsal spine may be fairly well protected by a full length corset, which the athlete should wear whenever he is participating in active competition. Adhesive strapping of the back to limit the motion involved in the activity is quite valuable. Since the strain is usually of the posterior muscles, the strapping should be applied so as to prevent forward and lateral flexion. I believe that parallel strips are very much more effective for this than criss-cross strips on the back. The back should be carefully prepared and shaved and the skin cleansed with ether before the strips are applied. One may use tincture of benzoin on the skin if one so desires. The most effective method of strapping is shown in Figure 354. Strapping so applied is much more effective in limiting motion of the back than is a corset and is of course much less expensive if it is to be worn a relatively short time. Elastic adhesive cross-stretch tape is considerably stronger than regular tape and may be substituted for it. Elastic adhesive with long-way stretch is not adequate in this instance, since its longitudinal stretch does not provide enough support. Heat can be applied right through adhesive tape. The tape is changed only when it becomes ineffective. Any adhesive that is dependent upon adherence to the skin for fixation will become ineffective if the patient perspires unduly. As the condition improves and less support is needed, one may shift to the use of long-stretch tape or a corset, but some protection of the muscles should be continued for several weeks to prevent re-injury.

The *chronic back strain* represents a major problem. It is frequently the result of an acute strain that was not adequately treated. Every recurrence of the condition makes the final cure more difficult. It is frequently cured only after the season's athletic competition is over. The best treatment is physical therapy and protection. One is quite prone to accuse a player with the condition of being "chicken" or "dogging it," since in these back strains there are few, if any, positive findings. Little is to be gained, however, by insisting on strenuous activity in the presence of a painful back unless this seems desirable to establish the diagnosis. In the chronic condition, there is usually not enough localization of pain to justify local injection. Frequently, the so-called fibrositis, which can be described as irritation of the fascial planes of the back, may be relieved by general therapy. We frequently use a combination of a muscle relaxant, salicylates and a cortisone derivative. Cortisone is well tolerated by the young athlete if the dose is small and is not continued too long. One should avoid long-continued use of any cortisone preparation. In the final analysis, since strain is basically overuse of the musculature, the ultimate relief must come from rehabilitation of the muscles. Dedication to long-continued rehabilitative exercises should pay dividends in diminishing and in finally eliminating the strain (see page 682).

Sprain

Many of the statements made previously about strain may also be applied to sprain. In the spine it may be difficult to distinguish between the two. The same force that causes muscular strain may tear some of the many ligaments of the spine. Many of these ligaments are deeply placed, such as those around the articular processes and between the lateral processes and those extending between the lamina and vertebrae. About the only ligament that can be palpated easily in the dorsal spine is the supraspinous, which extends along the tips of the spinous processes. Injury to this ligament can be determined by localized palpable tenderness either along the course of the ligament itself or at its attachment to the bone. Extension of the spine should be pain-free, but forward flexion will cause pain at the involved area if the supra- or interspinous or interlaminal ligaments are involved.

The direction of the motion that causes pain is the key to diagnosis of spinal ligament injuries. Given *right side* involvement, with damage to the capsular ligament, one would expect the local tenderness and spasm to be on the right side in an effort to prevent stretching of this involved ligament. Forward flexion, either active or passive, is painful. Backward flexion, either active or passive, is not. Homolateral flexion should relieve the symptoms and, indeed, the patient will stand pulled toward the injured side. Contralateral flexion will increase the pain unless it is prevented by the spastic muscle. X-rays are of little importance in the diagnosis of sprain, although x-ray examination should be carried out in a serious injury, if possible, in order to rule out bone damage. The one condition in which x-rays may be valuable is in aiding in the diagnosis of rupture of the supra- and interspinous ligaments. In this instance, as noted earlier, the tenderness will be right on the ligament. Sometimes a palpable defect may be felt. If the tear is complete, forward flexion may reveal greater separation of the affected spinous process than of the ones above and below. This is an extremely unusual injury in the dorsal spine.

Treatment of a ligament injury of the dorsal spine is the same as that of ligament injury elsewhere, that is, protection of the ligament

Figure 354. Six to eight strips of heavy 3 in. tape are cut long enough to extend from the base of the neck to the pelvis. The first strip is placed parallel with the spinous processes and just adjacent to them. A strip is placed on either side of the spine. It is anchored below by a circular strip placed just at the level of the trochanters and extending entirely around the trunk. The pubic hair is protected by a cotton pad. Transverse strips should be overlapped. It is important to get the first strip low enough to protect the inguinal canal. The second pair of vertical strips is then applied overlapping the first by one-half. The second horizontal strip is applied overlapping about one-third. This is continued until the strapping extends 4 to 6 in. on either side of the spine. This requires three or four pairs of vertical strips. It is not necessary to use cross-lap strips above. Cross-stretch elastic tape is good here. Long-stretch elastic tape is useless!

against stretch until it is healed. A period of bed rest may be necessary if the injury is severe. The back should then be strapped in a way to prevent the motion that causes the pain (Fig. 354). This is a good test of the effectiveness of the strapping. One should be extremely careful not to discard the protection too soon since recurrence is as likely in the spine as it is in the ankle or knee when the injury occurs in the latter.

Dislocation

The ultimate sprain is dislocation (Fig. 355). This is extremely unusual in the dorsal spine. Even in the mayhem caused by the modern automobile, the dorsal spine is infrequently dislocated. As mentioned in the discussion of the anatomy of the spine, the vertebrae are very securely bound together and have a good

Figure 355. *A,* Fracture-dislocation of D-12 on L-1. Note backward displacement of L-1 and complete dislocation of the articular facet. *B,* Reduced and held with wire around spinous processes and spinal fusion. Neurological symptoms in lower extremities completely disappeared. *C,* Fracture-dislocation of D-11 on D-12. Paraplegia. *D,* Postoperative film showing internal fixation and graft. *E,* Complete dislocation of D-11 on D-12, without apparent fracture which resulted in complete paraplegia.

deal of bony as well as ligamentous stability. If there is dislocation, the injury will obviously be a major one. I do not comprehend the so-called "dislocation" of the "manipulators," who will make an x-ray film and glibly describe a dislocation in a normal-appearing spine. Following manipulation, this "dislocation" is reduced. Anatomically and physiologically such a thing is virtually impossible in the dorsal spine.

Fracture

Fracture of the dorsal spine is more common than dislocation but rarely occurs in ordinary athletic competition, such as football, basketball, baseball and track. On the other hand, it occurs more frequently in some of the more violent sports, such as automobile racing, polo playing and the like. The fracture may be of the body or of the arches or of the spinous or lateral processes.

Compression Fracture of the Vertebral Body

Fracture of the body of the vertebra is usually caused by sharp forward flexion, the so-called compression fracture (Fig. 356). The patient will give a history of sharp forward flexion such as falling violently on the buttocks or of having his head forcibly pushed between his knees. This tends to flex the very rigid dorsal spine; the posterior ligaments hold, and the force is taken by the anterior portion of the body of the vertebra. This cancellous bone gives way to a greater or lesser degree. The

anterosuperior corner of the vertebra may be broken off, or more commonly there is compression of the vertebra, so that the cancellous bone is impacted into itself.

There is nothing about the ordinary compression fracture of the dorsal spine that will prevent ambulation and therefore, the patient may actually be up and around in spite of his back complaint. On examination, although it may be difficult to determine the exact degree of injury, forward flexion will ordinarily cause considerable complaint. This may be elicited by having the patient lie supine. When the examiner flexes the patient's neck to force the chin against the chest, there will usually be localized pain at the fracture area. The results of this test will also be positive for ligament injury. Motion in any direction will probably cause pain, even in an impacted fracture.

Careful x-ray study will usually reveal this lesion, although it may be easily overlooked if the deformity is mild and the x-ray film inadequate or inadequately studied. In the x-ray the vertebrae should be carefully measured anteriorly to determine whether a single vertebrae is narrower than its fellows. This may be extremely misleading, however, since frequently one or more dorsal vertebrae will be of smaller size than the others. Of more importance is the appearance of the bone itself. A fracture line may be visible. The bone may be compacted, so that this particular vertebra not only appears smaller but seems more dense than its neighbor.

Treatment. In the young athlete if the compression is definite and amounts to as much as 25 per cent of the height of the body

Figure 356. A spinal injury with compression of D-9. The patient suffered persistent localized pain. *B*, Careful study of D-9 reveals unilateral compression on the right. This can also be seen in the lateral view (*A*). Note that the superior surface of D-9 presents two cortical shadows, whereas the inferior surface shows a single shadow.

Figure 357. *A*, Severe compression fracture of L-1, preoperative view. *B*, Correction by the jack method. The "X" marks the head of the jack, which actually is one vertebra above L-1. These x-rays were made with a surgical portable machine without a Bucky diaphragm, which accounts for their fogginess.

of the vertebrae, I think an attempt should be made to reduce it. In the older person this amount of compression may be accepted in order to speed up healing, but I do not believe this is acceptable in the youngster. The exact area involved is determined, and an effort is made to correct the vertebra by manipulation. This will not correct with the use of a simple convex bed if the bone is impacted. The usual methods of hyperextension in which the entire back is extended are needlessly handicapping to the patient, since the extension must proceed to the point where all of the anterior ligaments are taut before there is any effect at all upon the broken vertebra. Local hyperextension is much more effective.

For local hyperextension, I think the various modifications of the "jack method" are by far the best. In this method, with the patient supine on a suitable fracture table, the jack, with suitable protective cap, is placed directly under the spinous process of the vertebra involved. By elevating the jack, the corrective pressure is applied to this vertebra alone and the back is locally extended (Fig. 357). This causes some local hyperextension of the adjacent vertebrae, but it is not necessary to hyperextend the entire spine. Once the vertebra has come up to its normal height, a suitable plaster jacket can be applied, again without generalized hyperextension but with local extension, the pressure points being the pubis and sternum in front and the fracture site behind.

It is very difficult to keep athletic patients at bed rest, even though this treatment probably offers the best chance of maintaining the

degree of correction obtained by manipulation. If the cast is applied with great care and if the spine is extended enough to place the entire weight on the articular processes, little is to be gained by enforced recumbency.

In any event there may be some loss of correction—a fact that prompts some surgeons to believe that no attempt should be made to correct a compression fracture. The cast should be worn for six to eight weeks, to be followed by an adequate brace. In unusual circumstances, a brace of the three-point hyperextension type, with pressure on the pubis and sternum and over the involved vertebra posteriorly, may be substituted for the cast. X-ray examination will determine when union is complete, but athletic competition should not be permitted for at least four months and probably six would be better. There is some danger of late aseptic necrosis of this vertebra if weight-bearing is permitted too soon.

In minimal compression fractures of the vertebral body, rehabilitation can be much more rapidly carried out if the compression deformity is accepted. In these cases a protective brace needs to be worn only a few weeks until the fracture is well consolidated. In fracture of the anterosuperior corner of the vertebra, a differentiation should, if possible, be made between a snubbing fracture caused by flexion and an avulsion fracture caused by hyperextension, since in the latter, protection should be with the spine in flexion rather than in extension. Often the history of the injury will provide a valuable guide as to the diagnosis. The increased pain on backward bending as compared with that on forward bending will also be significant. Sometimes the x-ray film taken on backward bending will show actual separation of this fragment.

Arch Fracture

Fracture of the lateral processes of the dorsal spine is extremely infrequent, since they are well protected by the ribs. If it does occur, a corset, brace or body jacket may be worn until union has taken place. Fractures of the laminae or interarticular portions of the bone or of the articular processes themselves require very careful examination using x-rays to aid in the diagnosis. Adequate support by brace or cast should be worn for six to eight weeks to prevent painful excessive formation of callus or nonunion. In fracture of the spinous process, protection should be against forward flexion. If there is separation of the fragment, rather than waiting for nonunion and then removing the fragment if there is resultant pain, the fragment should be removed early (Fig. 358) as a primary procedure. This will result in a shorter period of disability. Separation is much more frequent in the upper dorsal spine and may be the result of avulsion of the tip by sharp forward flexion of the neck and upper spine or by a direct blow. It is occasionally caused by muscle jerk, the so-called "clay shoveler's fracture". The "clay shoveler's fracture" is caused by the jerk on the handle of the shovel when the worker forcibly tries to throw the dirt off of it. When the wet clay sticks to the shovel, this jerks the handle of the shovel and may cause avulsion of a fragment of the spinous process.

LUMBAR SPINE

Anatomical Considerations

Whereas the dorsal vertebrae have a good deal of inherent stability as indicated earlier, the lumbar spine (Fig. 359), lying between the rigid pelvis and the thorax, is so designed as to permit greater mobility and yet provide inherent stability. The vertebrae in this area are massive. The convexity of the front part of this area of the spine is caused by vertebral bodies which are taller and slightly wider in front than behind. The entire arch is massive, with heavy lateral processes extending well away from the midline to add additional leverage for muscle attachments. The laminae are heavy. The articular processes, which in the dorsal spine angulate to form a diagonal line with the body, in the lumbar spine are much more in the sagittal plane. Although the processes on the vertebrae above do lock behind the one below, they are at a much flatter angle. Hence, the mobility in the spine is largely in flexion and in extension, in which the intervertebral joints serve more or less as an axis, with motion permitted by compression and expansion of the discs and by separation and apposition of the spinous processes. There is little rotatory motion in the lumbar spine.

The muscles of this area of the back (Fig. 360) are very massive. The sacrospinalis group interdigitating up into the dorsal spine consists of heavy muscles arising from the pelvis to attach to the spinous processes and to the vertebral bodies. These muscles act as firm stabilizers of the trunk over the pelvis. The

Figure 358. "Sprain" of the upper dorsal spine, with persistent complaint. Early x-ray studies had not adequately visualized this area. More careful x-ray technique revealed the ununited fragments of the D-1 and 2 spinous processes. Uneventful recovery followed removal of the fragments, but months of disability might have been prevented by more careful early treatment.

Figure 359. Skeletal view from the front and from behind. In both figures, certain of the ligaments of the trunk and extremities are shown. (From Anson, Atlas of Human Anatomy.)

Rectus capitis posterior
minor

Rectus capitis posterior
major

Obliquus capitis superior

Splenius capitis

Obliquus capitis inferior

Semispinalis cervicis

Semispinalis capitis

Splenius cervicis

Longissimus capitis

C 7

Iliocostalis cervicis

Longissimus cervicis

Longissimus cervicis

Iliocostalis cervicis
and thoracis

Iliocostalis thoracis

T 6

Spinalis thoracis

Semispinalis
thoracis

Longissimus thoracis

Iliocostalis lumborum

L 1

Multifidus

Erector spinae

Figure 360. The chief muscles of the back (From Hollinshead, Functional Anatomy of the Limbs and Back.)

muscles of the abdomen complete the stabilizing effect in front. These muscles extending from the pubis to the ribs serve as anterior guy wires to provide active forward flexion and to prevent overextension. The heavy mass of spinal muscle also serves to protect the posterior portion of the abdominal cavity and prevent injury to the kidneys, spleen and liver.

Contusion

This area of the spine is frequently contused, but fortunately the injury is usually not particularly severe. The only subcutaneous bones in this region are the tips of the spinous processes. These lie in a sulcus between the two erector spinae muscles, so that the muscle ordinarily will absorb a blow unless it is by a relatively small object. Contusion of the muscle results in the same complications as contusion of muscle anywhere. The history is of a blow, with localized tenderness at the area of the blow, and moderate pain on function. After a few hours, muscle spasm supervenes, which tightens up the whole group of muscles on that side, apparently in an attempt to prevent painful motion. At this time, differentiation from strain may be very difficult. In a simple contusion, active muscle contraction is not especially painful.

If any *treatment* is necessary, application of ice followed by heat is indicated. If a massive hematoma appears to be present, an attempt can be made to aspirate it, although the location is difficult to determine in these heavy muscles. If the contusion seems to be severe, attention should be paid to the underlying structures to determine the possibility of a fracture of the lateral or spinous processes.

Strain

Muscular strain results either from overstretching or from overuse of the muscle. It may be difficult to distinguish from sprain. Fundamentally, any active motion of the. involved muscle against resistance will cause pain. For example, if you have the patient stand erect and ask him to bend sideways and you resist this motion so that he does not actually bend, he should have pain if the involvement is in the muscle but no pain if the involvement is in the ligament. The muscle involved is palpably tender, and passive stretching of the muscle will cause pain. If the strain is on the right side of the spine, active flexion to the right against resistance will be painful, whereas in ligament injury it should not be. Passive flexion to the opposite side will be painful as soon as the injured muscle is put under stretch. Backward bending against resistance will be painful, and forward flexion will become painful only when the excursion is sufficient to stretch the muscle.

The *treatment* of the acute strain is quite similar to that of sprain; that is, rest, protection and application of heat locally. Protection is necessary against active use of the muscle rather than against excessive motion. The former is a good deal more difficult to accomplish. The patient should be instructed not to make any movements causing pain. If the area can be treated promptly and adequately, recovery will be rapid.

Unfortunately this condition is often inadequately treated, and chronic strain supervenes with all of its implications. The only cure for chronic strain is prolonged rest until recovery is complete, after which gradual rehabilitation of the muscle can be carried out. If rehabilitation is too rapid, the pain will recur. If athletic participation is begun during the recovery period, a single excessive motion may start the whole cycle over again. Localized trigger areas in the muscle may be present and, if so, injection of long-acting anesthetic, along with injection of a corticoid preparation into this area, will be of benefit. This treatment is of little value in the case of diffuse muscle involvement, however. Muscle relaxants are useful, particularly in conjunction with physical therapy. Rehabilitation must be gradual, persistent and within the limits of pain.

The actual protection of the back can be accomplished first by bed rest, later by a cast or brace and finally by taping (see Fig. 354). It is important to bear in mind, however, that taping is not as effective in strain as it is in sprain because whereas taping protects against overstretching of the muscle, it will not protect against muscle contraction.

A chronic strain tends to recur and can be extremely troublesome to the athlete. In many cases I advise the use of a lumbosacral corset to help support the back and protect against overstretching—the same measure that is used in a case of chronic sprain. This is more effective than adhesive tape, since repeated applications of tape tend to irritate the skin. The corset should extend well up over the lower ribs, particularly posteriorly, and well down on the sacrum if it is to provide much protection (Fig. 361).

Figure 361. The lumbosacral corset.

Rehabilitation

As indicated in the section on the dorsal spine, rehabilitation is extremely important, both for complete recovery from strain and for prevention of recurrence. Proper exercises faithfully continued for many months may well prevent the recurrence of the strain, since strain is, indeed, the result of using a muscle beyond its capacity. Hence, the greater the capacity of a muscle, the less likely it is that it will be strained. (See page 682.)

Sprain

Sprain is frequent in the mobile lumbar spine, which has many ligaments giving support to the various joints. The supraspinous ligament, which extends along the tips of the spinous processes, is particularly susceptible. Sprain of the supraspinous ligament can be diagnosed by tenderness over it or over the tip of the spinous process where the ligament attaches. Active contraction of the muscle to pull the spine into hyperextension is pain-free, as is passive extension. Active flexion of the back, as in attempting to sit up from the supine position, is pain-free until tension is put on the process by forcing the head toward the knees. Passive hyperflexion of the spine will cause pain. This condition is treated by protection against overflexion by strapping. Activity can be permitted so long as the ligament is protected. Occasionally the ligament will be pulled in two or will be avulsed from the bone, and more extensive treatment will be indicated. In this instance, immobilization in extension in a brace or in a plaster jacket is in order. If the fragment of the spinous process does not unite, it may be removed. Primary early repair of the ligament would be advisable, but so infre-

quently is the condition diagnosed in the early stage that this is seldom practical.

Injury to the other ligaments of the back is much more difficult to determine with exactitude. The interspinous ligament is not frequently damaged because it has elastic fibers and is not readily overstretched. However, the articular ligaments around the apophyseal joints are frequently damaged, as in the anterior spinal ligament or the lateral spinal ligaments. Whether or not the ligamentum flavum is damaged by hyperflexion is problematical, since it, too, is an elastic structure and probably will allow as much motion without damage as the range of flexion of the back will permit. Diagnosis of these sprains is on the basis of tests that bring stress upon certain areas. In the diagnosis of sprain, it should be remembered that passive movements which put stress on the involved ligament will cause pain. For example, sprain of the capsule on the left will cause pain on flexion to the right or on flexion forward.

Treatment of the acute sprain is to place the ligament at complete rest. Unfortunately this is not often done, and a chronic sprain ensues. In the acute sprain, muscle spasm is a characteristic symptom. Ideally the patient should be put at bed rest and treatment should include the use of muscle relaxants and the application of inductive heat or an electric pad until the acute symptoms subside. At this time the area should be protected by elastic strapping or corset until the ligament is healed, and athletics should not be permitted. A sprain is easier to protect than a strain, since if the range of motion is limited, there is no stress on the ligament. For this reason, competition can be allowed much earlier in a sprain of the back than in a strain.

Dislocation-Subluxation

Sprain of the lumbar spine rarely leads to actual dislocation. There may be subluxation, which occurs when the interspinous ligament tears and the articular processes tend to disengage. If this is spontaneously relieved, it should be treated as a sprain. Unilateral dislocation in the lumbar spine is extremely rare and is not a common athletic injury. A frank dislocation of the lumbar spine occurs only after severe violence, such as a fall from a height or a motor accident. This is a serious injury. X-rays will reveal the deformity (Fig. 362), and in most cases, open reduction will

Figure 362. *A*, Complete dislocation of L-2 and L-3. This was treated by open reduction and graft. There were no permanent neurological sequelae. This is possible in spite of the intact lamina because the medullary portion of the cord stops just above this level, and the cauda will tolerate much more trauma than will the spinal cord. *B*, Results six months later. The distortion of the body of L-3 may well be due to damage of the epiphysis, since the original film does not show any compression here.

be required. This type of dislocation may cause severe neurological deficit. However, it is not as damaging in the lumbar spine as it is higher up because the cord proper does not extend into the lumbar area and so is not primarily involved. The peripheral nerves in the cauda will stand a great deal more trauma than will the substance of the cord.

Fracture

Fracture may occur in the body of a lumbar vertebra, in a lateral or spinous process or in some portion of the arch.

Fracture of the Body of the Vertebra

Fracture of the body of the vertebra (Fig. 363) is extremely rare as an athletic injury. It is a major injury and is readily recognized as such. X-ray examination will reveal the deformity, and anything beyond minimal deformity should be reduced as indicated previously in the section on the dorsal spine. Failure to correct the compression may result in disability (Fig. 364). Athletic competition will be limited for many months.

Fracture of the Lateral Process

Fracture of the lateral processes is quite common in athletes. It should be noted that the lumbar vertebrae have spikelike lateral processes, some of which are quite thin or have a narrow neck. These processes are ruptured by two different mechanisms—a contusion, as a complication of a direct blow, or violent exertion of the muscle—or by a combination of the two. There is a difference of opinion as to the relative frequency of the two causes, since the combination of a blow and exertion often occur simultaneously. However, I think it is quite possible that a direct blow will account for the breaking off of a single lateral process. Fractures of multiple processes are almost always of the avulsion type (Fig. 365). In any event, the significant aspect of the fracture is not the broken bone but the muscle injury. The distal fragment frequently separates quite widely, and nonunion is often the result. The patient reports a history of a blow on the back by the knee or foot, usually at the time of violent exercise during play. This causes immediate pain in the back, which may be quite severe or may be relatively minor. If participation continues, the pain increases and the muscles become more spastic. The player's

Figure 363. *A,* Severe compression fracture of L-4 following violent jack-knifing. *B,* Eight months later, note complete restoration of vertebral height by "jack" decompression.

A   B

Figure 364. *A,* Relatively mild compression fracture of the superior portion of the body of L-1 at eight weeks post-injury. *B,* Note persistent deformity following failure to correct compression. This relatively mild fracture has comparatively severe residual, whereas the very severe fracture in Figure 363 is pain-free.

Figure 365. Fractures of transverse processes of the left second and third lumbar vertebrae.

body will be pulled toward the affected side. This is more noticeable after a period of rest and then re-initiation of activity. There is localized tenderness over the area of injury. Stretching of the involved side by contralateral bending causes pain. Homolateral bending against resistance also is painful, as are passive forward flexion and active backward flexion.

Treatment depends almost entirely upon the symptoms present. If the patient is having severe pain and is seriously disabled, he should be placed at bed rest, with application of cold, followed by heat. In two or three days when the most acute symptoms have subsided (immediately if the primary symptoms are not too severe), some support should be applied to the back. Here again there is a great difference of opinion as to just what the nature of this support should be. I think this depends entirely upon the symptoms. If the patient is having severe pain and marked muscle spasm, a lightweight body jacket will give him good protection. He can wear this from ten days to two weeks and then substitute a corset. If the symptoms are not too severe, the back may be strapped or a corset applied, which limits the activity somewhat and gives some degree of support, although not as adequately as the cast. Ordinarily the symptoms will subside within three to six weeks. Infrequently in cases of nonunion, there will be persistent pain to the point that removal of the fragment becomes necessary.

The player may be allowed to participate in sports just as soon as the back does not hurt.

The pain level is a good indication for continuing or discontinuing the treatment. After recovery, there is no need for any restriction of activity, even if nonunion of one or more processes is persistent.

Fracture of the Spinous Process

Fracture of the spinous process in the lumbar spine occurs from three different causes: (1) Sharp hyperflexion that pulls off the tip of the process; (2) sharp hyperextension that impinges one process against the other and breaks one or the other, and (3) a direct blow that mechanically knocks off one of the projecting processes. The condition may ordinarily be diagnosed clinically by the sharp localization of pain and occasionally by the unstable spinous process. It can be confirmed by x-rays done with a technique to visualize the spinous processes (Fig. 366). If there is actual separation of the fragment in the distal 1 in. of the process, a great deal of time and trouble will be saved by removing this fragment, since it will be very slow to heal and the condition will likely terminate with pain on violent exertion. If the fracture is near the base of the process or in the arch, it will heal much more rapidly and completely, provided that the spine is immobilized in extension, preferably by a plaster cast. Athletic competition is forbidden until healing is complete.

Arch Fracture

Any fracture involving the arch of the vertebra is potentially serious because of the danger of neurological involvement. The fracture

Figure 366. Avulsion fracture of the inferior border of the spinous process of the third lumbar vertebra.

may be between the articular processes (Fig. 367). It may be through the arch at the base of the process. It may actually be of the articular process. In any event, once the fracture is recognized, the patient must be immobilized to permit it to heal, since painful function may result if union is imperfect. This is a serious injury and should be treated as such. Athletic competition is forbidden until healing is complete.

NONTRAUMATIC DEFORMITIES OF THE SPINE

Kyphosis Dorsalis Juvenilis (Scheuermann's Disease)

This condition is essentially a disturbance of the growth of the vertebrae. It is often quite extensive, as evidenced by the wedging of many dorsal vertebrae, with osteochondrosis of the bodies, which often goes on to fragmentation (Figs. 368 and 369). Occasionally only a single vertebra or adjacent ones may be involved, and this may cause some confusion in the early stages. There is usually no particular problem in diagnosis. There is no evidence that this condition is actually caused by a single injury. However, it seems quite apparent that malformation of the vertebrae is definitely increased by active or passive forward flexion and by exercise.

Figure 367. Vertical fracture through the lamina and articular process of L-5, visualized only on this right oblique view.

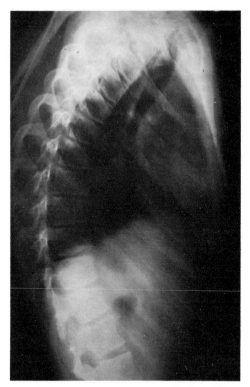

Figure 368. Generalized dorsalis juvenilis epiphysitis. Note wedging of all the dorsal and lumbar vertebrae.

The patient should be protected by a hyperextension brace to place the weight back on the arches and articular processes and to take it off the defective portion of the anterior body. The problem will be with that person who wants to continue athletic competition. Certainly in the active stage of this condition, athletics should be banned. As the replacement phase of the condition develops, as evidenced by improved density of the vertebrae, coalescence of the fragmented areas and absence of pain, the patient may be allowed to participate, although he should wear protection against flexion until the bodies are completely reconstituted. I recall one young man who was an ardent baseball player. Toward the end of the course of the involvement, we permitted him to play baseball in a body jacket. He was a catcher and used the cast for a chest protector, much to the detriment of the cast but apparently with no bad results to his back (see Fig. 369). These cases resemble Perthes' disease in that they cause very little discomfort and yet may give rise to marked deformity (Fig. 370). Patients with this disease are in a slightly older age group (12 to 15 years) than those with Perthes' disease, and *limiting* activity at this age may be extremely difficult when a patient is not actually having

Figure 369. Localized vertebral epiphysitis involving D-12, L-1 and 2. Note characteristic deformity, with interference of growth. *A,* The extreme involvement between L-1 and 2 may lead to erroneous diagnosis. *B,* Healing six months later. *C,* Final result six years later shows amazing restoration of architecture, with only minimal kyphosis due almost entirely to the wedging of L-3. This boy had prolonged protection against anterior weight-bearing, which I think was the prime factor in his good recovery.

many symptoms. Nevertheless it should be done.

Of more difficulty diagnostically is the localized manifestation of the same condition in which one or two or three of the vertebrae may be involved, with quite major changes, and yet be essentially pain-free, until an injury calls attention to this area or until the area becomes spontaneously painful. It may be that the injury is entirely coincidental. It should not be confused with an acute fracture. Adequate x-rays will help to differentiate the two. Here again it is necessary to reduce the patient's activity and by serial x-rays determine when the bone is repaired sufficiently to permit the stresses of athletic competition.

One does not add to one's popularity by refusing permission to these young men to participate in sports. Nevertheless a firm stand is vital, particularly if there is any major involvement, since increasing deformity may result in a persistent gibbus.

Congenital Deformities

Congenital deformities are much more common in the lower back than in the upper, specifically about the fourth and fifth lumbar and the first sacral vertebrae. These deformities are not caused by athletic injuries. However, they often become a problem to the athlete, since when recognized following an injury, a decision must immediately be made on the advisability of his continuing in athletics and, indeed, on the treatment of the acute condition. The great majority of these conditions do not affect the function of the spine enough to require restriction of activity.

Spina Bifida Occulta

The most common of these deformities is spina bifida occulta, in which there is failure of fusion of the arch of one or more of the vertebrae posteriorly (Fig. 371). This is a common finding and is ordinarily of no significance. The player should not be alarmed or be told

Figure 370. Untreated dorsal epiphysitis of only moderate severity, but note extreme deformity.

Figure 371. Spina bifida occulta in the first sacral vertebra. This is asymptomatic and of no significance.

that he has a dangerous condition of the lower back or that he should be careful the rest of his life. Exceptionally, a wide open spina bifida involving several vertebrae may be of sufficient concern to require the use of additional support or even the recommendation that some less strenuous activity be followed. A well-

placed sacral pad may provide some protection.

Spondylolysis or Spondylolisthesis

Spondylolysis (Fig. 372) is the failure of fusion of the arch of the vertebra, usually between the articular processes. Spondylolisthesis (Fig. 373) is spondylolysis in which there is displacement of the superior vertebra forward on the one below. This laminal defect does indeed cause weakness of the spine but to an extremely variable degree. Many people have spondylolysis or spondylolisthesis all their lives and never know it. However, if the athlete is having trouble in the lower back and spondylolysis is discovered, one may be justified in restricting him to some of the less active sports. Athletics basically should not cause serious damage to the spine, but the player probably will have discomfort to the point that he will not be very effective. After the pain is relieved, he should be advised to wear a lumbosacral support or sacroiliac belt during periods of active competition.

In actual spondylolisthesis there is separation at the line of defect, and here again it may be difficult to decide on the proper procedure. If there is sufficient pain, one should seriously consider treating the condition rather

Figure 372. Asymptomatic spondylolysis. Note (arrow) arch defect in the lamina of L-5 but no slipping. No present symptoms.

Figure 373. Spondylolisthesis. Note *A*, Grade I. Again the arch defect in L-5, with mild forward displacement of L-5 on S-1. Backache but no gross disability. *B*, Grade II. Note more forward slipping between L-4 and L-5, with collapse of the intervertebral disc. Definite symptomatic back with restriction of motion, muscle spasm and curtailment of activities. *C*, Grade III. More extensive slipping combined with a wide separation at the arch defect and degenerative changes of the disc. Grossly symptomatic. *D*, Grade IV. Vertebra slipped forward over halfway. Severe disability.

than forbidding athletics. However, if the pain occurs only on violent exercise, such as football, I think one is justified in discontinuing the football to see how the patient gets along with his condition. If he continues to have pain, treatment should be recommended. The person of 14 or 15 years of age with spondylolisthesis who is already having pain in the back almost inevitably will come to treatment at a later time in spite of any recommendation that he decrease his activities, since degenerative changes will certainly occur as the years pass. It is quite unlikely that he will become pain-free as he gets older. In such a case, one cannot assume that the simple banning of athletic competition will mean that the person is inactive. If he is an active, energetic type he will occupy himself with an equally strenuous occupation. If he is the indolent type, one questions the advisability of encouraging further indolence to protect a condition that might be remedied surgically.

Variations in Sacral Fusion

As has been noted previously, the sacrum originally is made up of five bones, which fuse into a solid mass during adolescence. Various anomalous conditions may arise as a part of this process. The lower lumbar vertebra may participate to some extent in the sacral fusion and, indeed, may completely fuse so that there is *sacralization of the fifth lumbar vertebra*

(Figs. 374 and 375). This is of no significance activity-wise. If the fusion is incomplete, with one side fusing and the other not, some imbalance may arise in the lower back, and occasionally pain will be present. The same can be said here as was said of spondylolisthesis, namely, that a person having pain in his early teens will inevitably have pain when he becomes older. One should therefore proceed to complete the fusion, after which unlimited activity can be permitted. A symptomfree unilateral sacralization is of no significance—and most of the cases are symptomfree. The same is true of *lumbarization of the first sacral vertebra*. If a portion of the sacrum fails to fuse, this is of no significance. Certainly the fibrous fusion is extremely firm and highly unlikely to be damaged by any type of athletic competition. I would not recommend the wearing of a belt or brace or other support. On the other hand, a sprain of the back in which there is a congenital anomaly may be somewhat more resistant to treatment than uncomplicated sprain, and protection should be given, not for the congenital anomaly but for the accompanying sprain.

Other Anomalies

Other conditions, such as hemivertebrae (Fig. 376), scoliosis (Fig. 377), kyphosis (Fig. 378) and increased lordosis (Fig. 379), must be managed on an individual basis. In many

Figure 374. Unilateral sacralization of the fifth lumbar vertebra. *A,* Note the massive formation of the sacral ala on the left side, with the relatively normal transverse process on the right. *B,* Lateral view showing the very narrow disc space and the massive arches.

Figure 375. Complete sacralization of L-5.

Figure 376. Hemivertebra of the lumbar spine (L-2).

Figure 377. *A,* Moderate scoliosis, asymptomatic. *B,* This asymptomatic scoliosis was found incidentally in a college athlete who had ruptured his cartilage while playing varsity football.

Figure 378. Moderate dorsal kyphosis, probably from asymptomatic mild dorsal epiphysitis, although it may be postural.

Figure 379. Typical adolescent lordosis in a 9 year old boy. The vertebral epiphyses have not yet ossified, but these vertebrae are normal for this age. Note that the separate pieces of the sacrum have not yet fused. This condition presents no contraindication to athletics. On the contrary, physical fitness should be encouraged.

disc is the pad lying between the two vertebrae. The periphery of the pad, the so-called annulus fibrosus, is the firm ligamentous and cartilaginous structure that forms a ring, within which is enclosed the softer nucleus pulposus. This arrangement acts as a hydraulic shock absorber between the bodies of the vertebrae. Infrequently the annulus may be subject to damage by excessive motion. Compression of the two vertebrae, forcing the bones together, puts pressure on the inner mass and causes it to bulge, so, theoretically, the disc could rupture. However, the normal annulus is so strong that excessive pressure in a single violent effort usually will break the disc into the body of the vertebra or will compress the vertebra rather than rupture the annulus.

Classic ruptured disc has its origin in a degenerative annulus. The disc commonly ruptures posteriorly, owing to the lordosis of the lumbar spine, which causes eccentric weight-bearing with an inordinate amount of weight placed on the back margin of the disc. It is probable that pressure on the disc causes it to rupture or herniate through an already defective area of the annulus. This pressure may be caused by anything that raises the pressure within the disc, such as leaning forward to tie the shoe, but is more likely to be caused by lifting—and particularly by lifting in a rather strained position, requiring the same sort of effort that would cause muscular strain. The athlete is not in the common age bracket for ruptured disc. In addition, his splendid muscular condition takes a good deal of strain off the disc itself.

The classic symptoms will not be reiterated here. One should suspect disc involvement in an injury in which the pain follows the root distribution in the leg and is increased by coughing or sneezing or by raising interspinal pressure by pressure on the jugular veins. The difficult case will be the mild one in which there are few nerve root signs. There is some stiffness in the back but not at a disabling level. Shall this patient be allowed to participate in sports? I think that each case must be viewed individually and some balance struck between the urgency for participation and the danger of it. If athletic competition will accentuate the patient's discomfort, he probably will require definitive treatment anyway, so he is probably doing himself no major harm by participating. Whether or not he is effective is a wholly different thing. Thus, although a ruptured disc must be considered in many conditions of the back, it is not really a major problem in the treatment of athletes.

conditions, such as extreme lordosis, athletic competition may be valuable from the standpoint of posture. It must be accompanied by instruction in the treatment of the primary condition. The patients must be judged symptomatically. The deformity itself is not necessarily disabling if it is not accompanied by signs of secondary involvement, such as nerve root pressure and muscle contracture. There is no justification for making a chronic invalid out of a patient because of an x-ray diagnosis of a spinal anomaly.

SPINAL DISC LESIONS

In recent years the diagnosis of disc rupture with attendant nerve root injury has been increasing in frequency and consequently must be considered in the treatment of athletes. In my experience this condition has rarely resulted from athletic participation. However, once a ruptured disc is present, it tends to be recurrent, and strenuous athletics should be banned until the condition is corrected. The

Injuries of the Pelvis and Hip

16

It is convenient to include the pelvis and hip under a single heading, since these areas are closely related anatomically.

ANATOMICAL CONSIDERATIONS

The pelvis is a uniquely devised mechanism designed to transfer the body weight from the single weight-bearing axis of the trunk to the bipolar weight-bearing lower extremities (see Fig. 359). It is designed to have a whippletree effect. Thus, the spine attaches to the pelvis by a single connection to the sacrum and for stability is anchored in all four directions by various combinations of ligaments and muscles. Through the bony ring of the pelvis the weight is transferred from the spinal column to the two lower extremities, so that of necessity the pelvic ring must be intact in order to give stability. The primary function of the pelvis, including the bones, joints, ligaments and muscles, is this mechanical transfer of weight. A secondary function of the bony pelvis is protection of the pelvic viscera. Enclosed within the pelvis are the bladder, the female genitalia, the rectum and the great vessels and nerves extending to the lower extremities.

At the lumbosacral level the spinal muscles descend to attach to the sacrum and the wings of the ilia. The hip joint is an extremely stable ball-and-socket joint—stable, that is, from the standpoint of dislocation. However, by virtue of the fact that it is a ball and socket, there is no bony restriction of motion in the hip as there is in other joints. The functional stability of the hip depends entirely upon the musculature about the hip. The strong capsule and capsular ligaments maintain the ball within the socket, but the stability of the thigh in relation to the pelvis and hence to the trunk is entirely controlled by muscle. There is no stable posi-

tion in the flail hip as there is, for example, in the flail knee. The knee can be locked in extension by the stabilizing effect of the posterior capsule and collateral ligaments, with no muscle action involved. Not so the hip. To effect stability the hip is surrounded by a great mass of muscle which must be adequate to support the trunk in the erect position and, indeed, in many other positions. The muscles must also serve to propel the trunk by action of the lower extremities and to give powerful impetus to the lower extremities in relation to the trunk, as in kicking.

The various muscles have wholly different effects as the relative position of the trunk and lower extremities is altered. Careful analysis of the types of forces involved will often give a valuable lead as to the injury to be expected.

CONTUSION

Contusions about the pelvis may be of almost any kind or degree, since in some areas the pelvic bone is subcutaneous and in other areas it is surrounded by masses of muscle. Contusions in general should be managed as are contusions anywhere, depending upon the degree of injury. The local area may be injected with a long-acting anesthetic agent plus hyaluronidase. Application of a compression bandage and cold compresses in the early stage, followed by heat, is useful. Protection against re-injury is by contact pads rather than by strapping.

Muscular contusion frequently involves the buttock and, if severe enough, may be quite disabling for a period. In a severe contusion with major local symptoms, careful investigation should be made for a possible fracture of the underlying bone. The contusion may result in a deep-seated hematoma, which is virtually impossible to diagnose in the early stages. It is not common for a hematoma in the pelvic muscles to lead to myositis ossificans. Occasionally a contusion of the tuberosity of the ischium will cause an ischial bursitis or an ischial periostitis, leading to actual spur formation. Of major importance in contusion is the ruling out of a more serious injury. Subcutaneous hematoma along the crest of the ilium may cause extreme tenderness and require protective padding all season. It can be distinguished from deeper injury in that functional movement of the muscles attached to the iliac crest does not cause increased pain.

Because the types of injury to the pelvis vary greatly, depending upon the anatomical structure of the area involved, they will be discussed on a regional basis.

INJURIES IN THE VICINITY OF THE ILIAC CREST

Contusion and Strain

An area of the pelvis that is particularly susceptible to injury is the iliac crest. This area extends from the anterosuperior spine in front over the crest of the pelvic bone (ilium) to the posterosuperior spine in back. Along its outer margin attach the large muscles going to the lower extremities and on its inner margin the group of muscles going to the abdomen and spine (Fig. 380). The area between is largely subcutaneous.

The vast majority of injuries about the pelvic crest are contusions that will respond promptly and well to the simple measures outlined previously. A definitive diagnosis should be made at the time of injury to rule out a more serious injury. Too often a more serious injury is detected only after ordinary measures fail to give relief. This results in a delay in definitive treatment for the serious condition, which may well prolong morbidity and cause greater permanent disability.

Injury along the pelvic rim may consist of a contusion of the bone of the iliac crest—the so-called hip pointer—a periostitis of the iliac crest, a strain, an avulsion of the muscles attaching to the crest or other abnormality. It is of considerable importance to determine the exact nature of the injury, because the treatment, particularly the protective treatment, and, also to a considerable extent, the immediate prognosis may depend a great deal upon the muscles involved. The injury frequently damages the attachment of the abdominal muscles along the anterior and inner portions of the iliac crest. This is caused by forceful con-

Figure 380. Drawing of the iliac crest, subcutaneous, but showing the hip muscles below and the trunk muscles above. (From Anson, Atlas of Human Anatomy.)

traction of the abdominal muscles while the trunk is being forced to the contralateral side. The result is some degree of detachment along the iliac crest, the separation varying from that of a few fibers to complete detachment of the entire muscle from the bone (Fig. 381).

I recall one case of a high school boy who threw himself in front of an opponent in making a block. He had immediate severe pain along the iliac crest with severe disability. When examined a few hours later he was able to walk only with the hand on the involved side dangling below the knee and the rib cage drawn down into the pelvis. Any effort to straighten him up from this position was strenuously resisted because of severe pain. Palpation revealed extreme tenderness along the entire iliac crest. When we were able to get him to relax a little, a palpable defect was found above the iliac crest. At operation an incision was made completely encircling the iliac crest. There had been complete avulsion of the aponeurotic muscle attachment to the crest of the ilium, so that the attachments of the iliacus and the abdominal muscles remained together but were completely pulled away from the iliac bone. The whole medial

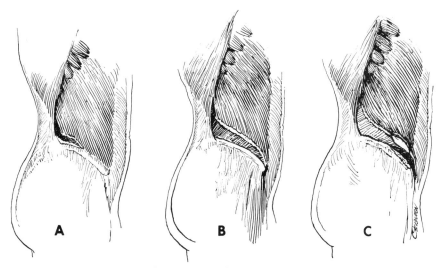

Figure 381. Drawings showing degrees of detachment of the aponeurosis at the iliac crest. *A,* Mild (first degree): a small tear. *B,* Moderate (second degree): an appreciable tear, with bare bone exposed. *C,* Severe (third degree): avulsion of the caput.

crest and interior surface of the ilium were denuded. The damage was easily repaired by placing drill holes along the iliac crest and pulling the detached cap snugly back into position on the crest. The boy had a good recovery and went on to play varsity collegiate football without disability. This is admittedly an unusual case, but it illustrates the variation in degree of injury and shows why results of treatment are so often disappointing.

At examination to determine the type of injury, certain findings are of extreme importance. Tenderness is not particularly diagnostic, since it is present in both contusion of bone and avulsion of muscle. In contusion, however, contraction of the involved muscle will not cause pain. On the other hand, if the athlete has pain on contracting his abdominal muscles or on flexing to the opposite side, one must assume some degree of damage to the muscle attachment. Similarly, if pain is caused by active abduction or extension of the thigh with the patient lying on his opposite side, one must assume some damage to the gluteal attachments or possibly to the tensor fascia femoris or to the lateral abdominals. Careful check must be made of the muscles that attach in the involved area. Once it has been determined that muscular involvement is present, the next step is to determine its degree. This may be extremely difficult. If there is complete avulsion, surgical repair should be carried out promptly. Fortunately complete avulsion of the iliac crest seldom occurs. I am sure, however, that it does occur more often than it is diagnosed. A great many of these injuries never actually reach the physician and are

treated by the athlete himself or by the trainer, often without true recognition of the nature of the pathological condition.

If the avulsion is less than complete, treatment should be the same as that for strain. The muscle should be put at rest. In the early stage one should use cold and compression, and after 24 hours, heat and protection. Since we are assuming some degree of avulsion of the attachment, local treatment may be of considerable value. Any hematoma should be aspirated first, and then a long-acting anesthetic agent is injected. Protection must be given to the muscles at the attachment of the iliac crest. Even though the trunk is strapped to hold it toward the involved side, which in itself is difficult, this does not prevent active forceful contraction of the muscle. It simply prevents overstretch. So if there is pain on active use of the abdominal or thigh muscles, a period of inactivity is necessary in order to restore normal function. Rehabilitation should be within the limits of pain, and this can be determined most readily by the patient himself. When activity is resumed, strapping of the flank, as described in Figure 382, may be undertaken, although its accomplishment is quite difficult. Properly applied, this strapping gives considerable restriction of motion. A good plan is to begin the strapping with cross-stretch tape and progress to long-stretch elastic tape as healing progresses and more activity is permissible. Indeed, if applied adequately enough to give good protection against overstretching, it probably will be a material handicap to athletic competition. Contact sports of any kind should not be permitted without very

Figure 382. Strapping of flank. The strapping is done with adhesive applied while the patient is in the erect position, with the trunk flexed toward the involved side. Broad strips of long-stretch or cross-stretch elastic tape are used. The former stretches on its long axis and allows considerable motion, whereas the latter stretches on its cross axis and gives more restriction of motion; so the one to be used depends upon the degree of fixation desired. Various methods can be used for application. A good method is by cross-hatching the strapping (B), one strip beginning in the region of the substernal notch extending diagonally downward and backward across the anterosuperior spine and over the trochanter to terminate on the back of the thigh, and another beginning in the back, starting at the lateral margin of the opposite lumbar muscle mass and crossing downward over the trochanter to end on the anteromedial thigh. These strips should cross at about the level of the crest. Successive parallel strips extending backward and forward form cross-hatching of the adhesive. The crossed strips begin at the trochanter and extend to the lower ribs. For additional support, the dressing can be given an underlying foundation of vertical strips, as illustrated in A. At the completion of the strapping, the tape should be secured by circumferential strips.

effective protective padding over the iliac crest, since the crest will remain extremely sensitive. This protection should be used for the remainder of the season.

A tendency toward recurrence of these lesions is disheartening. I am sure that the majority of them are undertreated rather than overtreated, since they are considered to be simple contusions when they are actually muscular avulsions.

Fracture

Fracture of the *wing of the ilium* is not a frequent athletic injury. It is usually caused by a direct blow against the wing of the ilium. In most sports in which such a force is likely, the iliac crest is protected by padding to prevent injury to the bone. The sport in which this

occurs most frequently is horseback riding, often in the manner described in Figure 383. This, as may be expected, is an extremely painful injury, not only at the time of the blow but also in the immediate period after the injury. It will ordinarily be recognized as a serious injury. Examination reveals extreme tenderness along the iliac crest and down onto the wing of the ilium, the area depending upon the extent of the fracture. The patient usually will not permit palpation deep enough to enable the physician to actually feel a defect along the rim, although this is occasionally possible. Any attempt at function of the involved muscles is extremely painful, and even involuntary spasm of the abdominal or hip muscles may cause acute distress. It is necessary to have the patient completely relaxed mentally and physically before a definitive examination can be done. If a lesion of this severity is suspected, an x-ray examination should be carried out. The fracture can be completely overlooked in the ordinary anteroposterior view of the pelvis. The fracture will be well delineated by an anteroposterior view of the ilium rather than the pelvis (Fig. 384). This view is obtained by rotating the pelvis 45 degrees toward the involved side. A lateral view may be obtained by directing the ray along the anterior iliac crest.

This fracture may be treated by complete bed rest, and with a tranquil patient, this is usually adequate. Even with some degree of displacement of the fragment, reduction is not necessary. Reposition would of necessity have to be by open reduction with internal fixation. This is a more formidable procedure than is usually justified. If simple bed rest does not provide adequate relief of pain, a pair of plaster pants extending from above the knees to above the rib margin may give substantial relief of discomfort and permit mobility of the patient in bed. A simple corset may suffice, or adhesive strapping may relieve the patient. It should be borne in mind that if there is real, measurable displacement of the fragment, a compression dressing with a corset or strapping may increase the pain and in fact increase the displacement. The duration of recumbency will vary widely, depending upon the severity of the injury and the equanimity of the patient. Ambulation may be allowed whenever the degree of discomfort permits. It will require six to eight weeks for the fracture to heal, but activity may be allowed as soon as the local reaction subsides and the pain permits.

Another injury in the region of the iliac crest is fracture of the *anterior superior spine of the*

Figure 383. A young female sustained a linear fracture of the ilium while horseback riding. The horse headed for the stable and turned through a gate so abruptly that the rider bumped the ilium on the center post. (For x-ray positioning, see Fig. 384.)

ilium (Fig. 385). This fracture is almost always an avulsion fracture, the fragment being pulled off by the sartorious and tensor fasciae femoris attachments. The patient's history is usually of unusual muscular violence in running or jumping—occasionally jumping down from a height. Examination reveals local pain and tenderness at the anterior spine. This can be distinguished from a contusion in this area by the fact that function of the involved muscle attachments is painful and active flexion of the thigh or passive overextension of the thigh will

Figure 384. Positioning for x-ray of the wing of the ilium. Place the patient in a supine position. Elevate the unaffected side about 40 or 45 degrees and support with sandbags or angle block. Center the anterior superior iliac spine to the midline of the table and center the cassette to the level of the anterior superior spine. Slightly flex the knees for comfort, but keep the hip fully extended. Direct the central ray to the center of the cassette.

Figure 385. Avulsion of anterior supine spine. A 14 year old athlete was knocked against a wall playing basketball. No symptoms developed until a month later, when he felt something pull while he was running. He continued to have pain for a month before seeking medical attention. *A,* X-ray two months after the injury reveals avulsion of the anterior superior spine of the ilium. Fragment was sutured back through drill holes. *B,* Four months postoperatively, the fracture shows good union.

cause pain directly at the area. If the physician examines the patient early, he may be able to palpate a separate fragment of bone which may be 2 to 3 cm. or more below the location of the attachment at the anterosuperior spine. X-rays should be taken. An anteroposterior view of the ilium rather than of the pelvis may be necessary if the fragment is not to be missed. An avulsion of the tendon may occur without a fragment of bone being displaced.

Treatment of this condition is primarily surgical. If it is diagnosed promptly, surgical correction is relatively atraumatic and not difficult. The fragment can be drawn back into position and fastened by whatever type of internal fixation seems most effective in the individual case. It may vary from a single screw fastening the fragment of bone to the pelvis to direct suture through drill holes. If the avulsion is incomplete or if for some reason surgery is inadvisable, treatment should be by immobilization with the thigh flexed. This can be accomplished by bed rest with the knees elevated or by plaster fixation in the appropriate position. I believe it is more simple and less traumatic to carry out prompt open reduction with definitive fixation than it is to immobilize the patient for the period necessary to permit healing to become complete. If nonsurgical treatment is selected, local measures will consist of aspiration of the hematoma, injection with local anesthetic, use of a compression bandage, and application of cold early and heat after 24 hours.

Following surgical repair, the degree of activity to be permitted will depend upon the security of the internal fixation. If firm fixation is obtained, I prefer to use a short single spica starting at the knee on the affected side and continuing around the pelvis, with the thigh flexed 30 degrees. The patient should be allowed up on crutches within a day or two, and rehabilitation should begin promptly. This includes isometric contraction of the involved muscles. At the end of two weeks, the spica is removed. The wound is dressed, and if it has properly healed, a spica of elastic adhesive bandage is applied with the patient standing and flexing the thigh and knee slightly by putting the foot on the involved side on a 4 in. block. This permits rehabilitation of the hip joint to proceed. Ordinarily active running should not be permitted short of six weeks, and in the case with less secure surgical fixation, a longer period may be required.

If at operation the fragment is found to be small or comminuted, it should be removed rather than repaired, and the muscle should be sutured to the bone. Indeed, there is some argument in favor of routinely removing the fragment and obtaining muscle-to-bone healing rather than waiting for bone-to-bone union. The latter may require considerably longer and may prolong rehabilitation. Unless I can get anatomical reposition and very positive screw fixation, I generally remove the fragment and repair the attachment to the ilium through drill holes.

INJURIES IN THE VICINITY OF THE POSTERIOR SPINES OF THE ILIUM

Injuries to the posterior spines of the ilium are not frequent, since the attachments here are such that there is no acute avulsive force applied. The most frequent injury in this vicinity is simple contusion of the posterior superior or inferior spine. Although this may be somewhat distressing, it is not particularly disabling and responds well to local treatment using heat and other means of physical therapy.

INJURIES IN THE VICINITY OF THE SACRUM AND SACROILIAC JOINTS, INCLUDING THE COCCYX

The sacrum is the keystone of the arch of the pelvis. The two innominate bones are attached to the sacrum at the sacroiliac joints. The sacroiliac joint has an extremely irregular contour, the bones fitting together with interdigitations much like the ratchets in the bracket of an ordinary desk lamp. There is no true articular motion between these two bones, but there is articular cartilage and often a synovial lined capsule, so it must be classified as a diarthrodial joint (Fig. 386).

Contusion

Contusion in the vicinity of the sacrum and sacroiliac joints is a common injury, occurring so frequently that sacral pads are a required part of the equipment for contact sports. The sacrum itself is largely subcutaneous on its posterior surface, as is the posterior inferior spine of the ilium. A direct blow to the unprotected sacrum may cause an extremely painful injury. Examination reveals tenderness over

the sacrum, which may be diffuse or may be sharply localized on the sacrum or on one of the iliac spines. If the injury appears to be acute, an x-ray should be made, since it is not unusual to crack the sacrum or to fracture one of the spines by direct trauma. If fracture can be ruled out, treatment should consist of early application of cold and compression followed by heat and support. Actually this injury, although it is quite painful, is not particularly disabling. As long as the sacrum is tender, it should be protected against direct contusion.

Fracture

A fracture of the sacrum is usually transverse or stellate in type and will respond quite well to conservative treatment (Fig. 387). This will require a period of bed rest followed by support. Ordinarily a corset will be adequate. Healing will usually be complete within four weeks, but residual tenderness and pain may last another month. If the displacement is gross or if angulation is severe, an orthopaedic consultant should be called. This force is not likely to injure the rectum, but a rectal examination should be routine. If blood is encountered, a proctoscopic examination is indicated. One should also be alert for irregularities of the inner surface of the sacrum.

Sprain

A sprain of the iliosacral ligaments is possible. It may be of the ligament extending from the posterior projection of the wing of the ilium to the posterior sacrum or of the ligaments within the pelvis. It should be borne in mind that many of the conditions that used to

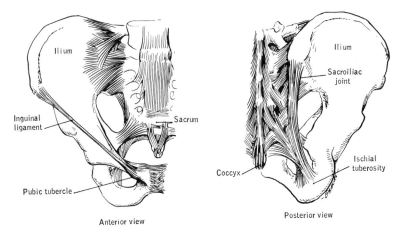

Figure 386. Anteroposterior view of the ligaments of the pelvis. Note the complete investiture of the sacroiliac joints by a continuous band of very heavy ligament. This includes also the ligament attaching the third lumbar vertebra to the ilium. Note that the entire pelvis is firmly bound down with strong ligaments. (From Anson, Atlas of Human Anatomy.)

Figure 387. Transverse fracture of sacrum just below the sacroiliac joint, caused by a forceful blow against the lower portion of the sacrum. *A*, Anterior view. *B*, Lateral view. This fracture is treated symptomatically. The patient probably would be more comfortable in a sacroiliac support for a few weeks.

be called sacroiliac sprain were actually other entities. It was a "wastebasket" term. The sacroiliac ligaments are so strong, particularly in the young athlete, that ordinary stresses will cause damage to the lumbosacral ligaments more readily than to the sacroiliac ligaments. One should, therefore, be very wary of the diagnosis of sacroiliac sprain.

Following injury in the vicinity of the sacroiliac joint, there will be pain localized about the joint. There also may be pain referred to the groin, hamstrings or back of the thigh. It will not ordinarily be along the sciatic distribution. If this condition is suspected, great care must be taken to localize the lesion to the sacroiliac joint. Many of the tests that will elicit pain, i.e., be positive, in the sacroiliac joint will also elicit pain in such conditions as ruptured disc, sciatic neuritis and lumbrosacral sprain, so that the mere fact that the tests cause pain is of little significance. Of greatest significance is the location of the pain. In an acute injury this may be extremely difficult to determine accurately. The common tests, such as straight leg raising (Fig. 388A and *B*), that put torsion force on the sacroiliac joint, or the similar test of forward flexion of the trunk with the knees straight, will cause pain in sacroiliac joint involvement but will also cause pain in many other conditions. Some tests are designed to stress the sacroiliac area particularly. The popular Gaenslen test (see Fig. 388*C*), in which the opposite thigh is flexed on the abdomen in order to immobilize the pelvis in

forward flexion and then the involved leg is pushed into hyperextension, causes rotatory stress on the sacroiliac joint. Obviously it would also strain other areas, so again the mere positive result of the test is not diagnostic.

Of more significance are tests designed to compress or separate the iliac crests (see Fig. 388*E* to *H*). With the patient lying on his back, simple compression force across the crests will put some stress across the sacroiliac joint. The opposite maneuver of forcing the crests apart can be applied in a thin individual by locking the heels of the hands against the inner portion of each anterior spine and attempting to separate the spines. A similar test is to have the patient lie on his side with the inferior thigh flexed to 90 degrees to fix the lumbosacral area. Compression downward against the upward iliac crest will throw stress on the sacroiliac joint.

If the sprain is acute, the pain will be relieved by bed rest. Local treatment consists of injection of the tender area with an anesthetic followed by application of compression, using a constricting elastic adhesive dressing wrapped around the pelvis or a sacroiliac belt or a simple corset. Heat will relieve the attendant muscle spasm. As in back injuries, muscle spasm may be relieved by oral antispasmodics. The duration of immobilization in bed depends upon the severity of the injury. The patient may be permitted to get up as soon as it is possible without pain. If the injury is actually an acute sprain of the ligament, five to six weeks will be needed for the ligament to repair, and the area should be carefully protected during this time.

Dislocation

Actual sacroiliac dislocation occurs only as the result of a massive injury that is ordinarily not athletic in origin, although it could occur by being thrown from a horse or similar severe trauma. The treatment, which is the same as that for a fractured pelvis, is not within the scope of this work.

Subluxation

Osteopathic physicians have called our attention to the dramatic relief which may be secured by manipulation in the sacroiliac joint. It is probable that in certain circumstances of relaxation of the iliosacral ligaments, some of the interdigitations of the joint become caught with a minimal degree of displacement, which is undectable by x-ray examination. In these cases manipulation may cause them to "snap back into place" and provide relief. This happens too frequently to be ignored, but I am sure that many times the relief by manipulation either is relief of the muscle tension or is psychic. The exact manipulation may vary. One of the most effective maneuvers is the forceful application of the Gaenslen test (Fig. 389A), in which one thigh is sharply flexed and the other hyperextended. Another manipulation (Fig. 389B) is carried out with the patient lying supine on the table. Instruct him to reach over and catch the left edge of the table with his right hand over his left shoulder. The left thigh is then grasped and, with the knee in

Figure 388. A, Straight leg raising. Note the extended right thigh. The left lower extremity is flexed with the knee extended. B, Straight leg raising test with dorsiflexion of the foot (Lasègue). C, Thigh flexion test (Gaenslen). Note the right thigh held in extension. It may be dropped off the table in hyperextension while the left thigh is flexed. D, The heel to knee test. The left pelvis is fixed by the examiner's left hand. With the right heel on the left knee, the right knee is pushed down toward the table. E, F, G, H, Iliac compression or separation. E, Lateral decubitus. With the opposite thigh flexed for stability, the right iliac crest is compressed toward the table. F, With the patient supine, the examiner's hands force the iliac crests apart. G, With the patient supine, the legs are widely abducted. H, Examiner forces crests together.

Figure 389. Sacroiliac manipulation. *A,* Forceful flexion of thigh with opposite thigh fixed. *B,* The patient fixes the upper trunk by grasping the edge of the table with the right hand while the left lower extremity is forced up into flexion and adduction, thus rotating the pelvis on the spine.

extension, the thigh is flexed 45 degrees and then adducted and internally rotated. This rotates the pelvis toward the left. This maneuver can be carried out in either direction. Sometimes it is rewarded by an alarming snap and dramatic relief, but alas, most often there is no result at all! Manipulation should not be attempted casually by the uninitiated and by no means with the patient under anesthesia. When the patient is awake, his muscular resistance will usually prevent any actual damage. However, when he is relaxed under anesthesia, the leverage applied may cause serious damage to the hip or spine.

As is frequent with a ligament injury, there is a tendency toward recurrence, therefore once the injury has been treated and the patient rehabilitated, a well-fitting sacroiliac belt should be worn when playing contact sports for the remainder of the season. It should be emphasized again that before diagnosis of sacroiliac sprain can be made the burden of proof remains with the examiner to show that the condition actually is a sacroiliac sprain and not some other injury.

Coccyx

There will occasionally be injury to the coccyx, although this too is not a common injury in sports. It usually occurs when the player falls in a sitting position or a blow (inadvertent) from a shoe. Although this is an extremely painful injury, it is not especially disabling and usually requires no specific treatment other than local application of heat. The pain may be severe enough to prevent competition for two or three weeks. Local protection is advisable in the form of a fiber pad, and some degree of constriction helps. Something like a panty girdle will be valuable for this purpose. A suitable pad can be inserted at the appropriate area in the girdle to give local protection. Ordinarily a moderate amount of displacement is of little importance, particularly in the male. The fracture will heal promptly.

There will occasionally be involvement of the sacrococcygeal joint by subluxation or trau-

matic arthritis. If pain is persistent and disabling, coccygectomy may be justified. Great care must be exercised to be sure that the coccyx is actually the seat of the trouble and that the condition is truly local. I cannot recall having to remove a coccyx damaged as a result of athletic injury. No disability results from coccyx removal.

INJURIES IN THE VICINITY OF THE BUTTOCK AND PERINEUM

Contusion

The most common injury to the buttock is from a direct blow. This does not usually cause injury to the skin because of the ample underlying padding. Contusion of the muscle is a common occurrence but usually is of little consequence. In most of the areas of the buttock there is a thick muscle mass, with relatively little danger of getting caught between two unyielding objects. As a result the condition is usually diffuse, without gross hematoma formation in the muscle. A tender, painful muscle mass results which may be uncomfortable but is not grossly disabling. The buttock is usually not protected in athletic competition by any padding other than that inherent in the anatomy, and so superficial contusion is relatively common here. One should be wary of the condition that appears to be unduly severe or that causes other than local symptoms.

A *contusion of the sciatic nerve* may result in pain in the buttock, extending down the back of the thigh into the calf and foot, which is similar to sciatic pain from other causes. This injury is nonradicular in nature and follows the whole distribution of the sciatic nerve rather than that of any single root. Straight leg raising causes pain in the area of the contusion. During the acute period, hyperesthesia of the skin may be evident in the lower portion of the extremity. This contusion is not frequent. The ordinary contusion of the sciatic nerve will require no particular treatment other than protection against stretch. Physical therapy may give considerable relief. A word of caution should be said about inductive heat. If deep therapy, such as short wave diathermy, causes an increase in the pain, it should be promptly discontinued. Sometimes local tension in the nerve will be increased by congestion due to the heat. This does not ordinarily occur with the whirlpool bath or infrared radiation.

Another area of the buttock in which a complication of contusion may arise is over the ischial tuberosity. Here the bone is essentially subcutaneous, although it may be protected by an overlying layer of muscle of greater or lesser thickness. A contusion here may cause a *fracture of the tuberosity,* in which case there will be severe localized pain. The pain is increased by straight leg raising or by any local pressure. More commonly the result of the blow will be periostitis or fibrositis over the roughened surface of the bone. In other cases there will be involvement of the ischial bursa. It may be impossible in the early stages to distinguish between these conditions. Treatment should consist of heat applied locally and rest. Usually the symptoms will subside promptly. In the case of periositis or bursitis there will be persistent pain and extreme local tenderness. In these cases local injection into the area in an attempt to aspirate fluid from the bursa is advisable.

If the injury seems severe or if the symptoms persist, x-ray examination should be carried out. A simple anteroposterior view of the pelvis may be unenlightening, and several views or subsequent films may be necessary (Figs. 390 and 391). The injury may occasionally result in spur formation or in calcification within the bursa (see Fig. 390). If there is calcification of the bursa and if this does not respond well to aspiration and local injection, surgical excision of the bursa is justified. Usually relief is prompt and complete following surgical excision. If the irritation results in ossification and spur formation which does not respond to treatment and which is constantly disabling, the spurring should be removed surgically. Completely atraumatic technique must be used. Access is readily obtained in this location by placing the patient in the lithotomy position, with a folded sheet beneath the sacrum. This presents the tuberosity of the ischium in its subcutaneous position. One is able to expose the tuberosity and the ascending ramus of the ischium or whatever area is primarily involved without extensive dissection. If careful attention is paid to hemostasis by proper coagulation, an extremely dry field

may be obtained and the exact pathological condition determined. If there is bursitis, the bursa may be readily removed and the underlying periosteum examined. If on the other hand there is irregularity of the bone or spur formation, the muscle attachments may be stripped away subperiosteally, the bone carefully smoothed off and hemostasis secured with bone wax. The incision need only be as extensive as is required for the lesion encountered.

Occasionally the ascending ramus of the ischium or descending ramus of the pubis will be injured by a direct blow such as a fall astraddle a bar. This may be an extremely painful injury, but ordinarily recovery is complete without specific therapy other than local measures. The treatment should depend upon the severity of the condition. Usually application of cold followed by heat and a period at rest will suffice. In the case of serious injury, x-ray study should be done to determine possible fracture. At the time of injury the patient will feel that a major disaster has befallen him, since the injury is painful and distressing—and often humiliating. He may try to avoid embarrassment over his ineptitude by appearing to be badly injured.

Injuries to the deeper structures of the perineum hardly fall into the scope of this work, since they are very infrequent in athletic pursuits. Probably the most common of them is contusion from falling forcibly on a hard ob-

Figure 390. Calcification within ischial bursa.

Figure 391. This 14 year old female fell astraddle the gymnasium rail, receiving a severe perineal contusion, immediate, severe pain and disability, with terrific adductor and hamstring spasm. The original x-ray was negative. Three weeks post-injury x-ray did show osteomyelitis of the ischium, the result of stagnation of blood from contusion. This was relieved by adequate drainage and antibiotic therapy.

ject, with resulting painful hematomas (see Fig. 391). In injury of any consequence, careful examination should be made to be sure that there is no serious damage to the underlyimg structures. In the male, the cavernous muscles and urethra may be damaged; in the female, the vulva. Suitable consultation should be obtained from a competent urologist or gynecologist, particularly if there appears to be subcutaneous bleeding or open laceration. So, also, damage to the anus and rectum may occur. If there is any question as to whether such damage exists, a rectal examination should be carried out immediately to determine if there is local tenderness, presence of bleeding or even the presence of a palpable defect in the sphincter or wall.

In discussing perineal-type injuries, one must not overlook the male genitalia. The almost universal use of the athletic supporter has been very valuable in preventing injury. Contusion is the most common type of injury. The penis in its relaxed condition is soft and pliable and is seldom injured by contusion. The testicles, on the other hand, which lack the protection of the abdominal walls, hang relatively free and unprotected and are very subject to injury. Their location between the thighs, however, provides a good deal of protection. Also, the instinctive recoil from a threatened blow serves to render the blow less

severe. Nonetheless, the testicular contusion is not uncommon. However, it is not often actually damaging. The immediate pain may be excruciating and thus disabling. The rebound is rapid and disability short.

Trainers have a favorite trick in which they pull the injured person to a sitting position. The operator grasps his hands in the patient's axillae, lifts him 10 to 12 in. off the field, then drops him hard on his buttocks. Why this is effective in counteracting the pain from a testicular injury is hard to understand. Possibly the pain stimuli from the testicles are short circuited by the new pain stimuli from the drop.

Occasionally bruising may occur, resulting in a swollen, tense and painful scrotum. In this case ice packs should be applied for 24 hours, followed by use of a whirlpool and sitz bath. Warm packs are also effective. Complete recovery may be expected, although it may be hard to convince the victim of this.

Other types of injuries such as avulsions and lacerations are very uncommon and obviously will require immediate transportation to a hospital for special care. Skin conditions such as jock itch, excoriation, eczema and furunculosis will require great care and patience. Cleanliness is imperative. One should shower daily, taking care to rinse off all the soap, which in itself may be irritating. Application of a bland,

Figure 392. A 21 year old football player faked to the left. He had severe pain and fell as he cut sharply to the right. After a few days, local symptoms subsided. Three months later, during a squatting exercise requiring sudden strain, he had recurrence of the same pain in a more severe form. A, X-ray following the second episode showed a stress fracture across the top of the ischium, with callus formation. This undoubtedly occurred at the time of the original fall. B, Uneventful healing four months later.

lubricating cream will lessen the friction and the discomfort.

Strain

This same ischial area is quite subject to muscle strain (Fig. 392), a common one being strain at the origin of the long head of the biceps and the semitendinosus on the tuberosity of the ischium. This may result in avulsion of the ischial tuberosity, particularly if the epiphysis in this region is not yet closed. It usually occurs as a result of forcible flexion of the hip with the knee extended, as in the leading leg of the hurdler (Fig. 393). Extremely forceful straight leg raising is the same mech-

anism and it pulls heavily on the origin of the long head of the biceps. The result may be irritation at the attachment of the muscle or complete avulsion from the bone (Fig. 394). Symptoms are localized pain on pressure over the ischial tuberosity, pain on flexion of the thigh with the knee extended and pain on active forceful contraction of the biceps muscle. X-ray examination may or may not reveal the nature of the injury.

Treatment is the same as that for avulsion anywhere, except that replacement of the avulsed fragment may not be necessary. It should be replaced if the separation is wide and complete (Fig. 395). Immobilization of the leg with the knee flexed and avoidance of thigh flexion will usually suffice for protection. In

Figure 393. Avulsion of a portion of the ischium by the attachment of the biceps muscle. Following a relatively acute period of two or three weeks, subject had recurrence of pain on running or jumping. The fragment was removed and the muscle sutured to the bed with a good recovery. Recent studies have suggested that even with wide displacement, firm fibrous scar may result in a normal hip. Nevertheless, I personally prefer open reduction if the displacement is marked A, Preoperative, B, Postoperative

Figure 394. *A*, A high school baseball pitcher who injured his kick-off leg while throwing left-handed during a game. He had pain and soreness but was able to complete the game, pitching a one-hitter. Subsequently he was unable to play. Now (eight weeks later) his recovery is proceeding well. The injury represents an avulsion of the attachment of the semitendinosus. *B*, An 18 year old male two years after a skating injury that remained untreated. The x-ray shows tremendous overgrowth of displaced ischial epiphysis. Removal of excess bone and repair of the tendon to the ischium was advised to relieve the symptomatic condition.

fact, in many instances, simple elimination of forceful activity is enough. If the symptoms are persistent, local injection and physical therapy are of value. A painful nonunion of the fragment may be relieved by removal of the fragment, although this is seldom necessary. As is true of many avulsions, this one is not compatible with athletic competition. A period of rest from strenuous activity is imperative, but under ordinary circumstances there will be no permanent disability. The same surgical technique may be used here as that indicated previously for ischial bursitis. In some instances, however, the lithotomy position may be inadvisable because it may overstretch the hamstrings. This can usually be minimized by extending the thigh somewhat from the acutely flexed position. The same approach can be utilized with the patient lying prone with a large pillow under the pelvis of the involved side and with the knee flexed.

A straddling injury caused by forceful abduction of the thighs may cause damage to the adductor muscles. They are particularly vulnerable at their attachments to the ischiopubic rami. Following this type of injury the symptoms are readily recognizable, since there will be localized tenderness along the subcutaneous edge of the ramus and to the lateral side. The diagnostic sign is pain on forceful passive abduction of the thigh and on active adduction against resistance, each of which causes pain localized at the origin of these muscles along the puboischium. This same force will occasionally cause avulsion of one of the adductors, usually the adductor longus (Fig. 396), in

Figure 395. This 14 year old girl was learning a new dance step when she did an anteroposterior split, with immediate, severe pain in the buttock with disability. X-ray revealed complete avulsion of the semitendinosus origin. Treatment by surgical replacement of the fragment resulted in complete recovery.

which case the symptoms are more pronounced, and there may be a palpable defect between the bone and the muscle belly. I have seen instances in the athlete in which the longus muscle has been ruptured at a distance from the insertion, usually about 5 cm. from the attachment of the pelvis. This may simulate a contusion and is often difficult to distinguish from one. If the condition can be recognized, prompt surgical repair of the rupture of the attachment or muscle is indicated. Detachment or rupture may be recognized by the bunching up of the adductor longus muscle a short distance away from the pelvis and by a tender, firm mass which is most noticeable on active adduction of the thigh against resistance. If several weeks have passed, any attempt at repair is doomed to failure because it will not be possible to get secure enough sutures within the muscle substance to overcome the shortening of the muscle. In this instance the condition should be carefully explained to the

Figure 396. Partial avulsion of the attachment of the adductor longus and gracilis from the pubic ramus. This gave chronic pain and terminated the player's basketball season. Local injection and physical therapy relieved the symptoms.

Figure 397. Injury of the mons pubis by a fall on the ice, with resulting hematoma.

patient, pointing out that the mass is of no consequence in itself. In most instances the athlete will accept this without insistence on further treatment. Should the pain be persistent and to some extent disabling, late surgery may be justified. At this time the fibromuscular mass should be removed and the remaining muscle belly sutured to the adjoining adductor magnus. An injury of this severity is rather unusual, but prompt relief may be obtained by definitive treatment. It is important to point out to the athlete that this treatment will not add to his muscular strength or ability or agility but is simply designed to relieve his pain.

As indicated previously, by far the most common injury to the ischial area is a strain at the muscle attachment. In this instance the symptoms are similar to those of this condition anywhere and are relieved by the same measures. If the patient is seen immediately after the injury, there may be some virtue in application of cold. Ordinarily the symptoms are not called to the physician's attention for several days, when the patient is seen because of persistent pain and discomfort. At this time local measures should consist of local injection of a long-acting anesthetic, application of heat using sitz baths, whirlpool, and diathermy and rest. Injudicious exercise in an attempt to improve the range of abduction will only prolong the symptoms. Constant effort should be made to avoid forcible abduction of the involved thigh.

Pubic Symphysis

Damage to the pubic symphysis is not frequent except in major accidents involving the pelvis. However, one may get a painful contusion over the subcutaneous anterior surface of the symphysis. This may result in considerable local swelling and even hematoma formation, but it is not a dangerous or crippling injury. I saw a girl who fell heavily forward on her mons pubis while ice skating (Fig. 397). The result was the prompt development of a hematoma the size of a small orange, which was alarming and distressing to the patient. The actual disability, however, was minimal, the pain being present only on direct pressure. Because of the unsightly swelling, an attempt

was made to aspirate it. This was unsuccessful because of infiltration of blood through the fibrofatty pad, and ultimately it was necessary for the gynecologist to evacuate the hematoma. This case is mentioned particularly because the condition may seem quite alarming and drastic remedies may appear in order, whereas it is a relatively superficial hematoma and ordinarily will respond to the local measures used for treatment of hematoma elsewhere.

In the adolescent the pubic symphysis is not nearly as firmly fixed as it is in the adult, and sprain of the ligaments connecting the two pubic bones can occur by forceful abduction of both thighs. This must be distinguished from a contusion, which is considerably more common, because in a strain of the pubic ligaments, the force applied is one that separates the pubic bones rather than a direct blow to the local area. The treatment is quite different in the two instances, since the treatment of sprain of the pubic ligaments must be designed to hold the pelvic ring together and to prevent wide abduction of the thighs. This can be accomplished by circumferential adhesive strapping or by a well-fitted lumbosacral corset. Early treatment should consist of local injection, application of heat and rest. As with any sprain, several weeks are required for healing, and protection should be continued for many weeks, particularly if there is participation in any sport that causes tension on these ligaments, such as horseback riding or water-skiing. The prognosis is quite favorable if the condition is recognized and treated adequately.

INJURIES IN THE VICINITY OF THE GROIN

Contusion

In this area we find the tunnel formed by the bridging of the anterior pelvis by Poupart's ligament, which runs from the pubis across to the anterior superior spine on either side (Fig. 398). Under this ligament pass the vascular sheath, the femoral nerve, the inguinal canal, the cord and some muscle groups, particularly the iliopsoas. A direct blow over this area may

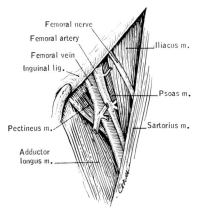

Figure 398. Note compartment formed by the inguinal ligament above, the iliopsoas laterally, and the adductors medially. This compartment houses the femoral artery, vein and nerve. The sartorius and rectus attach to the anterosuperior spine, whereas the adductor muscles attach along the pubic ramus. Note also how the psoas and iliacus blend to form the iliopsoas tendon, which attaches to the lesser trochanter of the femur. (From Anson, Atlas of Human Anatomy.)

cause damage to any of these structures. This is ordinarily not severe but may be relatively painful. It may cause a few minutes or hours of disability, but there should be a good and complete recovery.

Permanent vascular damage after a blow to the groin is infrequent. Traumatic phlebitis and even phlebothrombosis from a direct blow over the femoral vein can occur. Trauma to the femoral nerve may cause paresthesia along the front of the thigh, which is worrisome to the patient but of little significance from the standpoint of disability. The well-trained athlete has been taught to protect his abdomen and groin by flexion of the thigh; therefore, injury in this area is not as frequent as might be expected considering its relatively exposed position.

Strain

Muscular strain in this area is relatively frequent, the most frequent being *strain of the iliopsoas tendon*. This may occur at its attachment to the lesser trochanter of the femur or in the musculotendinous junction. It is not caused by a direct blow to the groin but by overactive contraction of the iliopsoas when the thigh is flexed and then forced into extension. The patient complains of severe pain in the groin and holds the thigh in a flexed, adducted and externally rotated position. Any attempt of the examiner to extend or to internally rotate the thigh causes severe pain. So

does active contraction of the iliopsoas muscle. Tenderness will be found at the area of the injury. If it is at the lesser trochanteric attachment, the tenderness will be below the groin, along the upper anteromedial aspect of the thigh. Careful x-ray study should be done of the lesser trochanter to determine whether there has been an avulsion of the bone (Fig. 399). This is particularly necessary in the adolescent in whom the epiphysis of the lesser trochanter has not yet united with the shaft. Even if the avulsion is complete, surgical repair is rarely indicated. The trochanter reattaches with fibrous union and usually is not painful. Protection should be carried out by immobilization with the thigh flexed and externally rotated. If a painful union occurs, the attachment of the iliopsoas tendon to the lesser tuberosity may be transferred to the anterior femur. If the lesion is incomplete, as it most frequently is, treatment should consist of bed rest, with the thigh flexed and externally rotated and application of cold compresses in the early stage followed by application of heat locally. After a few days, better determination can be made as to the severity of the injury. Duration of treatment will depend upon the symptoms. This is an extremely disabling condition, since any effort to run or jump causes excessive strain on this tendon, with resultant pain. The patient's athletic endeavors must be terminated for whatever period is required for the symptoms to subside, usually several weeks.

Because of the complexity of the various flexors of the hip, it is sometimes difficult to

Figure 399. Avulsion of the lesser trochanter.

determine whether or not complete avulsion of the tendon has occurred. In case of persistent pain with chronic irritation, treatment by local injection into the tender area may be tried. This area is relatively inaccessible, and skillful manipulation of the needle is needed to reach the involved area. The iliopsoas is an important flexor of the thigh, and complete recovery is necessary before unrestricted function can be permitted. Strapping that holds the thigh in slight flexion will prevent overstretching of the muscle but does not prevent overactivity and so is relatively ineffectual. Plaster fixation is ordinarily not necessary, since the thigh readily assumes the position of flexion, which puts the muscle at rest. This position is all too often held even after the lesion has healed, so that troublesome flexion contracture of the thigh may be the result. In order to minimize this danger, the patient should be encouraged to extend the thigh actively within the limits of pain several times each day. After the acute symptoms subside, a daily period spent lying prone in bed is desirable.

Also susceptible to damage in this area is the abdominal muscle group which attaches along Poupart's ligament. Strain of these muscles must be treated by rest, by application of heat and by protection—the same type of treatment necessary for similar injury along the iliac crest. Occasionally there will be a painful strain of the conjoined tendon of the abdominals at the attachment to the pubis at the inner end of Poupart's ligament.

Great care must be taken to eliminate other conditions which may be present in this general area, such as hernia, involvement of the spermatic cord, lymphadenitis and phlebitis, since all these conditions may well become symptomatic after trauma or overactivity. In case of doubt, treatment should be essentially the same except that no injection should be administered.

INJURIES IN THE VICINITY OF THE TROCHANTER

Contusion

The significant area of contusion in the vicinity of the hip is over the trochanter. In this area the bony trochanter is covered only by the trochanteric bursa, the iliotibial tract and the skin. The tract is separated form the trochanter by the trochanteric bursa, which is a constant structure of considerable size lying beneath the muscle and tendon of the tensor fasciae femoris. Contusion may result in damage to the muscle or to the bursa. The symptoms are the same as in those of contusion elsewhere, and the treatment presents no unusual elements.

A trochanteric *bursitis* may be caused here by a direct blow, by infection or by friction between the adjacent bursal walls. In many instances contusion of the trochanter may result in bursitis, and the symptoms will gradually change from those of a contusion to those of involvement of the bursa. In this instance there will be tenderness over the trochanteric area with pain on forcible activity of the thigh. In the course of flexion and extension of the hip or of rotation of the extended thigh, the tensor fasciae femoris slides backward and forward over the trochanter, and in the presence of an inflammatory reaction, this will cause pain.

On examination there is local tenderness over the bursa, often with crepitation on motion. Pain is elicited by adducting the thigh with the knee extended, which puts the tensor under strain as it passes over the trochanter. In this position, internal and external rotations of the extremity will cause the trochanter to slide back and forth under the tight tensor, and pain will be caused on this maneuver which would not be present with a simple contusion.

The so-called snapping hip should be mentioned in this connection. This is due to chronic bursitis with thickening of the bursal walls and spasm of the tensor, so that on each step, as the tensor slides back and forth over the trochanter, an audible and palpable snap will occur. This is quite distressing. The condition is much more common in females, since they have wide pelves and prominent trochanters and the tensor bows over the trochanter at a more acute angle than in the narrower pelvis of the male. X-ray examination is ordinarily of little value, although it may occasionally show calcification within the bursa.

Treatment of the acute bursitis consists of rest and application of heat locally. Early injection of a local anesthetic into the bursa may give prompt relief. There is a decided tendency toward recurrence. In the occasional patient with chronic recurring bursitis that is resistant to treatment, excision of the bursa may be necessary. If the chronic bursitis is accompanied by a snapping tensor tendon or by undue tension between the tensor and the trochanter at the time of operation, it is advisable either to divide the tensor and make suitable repair or to shift it anteriorly or posteriorly. The indication for this operation is extremely uncommon in the male but is relatively frequent in the female, although not ordinarily as the result of athletic injury.

The technique for surgery will not be described in detail here other than to say that the whole aim of surgery is to release the tension on the tensor fascia femoris muscle in the iliotibial tract so that it will not be snapping back and forth over the trochanter. This can be done by dividing half of the band and transferring it either posteriorly or anteriorly so that on ordinary stride the band does not snap over the trochanter. This is probably preferable to the operation which divides the iliotibial tract, since the tract does have a definite function in the thigh which may be handicapped to some degree by this transection.

Strain

There may be strain of the muscles attaching to the trochanter, particularly the gluteus medius (Fig. 400). This is ordinarily caused by overactivity of the gluteus medius and is usually chronic rather than acute. A symptom in such a case will be pain on active contraction of the gluteus medius against resistance.

Functional tests are of considerable importance in finding the exact muscle involved, since active use of the muscle should not cause pain if the involvement is in the bursa alone. To examine the abductors, have the patient lie on his side and actively elevate the leg, putting stress on the gluteus medius and the other adductors. In particular, if this is done against resistance it will be painful. Passive motion through this same arc with the muscles relaxed will be pain-free.

Similarly if it is the external rotators which attach at the back of the trochanter that are involved, pain will be elicited when the thigh is actively externally rotated against resistance, whereas passive external rotation without resistance will not be painful. In order to distinguish injuries to the psoas muscle from other conditions in the groin, flexing the thigh against resistance, particularly flexion and external rotation, will cause pain, whereas passive movement will not. In a similar manner one can determine a suitable test for any muscle which will serve to determine whether the trouble is in the muscle itself or somewhere else. Forced passive motion beyond normal range in any of these directions will cause pain on the opposer. In other words, forcible, passive adduction of the thigh may cause pain in the abductor muscle. Forced internal rotation may cause pain on the external rotator. Forced external rotation may cause pain on the internal rotator, and so forth.

Such contraction will not cause pain if the involvement is of the bursa alone. Similarly, a tendinitis of the rotators of the hip joint attaching along the posterior margin of the trochanter will cause local tenderness at the area of their attachment, with pain on active exter-

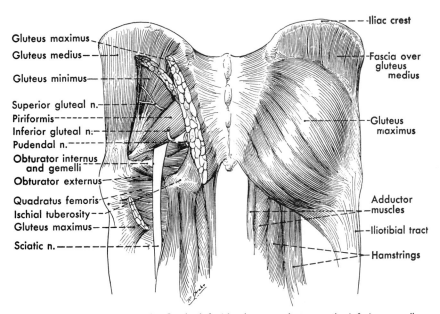

Figure 400. The musculature of the buttocks. On the left side, the space between the inferior gemellus and quadratus femoris is exaggerated so that the insertion of the obturator externus can be shown. (From Anson, Atlas of Human Anatomy.)

Figure 401. Avulsion of the anterior portion of the greater trochanter six months after injury, with nonunion.

nal rotation or passive forceful internal rotation of the hip. These conditions are treated by application of heat locally, some sort of inductive heat being necessary to reach the area of involvement (diathermy or microtherm). Local injection is relatively simple here, and the use of a long-acting local anesthetic plus a suitable corticoid will frequently give very good results.

In the adolescent in whom the greater tro-

chanteric epiphysis is not united with the shaft, an *avulsion* (Figs. 401 and 402), complete or partial, of the trochanteric epiphysis is not infrequent. This is a relatively serious injury and is analogous to complete avulsion of the tendon attachment. If the avulsion is incomplete and the epiphyseal plate appears to be only a little bit wide, it should be treated by immobilization with the thigh in abduction and slight external rotation. This position is main-

Figure 402. Avulsion of the trochanter by violent, active abduction against resistance. This minimally displaced fragment held without surgery. This injury is borderline for internal fixation.

tained for at least six weeks and activity is resumed gradually. If the avulsion is complete, it should be treated by surgical replacement and fixation with a long wood screw or similar appliance. The same treatment is advisable if the trochanter is broken and displaced. Following firm internal fixation, support is needed only during the period when the wound is healing, but athletic activity should be eliminated for at least six weeks.

INJURIES TO THE HIP JOINT PROPER

From an orthopaedic standpoint and indeed from the standpoint of the traumatic surgeon, the hip is extremely liable to injury. Fortunately the hip joint is rarely injured as a result of athletic activity. This is in contrast to the knee, which is highly vulnerable. Owing to the extremely free motion of the hip joint, sprain of the ligaments of the hip is very uncommon. Strain of the muscles and tendons about the hip has been discussed previously, and nothing needs to be added here.

Fracture and Dislocation

Fracture about the hip is unusual in the adolescent and young adult. The bone is exceptionally resilient, and the hip is much more likely to dislocate than it is to break. For this reason we may see a *dislocation* of the hip in an athlete, but fortunately it is a great rarity. If it occurs, it is obviously a major injury and should be treated as a medical emergency. The patient is completely disabled at once. He has

severe pain in the hip and resists any attempt to manipulate the limb. The extremity is usually held with the thigh internally rotated and adducted, with the knee resting above and against its fellow on the opposite side (Fig. 403). The trochanter appears quite prominent. Any attempt to move the thigh from this position of flexion adduction and internal rotation causes severe pain. Diagnosis is confirmed by x-ray examination, and the film should be carefully studied to make sure that there is not an accompanying fracture. This is quite infrequent in youth. The posterior acetabular margin, which is so vulnerable in the adult, is seldom broken in the adolescent or young adult.

No attempt should be made to reduce the hip on the field. The patient should be taken immediately for x-ray examination, after which the dislocation must be reduced *under anesthesia* and *at the earliest possible moment*. Although these two requirements may seem incompatible, they are vital and there is good reason for both. The most important complication of dislocation of the hip is aseptic necrosis of the head of the femur. It has been shown definitely that the frequency and degree of aseptic necrosis of the head vary in direct proportion to the length of time that the hip was displaced. Even minutes are of vital importance prior to complete reduction. On the other hand, experience has shown that it is virtually impossible to reduce a complete dislocation of the hip without profound relaxation, and any effort to do so may cause considerable damage to the vulnerable cartilage of the femoral head.

A third consideration is that it seems unwise to attempt reduction of the dislocated hip until

Figure 403. Drawing showing patient with dislocated hip. Note that the leg is shortened, internally rotated, and adducted and that there is a tendency to rest the affected foot on top of the opposite foot. Also note prominence of the greater trochanter laterally. (From DePalma, The Management of Fractures and Dislocations.)

one can be reasonably sure that there is no other injury such as would be demonstrated by x-ray examination. Clinical examination must be made to determine whether the sciatic nerve has been damaged before and after reduction. It is very distressing to discover a nerve deficit that may or may not have preceded the manipulation. In spite of the patient's discomfort, a few simple movements of the foot will demonstrate an intact nerve. If active motions in plantar flexion, toe flexion and inversion are present, the tibial portion of the nerve is not severed. If the patient can actively dorsiflex and evert the foot, the peroneal division is intact. A rudimentary sensory check may also be made. If the nerve seems completely afunctional and remains so after reduction, an early exploration is advisable, since the traumatized area of the nerve may be readily exposed by the posterior approach. On the other hand, if the lesion is incomplete or if the deficit develops gradually, one may safely assume that the injury is a contusion and compression rather than severance. In this case watchful waiting is the best treatment. The deficit may recover in a few days or a few weeks. If there has not been definite improvement within three months, the sciatic nerve should be explored. During the waiting period it is important to protect drop foot or knee flexion by a suitable brace (Fig. 404). I should like to emphasize that if loss of sciatic function is complete and immediate, surgical exploration must not be delayed more than three weeks.

Following dislocation of the hip, it is imperative that the hip be immobilized for sufficient time to permit the capsule to heal. There seems little justification for overly prolonged denial

Figure 404. Short leg brace for drop foot. The spring is included in the Klenzak joint.

of weight-bearing, however. It has been recommended in the past that weight-bearing should not be permitted for at least six months in the hope that aseptic necrosis will not develop. Studies have shown conclusively that the die is cast by the time the hip is reduced and that weight-bearing itself is not a factor in the development of aseptic necrosis. Immobilization should be continued for four to six weeks and then active rehabilitation encouraged. Active participation in sports should not be permitted for at least three months following a complete dislocation of the hip.

It must be obvious that there are cases in which the hip dislocation is incomplete and goes unrecognized. The head either does not entirely leave the socket or is spontaneously reduced. The true pathological condition can be very easily overlooked. The patient usually complains of immediate severe pain at the time of the injury, which promptly subsides, and at the time of the examination there may be essentially no positive findings. Explanation for the lack of symptoms rests in the fact that by examination of the hip joint it is very difficult to detect strain of the ligaments of the hip. In the normal hip, subluxation or dislocation cannot occur without laceration of the capsule. This usually occurs posterosuperiorly. This capsule tear is not put under stress by ordinary manipulation of the hip. The significance of this condition is that if one can be reasonably sure subluxation has occurred, the hip should be put at rest for a period of about six to eight weeks in order to permit the capsular tear to repair (Fig. 405). If it does not repair or if it repairs with redundancy, this may well be the cause of repeated episodes of incomplete dislocation of the hip. A diagnosis of incomplete dislocation of the hip is extremely uncommon, especially in the athlete, but it is probable that many such cases are not diagnosed.

In the adolescent with an unfused capital femoral epiphysis, there is occasionally a fracture through the epiphyseal plate (Fig. 406). This is a serious injury and requires adequate treatment. The symptoms of this injury, if the displacement is complete, are those of a fracture of the femoral neck. There will be severe pain in the hip, shortening of the extremity, external rotation and abduction of the thigh. However, the dislocation is frequently not complete, and this characteristic position will not be assumed. This injury may even resemble dislocation of the hip, which is another reason for careful x-ray study before any manipulative measure is carried out. If this is an

Figure 405. This interesting patient was sent in at the age of four with synovitis of the hip and a history of having had an injury to his hip the year before. It was extremely painful and sore. Perthes' disease seemed one possibility but x-rays at that time were read as negative. He seemed to improve but a year later began to limp again. A, X-ray at that time showed calcification within the capsule. No specific treatment was recommended other than to keep the patient under observation. Six months later the boy's mother called to say he was again having trouble. B, X-ray at this time showed increased calcification. The caput looked normal, and there was no real derangement of the hip. Inadequate support had resulted in an increase of calcification within the capsule. One year later the calcification looked the same, and he had no symptoms. No treatment was recommended.

Figure 406. *A,* An acute epiphyseal dislocation analogous to fracture of the neck of the femur. Note that this patient has none of the stigmata of slipped femoral epiphysis. *B,* Uneventful healing followed reduction and fixation with a Lorenzo screw. The screw was used to avoid undue trauma to the head, which could result from driving in a nail. Multiple threaded pins are probably preferable to the Lorenzo screw. This picture was at one year, but the epiphysis had closed by four months after the fixation.

acute traumatic dislocation of the epiphysis, it should be treated as a fracture of the femoral neck, with reduction and internal fixation. If this is to be successful it must be done within days, not weeks. The displaced epiphysis fixes very early to the neck. The force necessary to break it loose and so permit reduction will very likely damage the epiphysis and cause necrosis. Therefore, such force should *never* be used in such a case.

Special Conditions

A related condition for which one must be on guard is a *slipped capital femoral epiphysis* (Fig. 407). An apparently minor injury may be the precipitating cause of the slipping, and careful study should be made of any injury about the hip to determine whether there is damage involving the epiphysis or epiphyseal plate. The treatment of slipped femoral epiphysis may be quite different from that of acute epiphyseal fracture. In any of these conditions about the hip, time is of the essence. If the diagnosis is uncertain, consultation should be sought at the earliest possible moment, since

disaster with loss of function of the hip frequently results from delayed diagnosis.

Slipped capital femoral epiphysis is most likely to happen in the Fröhlich type of individual, who has excessive deposits of subcutaneous fat, together with delay in development of sex characteristics, as indicated by the infantile penis and the underdeveloped testicles. In such an individual, one's index of suspicion should be extremely high if there is pain in either the hip or knee. Very frequently hip pain is referred to the knee, whereas findings at examination of the knee may be entirely negative. Careful study of the lateral hip x-ray, as indicated in Figure 407, will be rewarding, since the slip is most often detected in the lateral view. If the slip can be detected at this early stage, as illustrated in Figure 407, adequate internal fixation without forceful manipulation will result in excellent function of the hip. On the other hand if the injury is acute and displacement is more marked and there have been no symptoms prior to the injury, cautious manipulation may be attempted to reduce the displaced epiphysis, in the course of which the hip is rotated into internal rotation and abduction. If this manipulation without force successfully reduces the displacement, the caput should be held by internal fixation with some type of screw, such as Hagie pins, in order to avoid trauma to the femoral head by pounding one of the various types of nails. In this type of individual, namely, the Fröhlich type, prophylactic fixation of the op- posite hip by some sort of screw fixation is appropriate because of the high incidence of bilateral involvement and because prophylactic pinning almost always results in a normal hip. However, if one waits until the head has slipped off, it is very difficult for the hip to ever really approach normal again. In any

Figure 407. Slipped femoral epiphysis. *A*, In the anteroposterior view, the lesion is readily overlooked. *B*, In the lateral view, the degree of slipping on the left side is revealed. (Note the osteochondritis dissecans of the acetabular roof on the same side.) *C*, One year after reduction and internal fixation, with premature closure of the epiphysis. The osteochondritis dissecans had healed. It is too early to be sure that circulatory changes in the head will not occur, and this area should be observed.

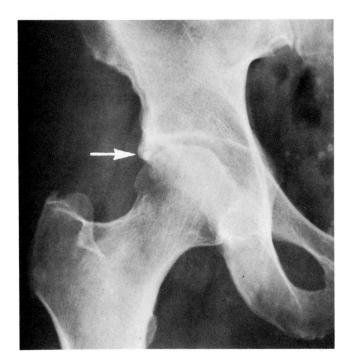

Figure 408. Typical osteochondritis dissecans of superior portion of the acetabulum. The osteocartilaginous fragment is surrounded by a radiolucent area.

event, a youngster with such a problem should be carefully checked by a competent orthopaedist, who may be able to prevent extreme and permanent disability in the hip.

Involvement of the acetabulum is not frequent in the athlete. Although chondral fractures can occur along the margin of the acetabulum, it is much more likely that the fragments seen on the x-ray are developmental. Careful study should be made of both hips before diagnosis is made of fracture of the rim of the acetabulum.

Osteochondritis dissecans (Figs. 407*B* and 408) is infrequent in the acetabulum or in the femoral head, or at least it is infrequently diagnosed. Even in a joint permitting ready x-ray visualization, such as the knee or ankle, osteochondritis dissecans may be extremely difficult to recognize. In the hip it is doubly difficult, not only because of the depth of the joint surrounded by soft tissue but also because of the fact that the head is enclosed within the acetabulum and there is superimposition of bone. Special x-ray studies may be required, such as stereoscopic pictures or laminograms. If x-ray study shows a specific lesion in the acetabular roof or the femoral head, careful analysis must be made as to whether this is really the cause of this patient's disability. If it is, surgical intervention may be indicated, but in the vast majority of cases nonsurgical treat-

ment will result in restoration of the configuration of the acetabulum and the femoral head.

The hip joint is frequently subject to *traumatic synovitis*. It appears that effusion of the hip is more common than is recognized, since it is rather difficult to determine whether there is actual distention of the hip capsule by fluid. One infrequently makes the diagnosis of synovitis of the hip. This again is probably due to the fact that the hip itself has such freedom of motion that it is not subject to the same forces that damage the knee and ankle. Many cases of limping and undiagnosed painful hips are very probably due to synovitis. In such a case diminution of activity or even complete rest is indicated. This condition may be very distressing because the patient has minimal symptoms, yet the symptoms may persist for a long time. It is hard to keep reassuring the parents that nothing is seriously wrong and that the condition will ultimately subside. If it is persistent and disabling, aspiration of the hip may be rewarding. A culture can be made of the fluid obtained from the hip joint, and if low-grade infection is determined by the laboratory report, specific antibiotic treatment may be of considerable benefit. This condition is relatively common in the pre-teenage group and fortunately almost always resolves without any major interference, just careful observation.

Injuries of the Thigh

17

This chapter covers injuries of the thigh proper. Injuries in the vicinity of the knee and hip are discussed elsewhere, under the appropriate headings. Anatomically the thigh consists of a single bone completely surrounded by very heavy muscle. One would expect the common injuries to be concerned with the muscle and such is the case. Injuries to the skin are not frequent in the thigh, since the skin is well protected by the resilient muscle pad beneath.

CONTUSION

Contusion of the thigh is a frequent injury in contact sports such as football, since the thigh often receives the brunt of a collision between participants. The thigh is extremely well suited for this, however, since its thick muscle surrounding smooth bone can absorb a tremendous amount of impact without apparent damage. Ironically, contusion of the muscle is often caused by the edge of a misplaced thigh pad, which is designed to protect the anterior part of the thigh from a direct blow. The thigh pad should be firmly strapped in place.

The *symptoms* of contusion of the thigh are much less localized than in the more subcutaneous areas. The patient is usually not disabled at the time of the blow. He is able to continue playing but at the end of the contest complains of aching and soreness within the muscle. There is disability and pain on passive stretching of the muscle involved. By far the most frequent area of involvement is some portion of the quadriceps, usually the lateralis or intermedius. The rectus is less frequently involved in a contusion, since it is protected by the muscles beneath it.

Upon *examination*, diffuse tenderness along the anterior and lateral portions of the thigh may sometimes be accompanied by muscle spasm, elicited by deep palpation. A point of sharply localized tenderness is not commonly present. Partial flexion or extension of the knee is not particularly painful, but forced flexion beyond a right angle will cause tension in the swollen muscle fibers and some distress. Active extension of the knee against firm resistance may cause rather minor and undramatic discomfort. Some degree of hematoma is probably present in any contusion of the muscle, although the bleeding may be more in the nature of an infiltration in the muscle than of pooled blood. Because it is so deep-seated, an actual hematoma of the thigh, unless it is quite extensive, can be diagnosed only with extreme difficulty.

Treatment will depend upon the severity of the lesion, and the same principles apply here as in other areas. If there seems to be infiltration of blood or hematoma formation, an attempt at aspiration under aseptic conditions is justifiable. A firm pressure bandage is applied. The bandage may be very snug and firm on the thigh of the athlete. If there is some concern about swelling distal to the pressure bandage, the bandage may be started at the toe, run to the knee and then applied with increased pressure above the knee. After the application of the compression bandage, the thigh should be carefully packed in ice and the extremity elevated and immobilized by bed rest. Since infiltration of the thigh may be quite extensive, I consider it important to encourage absorption of the blood by local injection of hyaluronidase into the immediate area. Intramuscular injection of an enzyme, 1 ml. for two to three days, is of value. Following this an oral enzyme is used. There is a wide divergence of opinion as to the value of these enzymes, since very few controlled series have been reported, and each of us is inclined to judge by his own experience. I believe that these enzymes help materially, and I use them freely when blood infiltration is a factor.

Examination the following morning will give good insight into the extent of involvement. If the thigh is tense, swollen and quite painful, immobilization should be continued along with the use of the pressure bandage. After 48 hours, heat should be substituted for cold on the assumption that any active bleeding has stopped and increased circulation is desirable. The degree of immobilization will depend entirely upon the location and extent of the area involved. A good rule of thumb is that no motion should be permitted which is painful. While the patient is in bed, a simple elastic compression bandage is adequate. When the patient is allowed to get up, the physician should immobilize the knee using a cotton cast or other similar type of dressing until the acute stage of the contusion and hematoma has passed.

Rehabilitation is extremely important and should progress as rapidly as possible but within the limits of pain. There is no excuse for forcible stretching of a contused muscle unless muscle healing is complete. On the other hand, the quadriceps muscle normally flexes functionally from its resting position, so that gentle active flexion of the knee up to the limit of pain does not necessarily put any stress on the injured area, and it will aid immeasurably in rehabilitation. *There is no place for massage in the early treatment of contusion of a muscle.* "Working it out" or "rubbing it out" simply increases the damage. On the other hand, after healing has progressed for 10 to 14 days, massage may be used as a rehabilitative measure, again within the limits of discomfort. The less extensive contusion creates a major problem in management. The player is anxious to continue his competition and practice, and one is hesitant to hold him out when he contends he can use the muscle quite well. Critical judgment is important, since a short period of complete inactivity will usually pay dividends in the long run.

MYOSITIS OSSIFICANS

The thigh is particularly prone to myositis ossificans. In my opinion this is due to the fact that the symptoms of muscle injury are often so mild that the player is allowed use of the muscle much beyond the limit set by his injury. This results in chronic irritation of the injured muscle, with the reparative response of ossification. Some degree of ossification is extremely frequent and I am sure this is increased by unwise early treatment.

Treatment. Overenthusiastic massage to "knead out the knotted muscle," forceful passive flexion of the knee, too early active use of the quadriceps, intensive exercise—all are important aggravating factors. Myositis ossificans in the thigh is not necessarily disabling when only a small plaque of bone is present in the muscle. However, it can be and frequently is extremely disabling, and the mass may reach an amazing size (Figs. 409 and 410). Once ossification occurs in contusion, the management requires even more patience than before.

Rehabilitation may progress within the limits of pain, but manipulation under anesthesia and similar measures are to be condemned (see Chapter 22 on Rehabilitation). *It can be stated unequivocally that early surgical removal of the mass of bone simply invites recurrence and magnifies the extent of the lesion itself and also the extent of disability.* This has been demonstrated too often to require further substantiation (Fig. 411). If the plaque requires removal because of disability, it should be excised only after the lesion is completely mature, as demonstrated by clinical findings and x-ray examination. It takes a minimum of six months for the lesion to mature, although frequently a longer time is needed, particularly if the lesion was overtreated in the interim. At the proper time, with the proper care, operative excision is extremely gratifying (Figs. 412 to 414).

At operation, an adequate incision that will expose the entire mass to view must be made so that the lesion can be removed without the necessity of scraping, curetting, etc. The mass is not ordinarily covered with periosteum, so I do not believe it necessary to carry out sharp dissection, leaving the capsule attached to the bone. This does not apply when the parent bone is reached, and great care should be taken not to strip the periosteum away from the femur as the mass is detached from the femoral shaft. The location of the lesion will determine the approach, and one should fit the approach to the lesion, not the lesion to the approach. I recently removed a mass from the anteromedial aspect of the femur (Fig. 415). This was readily removed by an anterior approach, whereas it would have been extremely difficult, if not impossible, to handle adequately by a more conventional anterolateral approach. In these conditions it is extremely important that surgery be atraumatic.

After the incision is made through the skin, meticulous hemostasis is obtained by electrocautery. A very careful atraumatic approach through the intervening muscle mass is important. If it is at all possible, the penetration

Figure 409. *A*, Ossification in the quadriceps lateralis. *B*, Radiograph shows it spontaneously regressed and disappearing. The patient was immobilized for six weeks, after which gradually increasing, pain-free exercises were instituted. He had complete recovery.

Figure 410. Typical extensive myositis ossificans, illustrating plaques in the muscle separated from bone. This case was treated by complete excision of the plaque, with some slight recurrence of the mass. This is quite likely to happen in an area which is this extensive.

Figure 411. Myositis ossificans. *A,* Preoperative. This mass was obviously immature at the time of the operation, which took place only a few months after injury. The surgeon succumbed to the urgings of the player, coach and parents, with the result (*B*) that the recurrence was more extensive than the original lesion. These masses must not be disturbed until they are completely mature.

should be muscle-splitting rather than muscle-dividing. The division of a muscle, if it must be done, should be by sharp dissection, obtaining careful hemostasis as the operation proceeds. Care is taken to coagulate only the vessels and not a great deal of the muscle mass. The method of making a small button-hole through the muscle and then proceeding to tear it open by so-called blunt dissection is to be avoided. In this method an index finger is placed at each extremity of the wound, and the muscle is forcibly pulled apart. This is much more disrupting and traumatic to muscle fibers than is sectioning them with a sharp instrument. It results in many torn blood vessels and muscle fibers, a condition very similar to that occurring at the time of the original contusion to the muscle.

As the bony mass is approached by careful division of the overlying structures, there is a temptation when reaching the mass to strip the tissues away from it. This temptation must be resisted. The whole purpose of the procedure is to remove the mass of bone in its entirety

and leave as little dead space, as little necrotic tissue and as little infiltrated blood as possible. After the mass is thoroughly exposed, it is divided from the femur by a sharp, curved osteotome, care being taken to leave the femoral surface smooth. In the ordinary case one can readily distinguish the line of division between the recent ossification and the femoral cortex. In the occasional case the ossification may surround the shaft and blend so intimately with the femoral cortex that no line of cleavage can be found. These cases are not ordinarily symptomatic. The femur is simply larger than normal, and surgical removal is not necessary. If attempted, it may only increase the pathological condition.

After the mass is removed, complete hemostasis should be secured, including the vessels on the femoral surface. As a rule this surface does not bleed, but if it does, the bleeding can be controlled by judicious application of bone wax. Any shreds of muscle should be carefully clipped away. At the end of the procedure the wound should be dry and

Figure 412. On the first day of spring practice this 19 year old football player, while running, started having pain in the back of the left thigh. This increased in severity, so that he had to discontinue running. Further investigation revealed that he had had trouble with both thighs since his sophomore year in high school. He had an injection in the thigh but no other treatment. Examination revealed tenderness along the semitendinosus, with a very firm area on the posterior thigh in the upper third. *A,* X-ray reveals the block of bone 9.5 cm long, 1.5 cm wide in the hamstrings. The mass appears to be very mature. Note also the mass in the adductor longus which is asymptomatic. *B,* X-ray, lateral view. Surgery revealed the mass to be in the biceps muscle right along its apposition to the semitendinosus. It did not invade the semitendinosus, however. *C,* Four months postoperative. No recurrence of fragment. No change in the fragment in the adductor.

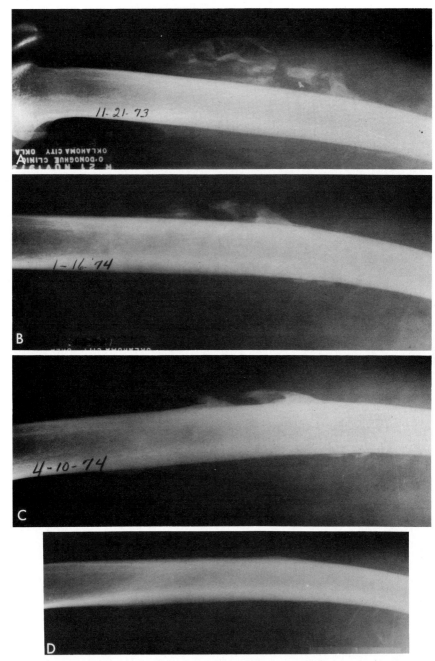

Figure 413. This 17 year old male was hit on the front of the thigh by a football helmet. He had severe pain following this for the next two or three weeks. He continued playing the rest of the game and two more games after the injury. He was told he had a bruised leg. His complaint was enlargement in front of the thigh, limited flexion of the knee, and inability to run. Examination showed a large mass which covered the whole front of the middle third of the thigh; knee flexion was 90 degrees; forced flexion was painful. A, X-ray shows the tremendous mass 19 cm. long by 4 cm. deep by 5.5 cm. wide. Since it was only two months post-injury, he was advised that the bone was quite immature, that he should definitely limit his activities and return in two months for recheck. B, Two months later note the marked diminution in size of the mass, with more definite maturity of bone but poor trabecular pattern. He was advised to wait further. C, Three months later (seven months post-injury) radiograph showing the mass quite mature, but there was still some of the mass in the muscle which was painful. Excision was carried out at this time. D, Two and one-half months postoperative, no recurrence.

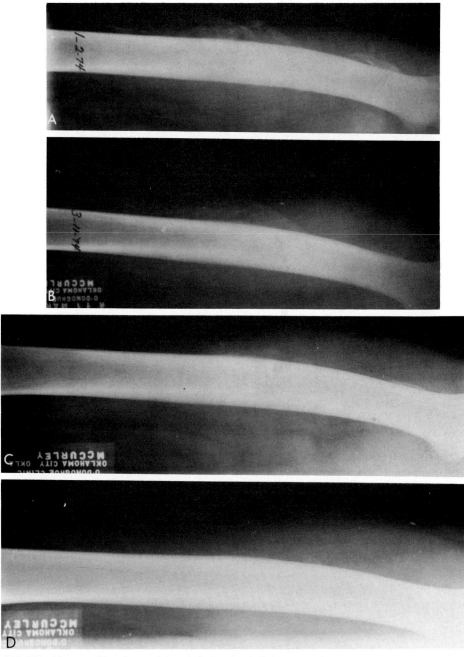

Figure 414. This 17 year old male was injured playing football three months prior to examination. *A,* X-ray shows the ragged, nonhomogenous appearance of the new bone. Note especially the smaller involvement proximal to the main mass. He was advised to let the growth mature. *B,* Two months later (five months post-injury) the mass is mature. Note the proximal mass has regressed. He was operated on at this time. The entire mass was resected with careful hemostasis. *C,* X-ray at two months postoperative shows a few remnants of ossification. *D,* X-ray one month later (three months postoperative) shows no remaining ossification. X-rays made at five months postoperative showed no recurrence.

Figure 415. *A,* Ossification of front of the upper femur (myositis ossificans), in this instance the result of partial avulsion of the iliopsoas tendon, with resulting hematoma and ossification. *B,* Six months postoperative, patient was asymptomatic.

clean looking, with well-defined margins. Closure is then carried out in layers. If possible the periosteum of the femur is sutured first. The muscle should then be carefully closed in layers, great care being taken not to leave dead space. In placing the sutures it is important that they not constrict large masses of muscle. After closure of the vaginal fascia and the skin, a firm pressure bandage is applied from the toes to the groin. It is my practice to utilize a heavy posterior plaster splint from the toes to the gluteal fold that is supported by a lateral stirrup running from high on the inner aspect of the thigh to under the foot and up to the trochanter laterally (see Fig. 452, page 482). This is bound snugly to the thigh and provides uniform pressure throughout the

lower extremity. The patient is placed in bed with the foot elevated. A suitable enzyme is given intramuscularly for three days. An oral enzyme is used post nauseam and continued for five to eight days. depending upon the degree of local reaction.

Active *rehabilitation* of the thigh is not initiated for at least three weeks. This does not prohibit isometric contraction of the quadriceps and hamstrings. We urge frequent periods of contraction of the calf and of the other muscles of the leg and foot. Unless the rectus femoris is primarily involved, we initiate active physical therapy of the hip on the involved side on the first or second day. It goes without saying that the rest of the muscles of the body are rehabilitated from the onset. The thigh and the wound are inspected at appropriate intervals. At the end of 12 to 14 days the stitches are removed and a long leg walking cast is applied, which should be worn for another four weeks, so that there has been a total rest period of at least six weeks. This may be continued for a longer period of time if there is still any evidence of injury to the muscles of the thigh. After removal of the splints at six to eight weeks, graduated active exercises are carefully begun and may need to be continued for three or four months before complete flexion of the knee is obtained. By this time the quadriceps should be of normal size.

Surgery for myositis ossificans of the thigh is not justified unless one is prepared to take the time and the pains required to make the necessarily rigorous regimen a success. This fact must be fully accepted by the surgeon and carefully explained to the player, his parents and the coach so that there can be no misunderstanding as to the time and effort required. Active participation in contact sports cannot be permitted until rehabilitation is complete.

The close resemblance of early myositis ossificans to osteogenic sarcoma has been the cause of constant apprehension and of all too frequent error. In early biopsy the gross pathological condition in microscopic specimen resembles tumor because of the immature growing bone. A little patience will reveal the different course of the two lesions. Lesions due to myositis ossificans rapidly mature and are sharply delineated as they mature. They do not invade the cortex or the medullary canal. Osteogenic sarcoma or Ewing's tumor is destructive as well as productive and tends to progress rapidly, with the destruction becoming more notable as the growth progresses. The malignant tumor may cause fever, malaise, pain and anorexia. The very unfavorable prognosis of even radical treatment of the tumor indicates that one should not panic into performing an amputation or prescribing extensive radiation therapy on the basis of the presence of immature bone. The unfavorable prognosis does not seem to be altered too much by a matter of two or three weeks' observation. In fact, some authorities say treatment is better after the malignant lesion is a little more mature. Although it may be nerve-racking, in the case of myositis ossificans a period of observation will be rewarded by subsidence of the symptoms and maturity of the lesion, at which time no further treatment may be indicated unless there is a physical mass of bone which will interfere with muscle function later. I must emphasize again the extreme importance of distinguishing myositis ossificans from osteogenic sarcoma. I have personally seen cases which, following biopsy of the lesion, have been treated radically for osteogenic sarcoma when actually the original lesion was ossification within the muscle. It is almost impossible to distinguish between the early growing bone of a myositis ossificans and the early osteogenesis of a sarcoma of the bone by pathological examination. I mention this again, although it is well covered in Chapter 4, since the majority of these lesions do occur in the thigh.

STRAIN

The muscles of the thigh are subject to the same stresses as muscles in other locations. Actually, these are extreme stresses because of the thigh's function of propelling the human body under various degrees of resistance. The strain may be mild, moderate or severe, and the treatment should be gauged accordingly. The mild, or first degree, strain simply will result in a painful muscle because of hemorrhage to a few muscle fibers. This will promptly resolve and result in no disability. Active treatment is really not necessary, and the vast majority of these cases never come to the attention of a physician. As in strain anywhere, one must resist the temptation to forcibly massage the muscle and stretch it beyond the pain-free range.

A more severe problem is the moderate, or second degree, strain in which there is definite damage to a segment of the muscle, which will definitely reduce the ability of this muscle to function. In this type of case it is important to determine the degree of the tear if possible. Although there is not a complete rupture of the muscle, the muscle may be quite severely damaged short of actual rupture. The early treatment should consist of rest and application of ice.

Resumption of muscle function must be within the limits of pain. Nothing is to be gained by forcing the painful muscle, since this just increases the spasm. As the acute symptoms subside, the danger point occurs because in a couple of weeks the subjective symptoms may be essentially gone; yet, the muscle will be materially weakened and may well rupture in its next stressful situation. Hence, it is important to decide if there has actually been definite loss of function of a significant percentage of the muscle. It is notable that complete muscle tear is frequently preceded by a less serious injury which has healed inadequately. Since the player wants to resume the very activity which caused the problem in the first place, there is a distressingly high rate of recurrence under these conditions. Take, for example, the "hamstring pull," so frequent in sprinting in either football, basketball, track or, in fact, any active sport. In this instance, the player, while running, feels a sharp pain in the hamstring muscle somewhere along its course, which is often sufficient to make him stop running. He goes through the classic stages of pain, muscle spasm, restriction of motion, and loss of strength. Yet, his impatience to return to competition means that he does not wait until the muscle actually heals; he simply waits until the symptoms subside. Then he goes back to the same activity, this time with repeated injuries. What started out as a relatively minor injury of the muscle may result in the complete loss of the season for the player. The only control of this situation is to insist on absolute elimination of stress in this muscle until it is entirely healed. This may be very difficult to do. Painless motion should not cause trouble, so that the player can be rehabilitated to a certain extent. But when he gets to feeling very good and starts that burst of speed again, the trouble returns and he is back to the doctor with a discouraging recurrence of his disability.

Various measures may serve to reinforce the muscle. Physical therapy, using inductive heat, is often good. The prevalent habit of strapping the thigh with snugly fitting adhesive seems to help, largely by virtue of the fact that it limits the action of the muscle to some extent. Careful adherence to the principles laid down in the section on Strain (page 51) will aid in solving this very distressing problem.

MUSCLE RUPTURE

The muscles of the thigh are sometimes ruptured. A particularly susceptible one is the rectus femoris, which extends from above the hip to below the knee. The injury often occurs as the result of a forcible blow on the muscle while it is in fixed contraction and the two ends of the muscle are firmly fixed. The muscle mechanism will tolerate considerable stress without rupture. If, while the muscle is under maximum stress, additional tension is caused by sharp flexion of the knee, the muscle gives way somewhere along its length. This is illustrated in the running athlete as he suddenly reverses the direction of the knee motion from extension to flexion by falling or by having his knee forcibly flexed. The additional force causes the muscle to give way. The most frequent sites for rupture are at the attachment of the rectus at the hip and the conjoined tendon above the patella.

If the tear is complete and is recognized early, surgical repair will be quite gratifying. Ordinarily the condition is diagnosed as a contusion or hematoma, and it is not until the local swelling and reaction subside that the true nature of the condition becomes apparent. By this time repair may not be possible if the rupture is within the muscle fibers. If there is actual avulsion of the attachment at the anteroinferior spine, it can be repaired even if the injury was recognized rather late. Frequently the muscle is torn off the tendon at the junction of the lower and middle third of the thigh or it may be separated at about the level of the lesser trochanter. In either instance the muscle bunches up on contraction and presents a definite tumor mass (Fig. 416). This swelling disappears when the muscle is relaxed. At-

Figure 416. Silhouette view of the front of the thigh while the patient is holding the quadriceps contracted. Arrow indicates bulging mass of the lower end of the rectus resulting from partial avulsion of the rectus attachment to the quadriceps tendon.

tempts at repair after several weeks may be very disappointing, since it may be impossible to suture the muscle down firmly enough to obtain the additional length required to bring the ends into apposition.

The typical patient will present with a painful swollen thigh, with rather localized tenderness in the muscle. Following treatment for contusion, the soreness will persist and the muscle mass will appear. There may be substantial disability for many weeks. After the local reaction disappears and the nature of the condition is recognized, the surgeon should carefully explain to the patient that the rupture will probably cause no actual disability, and that the pain and tenderness will completely disappear, but that the bunched-up mass of muscle will remain. He will notice that the muscle of this thigh is different from that of his other thigh. Usually careful explanation of the nature of the condition is satisfactory, and the athlete will condition himself to the asymmetry and will be little the worse for his lesion. Occasionally persistent pain will remain, apparently from chronic myositis or constricting fibrosis of the detached muscle ends. In this case, careful surgical removal of the detached portion of the muscle eliminates the mass and will relieve the pain (Fig. 417). One can only justify this procedure after a very thorough trial of physical therapy and rehabilitation. This type of surgery probably adds no strength to the thigh but serves only to reduce the muscle mass and to relieve the pain.

This same situation occasionally arises in the adductor muscles, particularly the adductor longus (Fig. 418). The signs will be present at some point between the pubis and the medial condyle of the femur. In this situation if it is the attachment that is avulsed, repair is quite satisfactory. If the tear is within the muscle itself, repair must be carried out within the first two weeks to have much chance for success. This same condition also occurs in the hamstring muscles, but avulsion of either origin or attachment is more frequent than tear in the muscle and so is more successfully sutured.

A good deal of acumen is needed to recognize an isolated muscle rupture. This is particularly true when the ruptured muscle is one of several muscles carrying out the same function; for example, the rectus femoris muscle (Fig. 419), one of the adductor muscles or one of the hamstrings. During the early stages of the acute injury, the telltale sign of bunching up of the muscle because it has lost its attachment

Figure 417. This athlete gave a history of running hard and receiving a "pulled muscle" in the thigh. No treatment was given other than advice to "work it out." He was examined six months after the injury. He had been sent in for a Baker's cyst, and the notation was that it was a little high. On examination, a firm mass was palpable in the posteromedial thigh just above the knee. This mass was nonpulsating, and on flexion of the knee against resistance, it moved downward and became more prominent. This was accompanied by aching pain. The patient's complaint was that on running hard he had pain of increasing severity in the back of the thigh. At surgery six months post-injury, this mass was found to be a muscle belly with a long tendon below and a spindle-shaped upper end, which was attached only by loose areolar tissue (A). Further dissection revealed the neurovascular bundle entering the mass in the posterosuperior aspect (B). The upper end detached (C). Note nerve entering muscle at superior end. The symptoms were caused by traction on the nerve in the neurovascular bundle as the semitendinosus muscle contracted. Muscle was entirely removed, relieving the symptoms.

is usually well screened by the associated local swelling.

The extremely heavy muscles of the thigh receive tremendous strain in almost any athletic competition. The very fact that the muscle ruptured in a given athlete would suggest excessive strain in the area involved. For this reason, athletic competition must be sharply

Figure 418. An 18 year old boy was injured at water-skiing when his ski turned outward throwing his thigh into forced external rotation-abduction. Severe knifelike pain occurred on the inner side of the thigh, with immediate disability. He was treated expectantly with application of heat and rest after a diagnosis of a ruptured vessel. He was seen four months post-injury because of a firm mass in the upper inner thigh. The mass itself was not painful but varied in size and was disabling because, when the youth would run, the mass would tighten up and strike the testicle. Running was interdicted. On examination there was a soft but firm mass along the adductor muscle just below the pubis extending about 5 in. distally. On contraction of the adductor, this mass would travel upward and become more prominent and more firm. Diagnosis was made of ruptured adductor, either adductor longus or gracilis. Surgery was recommended because of the disability.

A, The muscle at rest. B, With the adductor contracted showing impingement against the scrotum. C, The muscle dissected out, showing complete detachment of the lower end from its femoral attachment and rounding off of the end. Note the tendinous attachment of the avulsed adductor longus, with the intact gracilis lying inferior to it. D, Stimulating the branch of the obturator nerve to the adductor longus. Note contraction of the muscle into the spherical shape suggested in B. Uneventful recovery. Early diagnosis and surgical repair might have saved this muscle.

curtailed following such an injury. Certainly during the acute period no active use of the extremity should be permitted. As in so many instances of muscle damage, premature attempts at strenuous activity can result only in disappointment and prolongation of disability. A minimum of six weeks is needed for the healed tissue to even approach maturity, and even at this time, the scar is very susceptible to injury. Actually, the best criterion for active use is the level of pain experienced by the patient himself, since pain-free activity does not do any harm. The difficulty is that he may go along with ordinary pain-free activity and a sudden burst of exertion may cause reinjury. It would seem advisable to restrict activity sharply for at least six weeks. This is not to say that rehabilitation cannot be proceeding within the limits of pain. Protection of the muscle by padding or strapping is extremely difficult, since active contraction rather than passive stretching may cause the damage.

FASCIAL HERNIA

The muscles of the thigh are completely invested in one continuous sheath of fascia— the vaginal fascia of the thigh. Vagina means sheath, and this fascial sheath does indeed contain the voluminous muscles in a well-defined envelope. The fascia itself is inelastic but may change shape as the enclosed muscle mass shifts. Therefore, it is not easily torn, and a traumatic defect in the fascia of the thigh is not common. It may occur, however, and present as a fascial hernia, usually along the anterolateral aspect of the thigh, where the fascia becomes thinner anterior to the iliotibial band. The ordinary symptoms of fascial hernia may be present. There is a palpable tumor mass, particularly notable when the muscle is relaxed. In some instances, if there is not too much subcutaneous tissue, a linear defect in the fascia may be detected. When the quadriceps muscle is contracted to extend the knee, the tumor mass will disappear, and the defect will be less noticeable. If this rent is large enough, it probably will be asymptomatic. A small tear may cause some discomfort by pinching the areolar tissue or fat between the tight edges of the split fascia.

Treatment is usually not necessary. If the symptoms are too severe, the condition may be treated surgically by repair of the rent, provided that the edges are well defined and reparable. If repair of the defect is impossible, relief may be obtained by simply enlarging the slit to a length of 7.5 to 10 cm. This condition is ordinarily not disabling, and treatment can usually be postponed until a convenient time. Usually the patient becomes accustomed to the condition, and it becomes asymptomatic.

FRACTURE OF FEMORAL SHAFT

Fracture of the shaft of the femur is a very serious injury but fortunately is not frequent in athletes. The fracture occurs as a result of excessive force, usually rotatory in nature, applied to the lower extremities, and as a rule,

Figure 419. This 40 year old surgeon was playing football with his youngster, ran off the clipped lawn into tall grass, had a knifelike pain in the right groin and fell. Examination revealed local swelling in the groin, with severe pain on active flexion of the hip, less severe on passive flexion of the knee. Palpation revealed marked tenderness just in front of the hip, with the feeling of a defect above and a nodule below. Midline incision revealed the rectus femoris had been torn off the anterior inferior spine in a "Z" fashion, about half of the tendon tearing off the bone and the other half tearing off the muscle. *A* reveals the tendon avulsed from the anterior inferior spine, held in the left hemostat. Arrow, right, indicates the parallel portion of the tendon still attached to the muscle held by long Kelly forceps. *B,* Realignment with side to side apposition of the split tendon.

Figure 420. Traction splint for fractured femoral shaft, a half-ring splint with Jones' hitch. This type of traction should not be used for a long period, and care should be taken to preserve the circulation to the foot.

the ankle, leg or knee will give way before the femur does. If the fracture is complete, the disability is immediate, and usually there is little difficulty in recognizing the lesion. Incomplete fracture requires an x-ray examination for detection. In the presence of a serious injury to the thigh, the patient should be taken on a stretcher to the hospital, and if the fracture is not obvious, a definitive diagnosis should be made using radiography. For transportation a traction splint is applied, the most useful being a Thomas splint with half ring that rests against the ischial tuberosity, with the traction applied to the foot. For short periods this can be applied by a Jones hitch (Fig. 420) tied around the ankle and foot and twisted to tighten the rope. Great care should be taken not to constrict circulation of the foot for a long time with this apparatus. Treatment of fracture should be instituted at once.

It is not necessary here to define the various methods of *treatment* of fracture of the femur. It will be borne in mind that the athlete is usually young and healthy, that his healing potential is good and that he is very anxious to be rehabilitated promptly. He will of course lose the current season of competition.

Since this injury has happened to a young person with excellent general health, the very best method may be employed to restore him to normal activity. If open surgery is recommended, it should be balanced against the less hazardous, so-called conservative treatment. If conservative treatment requires traction for six to eight weeks, it must be demonstrated that this method is better than reduction and cast

or open reduction and internal fixation. The ingrown advantage of so-called conservative treatment is not valid in the young athlete. Again it must be remembered that the athlete is usually a young, healthy person, that his healing potential is good and that he is very anxious to be rehabilitated promptly.

Rehabilitation is extremely important in this type of fracture. The patient should be carefully instructed in exercise of the other extremities and in the use of whatever muscles of the involved extremity are available. If he is treated by traction he can keep the knee mobilized to a considerable degree. If he is placed in a plaster cast, isometric contractions will help, and he should be instructed to contract all the muscle within the cast, as by "shrugging" the patella and "setting" the calf. If he is treated by intramedullary fixation and this is successful enough to obviate the necessity for external fixation, rehabilitation can proceed much more rapidly.

One should emphasize again that although rehabilitation may proceed rapidly, active competition must not be permitted until the fractured femur is solidly united and the muscles of the thigh and calf are as large and strong as those on the other side. The range of the motion in all the joints must be normal. The strain on the fractured femur is magnified tremendously if there is any restriction of flexion of the knee, and re-fracture is certainly a distinct possibility due to the increased leverage. Knee motion must be essentially complete in range before any activity is permitted that could cause forcible flexion of the knee.

18

Injuries of the Knee

ANATOMICAL CONSIDERATIONS

The knee is probably the most vulnerable joint of the body from the standpoint of athletic injury. The articular cartilage of the femoral condyle at the lower end of the femur is divided into two areas in its posterior and distal aspect, the medial condyle and the lateral condyle. In front, however, the two become confluent to form the trochlear groove for the patella. Although functionally the knee joint is a hinge joint, physiologically it is a gliding joint, the femoral condyle rolling over the saucers of the tibial plateau, which are slightly deepened by the semilunar cartilages. The patellofemoral joint, particularly, is a gliding joint, the patella sliding up and down in the trochlear groove as the knee is flexed and extended. The posterior capsular ligament prevents overextension of the joint and, with the knee in complete extension, prevents medial or lateral instability (see Fig. 447). The lateral ligaments (see Fig. 446) prevent collateral motion. The lateral components also help to control rotation of the tibia on the femur. The medial components control slipping between the femur and the tibia on the medial side, whereas the lateral components control the slipping on the lateral side. Acting together, they control anterior and posteror displacement of the tibia on the femur. Anteriorly, support is given by the quadriceps mechanism, which provides constant tension on the ligamentum patellae, no matter what position the knee is in, so long as the quadriceps is normal.

The knee is enclosed in a capsule that is very closely applied to the ligaments posteriorly and laterally (see Fig. 447). In front it becomes more redundant, which permits flexion of the knee. It is tight anteriorly only with the knee in complete flexion. The superior fold of the knee capsule continues into the suprapatellar pouch, the two being divided to a greater or lesser extent by the plica semilunaris. When the knee is in flexion, this anterior structure is quite taut and when the knee is in extension, it becomes quite redundant. There is a cone-shaped fat pad which fills the gap between the patellar tendon and the joint. This is fastened back to the intercondylar notch by the ligamentum mucosa to give the fat pad some degree of fixation. The only intrasynovial structures in the knee are the semilunar cartilages and the popliteus tendon. The cruciate ligaments, the fat pad and all the other ligaments are extrasynovial.

The anatomically unstable joint is reinforced mainly by muscular structures. The quadriceps muscles covering the entire front of the thigh converge to attach into the patella, with some of the fibers of the aponeurosis extending medially and laterally as the patellar retinaculum to become continuous with the fascia of the leg. This provides extremely powerful extension to the leg. The anatomical position of the quadriceps is with the knee in extension. The muscle has to be extended from its resting position in order to function as an active knee extensor. The hamstring muscles arise from the back of the femur and the pelvis and extend to below the knee, where they attach on either side of the leg. These are powerful flexors of the knee. These muscles contract within their resting length in order to flex the knee. The fact that the internal hamstring tendons sweep around the medial side of the upper tibia to attach in front provides a lateral and rotatory stabilizing component to the hamstrings. These tendons also aid in preventing anterior displacement of the tibia on the femur.

The medial collateral ligament has many divisions, but from the standpoint of function there are essentially two layers. The short fibers run from the femoral condyle to the upper tibial margin and extend forward only to the midlateral line. Posteriorly these fibers blend into the posterior ligament of the knee. The more superficial portion of the medial collateral ligament extends down to attach to the tibia, 3 to 4 in. below the upper tibial

447

margin, passing under the pes anserinus. It lies under the fascia of the leg, blending with the deep fibers usually at about the line of the joint. The fact that this portion of the ligament attaches well below the tibial margin and anteriorly allows an arc of motion that permits the knee to bend while the ligament remains constantly tense.

The lateral ligamentous support of the knee has been generally misunderstood. True enough, the strong ligamentous band extending from the head of the fibula to the femoral condyle is called the lateral collateral ligament. A brief consideration of the anatomy indicates that lateral stability should not depend upon a band from the fibula to the femur. The fibula does not enter into the articulation of the knee joint and should not be considered as a major support of the knee. The iliotibial tract is a tremendous factor in the stability of the knee. As the iliotibial tract passes distally from the tensor fasciae femoris muscle, it becomes the vaginal fascia of the thigh. As it approaches the knee, it becomes a very dense fibrous band, which attaches to the distal femur through the intermuscular septum. Traversing distally across the knee, it attaches to the upper tibial flare at the tubercle of Gerdy. This structure is the true lateral collateral ligament of the knee. Whereas the short capsular fibers on the medial side usually blend with the long fibers of the medial collateral ligament, there is no such arrangement on the lateral side. The short capsular fibers laterally are relatively weak and have no connection to either the iliotibial band or the fibular collateral ligament. They may blend with the short fibular collateral ligament fibers, which run from the fibula to the femoral condyle, just adjacent to the capsule. The lateral meniscus attaches to these short capsular fibers by means of the coronary ligament.

With the knee in flexion, the femoral condyles are somewhat protected against a direct blow by the patella. The margins are quite vulnerable on either side of the patella, however. A direct blow may damage the articular cartilage of the patella or femur.

The medial and lateral menisci are intrasynovial and serve to deepen somewhat the fossa of the upper plateau of the tibia. They are minimally weight-bearing and tend to fill the crevice left by the lack of congruity of the arcs of the condyles of the femur and the plateau of the tibia. Only a relatively small area of the femoral condyle and a similarly small area of the tibial plateau are primarily weight-bearing. It should be noted that the menisci have bony attachments anteriorly and posteriorly, the me-

dial meniscus being "C" shaped and attached well toward the front and well toward the back of the upper surface of the tibia, whereas the lateral meniscus is more "O" shaped and attaches within the two attachments of the medial meniscus (see Fig. 510).

The anterior cruciate ligament arises from the nonarticular area on top of the tibia in front and extends upward, backward and outward to attach well posteriorly in the intercondylar notch on the medial side of the lateral condyle of the femur. The posterior cruciate ligament, on the other hand, attaches anteriorly in the intercondylar notch on the lateral side of the medial condyle, right at the cartilage margin. It extends backward, downward and outward, passing over the back edge of the tibia, through a well-defined groove, to attach to the posterior surface of the tibia near the midline (see Fig. 446).

The popliteus hiatus, which is an interruption of the short capsular fibers and the coronary ligament, permits the passage of the popliteus tendon. The tendon comes forward from the muscle origin on the back of the tibia to attach to the lateral surface of the lower femur, just superior to the chondral margin at about the midlateral point.

The entire front of the knee is subcutaneous. In many instances bursae lie between the skin and the underlying bone. Posteriorly, the gastrocnemius muscle and the hamstring tendons lie between the skin and the underlying bone. The vessels and nerves crossing the popliteal space are well protected by their deep position between the two femoral condyles, which project much further posteriorly than anteriorly.

DIFFERENTIAL DIAGNOSIS

The knee joint area presents a real challenge to one who treats its injuries. Anatomically the knee lacks the stability of the hip, with its ball and socket, or the ankle, with its mortise and tenon, each of which gives some degree of bony stability. At the knee joint the socket of the top of the tibia is so minimal that, indeed, the lateral tibial plateau may be flat or even convex. The little buffering by the menisci provides only a minimal increase in stability, since the menisci are unstable themselves. So, the stability of the knee must depend largely upon the soft tissue, namely, ligaments, capsule and muscles, aided by the fact that the lower end of the femur is like a bipod and one must lift or slide a condyle to develop instability. Hence, the extreme importance of making an accurate diagnosis as to the exact nature of the knee injury—this is doubly important because it is vital that the definitive diagnosis be made early so that treatment can be begun early. Examinaton must be determine two things: what part is injured, and how bad the injury is. The parts that may be injured include the following:

1. Ligaments.
2. Muscle tendon.
3. Capsule.
4. Menisci.
5. Cartilage.
6. Bone.
7. Bursae.
8. Any combination of these.

History

A complete history is vital in order to determine when the injury happened, how it happened and why it happened. What has been done since the injury? Was the player disabled? Did he come off the field by himself? Was he carried or helped off? Did he continue to play? Did he feel that he was badly hurt? Did anyone straighten out his leg? Did he feel something snap or pop? Did he have severe pain? Was swelling immediate? If so, where was it? Then study his present condition. Did he walk in without support or with crutches? Is the knee still sore? Does it give way or slip? Does motion hurt? Such information should be acquired before the knee is actually examined.

Examination

Examination should be done just as soon as the player can get to a place where proper examination can be carried out. A preliminary survey may be done even on the field in order to have some assessment as to the severity of the injury and how the player should be transported. As soon as possible, the player should be taken to a place where his clothes, pads, tape and the like can be removed from both legs. It is better that this is away from a crowd of players, fans and parents. You need to have the injured player's total attention. He should not be distracted by parents, coaches or teammates. It is always best to examine the opposite knee first. It allays the patient's apprehension and gives the examiner some guide as to what is the normal for this particular individual.

Observation. First, look at the knee. Observe contusions, swelling, discoloration and especially deformity. Compare one leg's appearance with that of the other. Is the patella displaced? Is there knock-knee or bowleg? Many times an objective look at the knee may give a genuine lead as to the pathological condition (Fig. 421). Position the legs at 90 degree flexion, with both feet flat on the table, and check the anterior profile of the injured knee. Does the tibia hang backward, suggesting posterior cruciate and posterior capsular redundancy? (Fig. 422). Is the patellar alignment normal? Note any difference between the injured and the normal leg. With the patient sitting with the legs hanging over the edge of the table at 90 degrees, check the position of the patella in relation to the patellar groove. Is there evidence that the patella angulates and faces laterally rather than straight ahead? Ask the patient to kick the leg up and down from 90 degrees of flexion to complete extension. Observe the path of the patella in the trochlear groove. Does it shift from side to side? Particularly, does it move into a lateral position as it comes toward complete extension? Ask the patient to squat if possible, and determine variation from the normal (Fig. 423).

Palpation. After observing the extremity, feel it. Note local heat, fluctuation and tension of the skin. Most important of all, locate any areas of tenderness exactly. Usually the tenderness will be at the site of the injury, whereas pain may well be away from this site. Determine if the swelling is actually in the knee. Is it hemarthrosis or effusion, or is it in the soft tissues? Careful palpation may indeed give an important lead to the proper diagnosis, for example, palpation of the tibial tuberosity can aid in the diagnosis of apophysitis or apophyseal fracture. Tenderness along the medial edge of the patella may suggest lateral luxation of the patella. The meniscus is likely to be torn where the tenderness is. In ligament injuries, tenderness is at the site of the tear. Palpation of a chondral foreign body in the knee may be the only objective clue to its presence when the x-ray findings are negative and there are no other physical findings.

Manipulation. *Manipulation should not be attempted until observation and palpation have been completed.* Manipulation may be defined as skillful use of the hands. It should be carried out on the normal knee first. It must be careful and gentle. If you grab the injured leg and shake it around like a terrier does a rat, not only will you make the patient very uncooperative but also you will get very little useful

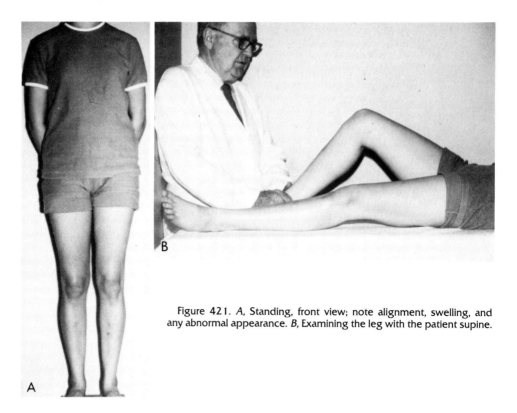

Figure 421. *A*, Standing, front view; note alignment, swelling, and any abnormal appearance. *B*, Examining the leg with the patient supine.

information. Check active motion first to note pain on motion, as from a muscle tendon injury, or limitation of motion by a locked meniscus or a foreign body. Check the knee carefully for crepitation under the patella as it is actively flexed and extended. Then add resistance to see if this increases crepitation or pain (Fig. 424). The same approach should be used for chondral damage in other areas of the knee. Compare active with passive motion, since passive motion may demonstrate a range not possible by voluntary contraction of the injured muscle.

Examine the patella for tenderness, pain, crepitation or instability as you slide it from side to side (glissement). The apprehension test (Fig. 425) to check for instability of the

patella should be done by flexing the knee to 30 degrees, with the patient in a supine position. Have someone hold the foot to permit the hamstrings to relax and then force the patella laterally. It may slip off or partially sublux. The patient's apprehension that it may slip off suggests a subluxing or a dislocating patella. Zero response indicates a stable patella. Grade 1 elicits mild anxiety, suggestive of some degree of instability. In Grade 2 there is more marked reaction as the patient moves the leg around, tightening up the muscles. In Grade 3 he grabs the physician's hands to prevent subluxation. In Grade 4 he takes a swing at the physician! Note also the "Q" angle formed by the intersection of the line of the quadriceps mechanism to the midpoint of

Figure 422. Note profile of two knees; the left (nearer) sags backward compared with the normal right knee, indicating posterior cruciate defect.

Figure 423. With the patient squatting, note position of patellae, depth of squat and location of pain.

the patella and the line from midpatella to the tibial tuberosity (see Fig. 477). An increased angle suggests a potential for subluxation (see Fig. 478).

Some of the tests for ligaments are as follows: The "drawer" test (see Fig. 458), which checks the anteroposterior motion of the tibia on the femur, indicates if there is damage to the cruciate ligaments. The drawer sign should be checked with the foot at neutral position,

medial rotation and lateral rotation to determine some possible involvement of the collateral ligaments. Collateral instability should be determined first with the knee in complete extension (Fig. 426). In this position the intact posterior capsule will prevent collateral instablity, even if the medial and lateral components are damaged. With the knee flexed 30 degrees (Fig. 427), the posterior capsule will not provide medial or lateral stability, and the defect in the medial or lateral ligamentous elements may be checked. Flexion-rotation tests are important to determine rotatory instability and also the possibility of meniscus damage. One should note the presence and location of the pain. If there is snapping or popping, is it constant or transitory? The foot is placed into internal rotation and the flexion test repeated to note variations from the straight position (Fig. 428). The foot is then placed into external rotation and the same tests are repeated (Fig. 429).

X-Ray. X-ray examination is an extremely important factor in the diagnosis of any knee injury. It is diagnostic in many conditions and often serves to rule out a suspected lesion. The position of the limb for x-ray is of considerable importance. An "as is" x-ray view may be the most revealing of all. For this view simply place the knee over the x-ray plate, without positioning the leg or holding the foot. The x-ray is then taken. (Fig. 430). The result may be quite dramatic and also quite revealing in complete or partial dislocation of the knee or in some fractures of the femoral condyles or tibial plateaus (see Fig. 539). After this, take "routine" x-ray views. I prefer to take a

Figure 424. Forced flexion to determine whether there is pain or snapping and where it is.

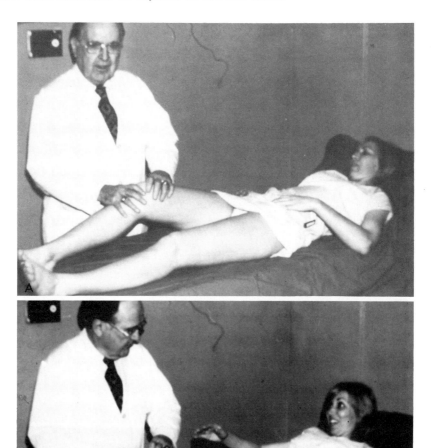

Figure 425. The apprehension test. *A*, The patient is positioned with the knee flexed at 30 degrees. The examiner grasps the patella between the thumb and index finger and forces the patella laterally. *B*, The apprehensive reaction of the patient indicates instability of the patella.

standing anteroposterior x-ray of both knees if it is feasible, since weight-bearing may show things not visible in a film with the patient supine. Then take a lateral x-ray of each knee. This may reveal an osteochondritis dissecans, osteochondral defects, degenerative changes in the patellofemoral joint, problems of the tibial tuberosity, patellar alta (see Fig. 481) and fractures or other injuries to the patella. A silhouette view also should be taken of each patella (see Fig. 491). This will help to reveal patellar subluxation, fractures of the patella, either of the bone or of the patellar cartilage, or irregularity of the undersurface of the patella. Multiple views may be necessary in case there is any doubt as to the findings on the

standard views. The oblique views visualize the individual condyles better and are particularly useful in determining damage to the anterior or posterior segment of either condyle. It may be necesssary to take a notch x-ray view that will show the presence of a foreign body or possible avulsion of the cruciate ligament with a segment of bone.

Only after these x-ray views have been obtained and examined should stress films be made (Figs. 431 and 457). The primary function of the stress film is to demonstrate ligament instability. However, it may be a false finding since in the acute injury if the knee has been examined repeatedly and has been stressed to determine instability, it may be

Figure 426. First, check lateral motion with the knee extended. In this position the posterior capsule is tight. Even with the medial collateral ligament gone, the knee will be stable in this position if the posterior capsule is intact.

very difficult for the x-ray technician to hold the knee open while an x-ray is made. There is often a dividend from stress films in that they may reveal some other condition. I have seen patients come in who were diagnosed as having a ruptured medial ligament when there was actually a fracture of the medial femoral condyle or of the upper tibia (see Fig. 537). Stress films are also of value in determining how thick the articular cartilage is on the side of the joint that is compressed. These tests, like all others, should be done carefully in order not to add damage to a part already injured. For this reason I do not like any of the mechanical ways of stressing the joint, since they can exert tremendous forces and may complete an incomplete ligament tear simply by overstress.

A further word about the stress films and ligament instability: I don't think stress films are needed to demonstrate ligament instability of the knee. They are helpful in determining whether the instability is medial or lateral, particularly in old injuries in which the element of acute pain is not present. However, in the acute injury I would accept the findings of a physicial examination showing instability of the knee, even though the x-ray did not show any actual separation. I would like to emphasize again that the reason for this is that if the knee

Figure 427. Second, check lateral motion with the knee flexed. In this position the posterior capsule is lax. Instability here indicates medial collateral loss.

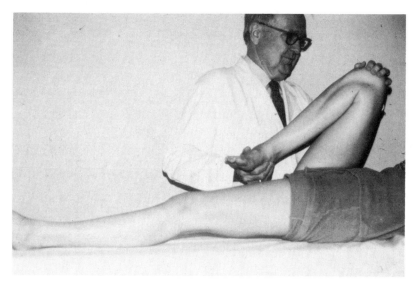

Figure 428. Forced flexion with the leg internally rotated puts different stress on menisci than straight flexion. Notice snapping and pain and location.

has been hurt, has been quite painful and has been examined by several people, by the time the x-ray technician gets around to holding the knee open while an x-ray is made, muscle spasm has taken over and the stress film findings may be entirely negative, yet there may be obvious clinical instability of the knee.

One should be very critical of x-ray films. It is no excuse to later say "it is a poor film, so I couldn't see the abnormality." If the film does not appear to satisfactorily demonstrate the area of interest, then have it done again. Nothing is more humiliating than having someone else make a picture which reveals a pathological condition that you should have discovered yourself. Demand adequate x-rays.

Arthrography

Arthrography is becoming increasingly popular in the differential diagnosis of pathological conditions of the knee. Ironically, the physician who needs it the most is likely to utilize it the least and to profit from the result of the study the least. It requires a radiology department with the know-how to make the proper views plus a specialist, either a radiologist or orthopaedist, who can properly interpret the films. This combination is most likely to occur in a place where many knees are examined. The irony of the situation is that in this circumstance one is least likely to need the more sophisticated diagnostic technique. Statistical

Figure 429. Forced flexion with the leg externally rotated, the opposite of Fig. 428. Note difference in pain or snapping.

studies are valid only if the conditions are properly controlled. To say that arthrography is 80 per cent correct as confirmed by surgery while clinical examination is only 75 per cent correct becomes valid only by definition of who is doing what. The experienced examiner will have a far different rate of success than will the occasional examiner. I see little excuse for routine arthrography. Not only is it expensive, but it also subjects the patient to another procedure. Even if it is shown that the danger of complication is minimal, it still cannot be a pleasurable experience to the recipient. If the result of arthrography is not going to change your management of a patient, I question its relevance. In the problem case it has its place and may be very valuable. If findings are positive, it certainly is comforting to the surgeon who has already decided on arthrotomy. But what about negative findings using arthrography in the symptomatic patient? One sees patients who have been examined previously and who were told that because the arthrographical findings were negative, nothing was wrong and therefore nothing could be done. This is small comfort to the patient who knows that something is wrong. A false negative result is probably worse than a false posi-

Figure 430. *A*, "As is" picture showing a complete anterior dislocation of the knee, with obvious ligament damage. *B*, "As is" view, *just as significant as A*, showing rupture of the anterior cruciate, medial collateral, and medial posterior capsule. *C*, The "positioned" anteroposterior view of the same knee as *B* showing no pathological change.

A   **B**

Figure 431. Stress films made with the knee flexed (A) and with the knee extended (B). Note the markedly greater amount of opening up when the posterior capsule is eliminated in A. This indicates major involvement of the medial collateral ligament, with a partial tear of the posteromedial capsule.

tive one. In regard to the value of arthrography in actually localizing the lesion, I say that in most instances a thorough examination of the knee at arthrotomy will reveal the occasional error made in locating the lesion by clinical examination. I certainly do not object to the use of arthrography, but I believe that it should not supplant careful, definitive clinical diagnosis. I examine many arthrographical studies but order them sparingly.

Arthroscopy

Arthroscopy seems to be a more formidable procedure than arthrography. It requires operating room surroundings and usually general anesthesia, but it can be done as an outpatient or ambulatory surgical procedure. However, it may contribute significantly to the preoperative diagnosis. Arthroscopy and arthrography are not duplicating procedures, although a good deal of the information may seem the same. Arthroscopy may be quite definitive in evaluation of lesions of the articular cartilage. It should reveal cruciate ligament conditions well, although a tear screened by synovial covering or a tear posteriorly may be difficult to define. My own experience with arthroscopy has been largely in postoperative evaluation of the progress of articular cartilage lesions treated by various methods, i.e., by shaving, trephining and drilling, or by leaving the defect alone. The difficulty is in recommending a somewhat formidable and expensive operation to a person who seems to be progressing nicely. However, if the procedure is confined to those

who are doing poorly, it becomes almost worthless as a means of evaluation of the relative merits of a method of treatment. Here, too, one is faced with the prospect of negative arthroscopical findings in a symptomatic patient. The method requires an experienced operator and observer to truly evaluate the pathological condition. The method is not for the occasional user, but in experienced hands it may be quite rewarding.

The techniques of performing arthrography and arthroscopy are not presented in detail, since they require more extensive study than is possible here. I can accept diagnostic arthroscopy much more easily than arthroscopic surgery. There is wide publicity of the procedure and exaggerated claims about the simplicity and quick return to sports. It is an expensive and invasive procedure.

CONTUSION

Basically, a contusion about the knee should be treated in the same manner as a contusion in any other location. There are certain characteristics of contusion of the knee joint, however, that deserve more detailed consideration. The knee is a highly vulnerable joint and is particularly liable to contusion either from a fall directly on the front of the knee or from a blow from the side, and one of the major considerations must be the differential diagnosis.

Diagnostically, we identify a contusion by local swelling, local tenderness, ecchymosis and overlying abrasion. Of greater importance, however, are the negative findings, since it is most important to distinguish major injuries from simple contusions. Thus, an injury along the medial side of the upper tibia may be called a contusion when actually it is a tear of the tibial attachment of the medial collateral ligament. An injury over the patella may be interpreted as a contusion, although there actually has been damage to the quadriceps mechanism in the nature of sprain or strain or even fracture. It is most important, therefore, in any given injury to check the function of the underlying structures carefully. Tenderness over the internal condyle of the femur may simply be the result of a blow from an opponent's boot. On the other hand, it may represent a serious injury to the femoral attachment of the medial collateral ligament. Careful attention to detail in examination will largely eliminate this diagnostic hazard. In case of doubt, the knee should be treated as if it had received the more serious injury until the actual pathological condition is evident.

If it is concluded that the injury is a contusion, *treatment* is basically the same whatever area is involved; aspiration for hematoma, local injection with hyaluronidase, application of cold packs and compression. In the ordinary contusion, splinting the part to prevent motion is not necessary. Usually motion itself is not an aggravating element. Athletic participation need not be prohibited, since under ordinary circumstances the part can be protected adequately. Protection should be designed to prevent repetition of a direct blow to the injured part. An additional knee pad, a doughnut made of sponge rubber or a plastic guard is ordinarily all that is necessary.

The conditions most likely to be confused with simple contusion are partial tears of the ligament attachments to either the tibia or the femur, strain of the attachment of the quadriceps tendon or patellar tendon to the patella, strain of the patellar tendon at its attachment to the patellar tubercle of the tibia and early apophysitis of the patellar tubercle (see Osgood-Schlatter "disease," page 572). A direct blow over the patella or femoral condyle may well cause contusion to the synovium, with resulting effusion, or may damage the articular cartilage or cause a chondral fracture (see Chondral Fracture, page 554). It bears repeating that should diagnosis be in doubt, the injury should be treated as the more serious condition. One should become quite suspicious of the contusion that does not heal promptly. The contusion may be the precursor of a bursitis or tenosynovitis or, more frequently, hematoma formation with later calcification or ossification.

STRAIN

Injuries to the Muscle-Tendon Unit

The vicinity of the knee is quite susceptible to injuries of the muscle-tendon unit, since violent muscular activity is involved in the normal function of this vulnerable joint. A few of the more common strains will be discussed in some detail, since they are particularly disabling to the young athlete. (See page 51.)

Quadriceps Mechanism

The quadriceps muscle attaches to the tibia by a succession of different divisions designed to transfer the multiple motors of the quadriceps, namely, the medialis, intermedius, lateralis and rectus, to the anterior tibia. These muscles converge on the patella. Their tendons completely invest the upper portion of the patella, and their aponeuroses extend down over the patella to be joined at its distal pole by the patellar tendon, which attaches to the nonarticular extension of the distal pole of the patella. The patellar tendon extends downward to attach to the tuberosity of the tibia and fans out over the crest of the tibia below. The stress may be at any point in this mechanism (see Fig. 517). It may avulse the quadriceps tendon from the patella; it may strain the medialis attachment along the medial side of the patella; or it may damage the lateralis attachment laterally or the rectus femoris on top. As the force is continued down into the patella, it is extended into the upper tibia by the patellar tendon, which runs from the distal pole of the patella to the patellar tuberosity of the tibia. The weakest link of this chain may be at any point along this complicated mechanism at any given moment. The injuries to these parts of the unit are essentially the same and require the same basic treatment. The diagnosis is made by the findings of pain, tenderness and swelling at the site, with pain on stress of the quadriceps unit.

Acute Fracture of the Patellar Tuberosity

Not to be confused with apophysitis (see Osgood-Schlatter disease, page 572) is an acute avulsion fracture of all or a part of the tuberosity epiphysis (see Fig. 37). In so-called Osgood-Schlatter disease there is usually not a specific, disabling injury that the young person can identify as the cause of his troubles. He may remember a fall on the knee or an incidence of overexercise, but there is no such acute condition as follows the avulsion. The history of avulsion will include a sudden burst of effort such as high jumping or pole vaulting (Fig. 432). The athlete has severe pain in the knee, and the knee collapses and he falls to the ground. He immediately recognizes that he is hurt and cannot extend the knee. The swelling is very local early and is right over the tuberosity. If the fracture extends into the joint, as it often does, hemarthrosis develops. If it does not extend into the knee, the swelling remains local. On examination the patient is extremely apprehensive. There is exquisite tenderness over the tuberosity and he cannot or will not actively extend his knee. Passive extension is pain-free. Passive flexion is painful. X-ray examination is confirmatory. It will show a loose fragment actually pulled away from the tuberosity rather than the usual fragmented condition of an apophysitis. This fragment may be just the central portion of the tuberosity (Fig. 433) or it may be the whole tuberosity, even extending into and including the top of the tibia (Fig. 434).

Treatment will depend largely upon the physician's evaluation of the situation. If the fragment is substantial and is obviously displaced, treatment must be surgical. In the case shown in Figure 435, the loose ossicle, which had been pulled off the patellar tuberosity, had folded under and was lying up in the infrapatellar tendon bursa, together with a substantial amount of patellar tendon. Other injuries, as I have said, may not disturb the attachment of the tendon at all, but the whole tuberosity may pull off, including the top of the tibia. In this case the fragment should be replaced and held by internal fixation (Fig. 434). Since there is an epiphysis under the tuberosity, if the fragment is the whole central part of the apophyseal side of the epiphysis, it may be better to take the fragment out and repair the tendon rather than to risk fusion of the epiphysis by replacing the fragment and expecting bony union (Fig. 433). In any event the patellar tendon should be securely fixed in order to restore active extension of the knee. In many cases there may be some active extension because the whole tendon may not be avulsed. In most cases there will be difficulty in locking the knee in complete extension, although it may be extended fairly well from 90 degrees to 45 degrees. If, on the other hand, it seems that the fragment is not of major importance and is not grossly displaced, a period of immobilization may permit the fracture to heal. However, this treatment is not very favorable

Figure 432. This 15 year old boy was high jumping and felt something give way in his take-off leg. He fell and had immediate swelling, pain localized over the front of the knee distal to the patella, and inability to use his extensors. *A,* X-ray shows the displacement of the recently closed apophysis of the tibia by avulsion of the patellar tendon. *B,* X-ray six months postoperative after removal of the fragment and reattachment of the tendon to the tibia.

Illustration continued on opposite page

for healing because the fragment is pulled away from the cartilaginous epiphysis and there may be some difficulty in getting firm union to the epiphyseal cartilage. I think in the majority of cases an avulsion is better treated by surgical repair. If the epiphysis is open and it is necessary to use internal fixation to hold the fragment down, this should certainly be removed as soon as union is secure in order to have minimal involvement of the circulation and to lessen the danger of epiphyseal fusion.

Knee Flexors

The biceps muscle-tendon unit attaches in the knee area to the fibular head, where it bifurcates to interdigitate with the bifid attachment of the fibular collateral ligament. In this area, strain must be distinguished from sprain of the ligament. Since the resultant tenderness is similar in both cases, the key to diagnosis is stress. Active pull of the biceps or passive stretch against the biceps will cause pain in a strain, whereas lateral stress of the leg and the thigh will cause pain in a ligament injury. On the medial side of the knee, hamstring strain may occur at the pes anserinus and may well go on to tenosynovitis or to bursitis in this area. The calf may be strained at the aponeurotic attachment of the gastrocnemius to the posterior capsule or to the femoral condyles. The popliteus may occasionally be strained at its attachment to the femur or in the muscle-tendon junction.

Figure 432 *Continued. C,* Surgical view showing, in the tenaculum, the avulsed patellar tendon reflected upward toward the knee, the raw bed below. *D,* Process of repair: mattress sutures through drill holes, suturing this patellar tendon down to the denuded top of the tibia. This boy had a good recovery.

Figure 433. This young female basketball player made a tremendous leap for a rebound. She fell to the floor with immediate, extreme pain. Complete disability resulted—she could not bend her knee or bear weight on the leg. *A,* X-ray showing the central portion of the epiphysis torn from its bed. *B,* The normal leg for comparison. *C,* Surgical view shows the avulsed patellar tendon with a square block of bone. Lifted up by the hemostat in the light area beneath is the epiphyseal cartilage. The fragment was removed to prevent possible closure of the epiphysis. No growth disturbance was noted.

In moderate (second degree) strain there is definite damage to the unit and some weakness as a result of this. It is sometimes very difficult to distinguish between the mild injury, which really does not require too much treatment, and the moderate injury, which requires protection. In general, the symptoms are more severe in moderate than in mild strain, particularly in relation to disturbance of function. For instance, if the hamstring muscle is partially torn, it will be ecchymotic and full of blood and very tender and sore. It obviously is a much more serious injury than mild strain.

As in most of these instances in which the mild condition does not require too much treatment and the severe condition requires repair, the moderate condition requires a good deal of insight in order to diagnose what exactly has happened. It may easily be confused with a contusion and hematoma, the classic example of this situation occurring in the thigh.

Around the knee the most critical areas are probably at the top of the patella in the quadriceps mechanism or along the muscle-tendon junction in the hamstrings. The importance of the diagnosis is that a substantial period of rest is required to protect these incomplete tears so that they can heal properly with normal length and without calcification or ossification.

Severe (third degree) or complete strains predicate a complete separation of some component of the muscle-tendon unit. This may be avulsion of the muscle from its origin, rupture of the muscle itself or rupture at any point in the tendon. In the area of the knee, these injuries almost always involve the tendon, the exceptions being injuries of the popliteus and the gastrocnemius, and even these are sometimes tendinous ruptures, either in the tendon itself or at the attachment of the tendon to the bone. In severe or complete rupture of the muscle-tendon unit, function is disrupted, and the diagnosis can often be made by the bunching up of the involved muscle on active contraction. Localization of the injury can be defined by the area of the tenderness. It may be difficult to diagnose a complete rupture of a muscle in the acute stage (Figs. 436 and 437). Nonetheless it is extremely important, since the time to initiate treatment is very much more abbreviated in a muscle-tendon injury than in a ligament injury.

Mild and moderate strains of the knee should be treated as indicated, the exact period of treatment depending upon the degree of damage present. The main error is to assume that the condition is less severe than it actually is. In a mild (first degree) strain, treatment is symptomatic; in a moderate (second degree) strain, it calls for protection until the lesion heals, whereas in a severe (third degree) strain, restoration of the unit is required.

Treatment of moderate (second degree) strain of the knee requires complete rest in order to prevent active function of the muscle involved. In some cases this will require the use of a splint and in others merely the avoidance of strenuous activity. In either instance,

athletic participation is incompatible with proper treatment. Direct therapeutic measures consist of injecting a long-acting local anesthetic into the area. Direct injection into the tendon should be avoided. After 48 hours, use of local heat, such as diathermy, is in order. Whirlpool baths, hot packs and analgesic balm may all be useful. The treatment of each degree of injury is fundamentally the same, the amount depending upon the extent of damage to the unit.

In the final analysis, for *mild (first degree) strain* some rest is indicated, at least enough to avoid all painful motion, so that the acute stress does not develop into a chronic stress. No appreciable weakness is present, and disability will be confined to those activities which repeat the stress that caused the condition. So rest, heat and mild exercise are useful; stress is not. Recovery should be prompt and complete.

In a *moderate (second degree) strain* of the tendons about the knee, the knee should be put at complete rest in a splint for a long enough period of time to permit the acute symptoms to subside (three to four weeks).

Figure 434. This 15 year old male athlete caught his heel as he took off on a high jump. He had severe pain, fell down and could not walk or actively extend the knee. Examination at 24 hours showed a badly swollen knee anteriorly with hemarthrosis. The tendon was not palpable. *A,* X-ray showing avulsion of the apophysis extending right up into the joint. Note the high patella. *B,* Postoperative x-ray showing repositioning and internal fixation. No notable growth disturbance, since the epiphyses were closing. The epiphysis seems more vulnerable just before it closes.

Figure 435. Six months before I saw him, this 13 year old male injured his knee playing football. He was seen by an orthopaedist who told him he had Osgood-Schlatter disease, injected the area and applied a cast. *A,* X-ray brought in with the patient shows a loose ossicle at the apophysis. When I saw him six months later he said that he had had persistent pain throughout this time with limited activities. He could not run, play basketball or do anything else very active. He had pain on hyperflexion of his knee and pain on extension against resistance. He was tender over the tuberosity of the tibia but also quite tender over the central portion of the patellar tendon. *B,* X-rays made at this time (six months post-injury) reveal a fragment of bone lying apparently under the tendon, possibly in the infrapatellar tendon bursa. This was diagnosed to be the ossicle now missing from the tuberosity but showing up in the tendon above. At surgery, on splitting the tendon we found an area of old granulation tissue at the apophysis where the bed of the fragment was, but the tendon seemed to turn back on itself and pass under the main portion of the tendon into the area of the patellar tendon bursa. *C,* In extracting this tendon, it was found that the tendon carried down the loose fragment of bone and cartilage that had been displaced off the apophysis and under the tendon. Removal of the fragment and repair of the tendon gave good results and now, three years postoperative, he is having no problem. This fortifies my opinion that many diagnoses of the so-called Osgood-Schlatter disease or apophysitis of the tendon are really fractures that fail to heal in this particular area because of the avascular tendon on top and the avascular epiphyseal cartilage underneath the fragment.

On removal of the splint, active motion should be carefully started, always within the limits of pain. Complete nonparticipation for an interval long enough to permit definitive treatment may well return the player to active sports, whereas continued participation in sports may render him quite ineffectual for the season. The danger is in recurrence, since it is difficult to eliminate the cause of the strain if the athlete is not grounded. Once recovery is complete, recurrence need not be anticipated. Straps, wraps and pads will have little effect in preventing re-injury.

In a *severe (third degree) strain*, a complete tear of the quadriceps from the patella or an avulsion of a rim of bone requires restoration of the unit by surgery. If the avulsed segment of the patella includes the full thickness of the bone, the fragment should be removed whether it is of the superior pole, inferior pole, or medial or lateral margins of the patella. The tendon may then be sutured to the patella through drill holes, with care being taken not to drill through the articular cartilage. If the avulsion is just a skin of bone, it may be replaced in the same manner, without removing the thin avulsed layer of bone.

The degree of aftercare depends upon the extent of the rupture and the security of the repair. It will require at least eight weeks to obtain reasonably good union of tendon and bone. With a complete tear of the patellar tendon or the quadriceps tendon, two weeks in a posterior stirrup splint followed by six weeks in a long leg walking cast will be required before rehabilitation can proceed to active resistive exercises. Isometrics can be begun almost at once.

The time spent by the patient in a plaster cast may be shortened by the use of a double bar caliper brace with heel socket or a hinged cast. Use of a dial stop at the knee will permit motion earlier and will allow flexion within the limits of tolerance. It will not protect against active resistive motion, however. In the young athlete the brace is not desirable. If the defect is medial or lateral, with or without a fragment of bone, the period of immobilization can be much shorter—two weeks in a splint and three weeks in a cast.

Complete rupture of a hamstring tendon is quite rare in athletes. The muscle-tendon junction is much more vulnerable. If a tendon rupture occurs and is recognized, the same treatment as that just mentioned is recommended. After a complete muscle-tendon rup-

Figure 436. This 16 year old male, while convalescing from knee surgery following a football injury, fell down the stairs, injuring his knee. He had gross swelling. An x-ray was made (*A*), which did not show avulsion of bone but did show some upward tilting of the proximal end of the patella when compared with the normal opposite knee (*F*). Successive pictures show (*B*) early ossification in the quadriceps tendon three months post-injury.

Illustration continued on following page

Figure 436 *Continued. C,* Six months post-injury, note the massive ossification. *D,* Ten months post-injury, continued ossification. *E,* Sixteen months post-injury, at which time he was examined here. Meantime he had continued to try to run and play, without success. Examination revealed the tremendously large mass of patella. He complained on flexion and extension. He also complained that the patella tended to slip sideways when he tried to cut. Poorly developed medialis and marked atrophy of the whole quadriceps. It would be difficult to remove this mass of bone without destroying the quadriceps tendon mechanism. Early repair of this avulsion of the quadriceps tendon probably would have prevented this result.

Figure 437. This 18 year old male suffered a football injury that required surgical repair one month later consisting of repair of the avulsed attachment of the quadriceps medialis to the patella. He was progressing very well when at two months postoperative he slipped in a wet shower and fell, hyperflexing the knee. At this time he was examined and had obvious damage to his quadriceps mechanism. He had a palpable defect above, with the rectus detached from the patella. He was operated on and the quadriceps mechanism was attached to the patella. *A,* The original radiograph showed a phantom profile of the superior border of the patella, with the patella somewhat low. *B,* Four months postoperative. *C,* One year postoperative showing the union of the rectus to the patella, with a lot of exogenous bone produced but with excellent function.

ture, under no circumstances should competitive athletic activity be allowed before three months have elapsed.

Rehabilitation

Rehabilitation following any degree of strain is quite different from that following sprain, since in sprain the injured ligament can be protected and active, and even stressful motion can be continued. In strain, the injury is to the motor unit itself, so that active contraction of the unit must be carefully controlled until the healing is complete.

Calcification or Ossification

Calcification after strain about the knee usually follows chronic strain with repetitive injury. Ossification usually occurs after acute injury. Calcification is most common at the attachment of the patellar tendon to the tubercle of the tibia. Treatment is the same as for chronic strain—rest, application of heat and local injection. It may be necessary to immobilize the knee in splints or a walking cast. Serial injections of a long-acting local anesthetic, plus a corticoid, around the area may be valuable. If the injections give complete relief, they need not be repeated. However, if symptoms begin to recur after 7 to 10 days, the series should be repeated. If necessary, the injections may be administered again up to three or four times. Injection must not

be made into the tendon. This treatment is much more effective if accompanied by immobilization and physical therapy. Occasionally ossification may have to be removed surgically. If this involves detaching any tendon, the appropriate degree of protective immobilization must be carried out, since the lesion may well recur.

Dislocation of the patella is another relatively common cause of damage to the muscle-tendon unit at the knee because of the frequent involvement of the quadriceps medialis attachment to the patella. (For details of this, see page 510.)

It is worth emphasizing again that one should spare no effort in making a specific diagnosis in these conditions about the knee. Proper diagnosis is the antecedent to proper treatment. Watchful waiting is usually watchful neglect!

BURSITIS

It was noted in the general discussion of bursae that many of them are relatively constant while many others are adventitious. Basically, a bursa develops in order to permit friction-free motion between contiguous moving parts. There is a wealth of bursae about the knee (Fig. 438) and a detailed anatomical description of all of them is not pertinent here. With a few exceptions, only those which are consistent in their formation and are particularly prone to inflammation in the athlete will be discussed.

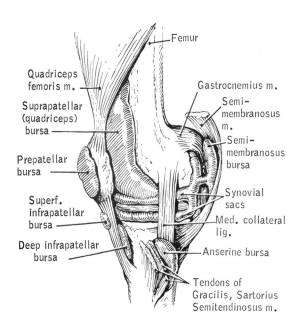

Figure 438. The bursae about the knee. Medial aspect.

Bursitis on the Anterior Aspect of the Knee

Prepatellar Bursa

Anteriorly the bursa most commonly involved is the prepatellar (see Fig. 438). This bursal sac lies between the skin and the anterior surface of the patella and serves to permit free sliding of the relatively thin skin over the underlying subcutaneous bone. This bursa is particularly susceptible to damage by direct trauma, as by falling on the flexed knee. Whereas in its normal state this bursa is somewhat smaller than the underlying patella, it may reach an amazing size when its sac is distended. Involvement of this bursa may be acute or chronic.

Acute Prepatellar Bursitis. Acute involvement will usually begin as an area of tenderness, reddening and inflammation directly over the kneecap. The skin becomes red and warm and sensitive to touch. If the knee is examined very early, snowball crepitation can often be elicited between the walls of the bursa as the skin is moved over the patella. This inflammation progresses rapidly to the formation of effusion, so that there is tense, hot swelling localized directly over the patella (Fig. 439). Ordinary motion of the knee is pain-free, but flexion to the point of skin tension will cause pain. This condition can be readily distinguished from involvement of the knee joint by its definite localization in front of the patella.

Treatment in the acute stage is that of any acute inflammatory reaction. Immobilization of the knee in a posterior splint (see Fig. 452*A*) and application of a warm saline dressing will usually suffice. If there is definite fluid in the sac, aspiration will distinguish between gross pus and bursal fluid. A culture of the fluid, if any is obtained, should be made. Ordinarily the inflammation will subside quickly, with only a slight residual thickening of the lining, the period of disability being only a few days. It is unusual for acute bursitis to go on to acute suppuration, but if this occurs, drainage is carried out through a short (4 cm.) incision through the skin on either side, parallel to the patella, about 1 cm. away from its border. Great care is taken to restrict the incision to the skin and bursa to avoid any possibility of opening into the knee joint. Use of through-and-through rubber tissue drainage together with moderate pressure and continuation of the hot pack will suffice in most local situations. A broad-spectrum antibiotic is given until definite sensitivity of the organism to a specific antibiotic can be determined.

Following acute bursitis, adequate protective padding over the knee should be used, since recurrence is a strong possibility owing to the extremely vulnerable location of the bursa.

Chronic Prepatellar Bursitis. A much more frequent involvement of the prepatellar bursa is chronic bursitis. This may develop as a sequel to repeated attacks of acute bursitis but is more likely to be the result of repeated mild trauma, which causes thickening of the bursal

Figure 439. Prepatellar bursitis of the patella in its normal position with swelling between the patella and the skin.

Figure 440. This 47 year old housewife has a prepatellar bursitis of 10 months' standing. Picture shows the very localized, discrete, swollen bursa. This was treated by excision of the prepatellar bursa with excellent results. Many times, particularly in the athlete, the bursa is much flatter than this because it has been subjected to repeated trauma, which spreads the bursal wall out until it sometimes may be 15 to 20 cm. in diameter.

wall, oversecretion of fluid and gradual filling of the bursal sac. Early examination of the knee will be unrewarding, the only finding being the well-outlined discrete sac of fluid, which is very obviously subcutaneous. It does not involve the knee joint (see Fig. 439).

Treatment at this stage should consist of aspiration of the fluid, injection of a corticoid and application of a firm pressure dressing. Since the condition is not disabling and since a pressure dressing is not consistent with active participation in sports, it is unusual for the player to seek or accept this particular plan of treatment. Usually the condition is allowed to continue, and as the athlete falls repeatedly or kneels on the distended bursa, pressure on its wall causes it to stretch and the sac to expand. A bursa which actually is much smaller in diameter than the patella may distend to cover the whole anterior surface of the knee, not infrequently reaching 15 to 20 cm. in diameter. It is seen as a loose, floppy, fluctuant tumor mass, causing symptoms largely by its very bulk (Fig. 440). Once a bursa has reached this stage, no treatment short of surgical excision is adequate. Surgical excision is relatively simple. A transverse incision is made slightly above the midline of the patella, extending from 8 to 15 cm., depending upon the size of the bursa. The bursa is carefully dissected out.

This is particularly difficult directly over the patella, where the skin is very thin. Care should be taken not to buttonhole the skin. It is important to remove the whole lining of the sac, and this is facilitated by opening into the sac and using the finger within the bursa to determine its limits. Following excision, it is advisable to tack the skin to the underlying fascia over the patellar retinaculum and the quadriceps in order to prevent development of dead spaces. If the bursa is quite large, the two angles of the wound should be drained for 48 hours by strips of rubber tissue. Recurrence of the fluid postoperatively is to be avoided if possible, since an adventitious bursa may develop that may have all of the characteristics of the original one.

Following excision of the bursa, the knee should be supported in a dressing such as the cotton cast (Fig. 441) in order to prevent excess motion between the skin and the patella until the space is completely obliterated. This usually requires about four weeks. It is important that the knee be inspected at frequent intervals during the early postoperative period, since any fluid that accumulates must be promptly aspirated. It is discouraging to the surgeon, and I dare say even more to the patient, to have the bursa recur. Those most likely to recur are the large ones. For this reason, it is recommended that the bursa be removed as soon as it can be definitely determined that irreversible chronic bursitis is present. The removal of a small, sharply localized bursa is relatively simple and very effectual, whereas the removal of some of the larger ones may present a major problem.

I recall a football player who insisted on playing without knee pads. He endured a prepatellar bursitis for an entire season, being treated only with repeated aspirations and some feeble attempts at pressure. At one time over a quart of fluid was removed from the bursa. At operation the bursa was found to be of tremendous size, extending as high as mid-thigh and down to about 10 cm. above the ankle. The player was cured by surgical excision of the sac (which could hardly be called a bursa) and suture of the skin to the underlying fascia. In spite of care at the original operation, there was a small area of recurrence, which required a second excision. The player had remarkably little disability, even during the period of extreme distention of the sac. One of the complaints was that the contained fluid sloshed up and down as he ran.

Characteristically, on examination the wall

of an extremely expanded bursa will present the picture of a very chronic synovitis, usually without villous thickening. It has a shiny, almost plastic-appearing surface interspersed with areas of petechiae the size of the end of the finger. The superficial appearance of these areas is similar to that of psoriasis on the skin. The pathological report uniformly is "chronic synovial inflammation." During the chronic stage of this noninflammatory type of bursitis, it may be necessary to aspirate the sac repeatedly, continue use of pressure bandages and allow athletic participation until a more convenient time for surgical removal. However, if the sac is widely distended, it is not desirable to permit competitive athletics for the reasons noted previously. In carrying out aspiration, it must be remembered that the sac is just beneath the skin, and great care should be taken to insure that the aspirating needle does not inadvertently penetrate into the knee joint. This is more likely to occur if there is an acute inflammation, since there will be edema, tension and considerable inelasticity of the tissue. Prepatellar bursitis treated nonsurgically is prone to recur; hence, adequate padding of the knee is mandatory in order to prevent direct trauma over the patella. After surgical excision also, even if cure appears to be complete, it is wise to insist that a player wear knee pads whenever he is engaged in competitive or contact sports.

Infrapatellar Tendon Bursa (Deep Infrapatellar Bursa)

The infrapatellar tendon bursa lies behind the patellar tendon and in front of the infrapatellar fat pad (see Fig. 438). It does not ordinarily communicate with the knee joint, being separated from the knee by the fat pad. The etiology of infrapatellar bursitis is quite different from that of prepatellar bursitis. The prepatellar bursa is frequently traumatized by a direct blow upon the hard patella, which makes up its floor, whereas the infrapatellar bursa is not particularly subject to direct trauma, since it lies behind the thick patellar tendon and in front of the soft fat pad. Occasionally the lower part of the bursa, which extends down over the front of the upper end of the tibia, may be traumatized. However, inflammation of this bursa is ordinarily due to friction between the patellar tendon and the structures behind it (upper tibia and fat pad), which is the result of overactivity.

The *symptoms* are usually pain on complete passive flexion and on active complete extension of the knee. Tenderness surrounds the patellar tendon and is particularly notable under its edges. If the tendon is picked up between the thumb and the forefinger and the thumb and forefinger are permitted to slip behind it, direct pressure will cause pain.

Diagnosis. Infrapatellar bursitis must, if pos-

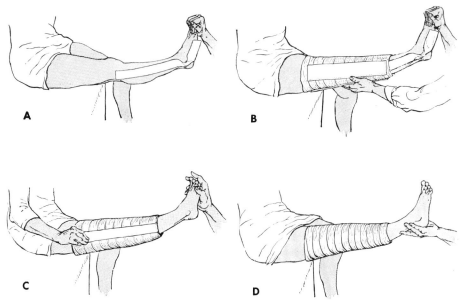

Figure 441. Cotton cast. *A*, The leg is shaved from the knee to the ankle and 8 cm. adhesive strip is applied to either side. *B*, The knee is wrapped in regular sheet wadding, usually five or six rolls, slightly longer than the length of the yucca board. A moistened yucca board splint is applied on either side and posteriorly, centering at the knee. *C*, Yucca board splints are wrapped snugly in place with 8 cm. gauze. The two adhesive strips are pulled back firmly over the ends of the two lateral boards. *D*, The finished cotton cast, the adhesive strips having been wrapped down snugly with gauze, and the whole protected by spiral elastic bandage.

sible, be distinguished from involvement of the infrapatellar fat pad, which lies directly behind it. In inflammation of the bursa which has proceeded to the point of fluid formation, it may be possible to demonstrate fluid in the sac lying directly behind the patellar tendon, which bulges out on either side. Pressure on one side will cause it to bulge out on the other. Similarly, flexion of the knee will cause the patellar tendon to compress the sac and make it balloon out on either side. Inflammation of the infrapatellar fat pad, on the other hand, will seem to be deeper and more posterior. Passive extension of the knee should be pain-free in infrapatellar tendon bursitis, whereas if the fat pad is inflamed and swollen, complete passive extension may be impossible or will cause pain. Complete flexion of the knee will cause pain in either instance. An attempt at aspiration may be quite rewarding if results are positive. The needle should be slipped along just under the patellar tendon. Once it enters the fat pad, all is lost and the results of the aspiration will be negative. An aspiration attempt in which the findings are negative does not rule out infrapatellar tendon bursitis. One distressing symptom of both conditions is the sharp twinge of pain on pendulum extension of the knee. This is particularly distressing to the place kicker, since in completing the kick there is a snap extension of the knee, whereas in punting or in running there is much less of this particular motion. If the involvement in infrapatellar bursitis is severe enough, it will seriously interfere with active motion of the knee, particularly in extremes of either flexion or extension. The condition must also be distinguished from apophysitis of the patellar tubercle (see page 572). In this condition the pain and tenderness are more specifically in the tendon or in the patellar tubercle. However, the same clinical tests, namely, extension of the knee against resistance, overflexion of the knee and direct pressure over the area will cause discomfort.

Treatment. The *treatment* of infrapatellar bursitis is that of bursitis anywhere. In the early stages, applying heat locally and splinting the knee in extension will reduce the inflammation. Aspiration of the bursa, with removal of any fluid encountered, followed by injection of a corticoid, is particularly effective if done early. If effusion is recurrent and resistant to local treatment, the bursa may readily be excised, the incision being made usually on the inner side of the patellar tendon. The bursa can usually be removed entirely through the single incision. If the bursal mass should ap-

pear to be more extensive laterally, incision may be made on the outer side of the patellar tendon. Following careful removal of the entire bursal sac, the fat pad is sutured to the back of the patellar tendon to obliterate the dead space. The knee is splinted in extension with a type of dressing that provides both immobilization and compression (cotton cast). The dressing must be maintained for at least three weeks.

Suprapatellar Tubercle Bursa (Superficial Infrapatellar Bursa)

Another bursa on the anterior aspect of the knee that may become symptomatic lies between the skin and the patellar tubercle of the tibia (Figs. 438 and 442). This is not a consistent bursa nor is it frequently involved. In a young individual there may be some difficulty in distinguishing inflammation of this bursa from early apophysitis of the patellar tubercle (Osgood-Schlatter disease). Indeed, many of these cases of apophysitis of the patellar tubercle which have apparently been relieved by local injection may well have been involvement of this pretibial bursa.

Symptoms of involvement of this bursa are sharply localized pain and tenderness directly over the patellar tubercle. They vary from those of infrapatellar bursitis in that active function of the knee does not cause pain, since the attachment of the patellar tendon is not involved. In the acute type, local inflammation will be the characteristic finding. I have yet to see an extensive collection of fluid in this bursa.

Since active function of the knee is not affected, protection against direct trauma is the most pertinent factor in prevention of recurrence. Following local treatment, there is no particular indication for immobilization of the knee, hence the importance of distinguishing this condition from patellar tubercle apophysitis, strain of the patellar tendon attachment, infrapatellar bursitis and other neighboring conditions which do require immobilization and do cause disability.

Bursitis on the Medial Aspect of the Knee

Anserine Bursa

Another bursa consistently present but not so frequently involved is the anserine bursa (see Fig. 438). Although this bursa may have the usual variants and may be single or multiple, it ordinarily lies between the aponeurosis of the attachment of the internal hamstrings (pes anserinus) and of the long fibers of the medial collateral ligament and the underlying anteromedial face of the upper end of the tibia (see Fig. 438). Under normal circumstances the pes anserinus and the long fibers of the collateral ligament attach to the anterior border of the tibia some 3 in. below the superior articular surface. The bursa serves to separate these freely sliding portions of the tendon from the periosteum of the tibia and the medial collateral ligament. Bursitis in this area is typically caused by friction, although it may be initiated by an external blow impinging the bursa against the hard tibia beneath. The resulting congestion and inflammation cause the same reaction that occurs in tenosynovitis or any friction bursitis.

Initial *symptoms* are pain from the contusion, which is persistent and rather sharply localized. Symptoms are aggravated by flexion and extension of the knee. Since the symptoms will be located on the upper anteromedial face of the tibia, they may be confused with those of injury to the medial collateral ligament. However, they are quite distinguishable by means of careful examination, the tenderness being located not at the attachment of the tendon and ligament but under their unattached portion. Crepitation, if it can be elicited, is diagnostic.

Treatment consists of application of local heat and immobilization of the knee. Recovery can be expedited by injection of a corticoid into the bursa. Although this condition may be quite acute, it seldom causes suppuration. In fact, I have never seen a case of acute suppuration in this bursa. The involvement does tend to be chronic, particularly if full activity is allowed too early. Protective pads against contusion are of little value, since real protection requires elimination of motion of the knee joint and so will demand nonparticipation in athletic activity. One is seldom able to aspirate fluid from this bursa successfully or see fluid develop to the point that it could be demonstrated as fluctuation. I think one explanation of this is that the tension that exists between the tendon and ligament structures and the tibia allows for no redundant fold of bursa that can be filled with fluid.

Other Bursae

Other bursae may be present in this area but are not frequently involved. Further posterior on the medial side is the semimembranosus bursa (see Fig. 438) lying between the attachment of the semimembranosus muscle to the upper tibia and the medial capsule of the joint. This position is slightly posterior to the midline of the tibia and extends about 1 in. below its upper end. Further posterior is the gastrocnemius bursa, lying between the

Figure 442. Ossification of the patellar tendon attachment. *A,* Silhouette view of patella, apparently showing an osteochondritic fragment in the joint. *B,* Lateral view showing the calcification in the patellar tendon attachment. Although in the silhouette view this appeared to be under the patella, it was actually some 10 cm. away. This illustrates the value of very careful interpretation of the film. The fact that this fragment did not show under the patella in the lateral view was suggestive. (Note the normal fabella, a sesamoid bone lying within the gastrocnemius and articulating with the femoral condyle.)

Figure 443. Baker's cyst showing the semimembranosus bursa lying between the semimembranosus and medial head of the gastrocnemius. The actual enlargement of the sac may be palpable at any level. If it protrudes proximally, it will appear in the midline. If it protrudes in its distal portion, it will appear medial to the midline. The medial gastrocnemius bursa (not labeled) lies under the tendon.

tendon of origin of the medial head of the gastrocnemius and the semimembranosus tendon. There may also be bursae between the tendons of the semimembranosus and the semitendinosus and the gracilis muscles. All these are subject to inflammation, the symptoms depending upon the location and the degree of involvement. Inflammation of the semimembranosus bursa may be confused with damage to the medial collateral ligament but is distinguished by the fact that tension on the medial collateral ligament does not cause an increase in pain. The tenderness is localized over the semimembranosus tendon just short of its attachment.

Bursitis on the Posterior Aspect of the Knee

Baker's Cyst

Posteriorly, the most common involvement in athletes is the so-called Baker's cyst. The confusion which so frequently accompanies the use of eponyms is certainly evident here, since the term Baker's cyst has been extended to include almost any synovial hernia or bursitis involving the posterior aspect of the knee.

One type of "Baker's cyst" is bursitis of the semimembranosus or of the medial gastrocnemius bursa (Figs. 438 and 443), a bursa which lies between the medial head of the gastrocnemius and semimembranosus tendons. In-

volvement of the bursa causes expansion of its wall, usually posteriorly, since there is no particular obstruction to its expansion in this direction. It is seen as a large soft tumor mass in the popliteal space. The appearance of the mass is usually preceded by a varying period of chronic, aching-type pain in the back of the knee. Since the bursa frequently communicates with the knee, often by a valvelike arrangement, the swelling may come and go and present great difficulty diagnostically. As a consequence of the valvelike connection with the knee joint, sufficient fluid may collect to produce a sizable tumor. This fluid then concentrates to the characteristic jell contained in a synovial hernia. Later as a result of trauma or other cause, it may be discharged into the knee, where the concentrated fluid becomes an irritative factor and causes synovitis. I frequently have found a to-and-fro connection between the knee and the bursa, so that increased fluid in the knee will distend the bursa, and as the knee recovers, the bursal fluid may remain only to be discharged back into the knee and cause recurrence of the joint effusion. It has been my observation that this bursal involvement is frequently the result of chronic trauma and is too often related to posterior damage of the medial meniscus to be entirely coincidental. Whether the trauma actually opens up the space between the bursa and the knee or causes exudation of fluid that discharges into the bursa rather than into the suprapatellar pouch varies with the individual patient. The patient with a semimembranosus bursal cyst, therefore, may present with a perfectly benign, asymptomatic swelling in the back of the knee or he may have swelling incidental to internal derangement or to chronic synovitis of the knee. So it can be seen that the involvement of the medial gastrocnemius bursa and semimembranosus bursa may actually be several different conditions that can be called Baker's cyst.

So also may Baker's cyst be the result of a synovial hernia off one of the tendon sheaths, specifically, from the semitendinosus. Add to this the fact that the cyst may also result from a true synovial hernia from the back of the joint due to a defect or degeneration in the posterior capsule, similar to the formation of a ganglion anywhere, and we have several different etiological conditions that have the same final diagnosis. If at all possible one should avoid the eponym "Baker's cyst" and be more specific in the diagnosis, since specificity of diagnosis will aid in treatment.

Diagnosis. This condition must be distinguished from other tumor masses, such as aneurysm of the popliteal artery, arterial venous fistula or soft tissue tumor. Occasionally wholly benign conditions may present a confusing picture. I well recall my humiliation at confidently exposing the mass of a "Baker's cyst" only to find that in this singularly well-muscled individual the "cyst" was an unusually low lying belly of the semimembranosus muscle. The only pathological finding in this instance was a preoperatively diagnosed posterior tear of the medial meniscus. As a rule, a Baker's cyst presents no emergency, and time and patience will permit diagnosis. If it is necessary to operate upon the knee for some other cause, as in the case mentioned previously, exploration of this area cannot be condemned, since a second operation may thus be avoided. On the other hand, one would be quite chagrined to operate under a primary diagnosis of Baker's cyst and find only over-redundant fat or overdeveloped muscle.

Treatment. If the pathological condition is a synovial hernia from the joint, then dissecting out the mass and carefully closing the defect into the knee joint will ordinarily effect a cure. If it is an involvement of the bursa, with an open connection into the knee joint, removal of the bursa must include careful suture of the defect in the joint capsule. If it is a result of involvement of the medial meniscus, removal of the Baker's cyst or of the medial meniscus alone will be disappointing.

On many occasions I have been able to demonstrate the opening extending into the bursa in the back of the knee in the course of exposing the posterior compartment for complete removal of the medial meniscus.

If the Baker's cyst is primarily an irritative bursitis of the bursa lying between the semimembranosus and the gastrocnemius muscles, removal of the bursa should be followed by careful suture of the semimembranosus to the gastrocnemius. This eliminates the irritative friction point between these two muscles. I have done this on many occasions and have yet to see any untoward symptoms as the result of suturing these structures together.

If this discussion of treatment for Baker's cyst seems somewhat confusing, it is because of the heterogeneous group of conditions that are lumped together under this name. After careful analysis it will be seen that the treatment recommended is the treatment for the basic underlying condition: if bursitis, excision of the bursa; if hernia of the joint or tendon, repair of the hernia; and if a defect in the posterior capsule or medial meniscus, appropriate treatment for the underlying lesion. In this situation, as in many others, the proper treatment will depend upon accurate diagnosis. In many instances this diagnosis may not be made preoperatively, and one must be alert at operation to determine, if possible, the basic underlying pathological condition so that both the condition and the symptoms are treated.

Following surgical correction it is advisable to hold the knee in compression immobilization (see Fig. 441) for at least four weeks. As in synovial hernia or ganglion elsewhere, recurrence may be prevented by adequate repair. If the condition is a true bursitis, recurrence may be prevented by permitting complete healing of the structures involved. My experience with nonsurgical management of these swellings in the back of the knee has not been satisfactory. I have occasionally aspirated the mass for diagnostic purposes and at other times have seen the tumor disappear spontaneously, but I have been dissatisfied with treatment by aspiration, local injection and immobilization.

Bursitis on the Lateral Aspect of the Knee

Bursae About the Head of the Fibula

On the lateral aspect of the knee are several bursae, any one of which may cause symptoms. The most common are bursae about the upper end of the fibula. The bicipital bursa, which occurs rather consistently, lies between the fibular collateral ligament and the biceps tendon just adjacent to the fibular attachment. Since each of these strong, fibrous structures splits to encompass the other, there may be several bursae in this area to permit active motion between them.

Diagnostically, inflammation of these bursae may present a considerable problem, since they are consistent in neither size nor location. Characteristically, the pain is proximal to the head of the fibula, with tenderness around the fibular collateral ligament and the biceps. However, the same findings may be present in a strain of the biceps tendon or a sprain of the fibular collateral ligament. In many instances, it is impossible to distinguish between these conditions, and in other instances, they coexist. Only in the unusual case does synovial effusion develop in a sufficient amount to permit palpation of a fluctuant mass. However, local swelling in this area, even though it may be diffuse, is much more common in bursitis than it is in the other conditions commonly found here. Thickening of the bursal wall plus effusion with local irritation may become severe enough to cause pressure on the peroneal nerve as it winds around the back of the fibular head. Symptoms are of pain along the distribution of the nerve; on occasion an actual peroneal palsy develops. Bursitis in this location is not commonly prone to calcification. The presence of a hard, calcified mass contained within the constricting walls of the bursa may cause great pain and may indeed cause pressure on the nerve. In case of unexplained peroneal neuritis, one should suspect bursitis about the head of the fibula.

Treatment of bursitis in this area consists of application of heat locally, rest and local injection. It should be noted that this treatment is similar to that of strain or sprain, and in many cases, one may not have distinguished between these conditions. This is particularly likely because active motion of the knee will cause pain in all of them. Strictly speaking, active flexion against resistance should hurt more in a strain or tenosynovitis of the biceps tendon than it should in a true bursitis, whereas direct pressure or passive extension of the knee might be expected to be more painful in bursitis. Bursal pain may also be elicited by activity within a range of motion that does not cause strain on the tendon. It should be realized that these are more impressions than diagnostic certainties. Involvement in this area may be particularly disheartening, since it is exceedingly prone to recur because of the previously mentioned anatomical relationships of the two bifid attachments which interdigitate to make multiple friction points.

If pyogenic bursitis develops, it should be treated appropriately for the infection. If the response to antibiotic therapy is not reasonably prompt, the best definitive treatment for pyogenic bursitis is early drainage, with identification of the organism and institution of specific antibiotic therapy. If one succumbs to the temptation to treat the condition with antibiotics alone, it is very apt to terminate in excessive thickening of the bursal walls and painful scar formation, even if the acute infection subsides. The condition is much more likely to go on to chronic suppurative involvement, with a long period of disability. If calcification develops in the early stages, it may respond to aspiration and injection with a corticoid, whereas in the later stages it must be surgically removed. I recall one instance in which exceedingly distressing peroneal pain had been attributed to many other things, including psychoneurosis. The patient, a woman, had a very large calcifying bursitis, and at operation, the peroneal nerve was found to be tightly stretched over the firm, solid mass of the bursa, which was full of calcium. Excision of the bursa and saline neurolysis of the nerve gave prompt and complete relief (Fig. 444).

Popliteal Bursa

A little higher up on the fibular collateral ligament a bursa will be found lying between the popliteus tendon and the fibular collateral ligament, slightly above the line of the knee joint. Another relatively consistent bursa lies upon the lateral head of the gastrocnemius located slightly behind the biceps tendon. Any of these lateral bursae may connect with the knee joint, particularly the one between the lateral condyle of the femur and the tendon of the popliteus and the one between the popliteus and the fibular collateral ligament. In this area, too, a specific diagnosis may present great difficulty because of the variety of structures which present similar symptoms. Since its lesions are so infrequently diagnosed, it has been said that the popliteus muscle is the overlooked structure of the knee. Differentiation between popliteal bursitis, popliteal tenosynovitis, strain of the popliteus muscle or tendon and involvement of the adjacent bursae is difficult. It is sufficient to state that treatment of the lateral aspect of the knee consists of local treatment of the tender area: injection, application of heat locally and protection against any motion that causes pain. This whole lateral complex of lateral meniscus, fibular collateral ligament, popliteus muscle and biceps tendon may present almost insuperable obstacles to diagnosis. Fortunately, as has been mentioned, the basic treatment is essentially the same in the incipient case, and the more advanced cases will present more specific diagnostic points.

Other Bursae

As one proceeds posteriorly one encounters the *lateral gastrocnemius bursa* lying between the condyle of the femur and the lateral head of the gastrocnemius. Involvement of this bursa is infrequently diagnosed. As to its frequency or whether it occurs as part of another pathological symptom complex, I have no information. I have never been able to diagnose inflammation of the *bursa lying beneath the popliteus muscle,* since in acute conditions it is indistinguishable from other conditions in the back of the popliteal space, and in chronic conditions, I have never seen it sufficiently distended with fluid to provide a clue as to its existence.

SPRAIN

It must be remembered that a ligament is a fibrous structure designed to prevent abnormal motion of a joint. Any injury to a ligament caused by abnormal motion may be defined as a sprain. It should be obvious, then, that a sprain can vary from a complete dislocation of a joint with total loss of integrity of the ligament to a slight tearing of a few isolated fibers with no loss of function. Properly, it should include avulsion of the ligament from bone with or without a small fragment of bone (sprain-fracture) (Fig. 445), partial avulsion of the ligament from the bone or tearing of the ligament within its substance either transversely, obliquely or longitudinally. In the last instance, the ligament will be elongated, although it may appear to be intact. The function of the ligament depends not only upon its strength but also upon its length, and a ligament that is elongated does not carry out its function of preventing abnormal motion of the joint. Since we are primarily concerned clinically with the function of the ligament, what is important is not in what way this function is disturbed but to what extent. It is apparent that the severity of the injury is of much more significance than the exact location or type of the tear. It follows that the determination of the degree of loss of function of the involved

Figure 444. Calcification of bursa about the fibular head with nerve involvement. This patient developed soreness around the outer side of the knee, which was attributable to increased activity. The pain gradually became more intense and lancinating in character down the peroneal nerve distribution. Physical examination revealed inability to straighten the knee, with peroneal nerve pain on attempting to straighten it and palpable tumor in the vicinity of the head and biceps tendon. X-ray revealed calcification in the bicipital bursa. Excision of the mass resulted in dramatic relief with uneventful recovery.

Figure 445. Acute avulsion of fibular collateral ligament from the femur with a flake of bone.

ligament at the earliest possible moment is of prime importance.

Ligamentous Anatomy of the Knee

The anatomical drawings (Figs. 446 and 447) will serve as a review of the ligamentous structures of the knee. The knee consists essentially of two long bones meeting end to end without benefit of either the deep ball and socket of the hip or the mortise and tenon of the ankle. The bony stability of the knee derives solely from the fact that the femur is like a bipod, with two separate distal condyles, and lateral instability will be present only when one or the other condyle of the femur can be lifted from the tibia. This bipod-like structure provides lateral stability, with much less demand upon ligament strength than would be necessary if there were but a single condyle. Nonetheless, real stability of the joint depends to a major degree upon the intricately designed and ingeniously arranged ligaments of the knee.

The *lateral ligaments* (see Fig. 446) and the *posterior ligament* (or capsule) (see Fig. 447) actually are part of the great investiture of the joint consisting of ligamentous structures which are massive and very strong on each side and posteriorly but which become thinned in front to permit motion of the joint. These ligaments are supported and their strength greatly augmented by the *cruciate ligaments*

(see Fig. 446), which are very strong, fan-shaped structures, each twisted on itself to permit motion but to provide maximum stability. The anterior cruciate ligament, arising anteromedially from the tibial plateau in front of the tibial spines, extends backward, upward and outward to attach to the femur posterolaterally in the intercondylar notch. Its primary function is to prevent forward displacement of the tibia on the femur. The posterior cruciate ligament, on the other hand, arises from the back of the tibia, well posterior to the articular surface. It extends forward, upward and inward to attach to the anterior edge of the intercondylar notch on the medial side, just adjacent to the articular margin. A primary function of this ligament is to prevent backward displacement of the tibia on the femur. It is also involved in preventing overextension of the knee. However, although its position seems ideal to check overextension of the knee, actual stress comes first on the anterior cruciate ligament because of the shorter distance from its attachment to the tibia to its attachment to the femur. On overextension, the posterior capsule tends to give way, followed by the anterior cruciate ligament and later by the posterior cruciate ligament. Another important function of the posterior cruciate ligament relates to the position of the knee. With the knee in complete extension, the posterior border of the femur between the two condyles is essentially directly above the posterior border of the tibia. So in complete extension, the posterior cruciate ligament runs vertically from the back of the femur on the lateral side of the medial femoral condyle almost directly downward, to the back of the tibia. This provides a very firm check to hyperextension of the knee. With the knee in flexion as the condyles rotate forward, the ligament assumes a more horizontal position and so is most effective in checking backward displacement of the tibia on the femur.

All the ligaments of the knee—the collaterals, the cruciates and the posterior capsule—are taut in complete extension of the knee, and in this position, the knee is the most stable. Varying degrees of relaxation occur in the different ligaments as the knee is flexed. This is particularly exemplified by the posterior capsule, which loses its stabilizing function completely with only a few degrees of flexion. The knee ligaments act synergistically to support each other in preventing abnormal mobility of the knee while permitting normal motion. Functionally the knee joint is a hinge joint, although anatomically its motion is much

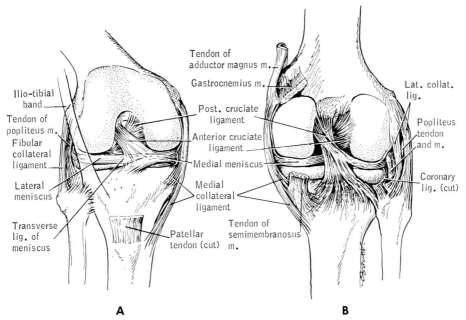

A
B

Figure 446. Anatomical drawings of knee. *A*, Anterior view. Patellar tendon is sectioned and the patella reflected upward. Knee flexed. Note that the cruciate ligament rises in front of anterior tibial spine, not from it. Note also that the medial meniscus is firmly attached to the medial collateral ligament. *B*, Posterior view, knee extended. Note that the posterior ligament has been removed. The two layers of the medial collateral ligament are shown diagrammatically, as is the tibial portion of the lateral collateral ligament. The posterior cruciate ligament rises behind the tibia, not on its upper surface. Observe the femoral attachment of the anterior cruciate ligament at the back of the notch.

more complicated than this. The ligaments of the joint are designed to prevent abnormal lateral motion, abnormal rotatory motion and abnormal forward and backward displacement of the tibia on the femur. The heavy posterior ligament serves to prevent overextension of the joint. The anatomy of the menisci will be described later in this chapter.

The ligaments, although providing good stability, are not strong enough to withstand the great stresses on the knee without active cooperation from the various supporting muscles.

Figure 447. Anatomical sketch illustrating posterior capsule of the knee joint. This is an extremely dense fibrous structure, attaching above the condyles clear across the back of the femur extra-articularly. It attaches below the knee all the way across the tibia and onto the fibula. This structure is tight in extension (*left*), at which time it adds materially to the stability of the knee in all directions except flexion. It is an extremely positive check ligament to prevent overextension. With the knee flexed (*right*) the ligament becomes redundant, so that it no longer has any stabilizing effect in any direction.

Figure 448. Photograph illustrating the forces causing "The Unhappy Triad," namely, sprain of the medial collateral and anterior cruciate ligaments and damage to the medial meniscus. (Permission to print granted by The Miami Herald, Miami, Florida.)

The ligaments must be considered as a first line of defense. Note the complete knee instability of the flail leg following polio, in which the muscle support is lost and the ligaments soon stretch.

Etiology

Sprain of the knee is caused by an abnormal motion of the joint that throws stress on the ligament or ligaments designed to prevent this motion. Forced motion beyond this normal limit will result in some degree of injury to the ligament primarily involved. This motion may be in any direction—adduction or abduction, overextension, internal or external rotation, forward or backward displacement—or almost any combination of these. Certain particular combinations are more frequent than others.

Although frequently it is not obtainable, detailed knowledge of the manner of the injury can be of great importance, since it may indicate the type of ligament damage and so permit early, definitive treatment. In the classic athletic injury of the knee, the foot is fixed to the ground, the thigh rotates inward and the leg outward, the knee is forced inward toward the opposite leg and the stress is primarily received on the ligaments on the inner side of the knee. The sprain is generally caused by the familiar lateral blocking or by the "cut-back" motion of the running athlete, when the foot is forced into external rotation and stress is exerted against the medial collateral ligament of the knee, the superficial layer of which takes the

strain first. As this stretches, tears or gives way, the force reaches the deep layer, to which is attached the medial meniscus. If the force continues, the anterior cruciate receives the stress and it, too, may fail. In severe injuries, the posterior cruciate, may also give way. In injuries of this etiology, one would expect to find sprain of the medial collateral and anterior cruciate ligaments and damage to the medial meniscus ("The Unhappy Triad") (Figs. 448 to 450). Obviously, the injury may stop at any point in this progression of events.

In a similar manner the adduction and internal rotation type of injury places the stress against the lateral ligaments of the knee, the lateral meniscus and the anterior and posterior cruciate ligaments (Fig. 451). If either medial or lateral stress is continued or if stress occurs with the knee extended, the corresponding part of the posterior capsular ligament will give way. Similarly, hyperextension of the knee throws initial tension on the posterior ligament of the joint, which is followed by stress against the cruciate ligaments and the posterior part of the two collaterals if the hyperextension continues. Direct forward motion of the tibia on the femur will injure the anterior cruciate, whereas the opposite motion will damage the posterior cruciate. Many different varieties of stress may cause damage to the knee ligaments. If the stress of the medial side is primarily rotatory, with less abduction force, one may find injury to the short capsular fibers (the deep layer) and to the anterior cruciate ligament, or to either alone, with the long fibers of the medial collateral ligament

Figure 449. Classic injury resulting from forces shown in Figure 448. Note superficial layer and deep layer of medial collateral ligament torn near tibial attachment. Medial meniscus is ruptured, and anterior cruciate ligament has torn completely.

left intact. The severity of this injury may be difficult to determine, since ordinary lateral stress will not reveal instability, yet the injury may be quite major. Aspiration of gross blood after what appears to be a relatively nondisabling injury should raise your index of suspicion that there has been some serious internal damage, particularly to the anterior cruciate ligament. It has been said that history of an injury in which there has been an obvious snap in the knee, followed by early swelling, with blood evacuated during aspiration, is prima facie evidence that there is damage to the anterior cruciate ligament. I do not believe these findings are quite that positive, but certainly such a situation merits investigation for anterior cruciate damage.

Diagnosis

Diagnosis begins with a general evaluation of the situation. Did it seem to be a serious injury? Was the player immediately disabled, or was he able to keep going? Did he himself feel that he had received a serious injury? Was he able to leave the field under his own power, or was he carried? Was he suffering extreme pain, or was it relatively mild? This general evaluation is subject to further modification

following examination but is often of considerable importance in determining the severity of the injury. Following this, an early, careful and complete physical examination of the joint is of great importance. The earlier this can be done the better because during early examination, findings are evident that will later be obscured by pain and swelling. Note whether tenderness is at the joint line, above the joint or below. Tenderness is a much more accurate localizing factor in diagnosis than pain. Pain may be almost anywhere in the extremity, whereas tenderness is very likely to be at the level of the injury. So if there is suspicion of medial collateral ligament injury, tenderness over the medial collateral ligament confirms the diagnosis, even though the patient may be more likely to complain of pain on flexion of the knee, particularly on rotation. Check the knee carefully for abnormal mobility in any direction, including rotation, lateral motion and anterior and posterior motions of the tibia on the femur. Observe the degree and the rapidity of swelling. Investigate whether the knee was actually locked at the time of the injury and whether it is actually locked at the time of the examination. All these findings are of extreme importance if they are obtained in the early stage before swelling, apprehension and pain obscure the true pathological condition. Often, in this initial examination, a definitive diagnosis can be made, including not only

Figure 450. "Unhappy triad." Classic injury with the medial collateral off the tibia and with the anterior cruciate pulled off the femur with a fragment of bone. This is very favorable for cruciate repair.

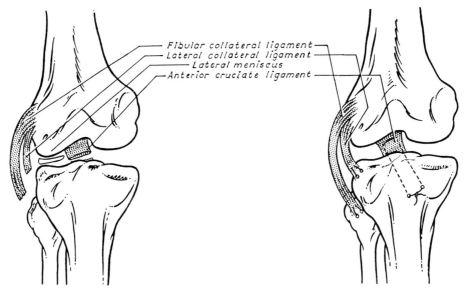

Figure 451. *Left,* Lateral side injury, the succession being fibular collateral, iliotibial band, lateral meniscus, anterior cruciate. The biceps tendon may or may not be avulsed, depending on the level of the injury. *Right,* Note the iliotibial band repaired to the tibia through drill holes and the fibular collateral ligament to the fibula through drill holes. The anterior cruciate is shown held by drill holes from the anteromedial face of the tibia. (From O'Donoghue, D. H.: J. Bone and Joint Surgery. *32–A:*735.)

the location but also the extent of a ligament injury. (For further discussion of diagnosis, see page 448.) A summary of what to look for when diagnosing a knee injury appears in Table 18–1.

For purposes of diagnosis and treatment, the various ligament injuries may be classified into three general groups according to their severity—mild (first degree), moderate (second degree) and severe (third degree) (Table 18–2).

Mild (First Degree) Ligament Sprain

In a mild ligament injury (Table 18–3), there has been some tear in the ligament fibers, but its strength has not been particularly impaired. There has been some degree of damage, either within the ligament itself or at one of its

attachments. The *symptoms* of such a tear are tenderness at the site of the tear, pain on active use of the knee, local swelling at the site of the injury and pain on forced motion or on attempt to duplicate the motion which caused the tear. Negative findings, such as no instability, no blood in the joint or infiltrated through the tissues, no effusion, no locking and no pain on normal motion are significant.

If the injury is indubitably mild—and fortunately the great majority of ligament injuries are—*treatment* is symptomatic and can be based on the premise that the strength of the ligament is actually unimpaired. Prolonged and extensive treatment is not necessary; in fact,

Table 18–1. The Diagnosis of Knee Ligament Injury

Demands early, careful, meticulous examination
Note particularly:
1. Apparent severity of injury
2. Degree of disability
3. Restriction or pain on normal motion
4. Presence of abnormal motion
5. Location and extent of tenderness
6. Amount and rapidity of the swelling
7. Location of swelling—intra- or extrasynovial
8. Deformity, either present or reported
9. Locking?

Table 18–2. Classification of Knee Ligament Injury According to Severity

A. Mild (first degree)—A few fibers of the ligament damaged
   No actual loss of strength of the ligament
   Little treatment necessary
   Treatment is symptomatic.
B. Moderate (second degree)—A definite tear in some component of the ligament
   Definite loss of strength of the ligament
   No wide separation of the fibers
   Treatment is primarily protective
C. Severe (third degree)—Ligament torn clear across
   Complete loss of ligament function
   Potentially wide separation of the fragments
   Treatment: Restoration of ligament continuity

Table 18–3. Symptoms and Treatment of
Mild (First Degree) Knee Sprain

1. Symptoms
   a. Positive
      (1) Tender at site of tear
      (2) Pain on abnormal stress
      (3) Local swelling
      (4) Pain on forced motion
   b. Negative
      (1) No instability
      (2) No blood in joint
      (3) No effusion
      (4) No locking
      (5) No pain on normal motion
2. Treatment—Symptomatic
   (Designed to relieve discomfort)
   a. Rest
   b. Local injection
   c. Compression
   d. Cold early
   e. Heat later
   f. Early, active use
   g. *No* immobilization
   h. Early activity permissible

the injured person seldom reaches the physician and practically never the specialist. The basis of treatment is, first, protection against further injury and, second, reduction of local reaction. Immediate application of a pressure bandage with an ice pack will minimize local swelling. These are the conditions in which apparently dramatic results may be obtained by local treatment. Application of a cold pack and use of the so-called ice cup for massage or ethyl chloride spray will tend to reduce the vascular spasm and will add comfort as well as reduce swelling when the injury is quite local. Local anesthesia inserted into the injured area will reduce pain and vessel spasm. Injection of hyaluronidase into the hematoma may speed absorption and reduce swelling and ecchymosis. Protective wrapping will permit prompt resumption of activity. Complete immobilization is neither necessary nor desirable. The patient may be rapidly rehabilitated without danger. *Warning!* Since the diagnosis may not be entirely certain at the time of injury, the player should not be permitted to participate in sports immediately if a local anesthetic has been injected. The injection may screen the symptoms and permit re-injury.

Moderate (Second Degree) Ligament Sprain

In moderate ligament injury (Table 18–4), it is postulated that the ligament has been partially torn. In this type of injury is included most of the sprains that require extensive treat-

ment, ranging from slight tears to tears with only a few intact fibers remaining. The strength of the ligament is impaired. The *symptoms* are very similar in pattern to those of mild injury but are greater in degree, one group shading imperceptibly into the other. The positive findings are as follows: pain in the knee; tenderness at the site of the injury; disability of a greater degree than in the mild type of sprain; swelling at first localized at the area of damage, later spreading to a diffuse swelling of the joint; fluid or blood in the joint; and pain on reproduction of the force and direction of the injury. There may or may not be locking due to meniscus damage. The findings *not present* in a moderate injury are excess lateral motion and increased anteroposterior slipping of the tibia on the femur with the knee flexed (positive drawer sign). Findings of these latter two tests and rotatory tests each indicate complete loss of function of a ligament, permitting abnormal motion, and are not positive if the ligament is only partially severed.

Treatment is protective and is based upon the premise that there has actually been significant damage to the ligament, with weakening of its structure and considerable loss, or at least potential loss, of function. Therefore, treatment for moderate sprain must be more comprehensive than that for mild sprain, and the emphasis is on protection from further injury. A firm compression bandage should be used and an ice pack applied. Following injec-

Table 18–4. Symptoms and Treatment of
Moderate (Second Degree) Knee Sprain

1. Symptoms
   a. Positive
      (1) Immediate disability to some extent
      (2) Swelling at first localized, later within the joint
      (3) Pain in and about the knee
      (4) Pain on lateral or rotatory motion of the knee
      (5) Local tenderness at the point of injury
      (6) Locking may or may not be present
   b. Negative
      No abnormal mobility in any direction
2. Treatment—Protective
   a. Complete bed rest with elevation of the leg
   b. Injection, local anesthetic
   c. Aspiration
   d. Compression—Cotton cast or elastic bandage
   e. Cold—Ice pack applied directly over compression bandage for 12 to 36 hours
   f. Later, heat (after 36 hours)
   g. Protection by long leg stirrup splints, to long leg cast, to cotton cast, to taping
   h. Rehabilitation

Figure 452. Stirrup splints. Note that the extremity is supported constantly by the foot and the thigh, permitting the tibia to drop backward and relax the anterior cruciate. *A,* A heavy posterior splint is applied first, wrapped with gauze and allowed to harden a little. *B,* The lateral splint is then applied and wrapped with gauze. After this has set, a single layer of sheet wadding is wrapped 15 cm. above to 15 cm. below the knee, and this is covered with a single roll of 15 cm. plaster (*C*). *D,* The completed splint. The circular plaster roll (*C*) is applied only during the postanesthesia stage in the operative case. It is not used routinely. The same type of splint may be used from below the knee to the toes if it is not necessary to immobilize the knee. This, of course, is not effective in any knee injury.

tion of a local anesthetic, aspiration of the local hematoma or of the knee joint is carried out. Since the exact degree of injury may not be readily apparent, one must protect the joint against further insult as long as symptoms persist. Bleeding is reduced by immediate compression with an elastic bandage and application of ice. Later, plaster splints are applied (Fig. 452), which are later replaced by a long leg cast (see Fig. 454). After this, plaster immobilization is discontinued and a cotton cast is applied (see Fig. 441). This is followed by the application of adhesive strapping (Fig. 453) and finally by the use of elastic wrap, as symptoms permit. This sequence of treatments will serve to promote healing and prevent further injury. If fluid in the joint persists, aspiration should be repeated as often as is necessary. Protection must be maintained and insisted upon long after symptoms disappear. Contact participation in athletic activity should not be permitted without firm adhesive strapping (see Fig. 453), which serves to protect the ligaments of the knee better than any available type of compression knee bandage or short brace.

Prime emphasis used to be placed on the treatment of the *complete* ligament tear. It is generally recognized by those treating knee injuries that the complete tear should be surgically repaired or, if not repaired, it should at least be protected for ten to twelve weeks in order for healing to occur. My own experiments with dogs have shown that a complete tear will require 12 to 14 weeks before it becomes firmly united. Similarly, a ligament which is cut *halfway* in two will require at least eight weeks before it becomes mature and approaches its original strength.

New emphasis must be placed on the treatment of the partial ligament tear, the second degree or moderate injury. This condition may be very well treated in the early stages by protection in a splint, pressure, compression, use of an ice bag and so forth. In two to three weeks the acute symptoms subside, and the patient becomes relatively asymptomatic. However, at this time the ligament is no stronger than it was the day of the injury. The symptoms have disappeared, but the ligament is not healed. The player returns to the game and re-injures his knee. The same cycle may be repeated three or four times during the season. At the season's end the knee injury which had caused no instability initially has terminated in complete instability of the involved ligament. This instability is recognized too late for primary repair, and reconstruction now becomes necessary. One must be extremely wary of accepting subsidence of clinical symptoms as a sign that there has been healing of the ligament. If activity is permitted too early, a moderate sprain may develop into a complete one. The physician must recognize that healing requires time. Function of and stress on the ligament before this time has elapsed results in re-injury from minor trauma. *It takes as long for a ligament to heal as it does for a fracture of similar degree.*

It is difficult to state positively just how comprehensive treatment should be in a given condition but it is quite apparent that the sprain which causes only moderate damage does not require as extensive or as prolonged treatment as one that is more severe. As a general rule, use of compression and an ice pack should be continued for several hours or even longer if the swelling is severe. Systematic use of one of the enzyme preparations may be of value—for the first 24 hours intramuscularly and then orally for a few days. With discontinuance of the use of the compression bandage and the ice pack, a decision should be made as to whether the injury is severe enough to require plaster splints from groin to toes or some type of coaptation splint (such as the cotton cast) from midthigh to midcalf. If the ligament is actually torn, at least eight to ten

weeks of immobilization will be required for complete healing, and there should be an additional period of protection using strapping. Here again the degree of the damage will be the governing factor, since if the greater part of the ligament is intact, the ligament remaining may serve to protect the injured portion, whereas if the defect is a major one, a longer period of external protection will be indicated to prevent re-injury. The posterior and stirrup long leg splints may be worn for seven to ten days and then be replaced by a long leg walking cast (Fig. 454) for several weeks. This may be followed by short splints and later by an elastic bandage, particularly if swelling or effusion persists. It merits repeating that the knee capsule should not be permitted to remain distended over a long period of time and that aspiration should be repeated as frequently and for as long as necessary. Also worth emphasizing again is the caution that this procedure should be carried out with the same aseptic technique that one would use if the knee joint were to be opened surgically. I prefer a thorough soap (hexachlorphene) and water scrub, and the use of protective draping and sterile gloves. One need not fear infection if its possibility is anticipated and if the proper preventive measures are taken.

Opinions differ as to the length of time the ice pack is beneficial. Since it diminishes bleeding and slows down metabolism, it should be continued as long as these two ends are desirable. In the ordinary case, bleeding will stop after a few hours. Later it is desirable to increase metabolism by the application of heat

Figure 453. A method for strapping the knee to support the medial and lateral collateral ligaments. The criss-cross straps should cross in the midline. Maximum support for this dressing is directly medially and laterally.

Figure 454. Long leg cast. Note that the extremity is supported by the thigh and the foot to permit the tibia to drop backward to relax the anterior cruciate. *A*, Posterior plaster slab. *B*, The completed cast with the foot in slight eversion, the ankle neutral, the knee at 20 degrees. *C*, The heel. *D*, Standing position. Note that the patient should have a shoe with heel of equal height on the good leg to balance the pelvis.

locally by means of an electric pad, diathermy or hot bath. If a well-equipped and well-controlled training room is available, the dressing may be removed daily for the application of heat and controlled physical measures, such as whirlpool therapy, massage and careful motion. This must be carried out under the protective eye of a qualified trainer. A typical set of rehabilitative exercises follows. There are obviously many that can be used (See also Chapter 22.)

Rehabilitative Exercises for the Lower Extremity

O'Donoghue Orthopaedic Clinic

Each of the following exercises should be done deliberately and to a particular count. In each instance, raise the leg slowly to the count of 3, hold to the count of 3, lower to the count of 3 and rest. Repeat this series ten times. Rest. Repeat this through three series of ten times each, 30 times total. The exercise should be repeated two or three times a day, depending upon your tolerance. Whenever you are able to complete this series of 30, add weight and start a new series, gradually adding weight as your strength improves. Build this weight up to 25 pounds if possible. Chart your daily prog-

ress and record it. Continue this until the involved thigh is *(a)* as large as the normal thigh and *(b)* as strong as the normal thigh and until *(c)* normal motion is reached.

The following exercises should be done as indicated previously, starting while the leg is still in the cast.

1. Lying on the back, raise the leg up with the knee straight and not flexing.
2. Lie on the unaffected side. Raise the leg up with the knee straight.
3. Lie face down. Raise the leg up with the knee straight.

(N.B. In each instance, increase weight as indicated previously.)

4. After removal of fixation, sit with the leg hanging and the knee at a right angle and go through the series of exercises with spring resistance or weight. If there is ligament damage, a spring or system of pulleys and weights is preferred to hanging the weight on the foot.
5. Lie face down with weight attached to the foot and flex the leg to vertical through the same series.

Exercises 1, 2 and 3 should be begun immediately postoperatively or even started preoperatively. Exercises 4 and 5 should be done after removal of the cast and should not be done if there is synovitis with effusion.

Active physical therapy, increasingly active use of the knee, protective strapping and re-education of the patient are all of importance.

Injudicious overuse or too early return to physical activity will interfere with prompt and complete recovery. Reduction of pain and swelling by local injection must not be permitted to cover up the true nature of the injury, since active stress must not be allowed until healing is complete. Ordinarily complete recovery should be expected, with no residual disability in the joint if treatment is adequate (Fig. 455). After complete healing there is no justification for limiting the activity of the patient. It is the unusual or the untreated patient who has permanent disability from a moderate sprain. The expression "once a sprain always a sprain" is sometimes used as an excuse to screen inadequate treatment.

Severe Ligament Sprain

In severe ligament injuries (Table 18–5), the *diagnosis* is based on the premise that one or more of the major ligaments of the knee are completely torn loose from their attachment or torn through their substance. The mechanism of this injury is that previously mentioned, namely, forcing the knee through a wide range of abnormal motion that is beyond the tolerance of the ligament. Symptoms in this type of injury are much more severe than those in moderate sprain. There is immediate disability, which is usually severe. There is the feeling that the knee has given way or dislocated. There is often extreme pain at the time of injury. Examination and evaluation reveal early disability, giving way of the knee joint, severe pain in the knee or leg, blood in the joint, blood infiltrating through the tissues (Fig. 456) and local swelling, first at the site of injury and then very rapidly into the knee itself. Confirmatory stress x-rays (Fig. 457) show abnormal lateral motion at the knee joint. Locking may or may not be present. Although these symptoms and signs strongly suggest a complete ligament avulsion, *the one single confirmatory finding is instability.* One should be able to demonstrate by examination the loss of function of one or more ligaments of the knee. It should be noted also that a torn ligament, particularly a cruciate, may be present without the signs of major injury indicated earlier. (See page 478.)

Increased abduction of the tibia with the knee in complete extension means loss of the medial collateral and anterior cruciate ligaments and at least part of the posterior ligament (see Fig. 457*A*). A knee that is stable in extension but not at 30 degrees indicates that the medial or lateral collateral ligament is gone

but that the posterior ligament is intact. Increased anterior-posterior mobility of the flexed tibia (90 degrees) on the femur indicates anterior or posterior cruciate ligament damage (drawer sign, Fig. 458). Anterior instability may be demonstrated with the knee flexed 15 to 30 degrees ("Lochman's sign"). The importance of these findings cannot be overemphasized. If surgery is indicated for some other reason, such as a locked knee or a knee with positive lateral instability and questionable anterior-posterior instability, the cruciate ligament can be checked at the time of the operation. Appropriate measures can be taken for repair at that time, without the necessity of a preliminary diagnostic anesthetic. In doubtful cases it is justifiable to induce anesthesia for diagnosis. Stress films are not always necessary to confirm instability, but they should always be taken to demonstrate other pathological conditions. Instability may be posterior or anterior, and a stress film may be necessary to demonstrate which it is, although physical examination will usually reveal it (Figs. 459 and 460).

Diagnosis must be early and be definitive in order to permit the proper decision as to treatment. If one waits three to four weeks until swelling and pain subside, instability becomes quite obvious. In the meantime the optimum time for treatment has passed. Although instability is necessary to confirm complete ligament tear, one must be sure that the

Table 18–5. Symptoms and Treatment of Severe Knee Sprain

1. Symptoms
   a. Immediate disability, usually severe; patient apprehensive
   b. Knee "gives way" on attempt at weight bearing, particularly with flexion
   c. Severe pain
   d. Blood infiltrated in tissues but may collect in joint
   e. Marked swelling, first local, later diffuse about the knee
   f. Pain on stress (lateral, rotatory, anteroposterior)
   g. *Abnormal mobility.*
   h. Positive stress x-ray
2. Treatment (Designed to restore continuity of the ligament)
   a. Surgical treatment should be given if at all possible
      (1) Make prompt diagnosis and decision as to surgery
      (2) Operate as soon as feasible
      (3) Repair each torn ligament
   b. Nonsurgical (not desirable)
      Same as for moderate sprain, but longer protection

Figure 455. This patient was first seen for his left knee at age 27 in 1970. He was originally hurt the previous fall and missed two games. He was hurt again one month later and has had several injuries since. Examination showed medial collateral and posterior cruciate instability. Note in view A the right and left knees show apparently very little difference between them, with essentially no degenerative change. He declined treatment. B, Four years later, his instability having continued, note the very gross involvement of the medial side of the joint. This is a good illustration of the fact that instability does lead to degenerative changes. Osteotomy and debridement were recommended. The patient was then 31 years old. Reduction of his instability by surgical reconstruction would probably have lessened or stopped his degenerative change.

Figure 456. Appearance of leg 48 hours after injury, with avulsion of posterior cruciate and posterior capsule from the tibia. Note extreme swelling, ecchymosis and hematoma formation.

instability is actually due to the injury to the ligament and not to a related injury to the bone which has given the *impression* of instability of the knee, even though the ligaments are actually intact (Figs. 461, 534 and 537).

Treatment. Treatment poses the question, Why is it essential that a diagnosis be made definitively and at once? The answer is basic in our approach to the problem of treatment. If all ligament injuries are to be treated by modifications of the same basic procedure, it may indeed be of academic interest only to define the exact pathological condition. It is agreed that certain basic measures are of value in the treatment of an injured knee ligament. We have seen that aspiration, local injection, compression, application of ice packs, immobilization, protection and rehabilitation are utilized to a greater or lesser degree, depending upon the severity of the injury. Using this approach, whether the sprain is moderate or severe, treatment will require only some variation of the extent to which these measures are utilized.

Obviously, if there is no effusion, aspiration will not be necessary. If effusion is recurrent, aspiration will need to be repeated. If the injury is mild, a compression bandage may well be the only protection applied, and it may soon be discarded. If swelling persists, so must compression bandaging, whether it is an elastic wrap or a cotton cast. If symptoms subside promptly, no protection by splint or cast is necessary. On the other hand, if symptoms remain severe, a cylinder for eight weeks may be required. The same approach applies to

rehabilitation, which can be perfunctory in the injury requiring only brief treatment but must be extensive if prolonged protection is required.

Why, then, do we demand "careful, tender but meticulously complete examination" of every sprain of the knee? If the treatment is to be the same whatever the injury, why not initiate this treatment first and then decide as we go along just how extensively the injury must be treated? Severity could be judged by the manner in which the condition responds to therapy.

Such specious reasoning insidiously undermines the physician's actual understanding of the condition which he is treating. It is easy to see how the habit of treating these injuries "by feel" rather than by diagnosis becomes fixed. If one is called upon to examine a knee injury and responds by directing that it be "packed in ice" until morning, the next time the trainer or team physician encounters this injury, he will "pack it in ice" himself. Indeed, if the treatment is to be standardized into a certain pattern, he is perfectly correct in doing so.

Many of us have found through years of observation that nonsurgical treatment is not always the best treatment. We may differ substantially on how frequently surgery is indicated and how complete it must be, but most would agree that many patients will require surgical treatment.

It has been shown that early operation (within two weeks) is distinctly more favorable than late operation (Fig. 462 and Table 18–6). In a series of 80 cases of knee ligament operations, the vital factor governing the degree of recovery was not the severity of the injury, the location of the tear or the age of the patient. It was the time of the operation. Almost without exception the patient who was operated upon within two weeks obtained a better end result than the patient with a comparable injury operated upon later. Indeed, a more satisfactory result was obtained in the severe case treated by early operation than in the milder case in which operation was late.

So if these two premises are granted, namely, that some cases need surgery and that early surgery is better than late, it follows that the decision whether to operate or not must be based on early, thorough, and careful examination, with the patient under anesthesia if necessary. All knee injuries must not be treated alike if they are to be treated in the best way. Attention to the exact diagnosis must be an integral part of the management of any knee ligament injury.

Figure 457. *A*, X-ray of injury to medial collateral ligament of knee. *Left*, Neutral anteroposterior view; *right*, position of abduction of leg on thigh; arrow indicates increased tibiofemoral joint space. *B*, X-ray illustrating damage to lateral collateral ligament. *Left*, Neutral anteroposterior view of knee; *right*, stress film showing rupture of fibular collateral and iliotibial band. Arrow indicates avulsion of tip of fibula.

These injuries provide classic examples of the importance of the precepts mentioned in the Introduction, which must be constantly kept in mind. The goal of treatment must be 100 per cent recovery. The best treatment rather than the most convenient one should be selected. The decision must be entirely objective, without consideration of extraneous influences. Above all, treatment must be prompt. A definitive decision as to the proper treatment must be made at the earliest possible moment.

Once the diagnosis of a complete ligament tear has been made, the method of treatment must be chosen. It will not suffice to try so-called conservative treatment first and then proceed to surgery. Early surgical repair yields so much better and surer results than late repair or reconstruction that surgery must not be reserved for only those patients in whom conservative treatment has failed. Modern anesthesia, operating room asepsis, highly skilled personnel and antibiotics have mini-

Figure 458. The drawer sign. The patient sits with her leg dangling from the table. The examiner is seated in front of her with the foot clasped between his knees, hands as shown. Forward pressure will demonstrate anterior cruciate instability; backward pressure, posterior cruciate instability. This motion should be made by slow, steady pull rather than by a succession of jerks, which will be painful to the injured knee. The inset shows a positive anterior drawer sign, the tibia sliding forward and downward in relation to the normal position. In my hands, the drawer sign has been a very reliable finding if it is properly elicited. It must be done with the leg hanging free. The ankle must be stabilized by the examiner's knees so that one cannot simply flex and extend the knee when pulling forward on the tibia. In this position, rotation takes place at the ankle joint as the tibia moves forward or backward. The Lochman test is done with the knee flexed only 15 to 30 degrees; the examiner grasps the calf with one hand and the thigh with the other, trying to displace the leg forward. I find the Lochman test very difficult to do in a strong, husky athlete, although it is a somewhat more sensitive test possibly than the standard drawer sign.

mized the hazards to the degree that in the well-run hospital with a competent surgical team, open surgery can confidently be placed alongside nonsurgical measures in terms of safety. In the absence of complicating factors, the management chosen must be that which will give the best chance of complete recovery in the shortest time.

I believe that when one can demonstrate complete severance of any single ligament or of any combination of ligaments of the knee, surgical repair is mandatory. The repair should include not only one ligament but all ligaments involved. It makes little sense to repair the collateral ligament and ignore the cruciate because it "adds to the severity of the operation" or is "too difficult" or "may not be essential." The cruciates are not vestigial. One has only to examine the splendid mechanism of the anterior cruciate, to note its size, to check its

Figure 459. Fifteen year old female fell while doing acrobatics and twisted her knee. She had a torn anterior cruciate ligament, with injury to medial collateral ligament and medial meniscus. *A*, Lateral view with posterior stress—negative. *B*, Lateral view with anterior stress shows tibia far forward, indicating loss of the anterior cruciate ligament.

Figure 460. Thirty-four year old male sustained hyperextension and valgus strain to the knee joint when he fell a distance of six ft. Had lateral collateral and posterior cruciate instability. A, Anterior stress—negative. B, Posterior stress shows marked posterior displacement. No anterior instability was present. Findings indicate loss of posterior cruciate ligament.

strength, to recognize its vital structure, in order to realize that it is not an evolutionary misfit ready to be discarded. The cruciates play a living, vibrant part in that ingenious mechanism that is the knee. We may argue about their exact function, but be assured they have a major one.

Even though it is agreed that the many interlocking ligaments of the knee act as a physiological unit and that a portion of this unit may be sacrificed without great disaster, it must be acknowledged that the knee without the cruciate is actually or potentially less than normal. Each of the various ligaments adds to the stability of the knee. One might make a comparison with the television aerial; one row of guy wires may be removed and the structure may not fall, but it may well collapse in the next high wind. The cruciate should be repaired, since in no other way may a normal knee joint be attained.

I examine many knees in which the only

Figure 461. Patient injured knee falling off a horse and landing on a rock. Came in with diagnosis of ruptured fibular collateral ligament. Note fracture-dislocation of fibular head, with instability of the fibula, simulating ligament injury. This is an illustration of the danger of assuming that the ligament is torn just because there is instability.

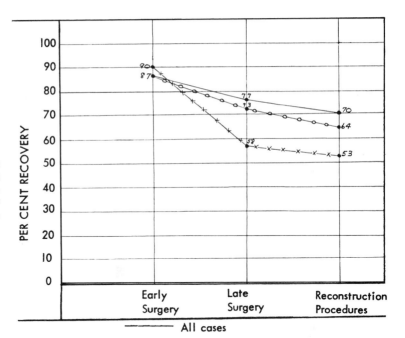

Figure 462. Showing end results of operations on ligaments of the knee. Note the time of operation, which is most important. (From The Journal of Bone and Joint Surgery, Volume 37-A.)

——————— All cases

-o-o-o-o All cruciates
-x-x-x-x "Unhappy triad"

detectable complaint is cruciate instability. These patients seek surgical reconstruction because to them the condition is materially disabling. This in itself is evidence that the cruciate in a given case may be vital for adequate function.

Late cruciate reconstruction is highly speculative and should be done only when the stakes are high, as for example in a professional baseball player who is unable to play because of anterior-posterior instability, or when the degree of anterior-posterior instability is such that late degenerative changes may be expected. Early cruciate repair is highly successful and should be done as a matter of

course. The operation, which is not unduly technical, is within the capabilities of any competent orthopaedist who properly prepares himself in the necessary technique.

In certain cases the ligament may heal spontaneously. This is particularly true of tears of the collateral ligaments. The real danger is in our inability to determine short of surgery which ligament will heal with normal length and which will not. At operation I have actually found the tibial end of the medial collateral ligament lying in the joint underneath the medial meniscus (Fig. 463). I have seen the ligament torn with the ends disengaged and retracted an inch or more (Fig. 464). I

Table 18–6. Follow-up Chart of 80 Knee Ligament Operations
(Comparison by Age Groups)

	EARLY SURGERY	LATE SURGERY	RECONSTRUCTION PROCEDURES	TOTAL
Under 20 years				
No. of Cases	21	12	12	45
Grade	89 (average)	75 (average)	66 (average)	79 (average)
Over 20 years				
No. of Cases	23	8	4	35
Grade	84 (average)	78 (average)	60 (average)	80 (average)

Note that the result was essentially the same whether they were under 20 or over 20. There were consistently poor results from surgery delayed over two weeks. In this table "early" is under two weeks, "late" is two to six weeks.

(From The Journal of Bone and Joint Surgery, Vol. 37A.)

Figure 463. Both cruciates off tibia. Tibial end of medial collateral under medial meniscus. Tendon widely separated. (From The Journal of Bone and Joint Surgery, Vol. 32-A.)

have located the femoral attachment of the medial collateral ligament lying in the joint on top of the meniscus (Fig. 465) and also the femoral end of the anterior cruciate lying over the lateral meniscus (Fig. 466). There are many other such situations which are unredeemable except by surgery. Anyone who has actually seen these or similar lesions at operation becomes very skeptical of the uniformly good results reported from nonsurgical treatment.

The results of surgical treatment recommend it. In 80 consecutive cases of ligament injuries, early repair gave positive results in approximately 90 per cent of cases (over 90 per cent in athletes), regardless of the severity of the injury.* It was demonstrated that the promptness of the operation and the completeness of the repair were much more important than the nature or severity of the injury; failure of cruciate ligament repair was the most common single cause of permanent disability in knee ligament injuries, and repair of the cruciate ligaments was highly successful when done early but very unpredictable when done late.

Operative Technique

I will attempt in this section to indicate some of the more common surgical procedures for ligament repair and to describe in detail those which I personally prefer. The exact pathological condition encountered may have many

---
*O'Donoghue, D. H.: An Analysis of End Results of Surgical Treatment of Major Injuries to the Ligaments of the Knee. J. Bone and Joint Surg. *37A*:1–13, 1955.

variants, but the diagnoses nevertheless fall into more or less definite categories. The procedures may be grouped on the basis of the diagnosis as follows:

1. Technique for repair of the medial collateral ligament, the medial portion of the posterior ligament, the anterior and/or posterior cruciate ligament, the medial meniscus and the medial hamstring tendons.
2. Technique for repair of the lateral components, namely: the iliotibial band (which is actually the strongest of the lateral components and is similar to the deep capsular fibers on the medial side), the fibular collateral ligament, the lateral portion of the posterior capsule and the cruciate ligaments; the lateral meniscus; the peroneal nerve; and the biceps tendon.
3. Technique for repair of the posterior components—the posterior approach for either the posterior capsule or posterior cruciate.

The *preoperative preparation* for all these procedures is the same, namely, meticulous preparation of the skin. In the presence of a specific skin contamination, this begins 48 hours before the operation, otherwise 12 to 24 hours before. If the operation must be delayed because of inability to obtain a hospital bed or for some other reason (such as irritative abrasions and cuts), I provide the patient with a hexachlorphene soap and instruct him to scrub his knee vigorously with very heavy lather at least ten minutes twice a day. If there is a lesion on the skin, it must have healed as completely as possible. However, I sometimes plan the incision to avoid an abrasion on the skin rather than postpone an operation unduly. Infected skin is a definite contraindication to surgical treatment.

Figure 464. Tendon and medial ligament widely separated from the lower attachment. (From The Journal of Bone and Joint Surgery, Vol. 32-A.)

Figure 465. Anterior cruciate torn from tibia. Posterior cruciate torn from femur. Medial collateral torn from femur and lying on top of medial meniscus. (From The Journal of Bone and Joint Surgery, Vol. 32-A.)

Figure 466. Anterior cruciate avulsed from femur and lying on top of lateral meniscus. (From The Journal of Bone and Joint Surgery. Vol. 32-A.)

The leg is carefully shaved from the toes to the groin in the immediate preoperative period in the surgical suite. I prefer shaving the leg just before the surgery rather than the night before. After shaving, the patient is taken directly to the surgical amphitheater.

On the day of operation the patient is taken to the operating room and anesthetized, after which the leg is suspended by a foot-holding apparatus (Fig. 467A), which relieves the nurse or other individual from holding the heavy extremity throughout the period of the preparation. This apparatus is a modification of that used to suspend fluids from a carrier and consists of a rather broad base with a vertical telescoping upright surmounted by a strong hook. The apparatus is placed on the operating table, with the base beneath the pad. A suitable loop is thrown around the foot, and the leg is suspended as high as it will readily go (preferably at least 45 degrees from horizontal). Use of the suspension frame is more difficult with the patient in the prone than in the supine position but is still easier than holding the leg manually. The tourniquet is applied as high on the thigh as possible, because one is never sure of the extent of incision required. The tourniquet is fastened with adhesive so that it will not roll down the cone-shaped thigh. Employment of the leg holder permits the nurse to use both hands in the preparation and encourages a full-length scrub time.

With the leg suspended in the apparatus, the surgical preparation is carried out with Betadine scrub (8 min.), followed by Betadine solution (2 min.). The preparer wears sterile gloves and, with compresses in both hands, works up a very generous lather. Scrub is continued for a total of 10 min. by the clock (see Fig. 467). It does not include the foot. It is my belief that when the foot is included in the preparation, an inordinate amount of time is spent in cleaning the toenails and foot whereas, if the foot is draped out, the entire preparation may be concentrated about the knee. At the conclusion of the preparation, the foot is grasped by the preparer and removed from the suspension apparatus (see Fig. 467D). The leg is held elevated at all times to help drain the blood from the extremity. Over the foot is rolled a combination of stockinette and plastic stocking (see Fig. 467), which will extend from the toes well up to above the knee. This stockinette, plus the plastic, is sterile, so that it can be rolled directly over the unprepped foot and up the leg. Meanwhile a barrier sheet is placed on the table beneath

the leg and up under the thigh. A folded sterile towel is wrapped around the tourniquet and held securely with a towel clamp. At this point a double fan sheet is placed under the leg and pulled up to the level of the top edge of the barrier sheet while the assistant holds the leg in an elevated position. A second double fan is placed on top of the double fan under the leg and not fanned out until a third double fan is placed on the thigh above the knee. The inferior edge of the upper sheet is clamped to the superior edge of the second double fan, which is placed beneath the leg. At this time the plastic and stockinette covering is pulled up over the sheets so that it completely covers the thigh and the draping sheets. The leg is held elevated all during this time. The combination plastic-stockinette sleeve is then split over the top of the knee, the edges are retracted to either side, and the Steri-Drape is pulled over this so that the area of the surgery is exposed, with only the Steri-Drape covering it. Then the leg is wrapped with an elastic bandage from the toes to the upper thigh. The pneumatic tourniquet is then inflated and the time carefully noted. From the moment of application of the tourniquet, no unnecessary delays can be tolerated, since the tourniquet time becomes all-important.

In certain instances when I need to reach a higher point on the thigh, such as in reconstruction operations or in repair of muscular conditions of the thigh, I use the sterile tourniquet as indicated in Figure 468.

1. Technique for Repair of the Medial Collateral, the Medial Portion of the Posterior Ligament and the Anterior or Posterior Cruciate Ligament

Exposure for Definition of the Pathology. A sweeping anteromedial incision is made beginning above the level of the superior pole of the patella (Fig. 469). It extends downward and forward toward the middle of the medial border of the patella, and continues downward along the anteromedial aspect of the joint, paralleling, and 2 cm. medial to, the patella and the patellar tendon. At the level of the patellar tubercle of the tibia, it curves backward to end at the posterior border of the tibia, about 8 cm. distal to its articular level. The medial skin flap is reflected backward along the superficial fascia to expose the entire anteromedial surface of the tibia, the joint and the femoral condylar area (Fig. 470A). All of the blood vessels and nerves in the subcutaneous area should be reflected with the flap, leaving the fascia of the leg entirely exposed with no fat. At this point ecchymosis may be noticed spreading through the fascial layer. It is quite unusual for the fascia to be torn. The medial collateral ligament is not exposed until the fascia is divided. If the fascia is not ruptured, the superior border of the pes anserinus is defined by observation and by palpation, and the deep fascia is incised along this line, care being taken not to cut through into the long fibers of the medial collateral ligament, which are immediately beneath. On reflecting this fascia, the long fibers of the medial collateral ligament will be seen passing under the pes anserinus, beginning at about the midmedial line of the tibia and extending well back behind its posterior margin. At this point the area of the tear in the long fibers may be defined. If it is obscure, rocking the leg open may serve to develop the defective area.

The incision is now carried through the patellar retinaculum along the edge of the patella and the edge of the patellar tendon, just below the patellar tubercle. An instrument then can be passed beneath the superficial portion of the ligament in order to better

Figure 467. Method of draping for knee operation not requiring use of sterile tourniquet. *A*, Notice leg suspended from suitable suspension apparatus to permit use of both hands in the scrub. The Betadine prep does not reach the tourniquet nor does it reach the unsterile stockinette over the foot. Scrub lasts ten minutes. (We now use Betadine scrub for the preliminary wash, followed by Betadine solution instead of Ioprep and alcohol. See text.) *B*, Note cuff of Betadine prep at each end to assure that prep does not reach contaminated skin. *C*, Betadine solution blotted with double sterile towel by preparer. *D*, Draping. Note the sterile towel wrapped around the leg just above the ankle at the junction of the prep and the foot to prevent any of the Betadine from oozing through the doubled sterile stockinetting which is applied over the foot and up the leg. Note the folded towel around the top of the prep. Note two double fan sheets, which will be clamped around the folded towel. *E*, Steri-Drape folded around the exposed, prepared area. *F*, Leg wrapped firmly with 15 cm. elastic bandage, knee flexed and tourniquet inflated. We now use barrier stockinette plus plastic instead of stockinette.

Figure 468. Method of draping for knee operation requiring use of sterile tourniquet. Leg is suspended for prep when it is necessary to use a sterile tourniquet. The purpose of the sterile tourniquet is to permit a much greater visualization of the entire leg, as is required in osteotomy for angular deformity, and also to provide a wider range of incision, such as in ligament reconstruction requiring exposure of the iliotibial tract. A, Note the double sterile stockinette which has been placed over the extremity up as high as the hip, following a shave, including pubis, and a soap and water prep the night before. This stockinette is rolled down, and the leg is suspended from the foot. Note the sand bag under the upper portion of the buttock, which permits the prep to extend under the buttock. The prep should also extend up on the thigh, including the groin and the lower abdomen as illustrated in B. B, Ten minute scrub of leg and thigh does not include the foot. If the foot is included, an undue amount of time is spent in preparing the foot and toes—time which could be better spent scrubbing around the knee. Note that the buttock rests on a sandbag so that the buttock is suspended away from the table and the Betadine is spread around the complete buttock. The towels underneath the leg are sterile. Care is taken not to touch the stocking covering the foot or any of the unsterile drape at the top. C, After the Betadine has been removed by a 2 minute scrub with Betadine solution, the prep nurse releases the foot and removes the standard. A surgical assistant has rolled a sterile double stockinette over the foot. Just above the ankle a towel has been wrapped around the leg, and the stockinette is rolled over this to prevent a seeping of contaminated preparation fluid through the stockinette. Note the squaring of sterile towels around the top of the thigh. The extremity is ready for application of the sterile tourniquet. D, Fan sheet is placed under the leg as high as the sterile towels at the buttock and another fan sheet above, and these are clamped around the thigh. Second lap sheet is placed under the leg and not fanned. Steri-Drape is now applied to cover the leg from the stockinette at the bottom to over the tourniquet above. E, The second piece of Steri-Drape is pulled over the upper thigh including the tourniquet. F, The whole leg is wrapped with an Ace bandage for exsanguination, and the tourniquet is inflated. Also split barrier drape is wrapped around upper leg and split Steri-Drape to exclude genitalia.

We no longer use double stockinette over the foot as a "preliminary day before prep," so the foot is fastened into the apparatus without the stockinetting. See text.

Figure 469. Medial incision for repair of the medial collateral ligament. Any part of this incision may be used. *a, b,* The portion of incision utilized for medial meniscectomy. It may be extended to *d* to further explore the knee joint or to treat the patella, and extend down to *c* for repair of the medial collateral ligament.

give way from the midline forward, since the medial ligament becomes very thin here to permit flexion of the knee and so has enough redundancy to permit the knee to "open up."

It is advisable at this stage to enter the knee by an incision through the synovium along the medial parapatellar line. In some instances this incision may be required to open the joint in order to specifically define the area of the tear, which sometimes can be better demonstrated from within out than from without in. At this point the deep layer of the medial ligament is reflected away from the tear. In other words, if the tear is along the tibial margin, it is reflected upward. If the tear is along the femoral margin, it is reflected downward. This gives ready access to the medial meniscus, which should be removed routinely to permit shortening of the medial collateral ligament. This is particularly necessary if the detachment is from the tibia below the meniscus. An effort is made to leave about 2 mm. of the cartilage intact to the medial ligament, since it provides a very firm area through which to place the plicating sutures.

After this exposure is made, the knee can readily be examined (see Fig. 470C). If the anterior cruciate ligament is torn, the knee will open up more widely and the pathological condition of the cruciate ligament may readily be determined. The posterior cruciate ligament should also be carefully examined.

If the anterior cruciate ligament is torn from or near the femur, it may be repaired by mattress sutures placed through two drill holes extending from the lateral epicondylar ridge into the posterior part of the intercondylar notch on the medial side of the lateral condyle. These holes are best made with a smooth pin the size of a guide wire for hip nailing (2.38 mm.). Guide pins are much better than twist drills, since they damage the bone less, make fewer bone crumbs and are in no danger of breaking. The holes should be placed at least 12.7 mm. apart where they exit into the notch, and they should be as far posterior as possible. If the knee will open up, particularly if a smooth wire is used, the drill holes may be made from within outward for more accurate placement of the drill holes within the knee. It may be necessary to use a sleeve on the 2.38 mm. guide wire. Two No. 1–0 cotton sutures, one blue and one white, are passed through the posterior hole into the knee with the aid of a ligature passer made out of a fine wire, with a knurled handle (Fig. 471). A curved needle holder and a stout, small (15.88 mm.)

demonstrate the area of the damage. The tear is defined usually either at the tibial attachment or just above this, but below the line of the joint, and the superficial layer is reflected proximally, with the fascia, to expose the deep layer. In many instances, the superficial layer may be reflected as a separate layer to a point above the line of the joint. At other times the superficial and deep layers will blend just below the joint. As this layer is detached and folded backward, the deep layer is exposed (see Fig. 470B). This layer must be inspected entirely across the line of the joint from front to back. Again rocking the tibia may give a clue as to the site of the tear. This tear is readily seen if the operation is done before healing begins.

Frequently, the ligament will be torn in an irregular fashion. A commonly found tear begins at the midmedial line on the tibial attachment of the deep layer and extends backward 2 to 5 cm. and then vertically upward across the joint and posteromedially across the femoral attachment. Another lesion frequently seen is a tear of the deep layer from its tibial attachment all the way posteriorly to include the medial one third of the posterior ligament. In other instances the ligament may tear at the joint line and the meniscus may be split, the upper part going with the femur, the lower with the tibia. Usually the ligament will not

Figure 470. *A,* The medial utility incision as drawn in Figure 469. *B,* Incision has been made through the patellar retinaculum and the superficial layer of the medial collateral ligament reflected upward in the tenaculum, revealing the joint line with irregular laceration of the deep layer of the medial collateral ligament, which in this instance is torn off the femoral attachment. *C,* The medial incision, the superficial layer of the ligament reflected upward, the deep layer reflected downward, the Russian forceps holding the anterior cruciate ligament, which is torn off the femur. *D,* The medial incision. A 3 mm. drill protected with a short sleeve (a 2.38 mm. guide wire is preferred) is drilled through the back of the intercondylar notch to emerge on the lateral epicondylar ridge. Two parallel holes are made. If the knee will not open up sufficiently to approach from within-out, the drill holes can be made from without-in. It is important to get the holes as far back in the notch as possible. *E,* Two sutures engaging the torn femoral attachment of the anterior cruciate ligament. *F,* The lateral incision along the epicondylar ridge showing the two No. 0 cotton sutures as they exit on the lateral side of the femur.

Illustration continued on opposite page

Figure 470 *Continued.* G, The medial incision. Drill holes are placed in the denuded medial femoral condyle, through which No. 0 cotton mattress sutures are placed to hold the proximal end of the deep layer of the medial collateral ligament. *H,* The deep layer is ligated to the lower femur by No. 0 cotton mattress sutures. *I,* A heavy No. 1 cotton stay suture is placed at the anterior edge of the reflected medial collateral ligament and is pulled snugly forward. This is about the level of the patellar tubercle. *J,* A No. 0 cotton mattress suture placed through the periosteum of the tibia beneath the pes anserinus. K, The superficial ligament is sutured into position. *L,* Wound closed with subcuticular wire or Steri-Strips, or both.

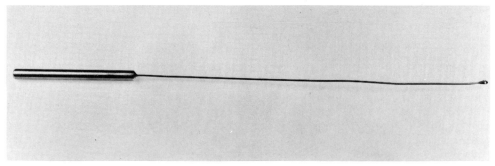

Figure 471. Ligature passer. The diameter of the eye must be less than 2.38 mm.

"knee needle" are used to separately mattress suture each thread into the torn stump of the cruciate ligament, care being taken to spread the ligament out at least 12.7 to 19 mm. rather than to pull it all together to one point. The suture is then pulled out through the second drill hole by means of a ligature carrier with a loop of thread to pull the two thread ends through. With this type of equipment, the holes can be very much smaller and thus will be less traumatic. The sutures are placed while the knee is still opened up, since this facilitates suturing into the cruciate ligament. It can readily be done with the knee entirely stable, but the drill holes must then be made from outside into the knee.

If the cruciate is torn off the tibial attachment, drill holes are made from the antero-medial face of the tibia up into the tibial origin of the cruciate ligament on the superior surface of the tibia. This repair is considerably easier than the other. Similar plication is done within the stump of the cruciate. If it is torn in the middle, I frequently make drill holes in both bones, and pick up the tibial stump through femoral drill holes and the femoral stump through tibial drill holes. I believe this, as a rule, is more successful than direct suture, although I sometimes utilize the latter, too. The important consideration is to get good contact of the torn ends. These sutures are placed but not tied. If the ligament is found to be redundant but not obviously torn, the most effective way to shorten it is to detach it completely from its tibial attachment, prefer-ably with a scale of bone. If parallel drill holes are made through the upper tibia, as described previously, the ligament may be advanced for-ward to get the proper degree of tension. Sutures on the epicondylar ridge should be extrasynovial. None of these procedures is formidable and, with proper tools, should add no more than 15 to 20 min. to the operating time. After the placing of the sutures, they are

not tied until the medial ligament repair is completed, the leg is positioned at 30 to 40 degrees of flexion and the wounds are ready to be closed.

Repair of the Medial Collateral Ligament. The immediate repair of the deep layer of the collateral ligament may be by one of several methods. If there is a direct tear in the liga-ment, with two well-defined margins, simple suture will suffice, with imbrication if feasible. If the ligament is avulsed from the bone, the best method of repair consists of making a series of three or four superficial drill holes about 1 cm. apart at the site of the attachment to the tibial margin or femoral condyle (see Fig. 470G), as the case may be. Suitable suture (No. 0 cotton) is then passed through the ligament into one drill hole, out of an adjacent drill hole and back through the ligament. When all these sutures have been placed, the knee is positioned at about 30 to 40 degrees of flexion, with the leg internally rotated, and all ligatures are tied (see Fig. 470H). As a rule, the superficial layer can be repaired by simple suture to its bed, overlapping the edges (see Fig. 470J) if possible. If this is not possi-ble, a similar procedure may be carried out using drill holes at the level desired.

In the repair of the collateral ligament, every effort should be made to obtain maximum shortening of the ligament, and its tibial at-tachment should be pulled forward as far as is possible (see Fig. 470I). All loose tags are carefully sutured down (see Fig. 470K).

Repair of the Posterior Capsular Ligament. With a rupture of both layers of the medial collateral ligament and one or both cruciate ligaments, there is, as a rule, damage to the posterior capsular ligament. Frequently the posterior capsule will simply split all the way around to the midline. At other times it will be pulled away from the tibia. It is seldom pulled off from the femoral attachment, since it blends together with, and is very firmly secured along, the gastrocnemius muscle origin. Care must be taken not to overlook the posterior capsular tear just because the synovial fold seems intact. Although the two blend very closely together in the posterior capsule, it is possible to have a tear of the capsule proper without an obvious rent in the synovium.

Since the posterior capsule does play a large role in the stability of the knee in general, both in preventing overextension and in stabilizing the knee in extension, it is vitally important that it be repaired. It is not adequate to assume that the ends will fall together. I recently did a delayed reconstruction on a young man who had such a tear in the posterior capsule, which in spite of six months elapsing had not healed at all.

With the knee flexed at 40 degrees, it is easy to pull the capsule together and make the sutures quite snug. To carry out this repair I use a smooth guide wire. The drill hole is started in the front of the tibia about 1 cm. below the articular margin and 1 cm. medial to the patellar tendon. This hole is drilled parallel to the top of the tibia and is drilled from front to back to exit at exactly the same point posteriorly; that is, about 1 cm. below the top of the tibia (see Fig. 504). With the medial collateral ligament torn and the posterior capsule torn, access can easily be obtained to this area. It expedites the procedure and adds materially to the accuracy of the drilling if a power drill is used. It is imperative that this drill have a variable speed because the hole should be drilled slowly so that the bone will not become eburnated. Three or four holes are made about 1 cm. apart, paralleling the first hole, and they are drilled from front to back so that there may be three or four holes, which would permit two or three mattress sutures. The number of sutures needed depends to a considerable degree on the extent of the tear posteriorly. With the use of the ligature carrier, as previously described—and it is important that this small carrier be used— a loop of suture is passed from front to back. A loop of No. 0 cotton blue suture and one No. 0 white suture are passed through this loop and as the ligature carrier is pulled out, it pulls one end of the blue and one end of the white cotton thread through the tibia and out the hole in front. A curved needle holder and a trocar needle the same size as the one which is used in the repair of the cruciate ligament is then used to place mattress sutures through the posterior capsule, with the mattress loop being placed in such a way that it is behind

the ligament. This pulls the ligament flush against the back of the bone. If the posterior tear is a direct one, it can be sutured by apposition sutures, with the knot placed outside the capsule. It is vital that the posteromedial "corner" be snugly secured, since this is very important for stability of the knee.

From this point on the procedure is similar for the different types of incision and has already been described. I will discuss the postoperative handling of the extremity at the end of this section. All apparent bleeding points are coagulated, and the wound is closed. Sutures used are No. 4–0 cotton for the synovium, No. 2–0 for the retinaculum, No. 1–0 cotton for the ligaments, No. 4–0 cotton for the subcutaneous tissues and No. 32 subcuticular wire and/or Steri-Strips for the skin. Color coding, with blue and white sutures being used for the front to back ligatures and for the cruciate, is simply a way of making it much easier to identify the sutures. It is not necessary but expedites the procedure.

Repair of the Posterior Cruciate Ligament Through an Anteromedial Incision. (See also 3. Technique for Repair of the Posterior Components, page 503.) If the posterior cruciate ligament has been avulsed from the tibia and if, additionally, the medial collateral ligament has ruptured, repair will frequently be possible from in front. A drill hole starts in front of the tibia about 1 cm. distal to the articular margin and proceeds directly backward, paralleling the articular surface to emerge posteriorly at the midline near the attachment of the posterior cruciate ligament. The drill holes for this repair are similar to the drill holes made for the repair of the posterior capsule, and if the posterior capsule is torn, both structures can be repaired through the same holes (see Fig. 504). It is important that the most lateral hole be located in the midline in order to keep the posterior cruciate ligament toward the midline. A similar drill hole is passed parallel to and about 1 cm. medial to the first. The suture can be passed, with a suitable ligature carrier, from front to back to emerge posteriorly. This suture is then placed in the knee needle, and since the knee will open up well, it is possible with some patience to plicate the ligature through the detached portion of the posterior cruciate ligament. The needle is then removed, and a suture is again threaded in the ligature carrier and pulled out through the second hole to be tied in front of the tibia after the other portion of the repair has been completed (see Fig. 463). It is important here also to use two sutures, one blue and one white, to make two mattress sutures of No. 1–0 cotton. Then, too, if one suture breaks when being tied, the remaining one can be used and the knee will not have to be opened again to replace the suture.

Repair of the posterior cruciate that has been torn off the femur is very easy through the anteromedial incision (see Fig. 465). The medial femoral condyle is already exposed. I simply denude an area extrasynovially along the medial epicondylar ridge and direct the drill holes from this area almost directly laterally to emerge at the chondral margin in the front of the knee on the lateral side of the medial condyle of the femur. To put it another way, the drill hole emerges on the medial side of the intercondylar notch as far forward as possible. A similar drill hole is made 1 cm. away, paralleling the first one. The two ligatures can be readily passed through this hole, plicated through the stump of the posterior cruciate and passed back out on the medial condylar margin, where each is tied.

2. Technique for Repair of the Lateral Components

With the patient lying on his back, with a sandbag under the buttock on the involved side to hold the thigh in internal rotation, the same meticulous preparation and draping are carried out as indicated previously. The incision begins at the level of the superior pole of the patella about 1 cm. lateral to its lateral margin (Fig. 472). It proceeds distally at this distance from the patella and patellar tendon to the level of the patellar tubercle of the tibia, and then swings downward and backward to terminate at the level of the fibular shaft about 2 cm. from its proximal end. The posterior flap is reflected backward to expose the lateral aspect of the knee, care being taken to take all the subcutaneous tissue with the skin flap.

Careful investigation is now made to determine the nature and degree of the injury. The upper end of the fibula should be carefully examined to see if there has been avulsion of the combined attachment of the biceps tendon and the fibular collateral ligament. If the lesion is in this vicinity or if the fibular collateral ligament is avulsed from its femoral attachment, the flap should be resected far enough so that the peroneal nerve may be examined and suitably protected either by leaving it under observation in its normal course or by dissecting it free and protecting it with a rubber drain retractor. My personal preference is not to strip out the nerve unless this is necessary

because of nerve injury. The attachment of the iliotibial band to the tibia should be carefully inspected. Frequently it will be found to be avulsed. The iliotibial band actually is analogous to the superficial layer of the medial collateral ligament. It becomes a ligament of the knee because of its firm attachment to the femoral condyle through the intermuscular septum, so that the section of the band from the femur to the tibia is a lateral tibial collateral ligament. One may easily overlook a rupture of the intermuscular septum which binds the iliotibial tract to its femoral attachment. It is important to be sure this is intact. This can readily be done as the operation proceeds by passing an instrument or a finger under the iliotibial band to see if the intermuscular septum is holding it down to the femur.

After the nature of the lesion is defined, the knee should then be opened along the line of the skin incision (lateral parapatellar) and the lateral meniscus carefully explored. If the knee will open up readily on the lateral side, this exploration is relatively easy. At the same time the popliteus tendon should be inspected. If there is serious ligament injury on the lateral side, it is advisable to remove the lateral cartilage for the same reason that we remove the medial one on the opposite side, namely, to permit more positive plication of the ligaments. The cruciate ligaments may be inspected from this incision and suitable repair carried out as noted on pages 497 and 501.

From this incision it is easy to make the drill holes to repair the anterior cruciate to the

Figure 472. Lateral incision for approach to the knee joint. This incision parallels the iliotibial band to within a fingerbreadth of the patella and then parallels the patellar tendon. This permits the iliotibial band to be split and reflected backward, giving good access to the lateral compartment. It must be extended downward and backward below the fibular head for lateral ligament repair or for treatment of peroneal nerve injury.

femur without a separate incision. If the anterior cruciate is avulsed from the tibia, there is no necessity for making a medial incision. Drill holes can be made from the lateral plateau forward, inward and upward to emerge on the medial side of the extraarticular portion of the superior tibial surface and a suitable suture is passed through these two holes as indicated previously. If it is necessary to repair the posterior cruciate to the femur, a separate incision on the medial side will be necessary to permit drill holes to be passed through the medial femoral condyle and into the medial side of the intercondylar notch just at its anterior edge. If the posterior cruciate is detached from the tibia, a similar procedure can be carried out as indicated previously for the medial repair, provided that the lateral components are badly torn.

After the sutures for repair of the cruciate ligaments have been placed, one then proceeds to the lateral repair. It should be emphasized that replacement of the fibular collateral ligament is in itself not adequate in repair of lateral ligament rupture, since usually far greater damage is present. The same technique is used to repair the posterior capsule as on the medial side, the posterior capsule being pulled downward to the back of the tibia, with every effort made to get it as tight as possible with the knee flexed about 30 degrees. Similar repair of the fibular collateral ligament is made, either of the femoral attachment to the femur or of the fibular attachment to the fibula. The latter frequently includes the biceps tendon attachment, which must also be replaced. The tibial attachment of the iliotibial band should be carefully replaced, even if this requires drill holes along the tibial margin. If the iliotibial band is detached from the femur, this should be carefully repaired. If necessary, the band can be divided and sutured down to the femur. After all the sutures are placed, the knee is positioned at about 30 degrees of flexion and all sutures tied. The leg is not permitted to externally rotate to beyond neutral and the thigh is kept in internal rotation by the sandbag under the buttock as the ligatures are tied. Closure is then carried out by usual methods.

3. Technique for Repair of the Posterior Components

The patient is positioned face downward, with the entire leg exposed and protected by a Steri-Drape, as previously illustrated. During a portion of the operation, a folded sheet may be placed under the knee to hold it in complete extension. The sheet may be moved beneath the foot to flex the knee when this is necessary to facilitate the operation. The incision begins about 8 cm. above the popliteal fold over the semitendinosus tendon, extends distally along the semitendinosus tendon to the level of the popliteal fold and then swings sharply laterally across the fold to the bicipital tendon and down the calf for about 8 cm. along the posterolateral surface (Fig. 473). This curvilinear incision has no sharp angles and, as it proceeds transversely across the back of the knee, is slightly oblique.

The posterior approach is utilized for repair of the posterior cruciate ligament when it is avulsed from the tibia and for repair of avulsion of the posterior ligament of the joint, which occurs as a result of hyperextension of the knee. The posterior ligament may be avulsed from the femoral attachment above the femoral condyles, but more frequently it is torn from the tibia. In this instance the whole attachment is peeled off the tibia as a cuff, leaving the upper end of the tibia denuded. It usually includes the posterior cruciate ligament. Although the posterior portion of the meniscus can be exposed by this incision, the approach is not proper for entering the posterior compartment to remove a foreign body or to complete removal of the posterior horn of either meniscus.

The popliteal fascia is exposed by reflecting both skin flaps. The classic landmark in this

Figure 473. Posterior incision. Note general line of incision. This can be extended proximally or distally or a shorter segment of it may be used. Two important points are that the vertical portion above the knee should be medial and parallel the semitendinosus tendon; the transverse portion should cross the skin folds behind the knee, with rounded rather than right angle corners. The vertical portion parallels the biceps tendon just slightly medial to it.

area is the posterior cutaneous nerve of the calf, which uniformly lies beneath the fascia, centered between the two heads of the gastrocnemius. The fascia may be split along the line of this nerve proximally as far as the fascial termination above the knee joint, where the nerve will be found to join with the tibial nerve. Following the tibial nerve proximally, one may locate the peroneal nerve as it comes off to the lateral side and extends down the lateral side of the popliteal space. This exposure is facilitated by the use of a tourniquet, but care should be taken to clamp and coagulate or ligate any vessel which may be damaged in the area. The tibial nerve is located posterior (and therefore superficial) to the artery and vein, so that it may be followed down across the posterior space to the bifurcation of the two heads of the gastrocnemius. It is ordinarily not necessary to dissect out the peroneal nerve so long as it is located and adequately protected. Since the peroneal nerve has a firm attachment, it is relatively immobile and will not tolerate forceful retraction, particularly toward the medial side. After these structures are located, careful dissection deeper into the space will reveal the popliteal artery and vein. These can be retracted toward the lateral side, which will expose the medial head of the gastrocnemius. The geniculate vessels crossing behind the knee in the popliteal space may be sacrificed as necessary, depending upon the pathological findings.

Having defined the medial head of the gastrocnemius by retracting the vessels and nerves laterally, the tendinous attachment of the medial head of the gastrocnemius to the femur is divided, leaving 1.3 cm. attached to the femur for resuture. It is extremely important that the approach be made from the medial side, for by sectioning the medial head of the gastrocnemius, the whole neurovascular bundle may be retracted laterally. The tibial nerve has much more retractability than the peroneal, and it is not as satisfactory to remove the lateral head of the gastrocnemius in an attempt to enter the area between the peroneal and the tibial nerves.

By this division and retraction of the medial head of the gastrocnemius and the vessels and nerves laterally, the posterior capsule of the joint is exposed. The posterior ligament of the joint is revealed and the pathological condition may be defined. If the posterior ligament has been avulsed from the tibia by hyperextension of the knee, a very heavy, firm rim of ligament will be found, with a free distal margin extending transversely across the lower portion of the popliteal space. This can be lifted up by a suitable instrument, and the posterior surface of the tibia will be found to be denuded. In most cases the posterior cruciate ligament is included with this avulsed posterior capsule. If not, it may be readily examined by reflecting the capsule or cuff proximally to inspect the posterior part of the knee. If the posterior capsule itself seems to be intact or possibly only stretched, access to the posterior cruciate may be obtained by a vertical incision in the midline, extending from the level of the femoral condyles to a point below the upper end of the tibia. By retracting the margins of the capsular incision, the posterior cruciate is exposed as it arises behind the tibia on its posterior surface and courses upward, forward and inward to attach to the lateral margin of the medial femoral condyle anteriorly.

The posterior ligament of the joint actually is made up of many structures, but usually it is torn en masse so that separate repair of each of these structures is not necessary. If it is necessary to carry out isolated repair of the posterior cruciate ligament, the exact procedure will depend upon the nature of the tear. If the avulsion is from the tibia, suitable drill holes are made in the back of the tibia, and sutures are passed through the drill holes and mattressed into the end of the ligament. This is a favorable type of repair. At this point the knee should be flexed to facilitate relaxation of the tissues in the popliteal space. If the tear in the posterior cruciate is anterior, it will be necessary to make a second incision on the medial aspect of the lower thigh in order to expose the subcutaneous border of the medial femoral condyle and permit drill holes to be made into the intercondylar notch as indicated previously. Although this seems quite formidable, it can readily be accomplished from the two incisions. Sutures are passed through the drill hole in the femur, using a suitable ligature carrier, and recovered in the posterior incision as they emerge in the notch. They are then plicated through the posterior cruciate and passed back out through the second drill hole. As tension is put on this suture, it replaces the posterior cruciate ligament against its attachment to the femur. If the posterior capsule is torn directly across, it may be repaired by direct suture. If torn away from the femur, it also may be repaired by suture to the attachment of the gastrocnemius. A certain amount of ingenuity may be necessary, depending upon the pathological findings.

I would like to emphasize that one cannot count on simple flexion of the knee to approximate the separate edges of the torn capsule. A recent case illustrates this very well. When the knee was hyperextended, the denuded part of the tibia was exposed, the whole posterior ligament and posterior cruciate ligament being torn away like a cuff. As the knee was flexed, this cuff did not slide down over the end of the tibia. Rather, it buckled into the back of the joint, so that even if union had occurred, it would have been with considerable redundancy of the ligaments. It is possible that with an intact posterior cruciate, the torn posterior capsule might well heal spontaneously by simple flexion of the knee. As in the case of other complete ligament tears about the knee, however, there is no means of ascertaining, short of operation, the exact nature of the lesion. Hence, surgical repair offers a much better overall prognosis. Granted, there are instances in which a good result is obtained by nonsurgical measures following complete rupture, yet the rate of success is substantially less than with surgical repair because some cases obviously cannot return to normal without surgical repair.

After all the ligatures are placed, the knee should be positioned at about 40 degrees of flexion and all the sutures tied. Closure is remarkably easy in this posterior approach. The gastrocnemius head is sutured back to its tendinous attachment. No other deep sutures are necessary, since as the popliteal fascia is closed, the whole area is snugly pulled together.

Postoperative Care

After closure of the skin, the management of the extremity varies according to the type of repair which has been made. Up to this time the leg has been positioned on the table at about 30 to 40 degrees of flexion, with the foot in internal rotation for medial repair, or neutral position for lateral or posterior repair. If there has been damage to the anterior cruciate ligament, the extremity must be supported above the knee and the upper end of the leg must be permitted to drop backward. Two attendants support the leg by the thigh and by the foot (see Fig. 452). This position is maintained until the dressing is completed. If in addition to the cruciate ligament, the medial collateral ligament is torn, the lower leg should be internally rotated in relation to the femur and held in this position until the external fixation is secure. If on the other hand the posterior cruciate ligament is involved, the support should be behind the calf rather than

the thigh in order to hold the leg forward and relax the tension on the posterior cruciate ligament. If both cruciate ligaments have been torn, a neutral position can be held by maintaining support under both calf and thigh. These measures are extremely important, since the simple weight of the leg may be enough to pull out the rather insecure suturing through the cruciate ligament. If both the anterior cruciate and lateral collateral ligaments are torn, the thigh and foot should be supported, with the leg in neutral rotation. If it is the posterior cruciate and posterior capsule that are injured and the incision is posterior, with the patient in the prone position, a heavy posterior plaster slab may be applied to the leg, extending from the gluteal fold to the toes. The lateral stirrup may be applied after this has set.

After this careful positioning of the extremity by the attendants, the knee is wrapped in sterile sheet wadding. We prefer to use Sof-Rol at the top of the thigh, since it does not fray so badly. A posterior slab is applied from the gluteal fold to the toes (see Fig. 452A). No matter how the leg is held, the foot must be placed in the weight-bearing position, namely, slight eversion and zero dorsal flexion. The plaster slab is wrapped in place with an 8 cm. gauze bandage and then supported by a lateral stirrup running from the perineum to the trochanter (see Fig. 452B). This is firmly wrapped in place with gauze.

At this point we have completed the stirrup splint (see Fig. 452C). However, the patient is usually an active athlete, and in order to obviate the possibility of his flexing the knee abruptly through the opening in front of the splint as he awakens following the procedure, a single roll of sheet wadding is wrapped around the knee from 15 cm. (6 in.) above the knee to 15 cm. below. Directly over this is wrapped a single roll of 15 cm. plaster of Paris bandage (see Fig. 452D). If the repair has been posterior and by a posterior approach, the splint may be applied with the patient lying face downward. Preferably the very heavy posterior splint is applied and permitted to set. Then the patient is turned on his back for completion of the dressing. The advantage of this type of stirrup splint is that as swelling occurs, it may be readily opened. As swelling regresses it may be tightened again.

When the patient is well awake, the plaster circular bandage is removed. If there is any doubt concerning the swelling, the entire dressing is split from the toes to the groin and the splint rewrapped. The dressing must not be split over the knee only. If swelling is severe enough to suggest an effusion or hemarthrosis, the dressing is removed under aseptic conditions, with the surgeon wearing cap, mask and sterile gloves and the knee is aspirated. This dressing is left for about two weeks, at which time under ordinary circumstances the size of the leg will be static. The dressing is then removed and the stitches are taken out and a lightweight, long leg plaster cast is applied with the knee flexed 15 to 20 degrees (see Fig. 454). The leg should be supported in exactly the same manner for application of this cast as for application of the original dressing, since union of the ligament is quite insecure at the end of two weeks. This plaster cast is worn for four to six weeks. Frequently a walking heel is used if the repair seems stable and if the patient is reasonably agile. He may use the heel for weight-bearing but is advised to continue using crutches. At the end of four weeks in the solid cast (six weeks postoperative), it may be removed and a cotton cast (see Fig. 441) applied. Aspiration is repeated as often as it is indicated. This splint is removed in two weeks (eight weeks postoperative) and an elastic bandage utilized as indicated. If effusion persists, repeated aspiration and injection may be done. Most cases do not require even one aspiration.

For *rehabilitation*, quadriceps setting and straight leg raising of both legs are encouraged from the first day (see page 484). The patient is in a wheelchair at 24 to 48 hours after the operation. He should be able to actively raise the leg, splint and all, by 72 hours and to walk on crutches in two to four days. Weight-bearing is not permitted, however. After the solid cast is applied (two weeks postoperative), he may walk with crutches on a walking heel if progress is good. In the meantime, exercise of all other available muscles is encouraged. (See chapter on Rehabilitation.)

After the cotton cast is applied at six weeks (postoperative), the patient is urged to walk and gradually decrease the use of his crutches. He is to continue his exercises. Two weeks later (eight weeks postoperative), the cotton cast is removed and quadriceps rehabilitation continues until the circumference of both thighs is equal. In recent years I have relented a bit about insisting on solid cast fixation for as long as eight weeks following an acute ligament repair. Various methods such as the use of the hinge cast, and early and well-controlled physical therapy, have been used to help regain motion earlier. If there is any possibility of damaging stress, it is better to continue the use of the cast. In some cases I have used a specially made brace with a very rigid bar running from the ankle to high onto the thigh, both inside and outside, held by Velcro straps. This brace has a controlled joint at the knee, so that it is possible to move the knee within the restrictions of the hinge. This brace can benefit a responsible person, but for a young person who has not yet developed a sense of responsibility, I prefer the relative security of the cast. The actual level of activity varies much with the individual patient. The agile, wiry person of relatively light weight may be allowed more freedom than the heavy lumbering giant whose ligaments are normally relaxed. Progressive resistive exercise in which the knee is flexed and extended should not be initiated if effusion or swelling is marked.

Running is permitted if synovitis is not marked. No contact is allowed until four months and not even then if the quadriceps is not completely rehabilitated. The knee must be thoroughly taped for every competition or every practice session for at least 12 months.

Naturally, each case must be strictly individualized as to both type of repair and postoperative management. A patient with a good, tight repair with intact ligament fibers can be permitted considerable liberty. Some patients need to be pushed in their rehabilitation, and the period of immobilization may be shortened. Other patients must be curbed (for example, 16- to 18-year-old athletes), and their knees will require a full eight weeks of protection. The elastic bandage should be discarded early in the timorous patient and retained as a reminder in the overbold one. If effusion persists, the usual treatment for effusion is carried out—namely, aspiration, repeated as needed, with injection of a corticoid and use of an elastic bandage—as long as moderate effusion persists. Some synovitis will ordinarily be present until essentially normal motion is recovered. In an occasional case there will be some difficulty in obtaining normal motion. This is made more probable by the fact that each ligament is sutured as snugly as possible, with the knee placed in the most relaxed position for that ligament. I would rather have some restriction of motion than any instability. Unfortunately the converse is more often true, more patients having persistent instability than limitation of motion.

Manipulation of the Knee. The necessity for manipulation of the knee arises when the patient is not developing a normal range of flexion in the anticipated period of time. This may occur owing to inadequate postoperative care or because of a lack of motivation by the patient. With any operation of the knee, particularly ligament reconstruction, a steady progressive improvement in the range of flexion is most important. If two to three weeks pass without an increase in flexion, manipulation is in order. This same rule applies in cases of total knee replacement. Manipulation should be successful if carefully done.

Great care should be taken in the exertion of force with the patient under anesthesia. It should be steady and even. It may take as long as 30 minutes before anything is gained. There usually will then be audible crepitation in the joint, but a sharp snap indicates that some major structure has actually been damaged. The extent of motion depends upon the resistance. If there is little resistance, there is no reason not to take the leg to normal flexion of 135 degrees. Otherwise flexion of 115 to 120 degrees must suffice, and another manipulation may be done in a couple of weeks.

This procedure is carried out with the leg suspended in an apparatus hooked to the fracture table, in which the thigh is fastened to the top of the table by a strap, with another strap attached under the calf. The first strap serves to fix the thigh, and the second strap permits traction to extend the leg, which makes the procedure much easier. When a satisfactory range of flexion is obtained, the flexed knee is carefully scrubbed. X-rays are made to be sure that there is no bone damage. The knee is injected with Marcaine (10 ml.) and with depromedrol (1 ml.), a cortisone derivative.

The knee is snugly wrapped in a single layer of sheet wadding, over which a 6 in. elastic bandage is firmly applied. The leg is extended and removed from the apparatus, and three ice packs, applied so that they encompass the joint, are held in place with elastic bandages. The outer bandages and ice packs should be changed every two to three hours. The inner elastic bandage is best left undisturbed, unless there is some problem with swelling of the foot. Physical therapy is ordinarily started the next day. Physical therapy *must* follow the manipulation in order to maintain the flexion obtained.

Early examination, prompt decision as to treatment and complete repair of all torn ligaments, followed by conscientious rehabilitation, will give increasingly gratifying results in the treatment of major injuries to the ligaments of the knee.

In our series of cases, 80 per cent of the patients are under 25 years of age (Fig. 474), 60 per cent are under 20 years of age. Since so many of these injuries occur in young people, we must try particularly to obtain the best possible recovery of function in the shortest time.

Following an injury to the ligaments of the knee, the question will arise as to whether or not the player should be allowed to compete in contact sports. The answer must depend entirely upon the individual circumstances. There is no reason why patients with *mild* (first degree) and *moderate* (second degree) sprains should not recover completely and be as strong as ever, provided they had proper management at the time of injury. Obviously, for one reason or another, complete recovery in other patients will not always be attained. In these patients the decision must be made as to whether or not the remaining ligament function is adequate to withstand the rigors of athletic competition. The same decision must be made following an injury that has been treated surgically. If the operation was early and adequate ligament repair was carried out, the player may usually expect a normally functioning knee. But if complete rehabilitation is not obtainable, the vital decision must be made as to what level of athletic participation should be permitted. If athletic activity has been an incidental factor in the patient's life and competition is truly not important to him, he may want to abandon contact sports out of fear that the injury will be repeated. This might happen even if good recovery has been obtained. I have seen many players return to competitive athletics with no apparent impairment following major injuries. The point I would like to make is that one must not be casual one way or the other. The case must be carefully studied and a considered opinion given, since this matter is of considerable importance to the people most concerned. If chronic irritation persists, with recurring synovitis, if there is slight instability and if there is pain on stress, these factors must be considered in advising the player on his athletic future.

OSSIFICATION OR CALCIFICATION

There is a distinct difference between calcification through the knee and ossification. Calcification as a rule is a sign of degenerative change, and it weakens the ligament. It has no function in the repair. Ossification is the laying down of mature bone in the ligament, which in some circumstances may give increased strength to the ligament, although it may also interfere with full range of motion. These

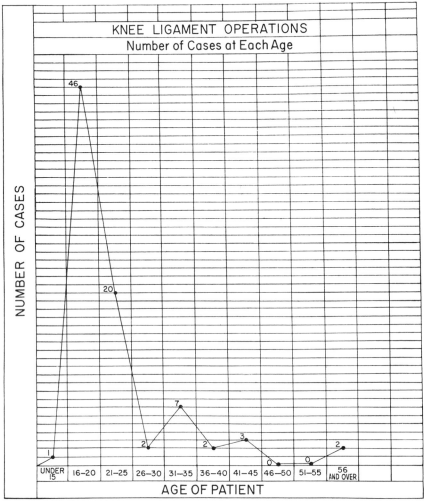

Figure 474. Note that 60 per cent of patients are under 20 years of age; 80 per cent are under 25 years of age. (From O'Donoghue, D. H.: J. Bone and Joint Surgery. *37–A*:4.)

conditions are not common about the knee, but they do occur and may have distressing sequelae. As with ossification elsewhere, I believe that one of its major causes is repeated irritation around the joint following infiltration of blood from an injury. In my experience, I have not seen gross ossification following early surgical repair of a knee ligament. I have seen it on many occasions after sprains that were not surgically treated, but it would be unfair to assume that surgical evacuation of the hematoma would have prevented ossification. It is my impression that ossification is more frequent following late operation that disrupts the organization of blood after it is well advanced (Fig. 475). This certainly has not been the rule, however, since in most cases, ossification does not occur.

A moderate degree of ossification in the medial collateral ligament may not be trouble-some. Major symptoms result from ossification in the part of the ligament that glides back and forth over the condyle of the femur or the upper end of the tibia. Ossification here actually seems to give more trouble than ossification in the ligament attachment itself, which is seen occasionally following a moderate sprain.

Treatment. A nodule of ossification that causes persistent symptoms may be removed, but one should be particularly wary of removing the bone when it is not symptomatic. A good test is the injection of a local anesthetic around the area to determine whether it relieves the pain. In removing the bony plaque, great care should be taken to split the ligament fibers longitudinally, even if more than one split is necessary to get all the bone out. Transverse section offers extreme difficulty in repair and will necessitate another long period of immobilization, whereas if the ligament is divided along the line of its fibers, a couple of weeks will be ample. There is a tendency to examine a patient, to take an x-ray which shows some ossification and to recommend removal of the bone without any real analysis of the symptoms. Disappointment will usually result, since there are, indeed, many areas of spurring in the body that cause no symptoms whatever. Many cases diagnosed as bone fragments in the back of the knee, using x-rays, have been referred to me for removal when actually the finding was a normal fabella that was perfectly innocent of any symptoms. Ossification of the lateral collateral ligament is infrequent. Ossification of the posterior ligament occurs but is usually not symptomatic, since this ligament does not slide directly over the condylar surface. Whereas ossification is relatively common to some degree, calcification is not. Calcification is more likely to be seen within the ligaments themselves than along the bone.

PELLEGRINI-STIEDA DISEASE

A condition commonly called Pellegrini-Stieda disease consists of the formation of a plaque of calcium or bone along the medial femoral condyle in the vicinity of the adductor tubercle, separated from the tibia by a band of radiolucency (Fig. 476). It is in some instances a reaction to a sprain in which there has been a forcible detachment of the medial collateral ligament at its attachment to the femoral condyle and, in other instances, to partial avulsion of the adductor longus tendon. The symptoms are those of sprain of the knee, with tenderness high on the condyle in the one case and of adductor strain in the other. The presence of the mass is not necessarily of any consequence, the significant factor being the degree of pain. Frequently the area remains painful even after the injury has healed.

Treatment. In some instances removal of the plaque is necessary. A word of warning is in order, however. If the surgeon is too eager

Figure 475. This 19 year old athlete with major injury to the knee was seen 24 hours after injury. He had tremendous swelling of the knee in the popliteal area extending down into the calf, with obvious severance of the medial collateral ligament. Any attempt to straighten the knee beyond 60 degrees caused immediate pallor of the foot and cessation of arterial pulsation for a period of minutes. Because of the extreme swelling, he was treated expectantly by aspiration of the hematoma, aspiration of the knee, elevation, ice pack, etc. He was operated on ten days subsequent to the injury. The medial collateral ligament was avulsed from the tibia, including the sartorius and semitendinosus; the posterior ligament was detached clear around the midline; the posterior cruciate was torn off the medial femoral condyle; the anterior cruciate off the femur. There was excessive hemorrhage into the popliteal space, with gross blood clot, which was evacuated. He had good stability following ligament repair but developed tremendous ossification. This was later excised. Now a surgeon, the patient still has restriction of motion of the knee. Before the ossification was removed he could not flex the knee 90 degrees. Three years postoperative he had 15 degrees restriction of flexion with a completely stable knee. This injury occurred almost 20 years ago. In a similar case I would now recommend immediate exploration of the popliteal space, with evacuation of the hematoma and ligation or repair of whatever circulatory damage had been done. A, Three years after injury. B, Three years after operation for bone removal. No attempt was made to remove the bone at the lower end of the ligaments, since this was not symptomatic.

Figure 476. Typical Pellegrini-Stieda disease caused by partial avulsion of the adductor muscle from the adductor tubercle of the femur and ossification within the hematoma. This particular case was persistently painful, and the ossification was removed. This ossification is not within the medial collateral ligament. Early treatment here should have been protection against abduction or any adduction stress, together with local measures.

and removes the mass before it is entirely mature, it will simply form again. If it is necessary to remove it, great care should be taken that there is no interference with the attachment of the ligament to the femur. In a preponderance of cases, removal of the plaque will not be necessary, since the condition may mature and become quite inert with the passage of time.

DISLOCATION

Dislocations of the knee are the end result of a severe sprain, since in order for any portion of a normal knee joint to dislocate, certain groups of ligaments must be disrupted. Two basic dislocations of the knee occurring as a result of athletic competition are the *patellofemoral dislocations* and *tibiofemoral dislocations*. In each instance we speak of the femur as being the stable bone with the other bone being displaced in relation to it.

Patellar Dislocations

Patellar dislocations may be classified as acute or recurrent. Recurrent dislocations may be subdivided into congenital and acquired.

Recurrent Dislocation of the Patella

Basically the true congenital dislocation implies an actual and constant dislocation of the patella, usually laterally over the femoral condyle. If fully developed, this condition will more or less prevent athletic participation and need not be emphasized here. Of much greater importance is the dislocation that occurs infrequently and under certain circumstances. It may be due to repeated episodes of acute dislocation in a normal knee. Quite frequently there is no true congenital dislocation, but there are certain physical characteristics that predispose to and set the stage for subluxation or luxation. One predisposing anatomical condition is an abnormally acute angle between the axis of the patellar tendon and the axis of the quadriceps mechanism, the so-called Q angle (Fig. 477). If the patellar tendon tends to angulate sharply laterally to reach its tibial attachment, this, combined with the fact that the quadriceps mechanism tends to angulate

Line of Quad Pull

Q Angle

Line from Patella To Tibial Tuberosity

10°

Figure 477. The "Q angle" is the angle formed by two intersecting lines. One is the line of the quadriceps pull, extending down the thigh to midpatella; the other is a line from the middle of the patella to the center of the tibial tuberosity. The angle illustrated is within normal limits.

Line of Quad Pull

Q Angle

Line from Patella
To Tibial Tuberosity

26°

Figure 478. This figure shows an increase of the "Q angle," which indicates a more lateral position of the tibial tuberosity. This predisposes to dislocation or lateral luxation of the patella.

medially at the knee, results in an increased angle (Fig. 478) between the patellar tendon and the long axis of the quadriceps, so that as the quadriceps muscle is contracted, there is a tendency for this angle to straighten by the slipping of the patella laterally. This action may be inhibited by the prominence of the lateral femoral condyle anteriorly, but the general tendency is for the patella to slide laterally with each forceful extension of the knee. The female with her wide pelvis (see Fig. 489) and internally angulated femora is thus much more prone to patellar subluxation or dislocation than the male. A similar situation arises in a person with knock-knee. A dislocated patella in a bowlegged individual is quite uncommon, since in such a person the axis of the patellar tendon and quadriceps is essentially parallel. However, in some bowlegged individuals, this bow is part of internal torsion of the femur, so that the femoral condyles are rotated toward the midline. Such a person often has an associated external rotation of the tibia in order to straighten the long axis of the leg. In this instance the "Q angle" may be markedly more

acute as the patellar tendon moves from the internally rotated patella down to the externally rotated patellar tubercle.

One may, therefore, expect recurrent dislocation of the patella in a person with a wide pelvis, knock-knee and a relatively flat lateral femoral condyle. This recurring dislocation may arise gradually, with the patella subluxating laterally, stretching the medial portion of the patellar retinaculum until the patella finally slips off either as a result of a relatively minor blow on its medial side or from a violent contraction of the quadriceps (see Fig. 479A). Ordinarily in the initial instance, the patella simply snaps off, and slips right back on, and there are few, if any, residual symptoms. The patient may describe the knee as having "given way." He may actually have fallen, since his proprioceptive mechanism has warned him of the impending dislocation and relaxed the knee to prevent it.

On examination, findings may be entirely negative. One must carefully distinguish between the giving way caused by the catching of the meniscus or by a foreign body in the joint and the giving way caused by impending or actual subluxation of the patella. Many a knee has been subjected to meniscectomy when the "giving way" was actually related to the patella. This is particularly pertinent because the same "cutting" movement of the athlete as he changes direction results in external rotation of the tibia on the femur, which may displace the involved meniscus. On the other hand, this same relationship with the femur rotating in and the tibia rotating out sets the scene for slipping the patella off laterally. One must always suspect patellar subluxation in the knee, which for reasons not understood by the patient simply gives away. In fact, a well-developed patellar subluxation and ultimate dislocation may occur with no actual tearing of the retinaculum. This patient soon learns that his activities must be curtailed and presents for treatment only when the recurrence becomes so frequent that it interferes with his ordinary activity. Surgical measures designed for correction of this condition must be carried out if the disability justifies them.

Treatment. One must carefully analyze the characteristics of the injured extremity. Frequently what appears to be recurrent dislocation of the patella may actually be repeated episodes of acute dislocation with no anatomical predisposition. This is particularly likely, since the most commonly accepted treatment for the acutely dislocated patella at the present time is nonsurgical. After replacement of the dislocated bone, the torn edges of the patellar

Figure 479. This 17 year old girl, seven weeks before, was playing basketball when she came down hard on the left leg, twisting the knee and falling to the floor. She had severe pain and swelling and could not extend her knee. Her history was that she had had recurrent episodes with the knee before this acute injury in which something "seemed to be slipping" and the knee would be quite painful. She had the feeling that the knee cap slipped to the side. It has been very much worse since the last injury. She cannot squat or go up or down stairs and feels that the knee cap slips off to the side. Examination in the sitting position revealed that the patellae seem to have a normal relationship. She gets a lateral shift as the patella comes to complete extension, much more severe on the left. As a matter of fact, it slips off every time she extends the knee. There was a 4 + positive apprehension test (see Fig. 425). *A,* Normally positioned silhouette view of the patella,* showing the patella slipping sideways and the fragment off the patella, indicating a recent tear of the medial retinaculum. *B,* The Hughston view,* showing the dramatic level of displacement in this position. Note the fragment remaining in essentially the same position as it did in the other silhouette *(A)* while the medial margin of the patella moves away. *C,* Lateral view of the patella showing the patellar index 6.4 cm. to 4.3 cm., a definite amount. (See Fig. 481 for discussion of patellar index.) Note also that the patella is above Blumenstadt's line, even though the picture is made at 45 degrees flexion rather than at 30 degrees flexion. If it were moved up to 30 degrees flexion, the disparity between the distal pole of the patella and Blumenstadt's line would be more marked. (See Fig. 481 for discussion of Blumenstadt's line.)

*For discussion of x-ray techniques, see Figures 491 and 492.

retinaculum remain more or less widely separated. After healing, this inevitably results in a relaxed medial retinaculum, so that as the knee flexes, the patella does not receive as much pull medially as it does laterally and any additional force applied to the patella on the medial side will snap it over the lateral condylar ridge. This may occur as repeated episodes of subluxation, with only an occasional complete dislocation. One must be on the alert, therefore, when examining a patient with such a history to determine whether or not there is actually a congenital (Fig. 480) or developmental defect, since the remedial measures may be quite different in the two conditions.

If the anatomical characteristics are normal, all that may be necessary will be medial plication of the patellar retinaculum, usually ac-

companied by division of the lateral patellar retinaculum and quad lateralis attachment, particularly if the condition has persisted over a long period of time. If on the other hand the angle of the patellar tendon is faulty, any of the capsuloplasty operations will give disappointing results, since the predisposing cause is still present. Many procedures have been designed to correct the basic anatomical condition causing recurrent displacement. One may expect excellent results from any of them if the proper indications are present. Once successful correction is carried out, activity need not ordinarily be restricted. I recall a figure skater with bilateral recurrent dislocation of the patella that was symptomatic to the point that she had to give up her skating. Following transference of the tibial attachment of the patellar tendon medially and capsuloplasty of the knee, she returned to her skating without further handicap. This particular patient was in her early 20's, and one knee required almost a year for complete rehabilitation. I mention this to deprecate the all-too-prevalent tendency to warn a person that he must permanently decrease his activity when carefully designed treatment may permit normal use.

As has been indicated earlier, many different techniques for transference of the patellar tendon have been recommended. I have tried most of them in the course of treating the dislocating patella. The one that I find the most satisfactory is as follows: A medial parapatellar incision is made beginning at the superior border of the patella. It follows along the medial margin of the patella, shifts over to parallel the patellar tendon and continues down to the patellar tubercle or tuberosity of

the tibia. It then curves medially to expose the medial face of the upper tibia. This skin flap is reflected to the lateral side. The lateral retinaculum is defined and incised, beginning at the level of the top of the patella or maybe slightly above, depending upon the degree of tightness, advancing along the lateral border of the patella and down along the lateral margin of the patellar tendon to the tuberosity. The tuberosity in most instances is found to be displaced laterally with an increased Q angle (see Fig. 478). Whether or not patellar alta is present should be determined by using the patellar tendon–patella index. The oblique cortical line extending across the femoral condyle (Blumenstadt's line) is used to estimate just about how high the patella is situated (Fig. 481). A block of bone is then outlined 2 cm. wide and 4 cm. long, beginning about 1 cm. above the attachment of the patellar tendon

Figure 480. This 76 year old female says her knee caps have been dislocating ever since her childhood, and now this condition is very much more severe. They do not actually dislocate, just slip sideways. She uses a cane so that she does not fall. Patellectomy may possibly be indicated if the symptoms are severe enough. *A* and *B* show the right and left patellae with very extensive osteoarthritis. *C* and *D* are the silhouette views (see Fig. 491). Treatment at an early stage would possibly have prevented this serious disability.

Figure 481. There has always been considerable concern about just how one defines patellar alta. Where should the patella normally be and how can one judge it? A simple way was recommended by Blumenstadt some time ago. He reported that with the knee at about 30 degrees flexion, the distal end of the patella ought to be at the level of the oblique cortical line extending across the femoral condyles as shown in A. More recently popularized is the patellar index; for this, take a measurement of the length of the patella, then a measurement of the distance from the distal tip of the patella to the dimple on the top of the patellar tubercle of the tibia. If the distance from the patella to the tubercle is over 1 cm. greater than the length of the patella, this would suggest patellar alta. The more the difference, the more the alta. This index can be made in essentially any position of flexion as long as the patellar tendon is tight. Therefore, the same film could permit both criteria (Blumenstadt line and patellar index) to be used. Obviously, neither of these tests is entirely accurate. Often in determining the patellar index it is difficult to determine just exactly where the dimple is on the patellar tubercle, and sometimes it does not seem to be present at all; so, it comes down to the fact that you just have to evaluate whether you think the patella is high and the patellar tendon is long. These two tests do help. A, Case demonstrating the patella situated higher than normal. B, Normal position of the patella.

to the tibial tubercle so that there is a block of bone about 1 cm. long and about 2 cm. wide, like a tongue, above the attachment. The saw cut is then continued down to about 4 cm. below the proximal transverse line, at which point an oblique cut is made extending at a 45 degree angle to make a "sled runner" toe on the block (Fig. 482). The block is then excised with the tendon attachment intact. The distal cortical part can be rather thin because its cortical bone is strong. The proximal cancellous part must be thicker, since it is very easy to break off the proximal extension, which is the key to the block.

The block with the tendon attached should be carefully removed so as not to break off the proximal extension. The patellar tendon is separated from the fat pad. The tendon and patella are reflected proximally to expose the underside of the patella. Whatever procedure is necessary for correction of the patellar pathological condition can now be done, as for example, chondroplasty by shaving, by trephining and drilling, or facetectomy.

Once the patella has been taken care of, it is then necessary to determine how far the patellar tendon should be transferred distally and how far medially. The medial displacement is determined by trial and error by simply holding the block against the proximal tibial face at different spots and flexing the knee. The tendon attachment should not be advanced distally unless there is a confirmable patellar alta, or else the patella will be pulled down too far toward the tibia (Figs. 483 to 485). The general plan followed is that if the patellar alta is in the range of 2 cm., advancement of perhaps 1 cm. should be made. It should be remembered when cutting the window that the length of the block that is above

Patellar Tendon

Patella

Patellar Tendon

Tibial Tubercle

Patellar Tendon

Tibial Tubercle 2 x 4 cm.
Fits into Opening
2 x 2 cm.

Tibia

Figure 482. Technique for transference of patellar tendon. See text.

4 cm.

2.5 cm.

A

4 cm

4.8 cm

B

Figure 483. This 35 year old female had surgery 18 months before this, at which time the patellar tendon was transferred too far distally. A, X-ray postoperative, showing patellar baja and actually an articulation between the patella and the top of the tibia, the index being 2.5 cm. to 4 cm. This was treated by patellectomy, since the patella was too badly damaged to salvage. B, X-ray of the opposite knee shows she does not have a patellar baja, the index being 4.8 cm. to 4 cm. (For discussion of patellar index, see Fig. 481.)

Figure 484. This 29 year old female was operated on at age 16, with transfer of the patellar tubercle distally. The tubercle was actually transferred 4 cm. distally, which pulled the patella down below the top of the tibia as shown in A. She has had recurring episodes of subluxation and dislocation of this left patella ever since. She cannot flex the knee more than 90 degrees. Examination at age 29 revealed gross subpatellar crepitation. At this time patellectomy and advancement of the tendon proximally were done. B, X-ray at three months postoperative showing the block transferred 2 cm. proximally. At six months postoperative the knee was doing well except it popped a lot. Mild extensor lag. She could actively extend to zero.

Figure 485. This 29 year old female has had recurrent subluxing patella since age 15, when she was active in ballet. There had been gradually increasing episodes until she was operated on at age 27—"Houser" procedure—with very long rehabilitation. She could actively extend her knee to 45 degrees. She would have to assist it by this point and then could extend on up to zero. The same thing occurred with the knee flexed. The patella slipped out of the groove at 45 degrees, and then it would flex further. Increasing pain and disability. A, Lateral view of the right "good" knee. B, Lateral view of the left knee, showing downward displacement of the patella. C, Postoperative film after replacing the patellar tendon attachment medially and shortening the patellar tendon. Marked improvement with no subsequent dislocation.

the tendon attachment must undermine the tibial cortex. If the extension is 1 cm., 1 cm. of advancement is lost by virtue of the proximal 1 cm. of the block being slipped proximally. The hole in the tibial face is made the same width as the bony block but is roughly half its length, so that the hole will be approximately 2 cm. square. The cancellous bone is cut out of this window to permit the block to be inserted, as illustrated in Figure 482. The distal end of the block is inserted in the hole and passed down along the medullary canal of the tibia far enough to permit the proximal end to be dropped into the hole, after which the knee is flexed and the proximal end of the block slides up into the excavation, which has been made proximal to the proximal end of the cavity created for the transference, and it locks there. The block in this way is completely strong and requires no healing to be secure.

The knee can be flexed completely to test the position to determine how much the medial side needs to be imbricated, the medialis advanced and the lateral side released so that the patella will glide freely in the groove without slipping laterally. Once it is locked in, cancellous bone can be packed around the block, although this is not necessary. It may leave somewhat less of an open space. The defect where the block was removed is covered with a thin layer of bone wax. The block removed in preparation for the transplant is not placed in the hole left at the tubercle. The closure continues by imbrication of the medial retinaculum to whatever extent is necessary, including advancement of the medialis. The lateral retinaculum is left open, this gap being filled by transferring the fat pad to fill the lateral hole, even if it is necessary to completely free the pad from its previous bed. I have noticed no difficulty when this has been done, except in two cases in which young female patients noticed that the fat pad was more lateral than normal.

In this type of repair the patient is kept in either long leg stirrup splints or coaptation splints for two weeks. These splints permit early ambulation, usually in one or two days. At the end of two weeks the splints are removed and the function and range of motion are tested. The knee is then put in either a long leg walking cast or long leg cylinder for approximately another two weeks. At this time full weight-bearing, straight leg raising and further exercises for the knee are recommended (see page 484). At the end of four weeks the external fixation can be removed

and the patient is advised to walk on crutches until obtaining 90 degrees of flexion. I recommend straight leg raising and active exercises from the first postoperative day, since the block is entirely secure at that time.

I have been gradually shortening the time of immobilization, depending upon the disposition of the patient and the condition of the surgical wound. If the knee is not swollen, the wound is healing well and the patient is quite responsible, I have on occasion removed fixation at 2 weeks rather than at 4 weeks. I do not believe this is advisable unless the knee can be flexed approximately 90 degrees at two weeks.

Admittedly there are many other techniques which may be equally adequate. In my own experience I have been able to mobilize the knee much quicker using this method, since all that is involved is the healing of the skin flap and recovery from the trauma of the operation. The transfer is secure once it is locked in.

It should be noted that this type of advancement should be done only when the epiphyses are closed or essentially closed. First, there is the possibility of premature closing of the anterior part of the tibial epiphysis, causing a recurvation. More importantly, however, if the tubercle is transferred below the upper tibial epiphysis, as the leg grows, the tubercle will grow farther and farther distally until in some instances the patella will be dragged down to or below the level of the top of the tibia (Fig. 486).

Although particular techniques are not described here, I should emphasize again that the technique must be matched to the case. The surgeon must not try to match his case to a predetermined or stereotyped procedure. If patellar alignment is at fault, it must be corrected. Capsulorrhaphy by release laterally and plication medially will certainly fail in this case. On the other hand, a patellar tendon attachment transfer is contraindicated if this alignment is normal. One must not transfer the tendon or the tubercle below the upper tibial epiphysis if growth is not complete. In the young person some means other than tubercle transference must be used. Plastic operations in the patellar tendon or the quadriceps tendon or in both may be effective. Transference of the attachment must be accompanied by release of the lateral retinaculum or the quad lateralis attachment, since alignment cannot be corrected otherwise. Careful attention to the undersurface of the

Figure 486. This 16 year old male was operated on at age 12, with bilateral patellar tendon transference distal to the proximal tibial epiphysis. As the leg continued to grow, the block that was below the epiphysis moved down the leg in relationship to the knee and pulled the patella down so that (A) the patella on the right knee was at the top of the tibia and (B) on the left the patella was well below the level of the top of the tibia. At age 16 he has severe symptoms, with swelling, pain, weakness, snapping and extension lag, which lately are much more severe. When he tries to extend his left leg, he has to lift it with his hand while the patella slips back into the groove. Treated by patellectomy and shortening of the extensor mechanism. This figure illustrates the result from transference of the tubercle below the growing epiphyseal plate.

patella is a must, since chondral damage is the rule in recurrent dislocation. There may also be damage to the cartilage on the lateral condyle. Recurrent dislocation of the patella may be very distressing to the athlete, particularly if it goes unrecognized. Many unsuccessful meniscectomies have been done because of an unrecognized subluxation of the patella. Correction of this underlying condition, if done before chrondral damage is irreparable, should result in the return of the player to active competition.

Acute Dislocation of the Patella

Although acute dislocations of the patella may occur with no predisposing anatomical condition, certain factors do predispose to this injury. Thus, a shallow patellar groove, an abnormal patella, an abnormally positioned patella, a laterally displaced patellar tendon attachment or some combination of these conditions is often present. The mechanics of the injury is as follows: As the person turns away from the externally rotating leg with the knee flexed, a violent contraction of the quadriceps may put intolerable stress on the medial retinaculum. The quad medialis is at a disadvantage, and the retinaculum tears, permitting the patella to snap over the lateral condyle. If the knee remains flexed, the deformity will persist, and the patella will lie against the outer side of the lateral condyle. If the leg is extended either spontaneously by the patient or by someone else, the patella will usually slip back in place.

On initial examination the patient will be in severe pain, with the knee flexed and the tibia apparently abducted. He resists any attempt of the physician to manipulate the knee.

Careful examination makes the *diagnosis* obvious if the patella is unreduced, since it will be found to be riding lateral to the lateral condyle of the femur. Much more frequently the dislocation is spontaneously reduced as the knee extends, so that the patient relates that the injury was accompanied by severe pain and often describes the knee as having been "dislocated" and then having slipped back into place. It should be noted that this history is quite similar to that obtained after injury to the medial collateral ligament and not too different from that after an acute meniscus tear, with locking spontaneously reduced. In describing the dislocation, the patient will often state that the distal end of the femur has displaced medially and is quite prominent in this position. This is explained by the fact that as the patella slips off, the anterior contour of the knee changes, and with the leg in external rotation and somewhat abducted, the medial femoral condyle becomes very prominent. The patient will describe the displacemnt as being medial when actually the patellar displacement is lateral.

If examination is done quite early, there may be a palpable defect along the medial border of the patella, with exquisite tenderness along the medial edge of this bone. The patient is extremely apprehensive of any attempt to push the patella laterally and will cry out and try to restrain the examiner's hand, particularly if manipulation is accompanied by a gesture toward flexing the knee (see Fig. 425). If examination is delayed, the knee joint will be filled with fluid and there will be diffuse swelling, which is more severe anteriorly, whereas in the case of a medial collateral tear, the swelling will be toward the medial side. On palpation of the knee one finds tenderness around the medial border of the patella, with pain on flexion of the knee, which is pathognomonic. The negative findings are of considerable importance, since there will be neither tenderness along the collateral ligaments nor pain on lateral motion of the tibia on the femur with the knee either extended or flexed. The patient who has had an acute patellar dislocation will permit a careful and considerate examiner to flex the knee a few degrees and externally rotate and abduct the tibia on the femur with no complaint, whereas in the acute case of medial collateral or indeed meniscus injury this will not be possible. If hours elapse before the examination is carried out, the findings become less specific, since muscle spasm tends to immobilize the knee, swelling becomes diffuse and tension within the capsule causes diffuse pain about the knee.

The lesion in acute dislocation is a rupture of the medial portion of the patellar retinaculum, which may be complete and may include a portion or all of the attachment of the vastus medialis. In fact, the vastus aponeurosis and patellar retinaculum may be peeled away from the medial border of the patella, leaving it bare or actually tearing off a portion of the bone (Fig. 487); the patellar retinaculum may be split, much as a piece of cloth tears, with the jagged tear extending anywhere along the medial aspect of the knee from the anterior edge of the deep layer of the medial collateral ligament to the patella.

X-ray examination is important (Fig. 488). Careful study of films may reveal an avulsion fracture or provide a clue particularly in regard to the general contour of bone, the anteroposterior view (Fig. 489), showing the increased tibiofemoral angle which predisposes to dislocation, and the silhouette view (Figs. 490 to 492), showing the shallow patellar groove. More specifically, the latter may show the fragmentation along the medial border of the patella, where there has been an avulsion of the ligament retinaculum (see Fig. 487).

Treatment. The treatment of acute dislocation of the patella in the athlete is surgical. One has only to see the damage to tissues to realize that there can be no real substitute for accurate repositioning of the torn fibers and adequate repair. Research work is confirming more and more the conclusions that have been reached clinically, namely, that ligament or tendon heals by ligament or tendon if good apposition is secured, whereas a gap that must be bridged in the healing process is likely to remain inadequate inelastic scar. I have seen separations of 2 to 3 cm. along the patellar retinaculum following acute dislocation, and there was no tendency for the split fibers to fall spontaneously into apposition. Indeed, even slight flexion of the knee tends to force them further apart, the only acceptable position being complete extension or indeed hyperextension of the knee. This cannot or at least should not be tolerated for the length of time required for tissue repair. The operation is relatively simple, since the lesion is essentially subcutaneous. In a well-conditioned athlete, if proper precautions are taken, the operation should pose no undue hazard. The reward will be a prompt and complete recovery.

Since the acceptable treatment is surgical, the general management is consistent with this approach. After a careful examination and diagnosis, a compression bandage is applied and ice is used, together with fixation of the knee, until the operation can be carried out. The ideal time for surgical repair is immedi-

Figure 487. Patellar dislocation with avulsion of patellar tendon and medial retinaculum. *A*, Anteroposterior view showing dislocation. *B*, Silhouette view. Arrow indicates avulsed retinaculum. Note also the shallow patellar groove, which tends to predispose to dislocation.

Figure 488. Dislocation of the patella. *A*, The anteroposterior view showing the patella locked laterally. *B*, The straight lateral view shows significant overriding of the patella and femur, indicating that there must be dislocation.

Figure 489. Note that because of the broader pelvis in the female, it is necessary for the femur to come inward at an increased angle in order to make the distal end of the condyles parallel with the ground. The quadriceps, patella and patellar tendon make an angle centered at the patella. As the quadriceps contracts, this angle tends to straighten, which forces the patella laterally.

Figure 490. A, Normal silhouette view of the patella. Note that the patella seats well in the groove, with configuration between the undersurface of the patella and the femoral condyles. The lateral edge of the groove serves to help hold the patella in its normal position. B, Shallow groove with flat patella. The lateral buttress is lost, predisposing to dislocation. C, Silhouette radiograph of acute complete dislocation of the patella. Note the relatively shallow groove but the sharply peaked patella. (For positioning of the silhouette view, see Fig. 491.)

Figure 491. Silhouette of the patella ("Sunrise View"). With the patient seated on the table, elevate the knees and support them with sandbags until the femur and tibia form an angle of about 45 degrees. Have the patient hold the cassette in a vertical position about 30 cm. proximal to the patellae. Direct the central ray to the patellofemoral joint space, forming about an 80 degree angle with the cassette. The angle of the knees and central ray may be varied according to the patient's tolerance. A centering light aids in directing the central ray just beneath the patella. A piece of art foam may be used to anchor the cassette if necessary. Both patellae, for comparison, are visualized on the film.

Figure 492. This figure shows the comparison between the Hughston view and the normal silhouette. This 34 year old female had a history of recurring trouble with her patellae as far back as she can remember. A and B, the silhouette views, could be interpreted as showing some lateral subluxation of the left patella (A), since the lateral edge of the patella is beyond the lateral edge of the trochlear groove, particularly as compared with the right side (B). In the Hughston view, C and D, there is definite tilting apparent on both patellae. I would interpret the Hughston view on the right (D) as being negative. However, if the left one (C) was not available for comparison, the right one might be considered to be tilted abnormally. I think one has to determine a normal in order to have a basis for accurate judgment of the Hughston view.

See Figure 491 for x-ray positioning of the silhouette view. The Hughston view is made with the patient prone with the plate lying under the knees, the knees flexed to about 60 degrees and the tube paralleling the tibia.

523

ately or at least as soon as proper preparation can be made. Although a day or two delay does not completely preclude a good result, increasing experience indicates that there is no time like the present for surgical treatment of the ordinary acute injury. Ideally it is best treated the day it happens, but in no instance should it be treated later than the following morning provided there is no contraindication to surgery.

The operative technique will vary with the pathological findings. As a general rule, a curved incision is made in the medial parapatellar area, beginning at the upper pole of the patella about 1 cm. medial to it, extending along the border of the patella and paralleling the patellar tendon. On retraction of the skin edges, the patellar retinaculum can be visualized and the nature of the damage ascertained. The incision may need to be extended higher if the vastus medialis has been avulsed or swung lower and somewhat posteriorly if the medial flap must be reflected to expose the retinaculum further toward the inner side. Usually the capsule of the knee will be torn open. The joint should be carefully inspected, particularly the undersurface of the patella and the lateral edge of the lateral femoral condyle. An osteochondral fracture may be present in either location (Fig. 493). If there is a chondral fracture or chondromalacia, it should be carefully treated by chondrectomy or other measures, the exact technique depending upon the severity of the condition. One may suspect chondromalacia in a knee with a dislocated patella, since the tendency for the patella to slide laterally on extention of the knee may be

quite traumatic to the cartilage over a period of time. Malacia along the medial and superior facets of the patella is quite common and should be corrected at the time of operation. Treatment of the dislocation itself is relatively simple. By approprirate suture, the defect is closed. If one is unable to suture to the edge of the patella, drill holes may be made along the edge of bone, carefully avoiding penetrating the patellar cartilage. Fixation is readily obtained in this manner. The lateral retinaculum and lateralis attachment along the margin of the patella should be incised if the patella is at all tight as the knee flexes.

Postoperatively the leg is placed in long leg posterior and lateral stirrup splints, with the knee slightly flexed (10 to 15 degrees), for seven to ten days, at which time the sutures are removed and the knee is further protected against flexion by an appropriate cast. Whether there should be weight-bearing depends upon the individual patient. Healing will be prompt. The long leg cast can be removed after another three weeks and a cotton cast worn for one more week (total six weeks). During this time activity is gradually increased, and the customary rehabilitative measures are initiated. A word of caution: If the patient has the anatomical characteristics that predispose to recurrent dislocation, these should be carefully analyzed and a definite plan of management instituted. Either his activity should be sharply curtailed or reconstructive measures should be carried out to reduce the tendency toward lateral slipping. This is particularly important if there has been damage to the patella. One should have no hesitation in recommending transfer-

Figure 493. Acute dislocation of the patella in the oblique view, with chondral fracture of the undersurface of the patella. Note the fragment lying just behind the femoral condyle slightly distal to the lower pole of the patella. Note also the defect on the underside of the patella. At operation an acute fracture with a fresh bleeding bed under the patella was found. The hooklike processes on the medial epicondylar ridge are normal variants. This type of trauma can cause apparent "patellar malacia" if not recognized early.

ence of the patellar tendon attachment from the lateral to the medial aspect of the tibia in such a case, since without this procedure, recurrent trouble in later life is almost inevitable, even though athletic activities are curtailed. If the anatomical alignment is normal and no predisposing characteristics are manifest, further protection after the completion of healing is not indicated. In this instance there should be no more predilection for trouble than there would be following a broken tibia, for example.

Tibiofemoral Dislocation

There seems to be general agreement that a recognizable complete dislocation of the knee is a rare injury. The recorded diagnosis seems to depend upon the dislocation persisting until it can be evaluated in the hospital by physical examination and by x-ray study. Very few patients reach the hospital with a dislocation unreduced. A New York hospital reported only two cases out of 20,000 admissions; one in Philadelphia reported only two cases out of 140,000 admissions. I think this gives a very

inaccurate picture of the actual number of cases in which the knee is dislocated. Certainly many of the dislocations are reduced spontaneously or at the scene and are never documented as dislocations (Figs. 494 and 495). The statements that "my knee slipped out of joint" or "my leg was off to the side and someone pulled it back straight" tend to be discounted and are considered to be descriptions of meniscus slipping.

I see many old cases for consideration of reconstruction in which both cruciates, often both collaterals and both sides of the posterior capsule are grossly unstable, some of them with peroneal nerve injury. This is not the place to document these cases in detail, but a relatively casual review of our cases reveals that those that have required two-stage reconstructions of the medial collateral, lateral collateral and both cruciate ligaments were determined, probably by careful history taking, to have actually had dislocations (Fig. 496). I mention this for two reasons: first, to state that this injury is not that rare and, second, to point out that in a severe knee injury one must always be on the alert for vascular damage whether or not there is an actual recorded dislocation.

Figure 494. X-ray showing late dislocation of the tibia posteriorly. This was a football injury, with gross swelling and complication of circulation to the foot and to the peroneal nerve. The x-ray many months later showed posterior displacement of the tibia on the femur and complete lateral instability. This was a posterolateral dislocation of the knee, sparing the medial components. At reconstructive surgery the patient had absent posterior and anterior cruciate ligaments, with complete lateral side instability. *A*, Posterior displacement. *B*, Showing lateral and cruciate ligament damage.

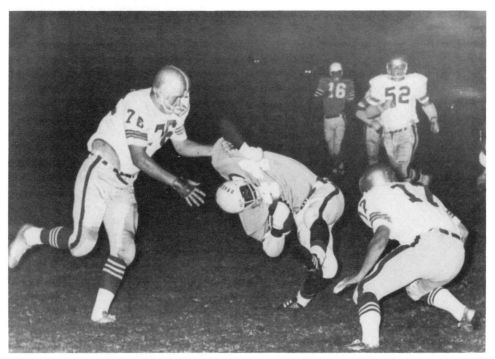

Figure 495. This 17 year old high school player with his weight on the right foot is being pulled the same direction so that his right knee is bent at 90 degrees. In this position the knee is completely dislocated. The medial side was completely torn with damage to the posterior capsule and both cruciates. The position was corrected on the field, which is proper. He had complete disruption of the anterior and posterior cruciates, the medial collateral and the medial posterior capsule. The lateral side was largely spared. Nerve and blood supply were undamaged.

Figure 496. This patient was seen several years post-injury. He reportedly had a dislocation of the knee, which was treated by reduction and cast; several days later bilateral meniscectomy was done with repair of the medial collateral, lateral collateral and both cruciates. Without subsequent injury he had increasing instability of the lateral side. We recommended and carried out lateral side, anterior and posterior cruciate ligament reconstruction, with marked improvement. A, Lateral stress x-ray several months post-injury shows wide opening of the lateral side, indicating the lateral collateral and both cruciates were completely afunctional, which I think confirms the fact that he did have a dislocated knee. B, Medial stress x-ray. Note the lateral slipping of the tibia on the femur, indicating redundancy of the medial structures as well.

Complete tibiofemoral dislocation is also very rarely recognized in the athlete. There is some separation of the tibia from the femur in any complete tear of the collateral ligaments. Usually this subluxation is spontaneously reduced, and by the time the patient is examined, it appears to be what it indeed is, a ligament injury. In some instances the displacement is so complete that it does not reduce spontaneously. At other times a frank dislocation has been noted before it is reduced by a fellow player or some other individual on the field. If the patient has a history of complete dislocation, one should investigate very carefully to determine whether it actually was tibiofemoral in character. A dislocation of the patella or indeed a dislocation of a meniscus with temporary locking may quite often be interpreted by the player himself as a dislocation of the knee.

The tibiofemoral displacement may be in any direction, and determination of this direction has important bearing on the surgical approach. Knee dislocations are classified according to the position of the tibia in relation to the femur:

1. Anterior dislocation–the most common.
2. Posterior dislocation.
3. Lateral dislocation.
4. Medial dislocation.
5. Rotatory dislocation.

Anterior Dislocation

The mechanism of injury has been much discussed in relation to the type of injury. Thus, hyperextension will cause anterior dislocation. Since hyperextension is a common injury, this is the most common type of dislocation. In this condition the force angulates the tibia forward until first the posterior capsule tears, then the anterior cruciate and then the posterior cruciate. Usually the medial and collateral components are damaged, but they do not necessarily have to be completely disrupted for the tibia to slip forward on the femur. As the overextension continues, the tibia slides forward and locks there (Fig. 497). This overextension may place intolerable stress on the popliteal artery, which is well tethered above and below the popliteal space. The artery is stretched and often large segments of the artery will show multiple ruptures, contusions and gross edema. This may require resection of such a large section of the artery that direct suture is not possible. The intima of the artery may rupture, whereas the outside wall may seem intact. Hence, delayed thrombosis may develop and the unwary physician will be unprepared.

Posterior Dislocation

Posterior dislocation cannot occur as a result of overflexion. The force must be directly applied to the front of the tibia with the knee semiflexed (Fig. 498). The tibia is driven backward and the posterior cruciate and posterior capsule rupture. Almost always one or both of the lateral components must give way, and there is a rotatory component, lateral to spare the medial ligament and medial to spare the lateral ligament. I am speaking now of movement of the tibia on the femur.

The vascular injury here is usually a frank rupture of the popliteal artery in the popliteal space. Suture is often feasible here. The peroneal nerve is usually spared.

The ligaments injured are the posterior capsule, posterior cruciate and medial and lateral collateral ligaments.

Lateral Dislocation

Lateral dislocation is caused by a force on the thigh driving the leg into wide abduction. The medial collateral components, the medial posterior capsule and the anterior and posterior cruciate ligaments give way, and the tibia slips laterally off the femur without serious damage to the lateral components, although they may also be torn (Figs. 498 and 499).

Vascular injuries are not frequent in this type of dislocation, although damage may occur if the dislocation is gross. The neurovascular bundle can move laterally with much more freedom than it can medially. Hence, it is more often spared.

The ligaments injured are the medial collateral, medial posterior capsule, anterior cruciate and posterior cruciate, with lateral injury less likely, although it may occur if there has been very major trauma.

Medial Dislocation

Medial dislocation is caused by a force driving the lower leg medially, a force not commonly present in athletic injuries. When the lower leg is struck directly laterally, as occurs when a car strikes a pedestrian from the side, the tibia is angulated medially, and slides medially on the femur, with rupture of the lateral components, the two cruciates and the poste-

Figure 497. This patient was struck from the rear by a car, resulting in compound anterior dislocation of his knee. Both cruciate ligaments were torn. He was treated elsewhere by early repair, which was successful except for residual posterior instability. A, Lateral view showing the anterior displacement. B, Showing superposition of the tibia and femur. Late reconstruction was required for the posterior instability.

Figure 498. This 19 year old female was involved in an automobile accident two years before. Complete posterior or posterolateral dislocation of the right knee. Critical general condition with ruptured spleen, etc. The dislocation was reduced under anesthetic; nothing else was done. Several weeks later she was operated on and the ruptured quadriceps tendon was repaired with a little suturing on the medial side. At 10 months postoperative she was operated on again with meniscectomy and an attempt was made to repair the posterior capsule. Three months later the dislocation was reduced but there was gross medial and lateral instability. Treatment here was by medial side reconstruction followed by lateral side reconstruction and reconstruction of the anterior cruciate. A, The lateral dislocation of the tibia on the femur. B, The posterolateral displacement is shown. C, Medial stress and (D) lateral stress at four years post-reconstruction. Excellent stability, with essentially no complaint of the knee, but note severe degenerative changes.

Figure 499. Football injury, with the player having been hit on the lateral side of the knee, forcing the femur inward and the tibia outward, causing a lateral displacement of the tibia on the femur. Six months post-injury he had complete medial and anterior instability, which was reconstructed. X-ray shows the stress film indicating the medial and anterior instability. Note the lateral subluxation of the tibia on the femoral condyle.

Figure 500. This 16 year old male was injured playing football the night before when he was struck on the lower leg, forcing the leg medially. It appeared to be off to the side and was straightened on the field. My examination revealed gross lateral instability, with the whole lateral side of the knee completely absent in flexion or in extension. X-ray shows the gross lateral instability even with the knee in extension. At surgery everything was torn off laterally, including the peroneal nerve, both cruciates, lateral collateral, popliteus and biceps. The medial side was ecchymotic and swollen but apparently stable. His immediate postoperative course was satisfactory. At four months postoperative the knee is laterally stable in extension and flexion; no anteroposterior instability; 3 + effusion; flexion to 130 degrees. Excellent result so far.

rior capsule (Fig. 500). The medial components may strip away from the femur and so not be ruptured. This medial dislocation is quite uncommon. Peroneal injury is often present.

Rotatory Dislocation

In posterolateral dislocation the force is anteromedial rotation of the femur on the tibia when the foot is fixed and the tibia dislocates posterolaterally off the lateral condyle (Figs. 498 and 501). The medial components may be spared, since the rotation point is on the medial tibial plateau. The cruciate ligaments are often torn, particularly the posterior cruciate. With extreme continuation of this force, the medial condyle may burst through the medial capsule in front and be trapped there. This type of dislocation usually requires open reduction.

In posteromedial dislocation the opposite is true. The rotation is on the lateral plateau of the tibia, the foot being rotated inward and the thigh outward, so that the tibia displaces backward off the femoral condyle. In this instance the damage is largely to the medial components, the anterior and posterior cruciates and the medial posterior capsule.

In any of these positions other injuries may occur. The menisci are usually damaged, often becoming completely loose. There may be chondral fractures, avulsion of the gastrocnemius attachment, rupture of the patellar tendon and fracture of a condyle or of the patella. There may be damage to the blood vessels and nerves about the knee, repair of which may take precedence over all else.

Diagnosis

If the patient is seen immediately, a careful examination will be highly informative. The first step should be to evaluate the circulation to the foot and the second to determine the state of the nerve supply. It is extremely important to know whether or not there has been

Figure 501. Rotatory dislocation caused by the foot being caught in a power take-off. Note residual posterior dislocation. At surgery both cruciate ligaments were torn and de-rotated. The posterior cruciate was torn off the femur, the anterior cruciate was torn off the tibia, the posterior capsule was torn, the iliotibial band was torn off the tibia, and the biceps and fibular collateral were pulled off the fibula. Following subacute repair, 17 days, he obtained good stability, since the two cruciate ligaments were torn off the bone rather than by their fibers.

immediate loss of innervation to any part of the foot. Late paralysis will suggest pressure intrinsic or extrinsic on the nerve and may well require different management than would early paralysis. The peroneal nerve is particularly vulnerable in dislocations.

After the preliminary survey of the condition of the leg and foot, attention is directed to the knee. Careful inspection will reveal any persistent deformity and its direction, thus providing a valuable guide to the pathology of the injury. If the deformity has been reduced either spontaneously or manually before the examination, it may be possible at this early date to determine the degree of instability of the knee. When examining the patient, the physician should be extremely careful, taking particular pains not to reproduce the dislocation. I remember one instance in which the patient had a complete dislocation of the knee that was spontaneously reduced and redislocated three times before x-ray films were made that showed the complete dislocation (see Fig. 430*A*). Obviously, redislocation is a serious

hazard and should be assiduously guarded against. After examination and some definition of the degree of abnormality, measures for treatment should be promptly initiated.

Primary Treatment

There may seem to be some disparity of opinion as to the treatment of acute dislocation of the knee. Actually, however, there is a surprising agreement on the basics of treatment. All agree that the primary consideration in knee ligament dislocation is the circulation to the leg. In cases of soft tissue injury or fractures, the viability of the circulation must also be a primary consideration. The essentials of treatment generally accepted are

1. immediate reduction,
2. evaluation of circulation,
3. arteriogram,
4. open surgery for vascular damage.

Reduction. There can be no doubt, and it has been well documented by many, that early, in fact, immediate, reduction is the very first priority. The end result may depend entirely upon this factor. Hence, reduction should be and ordinarily can be done at the scene of the injury. A prior knowledge of the force applied will help but is not essential. Careful, gentle traction in the line of the extremity will usually suffice to slip the tibia back under the femur. The more complete the disruption, the easier the reduction. If the femoral condyle is locked over the front of the tibia, simple extension of the leg will usually dislodge it. If not, flexion of the leg with forward pull on the calf will accomplish reduction. Usually this can be done under vocal analgesia, namely, calm reassurance and gentle encouragement.

In the lateral or posterior position it may be necessary to gently rock the tibia while continuing traction. Gentleness is the key to success. The longer the dislocation continues, the harder reduction becomes as muscle spasm fixes the displacement. Strenuous manipulation is never justified.

If the dislocation cannot be reduced without anesthesia, the emergency becomes more urgent, and the patient must be rushed to the emergency room, preferably where definitive treatment can begin. If undue delay of several hours is necessary to accomplish this, the patient should be taken first to the nearest available place in which the dislocation can be reduced. The only justification for x-rays showing the deformity is if they can be taken while other necessary arrangements are being made, such as calling the doctor, giving the anesthetic and so on. If atraumatic reduction cannot be carried out without anesthesia, anesthesia should be given. A spinal may be done because it may help circulation. If reduction cannot be carried out by gentle manipulation under anesthesia, open reduction must accompany inspection of the vessels.

Circulation. Circulation is the first priority after reduction! If the foot has been pale, cold and pulseless before reduction, this should promptly disappear, and a flush should be noted if the circulation is adequate. The dorsalis pedis and the posterior tibial pulses should return at once. The coolness disappears and is replaced by local warmth as circulation returns to the capillaries. Danger signs are

1. absent or diminished pulses,
2. continued pallor,
3. diminished sensation,
4. continued coolness.

One must not be misled, however, by questionable warmth on top of the foot. The top of the foot may be warm, yet the circulation may be quite inadequate. Simple absence of the pulses on this foot which are present on the other side is sufficient justification for exploration of the artery.

Watchful waiting here is disastrous. An arteriogram is helpful, although some say it may cause local irritation. If there is any doubt about the adequacy of the circulation, operation should be carried out. The following procedures are in general order of preference (see posterior approach to the knee, page 503).

1. Direct end-to-end anastomosis seems most successful, but one must be able to approximate the artery ends without tension.

2. Resection to normal artery with replacement by a reverse vein graft from the opposite saphenous vein has had considerable success and many prefer this method to use of any artificial prosthesis.

3. Replacement using an artificial prosthesis.

4. *Simple ligation is disastrous.* The leg will not ordinarily survive rapid loss of the popliteal artery.

After the dislocation is reduced, the extremity must be protected while further definitive treatment is considered. Use of a posterior slab is best, since it can be nonconstrictive, and it does permit observation. If there has been evidence of circulatory disturbance which has not required surgery, a suitable waiting period of 24 to 48 hours should ensue, de-

pending upon the condition of the leg. If surgical repair of the vessel has been necessary, the same conditions prevail. Observation must be constant and the patient's condition reported to the responsible physician. A few hours' delay from 2:00 A.M. until "morning" may be fatal for the leg. The same rules apply here. The appropriate surgeon should be on the alert, and if there is any doubt as to the condition, the vessel should be explored.

Treatment of the Injured Ligaments

Treatment of the knee injury includes the following:
1. Reduction.
2. Splinting.
3. Observation (24–48–72 hours).
4. Surgical repair of each torn ligament.
5. Postoperative immobilization (8 weeks plus).
6. Rehabilitation.

Although the treatment to this point has been generally accepted, there has been difference of opinion as to the treatment of the injured ligaments. My position is quite clear. If there is evidence that any ligament is completely torn and if the leg is safe for surgery, I think this ligament should be repaired at the time when there seems to be no doubt about the adequacy of the circulation. Although ligaments are better repaired at once, the elapsed time interval is not that important up to 7 to 10 days or even a little later if absolutely necessary. The pendulum seems to have swung toward repair of all torn ligaments. It has been documented many times that ligaments repair the best if they are placed end to end and immobilized until they heal. One only needs to see the inside of a dislocated knee to be impressed with the virtual impossibility of complete spontaneous repair. Indeed, I have seen the posterior capsule invaginated into the joint, the medial collateral ligament often lying on top of the tibia and various other combinations that seem impossible to recover by closed treatment.

Surgical correction should be done at the earliest safe moment, usually from 48 hours to 10 days. If the patient has been operated on for vein graft or arterial repair, I think one should wait at least 48 hours and preferably 72 hours to be sure the vessel is patent. This could also be confirmed by an arteriogram. Since immobilization must be continued for eight weeks from the day of the surgery, undue delay in initiating the surgery increases the total period of immobilization and so increases the time of rehabilitation.

If surgery is necessary for arterial damage, I would take advantage of this incision to get some indication of the location of the various injuries. This would help in the selection of the best approach for repair of the ligaments. If the posterior capsule is torn with the posterior cruciate off the tibia, I would quickly repair this if it did not require further dissection or trauma. I would not make another incision or unduly enlarge the one made for the vascular repair. Needless to say, if secondary operation is done one must wait until the first surgery is adequately dry.

Certainly in the athlete the treatment of dislocation of the knee is surgical, and adequate repair requires all the skill one can muster. True enough there have been cases treated nonsurgically that resulted in recovery of a useful degree of function of the knee, but I have never known of one so treated to end with anything approaching *normal* function. Immediate measures are the same as for any ligament injury of the knee. Following examination, aspiration of blood and application of a pressure bandage with ice are imperative. Then, without fail, the whole extremity must be protected with adequate splinting, since irreparable damage may be done to the leg by careless handling. The patient should not walk from the field with assistance or be carried, leg dangling, with his arms over another player's shoulders. He should be tightly splinted manually, placed on a stretcher and not moved from the stretcher until proper support is applied to the knee.

I cannot emphasize too strongly the vital importance of the circulation to the leg and foot. The popliteal vessels are well tethered in the popliteal space and do not tolerate much stretching. The injury may be to the arteries or to the veins. The artery may rupture, resulting in excessive bleeding and intolerable pressure in this area, with compression of the veins and the nerves. Venous bleeding will be less dramatic and more readily controlled by pressure.

A normal pulse in the early stages of the injury does not preclude arterial injury, since the intima may be damaged with no damage to the arterial wall. This injury may not be visible even on surgical examination of the outside of the vessel wall. The damaged intima encourages mural thrombus formation along the injured area. As the thrombus develops, it may completely obliterate arterial circulation. If there is *any* doubt about the integrity of the circulation, definitive surgery for repair of the ligaments should be delayed. If there is a serious question as to whether or not vascular exploration should be done, it should be done. Several days' delay in definitive treatment of the ligaments is a cheap price to pay for an intact circulation. Vacillation about the condition of the circulation, however, should not permit unnecessarily long postponement of any necessary surgical treatment.

After reassurance that the circulation is safe, plans are made for definitive treatment. This should not be interpreted as meaning that repair should "wait until the swelling goes down." It simply means that the physician should assure himself of the adequacy of the circulation of the foot, since if this is not adequate and does not respond to paravertebral sympathetic block and similar measures, the first step may well be exploration of the popliteal space. Rupture of the popliteal artery or vein is a distinct possibility. If it is necessary to explore posteriorly and if the circulation is not too disturbed, some degree of posterior repair may be carried out at this time. Repair of the posterior cruciate and posterior capsule may be feasible as part of this procedure. If the circulation of the extremity is intact, then a choice must be made between an approach to the knee from the medial or from the lateral side. This choice will depend upon where it is suspected that the major damage is located. One may obtain surprisingly good access to almost all parts of a badly torn knee with an incision on one side only. I have been able to repair the posterior cruciate to the tibia, the posterior capsule to the tibia, the anterior cruciate to the femur, and the medial collateral ligament to the femur and tibia, as well as carry out medial and lateral meniscectomy, using a medial approach. This is possible because the knee can be very carefully opened up in these circumstances to permit placement of sutures, which can be tied after the joint is reduced and positioned. Tourniquet time must be carefully guarded (90 min. maximum). Indeed, much of the closure may be carried out after the tourniquet is removed. Removal of the tourniquet before closure has the added advantage of permitting control of bleeding. It is good for one's peace of mind to know that no major vessel is the cause of the postoperative swelling, which is almost inevitable. The whole procedure may be done without tourniquet if deemed advisable. This does make for a long and tedious surgical experience, and use of a tourniquet is usually proper.

Following a suitable period of recovery from the initial injury and the reparative surgery, a second operation may be carried out if necessary. If the peroneal nerve has been primarily damaged, it should be explored and repaired within a relatively early period, say, within two weeks. There is a degree of urgency in the treatment of each of these structures and the priority is definitely in the following order: (1) circulatory embarrassment, (2) damage to the cruciate ligaments, (3) collateral ligament damage and (4) neurological deficit. Justification for this timing is quite evident after a little consideration. After the circulation I give second priority to the cruciates because the success of cruciate ligament repair varies inversely with the elapsed time after injury. It must be done within the first two weeks and the sooner the better.

A dislocation of the knee is an extremely serious injury. This is not sufficient justification for a negative approach to the problem, since the dislocation need not necessarily terminate in a major disability. Time is of the essence. The patient should be placed promptly in the hands of the specialist who will carry out the definitive treatment.

A recent personal experience involved a patient with complete anterior dislocation of the tibia on the femur, bilaterally. This 19 year old male was involved in an automobile accident and received multiple bruises and major injury to his lower extremities. He arrived at the hospital with both lower extremities dislocated at the knee joint. Figure 502*A* shows anterior dislocation of the right tibia on the femur. *B* is a stress film after reduction showing complete lateral side disruption. *C* shows complete anterior dislocation of the left tibia on the femur and *D*, complete lateral disruption in the stress film. X-rays were made while the patient waited for the anesthesiologist. The dislocated knees were reduced with the patient under anesthetic. Arteriograms of both extremities showed no disturbance of the vascular system. The patient was immobilized and observed overnight and then sent to me. With intact circulation 60 hours post-injury, the left leg was operated on, and complete disruption of the lateral side was found; the anterior and posterior cruciate ligaments were off the femur; the gastrocnemius was off the femur; the biceps and fibular collateral were off the fibula; the iliotibial band was off the tibia; and the

peroneal nerve was torn. Five days later the same findings were found on the opposite knee. Surgical repair was made of the cruciates to the femur, the gastrocnemius to the femur, the biceps and fibular collateral to the fibula and the iliotibial band to the tibia. Ten weeks postoperative the patient still had good stability. Delayed nerve suture was carried out. This case is unusual in that the patient reached the hospital with both knees dislocated. In spite of the long time interval before surgery, there was no vascular disturbance at any time, although there was complete peroneal palsy.

A partial dislocation or subluxation has been amply covered in our discussion of sprain. A chronically subluxing knee is a ligament reconstruction problem.

Summary

1. Many more dislocations actually occur than are diagnosed.

2. Any grossly unstable knee after injury should be considered dislocated until proved otherwise.

3. The first priority for treatment is circulatory damage.

4. As soon as possible surgical repair of torn ligaments should be carried out.

5. All torn ligaments should be repaired.

6. Rehabilitation is extremely important and should start at once while the patient is in the splint or cast.

RECONSTRUCTION OF THE KNEE

In previous editions I avoided specifics about the techniques of reconstruction. Originally this book was designed for the man "under the gun" (i.e., the primary-care physician). As the editions changed through the years and, I hope, improved, many of the subjects, such as reconstruction of the knee, became much more sophisticated. I have had many requests to discuss knee reconstructions because I have done many reconstructions. In fact, not too long ago I submitted a report on approximately 350 cases, with long-term follow-up, to the *Journal of Bone and Joint Surgery,* but it was too extensive to publish. However, it is difficult to describe a single typical situation, since each knee injury is different. Pressures from many of my peers finally convinced me to include some of this material in this book. The placement of this section, following that on dislo-

Figure 502. The case which is described on page 534 of the text. *A*, Right knee showing complete anterior dislocation of the tibia on the femur. *B*, The stress film made with basically no force shows medial subluxation of the tibia on the femoral condyle as well as wide open lateral side. *C*, The left knee showing essentially the same pathological condition as the right knee. *D*, The stress film showing even more medial shift of the leg.

cation, is appropriate because the instabilities that result in dislocation are the ones most likely to need reconstruction.

Reconstruction of the medial side is the operation in which I have the greatest confidence. I believe that it is possible to improve medial side instability, even if this instability also involves the anterior cruciate ligament. I have never been absolutely certain that the anterior cruciate is affected by the instability, but just tightening up the medial side decreases anteroposterior instability materially.

Therefore, I will discuss in some depth the technique and the indications for medial side reconstruction—that is, repair of the medial collateral ligament, the medial posterior capsule and the medial meniscus. Repair of the anterior cruciate is not specifically included, although it sometimes enters on the coattails of the other procedure. I have observed many instances of medial side instability; with the knee in extension this instability involves the medial posterior capsule. In these cases the medial structures can be tightened up, largely because this will not disturb their normal blood supply. The problem is that a graft has an inadequate blood supply as it traverses the knee joint because there are no connecting vessels. Eventually some sort of artificial replacement may be available. I do not have too great hope for this alternative, however, because the same problems will be present. It may be that microsurgery will be used to actually place blood vessels in the graft. Efforts have been made to do this by surrounding the graft with the fat pad. This has seemed to help because in some of my most successful cases I have been unable to find the anterior cruciate because it was completely incorporated into the fat pad. Incidentally, in these cases the ligament was very functional.

I must apologize for not being more specific about various reconstructions. I am not too happy about reconstruction techniques for the lateral side or for the posterior cruciate ligament. Some of my young colleagues will develop something dramatic to resolve the problem, but to get my attention they must find a way to supply some circulation to the knee joint. It ought to be easier to supply blood to the posterior cruciate than to the anterior cruciate because much of the posterior cruciate is on the posterior capsule and therefore does not actually run without blood supply through the knee joint. The information that follows is based on my experiences.

Reconstruction for Medial Instability of the Knee*

An unstable knee, whether or not it occurs in an athlete, presents a real challenge to the orthopaedist. Athletes are usually regarded as the prime candidates for salvage of an unstable knee, since without major improvement their abilities will continue to be seriously impaired and their athletic careers may be ended. However, currently, as more and more of our citizens participate in recreational activities that expose the always vulnerable knee joint to undue stress, orthopaedists are seeing more and more people past the so-called "athletic age" who have knee instability severe enough to prevent them from participating in sports such as golf, paddle tennis and water skiing and in the many other activities that may stress their knees.

It is not my intention to discuss in detail the philosophy of reconstruction of the knee, but certain comments are necessary. If the physician attempts reconstruction, he should have many strings for his bow in order to be prepared to perform these salvage procedures properly. He must balance the advantages of ligament reconstruction against other possible methods of treatment available in any given case. He must also decide whether it would be better to leave the knee alone and to simply reduce the person's activities to a level consistent with the instability. The possibilities include use of a brace, osteotomy for realignment, replacement of all or part of the joint by an implant or knee fusion. Obviously, the decision as to the procedure performed depends on the surgeon's experience with the various methods available to him and his appreciation of the result obtainable by any given procedure in a particular situation.

The questions to be answered are the following: Who should have a ligament reconstruction? Why should it be done? When should it be done? Where should it be done? Who should do it?

In making decisions based on answers to these questions, two factors are of major importance. The first relates to the current status of the patient. Is the instability sufficient to cause significant disability in the activities

---

*Reprinted in part from O'Donoghue, D. H.: Reconstruction for Medial Instability of the Knee. J. Bone and Joint Surg. 55-A:941–955, 1973.

which are important to him at this time? The second concerns the potential for future trouble. Is the instability severe enough that one may reasonably expect the condition to progress to increasing instability and, more important, to degenerative arthritis?

A provocative finding in our recent studies of the long-term results of knee ligament repairs in dogs was the almost constant relationship between instability and joint degeneration.* The dogs, followed for over three years after surgical procedures on one knee, showed a constant pattern. If the knee was stable, the degenerative changes were negligible. Almost without exception, however, the knees with persistent instability three to five years after operation showed degenerative changes paralleling the degree of instability. Eighty per cent of the knees with Grades 3 to 4 instability (on a scale of 0 to 4) had severe degenerative changes.

If reconstruction is to be successful, the patient must be healthy, well motivated and able and willing to carry out an extensive rehabilitation program. The knee itself must be in good enough condition to be salvageable. One must also visualize how good the knee would be if the instability was completely corrected in order to be sure that reconstruction of the ligaments is the appropriate procedure. Chronic degenerative arthritis, synovitis with effusion, angular deformity with degeneration on one side of the joint or malfunction of the quadriceps mechanism must be carefully evaluated, since other corrective measures may be at least as successful as restoration of stability. Upper tibial or distal femoral osteotomy to correct alignment may be in order. Similarly, it may be necessary to do a synovectomy, a complete debridement of the joint or a patellectomy. The ideal candidate for ligament reconstruction is the young person who has been disabled for a comparatively short time and whose knee is essentially normal except for the ligamentous instability.

Having decided that the patient is a fit candidate, the procedure should be done as soon as possible because further progression of the instability may make the knee unsalvageable by ligament reconstruction. The decision as to where the procedure should be

done and by whom is important. Obviously, the facilities and personnel of a modern hospital and well-trained competent assistants must be available. Since these reconstructions are salvage procedures and in many instances "last chance" operations, the surgeon must be prepared to do this type of surgery just as one must be prepared to do other specialized surgical procedures, such as instrumentation for scoliosis, total hip replacement and anterior spine fusion. If the surgeon does only an occasional reconstruction, the result is not likely to be good.

One of the most common types of instability involves the medial supporting structures of the knee: the medial collateral ligament, the medial posterior capsule and the anterior cruciate ligament. The combined laxity of these structures is quite disabling, since each supplements the others in preventing medial, anterior and rotatory instability of the knee and in preventing overextension of the joint. Many procedures have been proposed to correct this condition. I have had some experience with many of them. The method that I am presenting has evolved through the years in a constant effort to decrease morbidity and improve end results. However, there has been no change in principle in regard to reconstruction of the medial collateral ligament and medial posterior capsule during the period covered by this report. Any improvements have been technical in nature. They have facilitated the operation but have not had any appreciable effect on the end result. I am indebted to many people for their ideas and criticisms. This technique certainly is not a panacea, but I have found it to be the most consistently successful procedure to reconstruct the medial ligaments of the knee.

The approach is quite simple. Rather than attempt to isolate and advance or imbricate each separate ligament, I detach the whole medial capsular and ligament mass from the tibia, beginning at the midline in front and extending around to the midline posteriorly. A cuff is thereby developed without any effort made to identify particular ligaments. As a matter of fact, their identity often is lost in scar. This cuff is then advanced downward and forward on the tibia. By leaving all of these structures together as a single mass, their blood and nerve supplies are less likely to be disturbed. Also, one has a substantial mass of tissue available that will withstand considerable tension and will securely hold the fixation

O'Donoghue, D. H., Frank, G. R., Jeter, G. L., et al.: Repair and Reconstruction of the Anterior Cruciate Ligament in Dogs–Factors Influencing Long-Term Results. J. Bone and Joint Surg. *53-A*:710–718, 1971.

sutures. I often combine this procedure with reconstruction of the anterior cruciate ligament, using the iliotibial band. This is discussed in more detail in the next section. Since the ultimate instability is related to the sum total of the laxities of all the capsular and ligament structures of the knee, it is important to tighten each individual element to the greatest extent possible. One must recognize that not all reconstructions will correct instability completely, but that if each element of instability can be reduced partially, the resulting overall instability may become tolerable.

Surgical Technique for Medial Side Reconstruction

With the patient supine, the limb is positioned with the knee at about 40 degrees of flexion. A bolster is placed beneath the thigh, well above the popliteal space so that it does not displace the popliteal structures forward into the area of reconstruction.

A medial parapatellar incision is made. It begins at about the level of the center of the patella, directly adjacent to its medial margin, extends distally along the medial retinaculum, parallel to the medial edge of the patellar tendon as far as the tibial tubercle and then swings posteromedially at an angle of approximately 45 degrees to end at the posteromedial border of the tibia (see Fig. 469). The skin flap so outlined is then reflected posteriorly. In doing this, it is extremely important that all of the superficial tissues be included in the skin flap. Therefore, when the incision is made, it should be deepened immediately to the fascia, and then the dissection should continue medially along the surface of the fascia. By doing this, the superficial vessels and nerves remain intact in the flap being cut at the site of the skin incision rather than posteriorly at the level of the fold of the retracted flap.

After the flap has been reflected back to the posterior margin of the tibia, an incision is made through the medial retinaculum in the line of the skin incision and is extended distally to the top of the pes anserinus. The superior margin of the pes anserinus is quite readily palpated through the superficial fascia. This fascia is incised from the anterior border of the tibia posteriorly along the upper margin of the pes anserinus, care being taken not to cut the tendons of the pes anserinus. At about the middle of the anteromedial surface of the tibia, the long fibers of the medial collateral ligament are encountered. If the fascia and this ligament

are adherent to one another, no attempt is made to separate them. The incision is carried through the long fibers of the ligament at the level of the upper margin of the pes anserinus. Usually in addition to the previous injury there have been previous incisions, so that the fascia and the long fibers of the medial collateral ligament may be blended together. They should not be separated. Instead, the incision should be made right through them down to the periosteum, transecting the long fibers at the superior margin of the pes anserinus. From this point the incision through the fascia follows the upper edge of the pes anserinus, swinging proximally and posteriorly. The resulting capsular and ligamentous flap can then be reflected from the tibia extraperiosteally and be dissected free up to the joint, where, at about the midpoint of the medial side of the joint, the short capsular fibers are encountered. These are divided at their tibial attachment just below the articular surface of the tibia. As this incision is extended posteriorly around to the back of the tibia, the flap so formed includes the fascia, the long fibers of the medial collateral ligament and the capsular layer composed of both the medial collateral ligament and the posterior capsule with its associated ligaments (Fig. 503). If the anterior attachment of the semimembranosus is intimately bound to this flap, it is removed with the flap. On the other hand, if it is not adherent, the dissection is carried around it. It is important to extend the detachment of the capsule to the midline posteriorly. If the dissection is kept right at the capsular attachment to the tibia, there is no risk of damage to the deep structures behind the knee, since they drop backward with the knee flexed and with the thigh supported well above the knee. In order to get secure fixation of the advanced flap posteriorly, the surface of the tibia is exposed subperiosteally with an elevator or, if necessary, with an osteotome so that raw bone can be seen from the posteromedial corner to the midline on the posterior surface. This exposure does not extend distal to the level of the attachment of the posterior cruciate ligament on the tibia. By reflecting this flap, full access to the medial one half of the top of the tibia is provided. Any remnant of the medial meniscus is removed and indicated intra-articular procedures, such as removal of pannus from the medial femoral condyle, removal of osteocartilaginous bodies or chondroplasty, are performed.

Following this, the flap composed of the

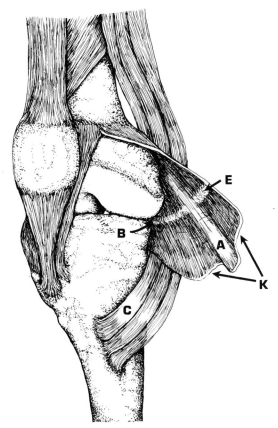

Figure 503. Medial capsular and ligament flap reflected upward and backward after division of the long fibers (A) of the medial collateral ligament and the fascia of the leg (K) along the upper edge of the pes anserinus (C). Note that the length of the flap decreases as the incision proceeds posteriorly. At about the level of the midpoint of the medial joint line the incision is about 2 cm. below the joint line. Here the incision transects the short capsular fibers of the medial ligament (E). Further posteriorly the incision is only 1 cm. below the joint line where it divides the tibial attachment of the posterior capsule (B). (From O'Donoghue, D. H.: Reconstruction for Medial Instability of the Knee. Journal of Bone and Joint Surgery. 55-A(5):944, 1973.)

medial and posteromedial components is advanced downward and secured to the tibia by mattress sutures along the tibial margin. In the posterior capsular segment parallel drill holes are made through the tibia for the sutures, using a 0.22 cm. guide pin as a drill (Fig. 504). This method has the advantage of compressing the bone rather than grinding it, so that the surfaces of the holes are smooth and will not damage the sutures. Another bonus from using the smooth pin is that no crumbs of bone are produced, which might promote ossification in the flap. Also, this pin will not break. The holes are drilled from front to back, beginning just at the medial edge of the patellar tendon

about 2 cm. below the articular surface of the tibia and emerging at the same level on the back of the tibia. Suitable protection is provided by an elevator or other instrument inserted posteriorly to prevent overpenetration of the pin into the popliteal space. Four, or sometimes five, parallel holes are made. In addition, at about the same level or slightly higher (1 cm.), four to six drill holes, about 1 cm. apart, are made around the medial margin of the top of the tibia, just through the cortex. Using a suitable ligature carrier, a loop of suture is then passed from front to back through the most lateral front-to-back hole. This loop is used to pull one limb of a blue No. 0 cotton mattress suture (previously placed in the posterior capsule) through the tibia into the anterior part of the wound. A similar procedure is carried out for the next (more medial) hole, using the loop to pull the second limb of the first blue mattress suture and the first limb of the next blue suture through the same hole simultaneously. This procedure is repeated until all of the sutures in the posterior capsule are in place. Usually these posterior sutures should be mattress sutured through the capsule at about the level of the bed of the excised medial meniscus. If they are in this position, the capsule can be advanced 1 to 2 cm. when they are tied. However, the amount of advancement must be determined by the degree of relaxation of the posterior capsule. With the sutures pulled taut, the capsule should be snug against the back of the tibia with the knee flexed 40 degrees (Fig. 505).

Before the blue sutures are tied, No. 0 white cotton sutures are placed through the more proximal holes in the cortex around the medial side of the tibia (Fig. 506). Beginning at the back, the first suture goes in through the most posterior hole and comes out through the second (more anterior) hole. The second suture goes in the second hole and out the third. Subsequent sutures are inserted in a similar fashion until all of them have been placed in the bone but not yet through the flap.

Prior to placement of the medial mattress sutures through the flap, tension is applied to the posterior capsular sutures. This maneuver should pull the posterior capsule snugly against the back of the tibia (see Fig. 505) and permit the surgeon to visualize where the medial white sutures should be placed in the flap to produce the desired amount of tension.

The medial mattress sutures are now passed through the flap in such a position that the flap is advanced downward and forward as far as

POSTERIOR CAPSULAR
LIGAMENT

Figure 504. Diagram showing method for placing sutures in the posterior capsule after parallel holes have been made through the tibia. The first limb (A) of the first mattress suture in the posterior capsule has been pulled through the first most lateral hole. The second limb (B) is being threaded through the loop (C–D) prior to pulling this limb through the second hole in the tibia. Before pulling this limb through, however, the first limb of the second mattress suture is placed in the same loop so that both limbs are pulled through together. (From O'Donoghue, D. H.: Reconstruction for Medial Instability of the Knee. Journal of Bone and Joint Surgery. *55-A*(5):946, 1973.)

possible (see Fig. 506). Usually these sutures are placed through the flap at about the level of the meniscal bed, but the position may vary depending upon the degree of relaxation of the medial ligament. Tenacula are placed on the bottom edge of the flap and used to pull it forward and downward as each mattress suture is passed through the entire flap, that is, the capsular ligament, the long fibers of the medial collateral ligament and the fascia. One must be sure that the most forward edge of the flap will reach the patellar tendon. It is very easy to tether this flap too far posteriorly by placing the mattress sutures improperly.

Once these sutures are placed, the posterior capsular sutures are tied in succession, starting with the most lateral one. In this way, if any suture breaks it can be replaced without taking the whole flap down again. Once the posterior blue sutures are secured, the more superficial white ones are tied. These should pull the flap forward. Therefore, tension must be maintained on the flap with the tenacula while the white sutures are tied.

At this point enough of the attachment of the pes anserinus is detached from the tibia so that the pes anserinus can be pulled up over the suture line in the distal portion of the medial flap (Fig. 507). If the ligament is very redundant, it may be necessary to divide the whole anterior attachment of the pes anserinus in order to place it in proper position. Once the pes anserinus is mobilized, it is retracted downward, and the distal edge of the flap containing the fascia and the long fibers of the medial collateral ligament is sutured snugly to the periosteum of the tibia and to the distal stump of the medial collateral ligament. The posterior edge of the flap must also be carefully

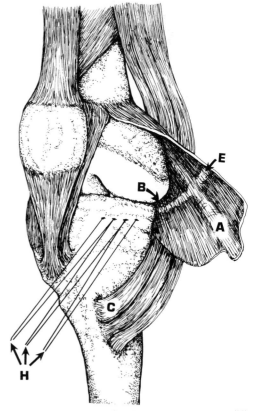

Figure 505. Diagram showing mattress sutures (H) in the posterior capsule (see Fig. 504) pulled taut. If properly placed these sutures pull the posterior capsule (B) downward against the tibia, so that the posterior capsule is taut with the knee in 40 degrees of flexion. Usually with the sutures taut the meniscal bed is well below the top of the tibia. These sutures extend medially as far as the posteromedial corner of the tibia. They do not include the short capsular fibers (E) of the medial collateral ligament. (A, Long fibers of medial collateral ligament.) (C, Pes anserinus.) (From O'Donoghue, D. H.: Reconstruction for Medial Instability of the Knee. Journal of Bone and Joint Surgery. *55-A*(5):947, 1973.)

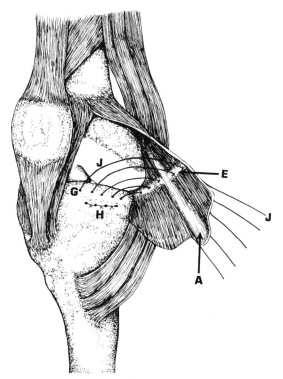

Figure 506. Diagram showing posterior capsular sutures tied (H) and the superficial mattress sutures (J) passed through the holes (G) in the cortex of the medial margin of the tibia. The holes are made at 1 cm. intervals. The most posterior hole is placed well behind the posteromedial corner of the tibia, about 1 cm. medial to the most medial posterior mattress suture (H). From five to seven holes are made progressing anteriorly as shown. The medial mattress sutures (J) are passed through adjoining holes and through the full thickness of the flap (E) at a level that will provide the desired amount of tension in the flap. As the sutures are placed the flap must be pulled forward and downward so that its anterior margin will reach the patellar tendon when all the sutures are in place (see Fig. 507). (A, long fibers of medial collateral ligament.) (From O'Donoghue, D. H.: Reconstruction for Medial Instability of the Knee. Journal of Bone and Joint Surgery. 55-A(5):947, 1973.)

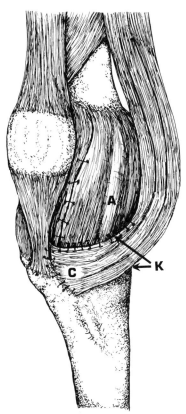

Figure 507. Diagram showing completed reconstruction. The pes anserinus has been detached from the tibia and reflected downward so that the entire ligament-capsular flap could be sutured to the periosteum and stump of the long fibers of the medial collateral ligament (A) beneath the pes. The pes was then sutured over the flap as shown (C). Note that the fascia of the leg (K) on the surface of the flap now lies beneath the pes instead of overlying it, as it did formerly. (From O'Donoghue, D. H.: Reconstruction for Medial Instability of the Knee. Journal of Bone and Joint Surgery. 55-A(5):947, 1973.)

secured to the underlying tissue. The pes anserinus is now pulled up over the suture line and securely sutured to the flap. The object of this procedure is to weld this whole mass into one homogenous fibrous supporting structure.

Tubes for suction drainage are placed, and the wound is closed. A long posterior plaster splint and plaster stirrup are applied and held in place with gauze bandages (see Fig. 452). This splint can be released if the limb swells and then tightened as the swelling goes down. It can also be removed with ease if aspiration is necessary. After the condition in the limb stabilizes, in approximately two weeks, a toe-to-groin plaster cast is applied. If the patient is quite active and has a relatively long mus-

cular leg, a walking heel is applied (see Fig. 454). If, on the other hand, the patient has a short, fat, flabby thigh, obviously the fixation by the plaster cast is less adequate, and a walking heel should not be used. This cast is worn for another six weeks, making a total of eight weeks.

The usual rehabilitative measures are carried out under supervision before and after surgery, active exercises being encouraged in the stirrup splint and also in the cast. A day or so after the operation, the patient is given a list of exercises, which are carefully explained (see page 484), which should be carried out both in the plaster splint and in the cast. He progresses to other exercises after the immobilization is discontinued. While in the cast, he is unable to bend the knee, so that when immobilization ends, knee flexion exercises are begun to develop a range of motion. If there is no marked effusion or swelling of the knee at this stage, progressive resistance exercises can be carried out, adding weight as indicated. However, the patient is not permitted to hang a weight on the foot while the leg dangles off the table. Resistance exercise should be done using a rope-and-pulley arrangement or some resistance apparatus in which the weight pulls the knee into flexion but does not distract the tibia from the femur. The patient is advised to walk with crutches until he can bend the knee 90 degrees, since until that time there is danger that he may catch his toe and fall. He can start trotting and running whenever the range of motion of the knee will permit and there is only minimum synovitis. No cutting to one side or the other or participation in contact sports is permitted until at least four months after operation. If the patient resumes playing football, he is advised to have his knee strapped with adhesive tape or to wear a well-fitted brace while playing. Each case must be viewed individually, since the timorous patient will need to be pushed whereas the overconfident one will need to be restrained.

Iliotibial Reconstructions About the Knee

Before going into a general discussion of the utilization of the iliotibial tract for knee reconstruction, some of the anatomical characteristics of this interesting structure will be described. Kaplan's masterful monograph,* which was published many years ago, presents an excellent, detailed study of this structure.

In the upper portion of the tract is the tensor fascia femoris muscle, whose function, as the name suggests, is to keep tension on the lower tract, but more particularly, on the vaginal fascia of the thigh, which encompasses the musculature of the thigh. The central, lateral portion of this fascia is somewhat thicker than the rest of the structure, the major portion of it being a thin, avascular, linearly oriented, fibrous sheath, with no transverse tensile strength but with considerable tensile strength along the line of its fibers. This structure is tethered along its whole length by the intermuscular septum that fastens the fascia to the femur. As the band approaches the knee, the fascial sleeve narrows and becomes much

thicker. It takes on the characteristic of ligament, with very great tensile strength. When this portion of the band crosses the knee joint to attach to the tibia on the tubercle of Gerdy, it is about 2.5 to 4 cm. wide. The attachment to the femur along the epicondylar ridge becomes very much shorter and stronger. Thus, the lower part of the iliotibial tract becomes a lateral ligament of the knee and, in fact, is the major lateral ligamentous support to the knee.

Two factors arise in a decision as to whether to use the band as a graft: (1) the effect of its absence at the donor site, and (2) its effectiveness as a transplant. The fascia lata portion can be utilized without fear of severe consequences at the site of its removal. This was learned when performing fascial arthroplasty was popular, and large strips of fascia lata were removed with no apparent functional disturbance. The material is very useful as a graft if it is exposed to an ample blood supply. It cannot provide its own. Hence, fascia is very good to reinforce the collateral ligament but is much less reliable within the knee, where its very extensive surface area is exposed to the synovial fluid.

The distal portion of the iliotibial tract is quite different from the fascia lata. It is thick, with relatively little surface compared with its mass. It also has some blood supply and great strength and so has a better chance to function in the knee, where relatively little of the graft is exposed to synovial fluid. Thus, this tract is my choice for utilization as a graft in anterior cruciate reconstruction, specifically in replacement of the anterior cruciate ligament. In this replacement, the very characteristics I have discussed permit utilization of the material in the most favorable way—namely, the heavy, ligamentous distal portion is used to traverse the joint as the anterior cruciate ligament and then the fascia lata replaces the lateral support, which is lost when the lower portion of the tract is removed. In this situation the fascia not only survives but actually enlarges and becomes a structure very similar to that which was removed.

Anterior Cruciate Replacement*

It is not my purpose to justify or to defend reconstruction of the anterior cruciate ligament. Moreover, there is still considerable

*Kaplan, E. B.: The Iliotibial Tract. Clinical and Morphological Significance. J. Bone and Joint Surg. 40-A:817–832, 1958.

*Reprinted in part from O'Donoghue, D. H.: A Method for Replacement of the Anterior Cruciate Ligament of the Knee. J. Bone and Joint Surg. 45-A:905–924, 1963.

difference of opinion as to the advisability of doing this procedure, since the results are frequently unsatisfactory. The occasional brilliant result hardly compensates for the many operations that have resulted in disappointment. I have tried different reconstruction techniques, and the majority did not seem to be worthwhile. Hence, I had the audacity to attempt to devise a different technique, which might represent some improvement over those previously available.

As noted previously, the selection of patient for this operation should be made carefully. This reconstruction should not be carried out in any patient with an acute injury, since I believe that many people can get along quite well without the anterior cruciate ligament, provided the collaterals are strong and the thigh muscles are fully rehabilitated. I do not think that reconstruction offers sufficient assurance of a completely stable knee to justify this extensive surgery just so the patient may play football again. An exception has been reconstruction for a professional football player who was unable to continue playing because of anterior cruciate instability and who was willing to gamble on the result since a successful reconstruction could mean many thousands of dollars to him and later a chance to establish himself in business.

My indication for anterior cruciate reconstruction is anterior cruciate instability sufficiently severe to interfere with the person's normal everyday living. This indication is an elastic one. Ordinary normal living for a person 50 years old may be quite different from that of the 20 year old. Reconstruction is indicated in females much less frequently than in males because females are better able to adjust to living with an unstable knee. Interference with ordinary living includes gross instability to the point that wearing a brace or arthrodesis is necessary; instability sufficient to cause the patient to fall frequently; inability to do such things as golf, bowl or play handball; and in some cases, pain that seems to be specifically related to the instability.

In every instance there was a frank discussion with the patient of the nature of his disability. It was pointed out that there was only a 50 per cent chance of success and that the operation was extensive. The procedure was then described to him. It was explained that the procedure might not improve his condition and that there was a small possibility that it could increase lateral instability. Only after such a discussion and explanation was operation agreed upon. In the great majority of cases the patient was requested to go home and discuss it with his family and his physician and was told that arrangements for surgery could be made at a later date. The exceptions to this were patients who came from a considerable distance and had been well sold (or perhaps oversold) on the operation before they arrived.

Operative Procedure

Here I will detail briefly how the lower end of the iliotibial band is utilized for reconstruction. The heavy, distal portion of the band is placed so that it traverses the knee, where it does not get the surface exposure that the fascia lata does. A section of the iliotibial band is excised (approximately 14 in. in length), which is about 3 in. wide at the top, tapering to about 1 in. wide as it crosses the knee and continues to the tubercle of Gerdy and into the fascia of the leg (Fig. 508). By trimming off a portion of the muscle attaching to the anterolateral face of the tibia, the bone is exposed and a drill hole can be made from this area into the top of the tibia, just into the attachment of the fat pad, using a guide pin to locate the exact position. A suitable twist drill is used (usually about 7/16 in. in size). The distal end of the iliotibial band is trimmed down, and then the band is rolled up to reduce

Figure 508. Diagram indicating the size and location of the graft from the iliotibial tract when used for reconstruction of the anterior cruciate ligament. (From O'Donoghue, D. H.: A Method for Replacement of the Anterior Cruciate Ligament of the Knee. Journal of Bone and Joint Surgery. 45-A(5):905–924, 1963.)

Figure 509. Diagram showing the graft from the iliotibial tract crossing the two drill holes. This portion of the tract actually crosses the joint space as the replacement for the anterior cruciate and is the strongest part of the whole iliotibial tract. (From O'Donoghue, D. H.: A Method for Replacement of the Anterior Cruciate Ligament of the Knee. Journal of Bone and Joint Surgery. 45-A(5):905–924, 1963.)

its volume, with stay sutures placed into its tip. The next step depends a little upon the length of the hard portion of the tibial band. If the band is relatively short and it is believed that it is not long enough to reach across the knee, it can be detached subperiosteally from the tubercle of Gerdy but left intact to the fascia. This is what is ordinarily done. The whole mass is passed through the drill hole in the tibia to exit on top of the tibia, right into the fat pad.

A tunnel is made through the fat pad and the graft is passed through it. Then a suitable hole is made in the femur posteriorly, into the medial side of the lateral face of the notch at the site of the anterior cruciate ligament attachment. Again, a guide wire is passed through and a suitable drill hole made, which exits on the epicondylar ridge above the knee joint laterally. The fascia is passed through this hole from within out. The entire graft is now through the knee joint and through the fat pad, and at no place is it freely exposed to the synovium (Fig. 509).

At this point there is a rather lengthy piece of iliotibial tract left (in this instance, the fascia lata) lying on the lateral face of the femur.

This is pulled very snugly and sutured to the rim of the hole through which it exits.

At this stage in the procedure there is a defect in the lateral collateral ligamentous structures of the knee created by transplantation of the iliotibial band. This band normally functions as a ligament extending from the femoral condyle to the tibial plateau and may actually provide more support to the lateral side of the knee than the fibular collateral ligament. The remaining 8 to 10 in. of the fascial graft emerging from the femur is used to replace this portion of the lateral ligament. This fascia lata from the thigh is thin, but the strip is about three times wider than the defect across the knee, and the edges of the graft can be folded over to either double or triple its thickness. It is secured firmly to the tubercle of Gerdy below. The fascia lata in this instance does have good blood supply and ordinarily should survive. Four to six inches of the widest portion of the fascia remain. This is then folded back on itself and sutured with moderate tension to the two cut edges of the iliotibial band.

The usual closure is carried out, making no attempt to close the iliotibial tract other than by the use of the residual portion of fascia lata, which extends down to fasten below the knee. This operation is described and illustrated in detail elsewhere.*

Other Iliotibial Procedures

The fascia may be utilized in other ways, although not with such uniformly successful results. If there is *lateral instability as well as anterior or posterior instability,* one can ill afford to remove the distal portion of the tract, since it is the major factor in lateral stability. Indeed, it could probably be used to tighten the lateral side, in which instance the lower portion of the band is left attached to the tubercle of Gerdy. The band is then attached firmly to the femoral condyle. This leaves a broad, long strip of fascia 10 in. by 3 in. as the residual graft. This may be passed through the femoral condyle into the back of the intercondylar notch and then passed across the knee and out through the upper end of the tibia in front. The residual portion exits along the lateral face of the upper tibia, where it can be utilized to add support to the lateral side.

If it is the *lateral side and the posterior*

---

*O'Donoghue, D. H.: A Method for Replacement of the Anterior Cruciate Ligament of the Knee. J. Bone and Joint Surg. *45A*:905–924, 1963.

cruciate which are unstable, the residual fascia can be passed through the lateral condyle to the front of the notch within the knee. It is then passed posteriorly through the knee to the back of the tibia and forward through the tibia to exit in front of the tibia. This structure may effectively replace the posterior cruciate ligament.

In neither of these instances is the result of the repair of the cruciate as consistently good as it is in the first instance, in which the lower end of the band was used. However, the results may compare favorably with those of other methods available. Some patients do exceedingly well.

It should be noted that whereas the lower end of the iliotibial band is readily available to replace the anterior cruciate, this part is not as available to replace the posterior cruciate, since it could only be used as a free graft. If the fascia is passed through the back of the tibia and then out through the femoral condyle, the heavy distal portion is largely within the tibia, leaving only the fascia to cross the knee.

In summary, I would say that using the *lower tract* to replace the anterior cruciate (the residual defect being replaced in turn by the fascia) has an excellent chance to reduce the anteroposterior instability. Reducing instability so that Grade 4 becomes Grade 1 or even Grade 2 (on a scale of 0 to 4) may seem very good to the patient with a very unstable knee. Using the *fascia* as the cruciate replacement is not as notably successful in either anterior or posterior cruciate replacement. Here again, however, some patients do very well. The results are certainly comparable with those obtained using other types of available substitutions.

In performing a *lateral side reconstruction,* I prefer to completely denude the femoral condyle, including the fibular collateral ligament and the popliteus tendon attachment. This whole mass is shifted posteriorly to remove the posterior capsular and the femoral attachment of the lateral head of the gastrocnemius, if they are together. The peroneal nerve is well posterior if the approach is intracapsular and is not subject to damage. This posterior mass is advanced upward by a set of parallel drill holes running from the front of the femur to the back, usually using three sets of parallel holes, each hole about 1 cm. apart.

The holes are placed linearly in line, so that the mattress sutures can be passed through them and then through the advancing flap and back out. Usually three loops of this will be adequate. Then the remaining anterior portion is pulled well forward and upward along the femoral condyle and epicondylar margin. Thus, the whole lateral cuff is advanced without dissecting out individual ligaments. This is then reinforced by the iliotibial tract.

Postoperative Care

The follow-up is essentially the same as that described for the medial side (see page 541). The patient's leg is placed in a long leg stirrup splint (see Fig. 452) with the knee flexed 30 to 35 degrees, depending to some extent on whether the anterior cruciate ligament has been reconstructed. This splint can be readily loosened if the knee swells and tightened up as indicated. As soon as the knee has stabilized, in approximately two weeks, the sutures are removed from the skin and a long leg cast is applied (see Fig. 454), with the leg in about the same position. With a responsible patient, a resting heel may be placed in the cast, and the patient instructed to "rest" the foot but not to walk without crutches. It is insisted that he walk with crutches for another six weeks because the cast does not completely immobilize the knee, particularly in the anteroposterior direction. On some occasions I have used the cast-brace, but I really do not feel that it protects the knee well enough in these young active people and it also is an additional expense.

Rehabilitative measures are the same as those for medial reconstruction, outlined on page 484. I would like to reiterate the importance of getting the cooperation of the patient and of explaining exactly what you want him to do. Carefully outline what should be done in the way of rehabilitation. A cooperative patient has a lot to do with the success of the operation.

Conclusions

I believe that ligament reconstruction of the knee is a worthwhile procedure, but that each case must be viewed individually and carefully evaluated before operation is recommended. None of my patients with medial instability alone was worse after operation and only one failed to show a decrease in medial instability. Increased stability and motion were not the only beneficial results. Even if there was considerable residual instability, if the procedure tightened up the knee sufficiently to enable the patient to dispense with a brace, cane or crutches, this difference represented a marked improvement.

Patients with knee instability may have emotional as well as physical problems. It is extremely important for the surgeon to be sympathetic, providing stimulation and encouragement when needed during convalescence and preventing overactivity when necessary.

It should be emphasized, however, that the results of medial reconstruction alone are not representative of those obtained with repair of other types or combinations of instability. The results in my whole series indicate that the more procedures required, the less likely is the outcome to be satisfactory. Still other factors that also must be considered are secondary changes, such as restriction of motion, degenerative changes and chondromalacia, which are more severe in knees in which multiple procedures were required. Therefore, one can proceed with considerable confidence when the goal is only restoration of medial and of medial posterior capsular stability, but when there are other components to be restored as well, the result is less predictable. It is very important to analyze the patient as a whole, with respect to his general condition, his needs and desires and to consider what end result may be expected in his particular case.

MENISCUS INJURY

Another common condition is injury to the menisci. This injury goes hand in glove with ligament sprain. The general structural anatomy of the menisci is well known, but it is well to recall certain significant differences between the two menisci in order to understand the damage one may expect from a given type of injury.

Medial Meniscus

The medial meniscus is "C" shaped (Fig. 510A). Its anterior attachment is on the top of the tibia near the midline and in front of the tibial spines. The posterior attachment is on the top of the tibia behind the spines. In each case the attachment is relatively near the periphery of the tibia, so that the two ends are quite widely separated from each other. The meniscus is attached by means of the coronary ligament (which has its origin around the top of the tibia) to the medial collateral ligament and hence to the tibia. This attachment is firm and although it does allow a little play, motion permitted in the normal medial meniscus is not very extensive.

In sprain of the medial collateral ligament, the tibia and femur tend to separate on the medial side, and stress is applied in the area of the attachment of the meniscus to the medial ligament. The cartilage may be forced to accompany either the femur or the tibia, depending upon the location of the ligament injury. Since the structure of the meniscus does not allow much bending stress, it will tear transversely or more commonly split around its periphery. If the tear is actually in the attachment to the ligament, it may heal. If it is within the substance of the meniscus, it will not. In my experience meniscus injury accompanies repeated sprains to the knee more frequently than it does the initial single sprain. I know of no way to determine in an acute injury whether or not the meniscus is torn unless the knee is actually locked. If the knee is locked and the ligaments appear to be stable and the episode is the first, one may be justified in attempting to reduce the displacement by careful manipulation or by traction. If the meniscus has been detached at its periphery,

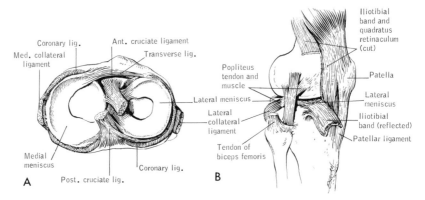

Figure 510. *A*, Drawing of the top of the tibia showing the menisci and the coronary ligament. *B*, Drawing showing attachment of lateral meniscus to tensor fascia femoris, which is frequently noted.

this attachment may then heal. This possibility is much more likely if the meniscus has slipped into the knee and locked and then immediately unlocked. Such an incident occurs when the player hurts the knee, and it is forcibly extended manually immediately following the injury and the meniscus snaps back in place. My own opinion is that if the knee actually locks even once, it should be operated upon, the meniscus examined and, if torn, removed. However, I have no particular argument with the surgeon who prefers to wait for the second episode. There is nothing to be gained by waiting for repeated episodes of locking. It has been shown that locking of the knee has a definitely deleterious effect upon the articular cartilage, not only on the condyles of the femur and tibia but also, more particularly, on the patella. Careful explanation to the patient of the undesirable effects of the locking episodes will ordinarily convince him that he had better have his knee operated upon early with the prospect of an excellent result rather than postpone operation until malacia has become advanced.

Lateral Meniscus

Where the medial meniscus is "C" shaped, with widely separated anterior and posterior attachments, the lateral meniscus is almost "O" shaped (see Fig. 510A), its anterior and posterior attachments being deep in the tibial notch and very close to each other. In many instances they are continuous with each other. The coronary ligament usually is much less firm and is more redundant than the coronary ligament attachment to the medial meniscus. This meniscus is not attached to the fibular collateral ligament. More motion is normally possible in the lateral meniscus than in the medial. Injury to the lateral side of the knee is less common than to the medial side. Furthermore, the lateral meniscus is much less likely to be damaged by acute lateral stress, so that a lateral meniscus tear in conjunction with an acute sprain of the knee is not frequently seen. On the other hand, by virtue of the looseness of the meniscus, particularly in its posterior portion, it is quite vulnerable to chronic damage, so that it is more likely to be hurt by chronic overflexion of the knee. Frequently the damage comes on insidiously as a result of squatting with the heel against the buttock for long intervals on frequent occasions. I have been so impressed with the vulnerability of the lateral meniscus because of redundancy of its posterior one third that I do not recommend deep knee bends or the so-called duck waddle as conditioning exercises. As the knee moves into complete flexion, the back of the meniscus may be caught between the impinging femoral condyle and tibial plateau and thrust forward, much as an apple seed gets pinched between the finger tips. This strains the posterior peripheral attachment until the meniscus may actually snap in front of the femoral condyle and finally progress to the typical bucket handle position and lie within the notch in front of and medial to the lateral articular condyle of the femur.

Although as a general rule the attachments of the lateral meniscus to the other lateral components of the knee are much less firm than is the case with the medial meniscus, this is not always true. In many instances there is a very firm attachment of the anterolateral section of the lateral meniscus to the iliotibial band. I have noted this to be almost always the case in partial or complete discoid menisci. Indeed, one often cannot distinguish a line of separation between the inner surface of the iliotibial band as it crosses the knee and the lateral margin of the lateral meniscus. This attachment of the meniscus is almost always bilateral and predisposes markedly to injury. In this instance the front of the cartilage is firmly attached, whereas the posterior part is relatively loose. As a consequence of this firm fixation, as the stress occurs to adduct the leg on the thigh, the cartilage is actually dragged forward and its whole posterior portion may catch in front of the femoral condyle. This anatomical variant has real significance in the fact that the lateral compartment is extremely difficult to expose until the cartilage is separated from the iliotibial band (Fig. 510B).

Diagnosis

If one never makes the diagnosis of meniscus injury until the knee has undergone repeated locking, many torn menisci are being overlooked! The diagnosis of meniscus injury may be made by history alone, and it is extremely important that the history be carefully and objectively taken. It is not wise to put words in the patient's mouth. If he gives a definite, detailed and reliable history of locking of the knee, the physician may assume meniscus damage until he can prove otherwise. More difficult to diagnose is the patient with chronic knee trouble, with recurrent effusion and recurring periods of disability but with no locking or "giving way." One suspects meniscus damage.

In this instance a very careful examination will be of extreme value. There is usually tenderness along the joint line in the damaged area. This may be posterior as a result of posterior tearing, or it may be midlateral or in front. The examiner should familiarize himself with the various manipulations that put stress on each meniscus. There are many manipulations described, such as McMurray, Ashly and so forth. None of these can be used to make a specific diagnosis, but many of them may be quite confirmatory. A positive reaction to one of these manipulations combined with other clinical evidence can be diagnostic. Sharply localized pain during these various tests may be as diagnostic as the click. The McMurray test is carried out with the patient supine; some others with the patient prone. With the knee semiflexed, lateral stress will usually cause pain in acute injuries but not as consistently in chronic meniscus damage. There is usually pain on rotatory stress. With the knee flexed, the calf is grasped firmly and the leg rotated laterally and medially. Pain will frequently be noted at the exact site of the injury to the meniscus. One should at least be able to determine which side of the knee is involved. Another test which I think is quite valuable is carried out with the patient supine. The knee is placed in complete flexion and then hyperflexed to determine whether this causes pain and where the pain is located. Many cases of posterior tear will give a definite cartilage click on this maneuver. In fact, this maneuver may actually cause the cartilage to slip forward and the knee to be locked. In this same completely flexed position, the foot is turned into external rotation and the knee flexed and extended a few degrees. The leg is then placed in internal rotation and the knee flexed and extended. Consistent clicking in these tests must be considered significant. Another similar test is conducted with the patient in a supine position. Bring the leg to complete extension while palpating the joint with the leg either externally or internally rotated. A similar test can be done with the patient standing and squatting, with the leg either turned in or turned out. In the final analysis, the knee that stubbornly resists conservative treatment and in which meniscus damage is suspected justifies arthrotomy. This is not to say that very painful knee should be operated upon meniscus damage. The weight of the evidence must point toward meniscus damage to ?y surgery under this preoperative diag-

Figure 511. This case is of interest from a diagnostic standpoint. The boy had an abduction injury to the leg with symptoms of medial meniscus pathology. He actually did have a bucket-handle fracture of the medial meniscus. Survey x-rays revealed a tumor in the femoral condyle. It proved to be a benign chondroblastoma. In this instance the solid tumor was an incidental finding. Treatment of the tumor designed to improve the condition of the knee would have failed. The tumor was removed at a second operation.

Treatment

I have previously stated that if the knee locks, this in itself is justification for surgical treatment. The locking may be due to meniscus damage, a foreign body in the joint, or displaced osteochondritis dissecans and so on. One must be particularly wary of pseudolocking, in which the patient cannot extend the knee completely and feels that the knee is locked. If this occurs several hours subsequent to the injury, hamstring spasm may well prevent complete extension, since the painful knee tends to flex and will resist extension. There are certain clues which help to distinguish among the types of locking. One is the history in which the patient has definite recollection that he could not extend the knee immediately after the injury. This is valid reason to conclude that it is probably actually locked. This is confirmed if the pain on extension is in the location of the meniscus. If, however, the patient is uncertain as to when he could not extend the knee because he actually did not try it and if when he did attempt to extend it, his complaint was posterior in the hamstring area, one would assume that the loss of motion is probably due to hamstring spasm and not bona fide blocking from internal derangement. At arthrotomy one must be prepared to treat whatever lesion is found. If the knee locks, some presumptive cause must be found if the operation is to be successful. Removing a normal meniscus will not stop the knee from locking! (Fig. 511).

Some general principles applicable to surgery are important. There is no justification for removing a normal meniscus just because one has diagnosed meniscus damage preoperatively. It is true that upon examination the front of the meniscus may appear to be normal, but there may be posterior damage that cannot be determined from in front; nonetheless it is pretty drastic to detach the anterior end of the meniscus in order to determine whether its posterior portion is torn. A better procedure is to enter the knee behind the medial collateral ligament so as to permit inspection of the posterior part of the meniscus. As stated, the removal of a normal meniscus is unjustifiable and particularly so because it does not eliminate the cause of the trouble in the knee. If upon inspection no abnormality is found in either meniscus, the knee must be carefully explored for other lesions to account for the symptoms. These may or may not be remediable, but they are not helped by removing a normal meniscus.

A question that must be answered is, "What constitutes a 'normal' meniscus?" This is an area in which surgical experience counts heavily. I have no hesitation in removing a meniscus that is yellow and sclerotic or in which there is redundancy of one or the other attachments, although there may be no obvious tear. However, I would feel extremely uneasy about removing a sclerotic meniscus in a knee in which there is a history of locking or giving way, since certainly a sclerotic meniscus could not be expected to cause these symptoms. Frequently at arthrotomy there will be found a rather marked redundancy of the fat pad, the posterior margin of which may appear grossly sclerotic. This can be symptomatic, usually causing pain on forced or rapid extension of the knee, such as in place kicking. However, once again I would feel quite uneasy about simply trimming away the fat pad unless I could assure myself that there is no other

pathological condition in the knee. Fat pad symptoms should be around the pad and are elicited by pressure on this area.

I realize that this is vast oversimplification of the meniscus problem, but I would like to state a few of my convictions:

1. A locking knee should be operated upon regardless of freedom from symptoms in the intervals between episodes.
2. Authentic "giving way" of the knee may be almost as diagnostic of meniscus damage as is locking.
3. The most constant symptom of meniscus damage is tenderness located at the site of the damage.
4. A careful history suggestive of meniscus damage, supported by pertinent findings, justifies arthrotomy provided that there is real disability of the knee. If the symptoms are so mild as to cause no effusion, instability or actual disability from pain, arthrotomy may be postponed, since the knee is not undergoing deterioration because of delay.

It seems we periodically go through the state of agitation about whether the medial meniscus should be entirely removed or partially removed. The present popularity of arthroscopy has made it seem more acceptable to simply snip off the abnormal part. I have seen this procedure carried out several times, and almost inevitably the patient ends up with a complete meniscectomy. Therefore, I would unhesitatingly recommend that the damaged meniscus be removed completely, including the residual rim of the bucket handle tear.

Technique for Medial Meniscectomy

The patient is placed in the supine position (see Fig. 467) and the usual meticulous preparation of the skin is carried out. The leg is draped and Steri-Drape is used. The footpiece (Fig. 512A) of the table is then dropped to permit the leg to dangle off the table at a 90 degree angle. The surgeon drapes a double fan sheet around the patient's body, extending from his waist to the floor. He is seated at the foot of the table with the patient's foot between his knees. I prefer a straight incision (see Fig. 512B), which begins about 1 cm. proximal to the lower pole of the patella and ½ cm. medial to the patellar tendon and proceeds parallel to the patellar tendon to terminate just proximal to the patellar tubercle. This is actually the central portion of the anteromedial incision which is used for knee ligament repair (see Fig. 469). The patellar retinaculum is split along the line of the incision, and the synovium is opened. At this

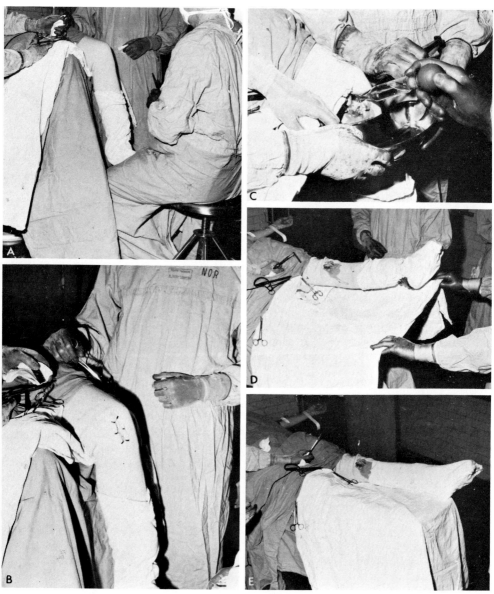

Figure 512. The author's general set-up for medial meniscus surgery. *A,* The leg is prepared and draped as shown in Figure 468, using Steri-Drape. (These pictures show sterile stockinetting, which we previously used.) Note the knee flexed to 90 degrees with the foot caught between the operator's knees. The surgeon is draped with an extra double fan wrapped around as a skirt. Note the white double fan lying under the knee and not fanned out. *B,* The short incision, which is actually the central part of the general utility incision on the medial side of the knee (see Fig. 468). This incision can be extended upward if it is desirable to expose the undersurface of the patella, downward if it is necessary to repair the medial ligament. *C,* At the beginning and termination of the operation, the knee is thoroughly lavaged with warm saline plus an antibiotic. The basin which catches the return flow will reveal many bits of foreign material which would be best out of the knee. *D,* As the anesthetist extends the end of the table, the double fan which has been lying under the knee is extended out over the end of the table, thus covering the whole end of the table which has been proximate to the floor. *E,* Position for exploration of the patella or any other procedure needed with the knee extended. The skin and capsular incisions are more readily closed with the knee in extension.

point the knee is carefully lavaged (see Fig. 512*C*) with warm sterile saline plus an antibiotic, particularly if blood is encountered. Through this short incision, a surpisingly good exploration of the knee can be carried out. The anterior attachment of the medial meniscus is examined. The anterior cruciate is checked. The posterior cruciate is noted. The knee is extended and the undersurface of the patella inspected by lifting it up with a toothed retractor and also by palpating it with the finger.

Should there be attendant damage, particularly involvement of the lower end of the patella, the incision is extended proximally at this time to permit better exposure. It is not necessary to enlarge this incision in order to carry out adequate repair of the anterior cruciate ligament. If there is damage to the collateral ligament which should be repaired, the incision is extended distally.

The meniscus is now carefully examined. If it is possible to spring the knee open on the medial side, the entire cartilage may be visible. This is the exception rather than the rule. The periphery of the cartilage may be palpated with a blunt Kelly forceps to determine whether there is a defect in the coronary ligament attachment or a split in the cartilage. I have devised a "feeler" for this purpose, which is a small rod curved in the arc of the femoral condyle with a 1 cm. right-angled blunt hook at its end (Fig. 513). The hook is used to avoid any possibility that the point of the forceps will be forced through the coronary ligament rather than be hooked into a defect. Anterior examination will ordinarily determine whether there has been damage to the meniscus. If the feeler hooks in the split in the cartilage or in its attachment, the presence of a posterior tear is assumed. With the knee flexed at 90 degrees, it is possible that the feeler may catch in a fold of synovium. This danger is obviated by bringing the knee to an extended position, at which time the synovium in back of the joint is taut and there is no recess in which the feeler may catch. I routinely carry out this maneuver in case the meniscectomy is going to depend upon the impression given by the use of the feeler that there is a posterior tear. Very often the feeler can be hooked into the torn meniscus either from the top or from underneath and actually can be pulled forward between the tibia and the femur to determine how redundant the meniscus really is. If the anterior part of the cartilage is friable, ecchymotic and redundant, it is assumed that the meniscus has been damaged somewhere. A very common finding in meniscus disease is a triangular-shaped overgrowth of synovium extending over the femoral condyle at just about the area where the anterior segment of the meniscus would impinge (Fig. 514). This finding is surprisingly consistent, and it often gives the physician a feeling of comfort to find this condition as he opens the knee expecting to find meniscus damage. If this examination leads to the conclusion that the cartilage is abnormal, it is removed as follows:

The anterior bony attachment is separated from the upper end of the tibia, and the periphery of the cartilage is carefully divided from the coronary ligament as far back as is convenient with the ordinary scalpel. At this point traction forward on the cartilage will confirm posterior damage. A cartilage knife or meniscotome is utilized to divide the meniscus from the coronary ligament as far back as possible. This instrument must be exceedingly sharp, and care must be taken that it follows the contour of the tibial rim, not the femoral condyle. If this instrument does not pass readily, it should not be forced, since damage can

Figure 513. Anteroposterior and lateral views of the "cartilage feeler." Note the curve corresponding to the curve of the upper end of the tibia and the short, blunt hook at the end. This can be deceptive if it is allowed to turn as it goes into the posterior compartment, where it can catch in the synovial sac, but it is a useful adjunct in the exploration. This synovial fold, which may catch the feeler in the flexed position, is eliminated as the knee is extended so that the catch should be confirmed by extending the knee and repeating the test.

Figure 514. Acute meniscus injury (two weeks), uncomplicated. Note the inflamed synovium growing out over the medial femoral condyle. Arrow indicates the fold of synovium, with the invasive edge going over the normal-appearing femoral condylar cartilage. Bucket-handle meniscus plus pannus. No other abnormalities.

be done to the femoral condyle, the upper end of the tibia, the medial collateral ligament or the posterior cruciate ligament by unwise instrumentation. When the straight, very sharp meniscotome is used, great care should be taken in making the dissection. The meniscotome is intended to be a dissector, not a guillotine. It should be held as a pen or pencil is held and not grasped in the fist. The crossbar on the handle of the meniscotome is not intended for pushing with the heel of the hand. It simply indicates where the blade is. Dissection should be carried out alternatively above and below the meniscus at about a 30 degree angle. It is seldom advisable to push the meniscotome around vertically.

At this point traction forward will tend to slide the cartilage under the femoral condyle. If it is detached peripherally posteriorly it will slide over into the notch. More frequently it slides part way over. Then, rather than dragging it over into the notch, which leaves the posterior attachment folded over, it is better to use the meniscus as a spreader. If it can be held between the tibia and the femur, it will permit the passage of the thin meniscotome posteriorly to complete the separation of the meniscus from the posterior capsule. A very thin straight meniscotome is used to divide the bony attachment, with care being taken to get all of the meniscus. The operation to this point has all been done through the anterior incision,

which means that the pathological characteristics were determined from in front, that the cartilage was readily divided by a meniscotome, and that all of the meniscus was removed when the posterior bony attachment was detached. If any of these steps has not been carried out, exposure of the posterior compartment of the knee must be made. This may be done in one of two ways. The anterior skin incision can be extended as for the ligament approach and the medial skin flap reflected subcutaneously. The posterior margin of the medial collateral ligament can be palpated as the curve of the tibial plateau swings posteriorly and a vertical split is made along the line of its fibers. Dividing through the synovium will provide access to the posterior compartment. This same area may be reached by making a short vertical incision through the skin, paralleling the ligament fibers just at the posterior edge of the medial collateral ligament. The posterior ligament is relaxed in this flexed position, and the posterior compartment can be readily visualized through this exposure. If no pathological signs are present in front, the cartilage is particularly examined for them posteriorly. If no signs of damage to the cartilage are found, it is not removed. If the removal from in front left a posterior tag or if the cartilage did not readily separate, the meniscectomy is completed posteriorly. Careful examination of this space is carried out to make sure that there is no other damaged tissue. The posterior cruciate ligament can be palpated readily. The posterior femoral condyle can be inspected, as can the upper end of the tibia. The wound is now thoroughly flushed with the saline and antibiotic solution and closed in layers, using No. 4–0 cotton in the synovium, No. 2–0 cotton in the ligament, No. 4–0 cotton in the subcutaneous tissue and No. 32 subcuticular wire for the skin.

Attention is next redirected to the anterior portion of the incision. The operative wound is thoroughly lavaged and the fat pad inspected. Any other morbid changes are noted and treated. If the patella is normal, the incision is then closed similarly to the posterior one. If it is necessary to treat the undersurface of the patella, the knee is then extended, the end of the table raised and draped as indicated (see Fig. 512D) and appropriate chondroplasty of the patella carried out by trephining and drilling (see page 580), shaving or partial or complete patellectomy as the case may be. At the conclusion of the operation a cotton cast (see Fig. 441) is applied and the tourniquet removed.

Technique for Lateral Meniscectomy

The lateral compartment is more difficult to expose than the medial. The leg is prepared and positioned as indicated previously. The incision I prefer at present has a horizontal and a vertical component. The horizontal limb begins about 3 cm. proximal to the lower end of the patella and level with it, extends straight forward along the line of iliotibial tract to the edge of the patellar tendon and then parallels the edge of the patellar tendon to the tubercle of the tibia (see Fig. 472). The decussating fibers of the iliotibial band, which swing forward to attach to the margin of the patella, are split parallel to the incision as far down as the patellar tendon. This permits the iliotibial band to be reflected backward without impairing its strength. The fat pad is troublesome but is incised to expose the knee. Electrocoagulation is used to seal obvious vessels. The lateral meniscus is now visualized. It is usually considerably more redundant than the medial. The same general rules are applied laterally as medially. There is one notable difference, however. This is in respect to the popliteal hiatus. There is normally a defect in the coronary ligament at the midlateral line of the meniscus through which the popliteus tendon traverses. One must not be misled into interpreting this as a tear. There is frequently a tear, sometimes difficult to detect, of the meniscus attachment from the popliteal hiatus back to the posterior meniscal attachment. If the cartilage is found by anterior inspection to be pathological, it should be detached in front and pulled forward, whereupon the posterior characteristics can be readily determined. If the anterior part appears to be completely normal, a second incision must be made similar to that on the medial side, the approach being just behind the fibular collateral ligament and in front of the popliteus tendon. This is somewhat more difficult to carry out on the lateral side than on the medial side, since one encounters the popliteus tendon as it crosses the back of the knee laterally, and care should be taken not to damage it. I cannot emphasize too strongly that excision of the meniscus should be a delicate dissection. It is not necessary to drag the meniscus out. It is undesirable to use a curved meniscotome and slice around the back of the joint in order to cut the posterior portion of the coronary ligament. All these maneuvers result in damage to other parts of the knee, with a corresponding delay in recovery and the possibility of permanent damage. The instruments must be very sharp, and one must resist the temptation to force the knife.

Postoperative Care

The postoperative care really should begin prior to the surgery. The patient should be instructed to walk with crutches and taught to walk with a normal weight-bearing gait. He is handed an exercise sheet (see page 484) which describes in considerable detail exactly what exercises should be done and when they should be initiated. I like to have the patient practice straight leg raising before the surgery, so that he will know exactly what to do when he starts straight leg raising in the splint.

Postoperative care for meniscus injury is as follows: A cotton cast is applied and the tourniquet removed. An elastic bandage is placed from the toes to the bottom of the cotton cast. Rehabilitation is started immediately. The patient is expected to raise his leg that night; exercise all of his muscles the next morning; be up in a chair the first postoperative day and be up on crutches with direct weight-bearing the second postoperative day. Weight-bearing without crutches is discouraged, however, because of the tendency to lurch and so strain the knee laterally. Since the cotton cast loosens up in a few days, the elastic bandage is removed from the foot and wrapped around the dressing.

The patient is allowed to go home in a few days and is instructed to rewrap the elastic bandage over the cotton cast every few days to keep it snug. When he reports back two weeks after the operation, the cotton cast and stitches are removed. If there is effusion, the knee is aspirated and an elastic bandage provided. If there is no effusion, rehabilitation is continued. At this point no effort is made to force motion of the knee other than by the patient's voluntary effort. In the uncomplicated case, recovery is rapid. Aspiration is repeated as often as indicated by effusion. It usually is not necessary at all. Athletic participation will be permitted as soon as the range of motion is normal and the strength of the operated leg is equal to that of the good leg. This may be at four weeks or may be later, depending upon the many factors that influence recovery, such as the duration of symptoms prior to the operation, the degree of synovitis of the knee and postoperative bleeding or effusion. There are specific exercises which are recommended for rehabilitation after operations on the knee, and in the case of meniscectomy, these may be started on the night of the surgery. They are first done with a splint on so that the knee does not move. In the occasional patient in whom there has been previous synovitis or in whom there were complications of other conditions of the knee with synovitis and effusion, isotonic exercises should not be done. Actually walking does little damage to inflamed synovium, but stair climbing, running and squatting do cause injury. I do not allow any exercises which bend the knee if there is painful synovitis or extensive effusion. I would like to emphasize again that persistent effusion is contributed to by irritation of an already irritated joint. Therefore, I urge the patient not to do knee flexing exercises with weight on the foot, since this tends to force the synovial membranes together and increase effusion. He may, however, rapidly increase his isometric exercises done with the knee straight. (See also Chapter 22.)

CHONDRAL AND OSTEOCHONDRAL FRACTURE

A chondral fracture is a fracture involving the articular cartilage and is particularly prevalent at the knee, owing to the direct stresses and strains applied to the knee joint. A chondral fracture may be extremely difficult to diagnose and in many instances may be determined only after arthrotomy of the knee. If there is no fragment of underlying bone involved, the x-ray findings will be entirely negative. The reader is strongly urged to refer to Chapter 4, page 76, for a more complete discussion of this very interesting, distressing and even frustrating condition.

The *diagnosis* must rest on the patient's history and clinical symptoms. If the fracture is complete and if a piece of cartilage is loose in the knee, the symptoms will be the same as those caused by a foreign body within the joint. Although this fracture may be quite difficult to distinguish from a tear of one of the menisci or from osteochondritis dissecans, early differentiation is somewhat academic, since in any case arthrotomy is indicated. Many chondral fractures go completely unrecognized, particularly when they are incomplete, so that the fragment is not actually dislodged. I feel quite sure that many cases of osteochondritis dissecans are in fact initiated by fractures of the cartilage. The most vulnerable areas in the joint are, first, the patella and, second, the two femoral condyles. The patella is particularly vulnerable because it is so common for the athlete to fall upon the flexed knee. The result may be a contusion of the articular cartilage, an actual fissuring of the cartilage or, in other circumstances, a complete chondral fracture with a piece of cartilage separated from the bone (Figs. 515 and 516).

The symptoms are the same as those caused by damage to the undersurface of the patella, i.e., pain on flexion and extension, particularly against resistance, and pain on manual pressure of the patella against the femoral condyle, particularly on "rubbing" the patella against the condylar groove with the knee in complete extension (glissement). Such a fracture may cause actual catching or locking of the knee by an interruption of the normal glide pattern of the patella in the patellar groove.

I operated on a patient diagnosed as having intrinsic injury to the knee, with chondromalacia of the patella, and was surprised to find that two thirds of the cartilage of the patella had been completely broken away and could be lifted up from its bed as a flap, exposing raw bone beneath. Another frequent chondral injury is an avulsion-type fracture of the cartilage and bone along the lateral margin of the medial femoral condyle at the femoral attachment of the posterior cruciate ligament (see Fig. 543). I have seen many patients at operation whose injury had been diagnosed as osteochondritis dissecans of the medial femoral condyle, in which the loose body was actually attached to the anterior end of the posterior cruciate ligament. Some conditions have been encountered in which the chondral body was completely free except for the fact that it was still attached to the posterior cruciate ligament. These are, in my opinion, chondral fractures rather than osteochondritis dissecans.

The primary problem in diagnosing chondral fracture is to differentiate it from other intrinsic conditions of the knee. It should be suspected if there is persistent pain and persistent dysfunction around an otherwise normal-appearing patella. This is particularly true if acute symptoms have followed immediately after an injury. The orthopaedist will see these patients relatively late, since they are usually treated for a contusion or a sprain, and the question of chondral fracture may arise only after the knee has failed to respond to ordinary therapeutic measures.

Proper *treatment* depends largely upon a proper diagnosis. If there is definitely a subchondral fracture, it is possible that protective

Figure 515. Acute chondral fracture of the patella with x-ray interpreted as negative. The patient had a history of falling on the flexed knee with more than the usual amount of symptoms including hemarthrosis. Surgery revealed (*A*) acute chondral fracture of the patella with multiple fragments of cartilage. Definitely not degenerative. *B*, The fragments may be lifted up, revealing the hemorrhagic bleeding bone beneath an acute injury. *C*, Further removal of the fragments and *D*, fragments all removed and the vascular bed of the bone exposed. Note the apparently normal cartilage surrounding the defect with no evidence of fibrillation or malacia. This would later have been described as a typical osteochondritis dissecans or chondromalacia; either of these diagnoses would have been wrong. This patient went on to a good recovery with no patellar symptoms at present.

Figure 516. This is a case similar to that of Figure 515 seen much later. Note the typical osteochondritic fragment. Note also the defect under the patella.

immobilization will permit it to heal. However, if the cartilage itself is broken without subchondral bone, the healing potential is so poor that it probably will not heal in any event. As a rule the exact condition has not been diagnosed previously, and one must be prepared to carry out whatever definitive measure is indicated at the time of the arthrotomy of the knee.

When a fragment of cartilage with some subchondral bone has been torn away, including a portion of the posterior cruciate attachment, the treatment is removal of this fragment and suture of the posterior cruciate to the cartilage bed through drill holes. This will successfully restore posterior cruciate integrity. In other cases in which the amount of cruciate ligament involved has been relatively small, I have simply sutured the torn ligament to its uninvolved portion. The loose fragment of bone and cartilage should be removed in any event and appropriate measures carried out to minimize the potential damage to the mechanism of the knee. Most of the young patients tolerate partial chondrectomy very well. One may smooth the margins of the bed either on the patella or on the femoral condyle and expect a considerable degree of filling in as healing proceeds. If the lesion is relatively localized and surrounded by healthy-appearing cartilage, it is much better to treat it by trephining and drilling (see page 580) than by chondral shaving, since trephining does not extend the area involved in the lesion. Indeed, in many cases the fossa has pretty well smoothed itself out before arthrotomy has been accepted by the patient. I am extremely loath to sacrifice the patella in a young athlete. I would oppose even more the use of a metallic prosthesis. In either case the femoral condyle is exposed to considerable direct trauma. The small metallic prosthesis serves to concentrate the force in a small area and is potentially more dangerous than any direct trauma to the condyle protected by the quadriceps aponeurosis only, after the removal of the patella.

FRACTURE

Fracture about the knee is not a frequent injury in the young athlete. The ordinary fracture is treated in the same manner as a similar fracture in any other patient, bearing in mind the general principles for treatment of the athlete, particularly in reference to prompt diagnosis with the aid of x-rays. The aphorism in fracture treatment that "the nearer the joint the more perfect the reduction" is doubly true for the knee, since the normally functioning knee joint will not tolerate any gross irregularity of its articular surfaces. This discussion will be confined to the treatment of those fractures about the knee which are most common in the athlete.

Fracture of the Patella

Fracture of the patella occurs in athletes but is not as common as chondral fracture of the patella. Fractures of either the upper (Fig. 517A) or lower pole (Fig. 517B) or along the medial or lateral margin (Figs. 517C and 518) usually are actually either strain fractures or sprain fractures and should be treated as such by removal of the fragment of bone and suture of the ligament or tendon to the patella. This should be done promptly, and a perfectly functioning knee may be expected. It should be emphasized that there is little place for bone repair in the treatment of fracture of the patella, and I can think of few circumstances justifying the securing of bone-to-bone apposition and waiting for patellar union. The exception is in the incomplete fracture or possibly in the linear fracture extending from the upper to the lower pole of the patella. One should particularly suspect chondral fracture to accompany stellate fracture of the patella without displacement. It is not wise to carry out patellectomy in the athlete if it can be avoided, since complete patellectomy is not compatible with such strenuous sports as soccer, football and the like, not because of failure of the quadriceps mechanism but because of the extreme vulnerability of the femoral condyles after removal of the patella. I would be even more fearful of permitting athletic participation following replacement of the patella by a metallic prosthesis, since this concentrates the force and in my opinion is more dangerous than complete patellectomy.

Fracture of the patella by direct contusion is not infrequent. The fracture usually involves the lateral portion of the patella, since the bone is thinner in this area (Fig. 519). This fracture differs from the avulsion type, in which the fragment is torn away by the tendon or the fragment. The avulsion fracture is usually on the medial side and occurs as the patella is forced laterally. It also differs from the explosive type of fracture caused by a forceful blow against the patella with the quadriceps in

Figure 517. *A,* Avulsed quadriceps tendon and fragment from superior pole of patella. The shell of bone makes the diagnosis simple, but the lesion is really a tendon avulsion rather than a fractured patella. Treatment by repair of the quadriceps to the patella. *B,* Avulsion fracture of lower pole of patella. In effect, a rupture of the tendon. Note that after removal of the fragments and repair of the tendon to the patella, there is essentially normal-appearing patella remaining. *C,* Fracture of lateral margin of the patella by a direct blow. This should be treated by removal of the fragment and suture of the lateral retinaculum to the patella.

Figure 518. Patient fell directly on the flexed knee, fracturing the patella. *A,* Preoperative radiograph. *B,* Operative picture showing linear fracture across the medial one fourth of the patella. *C,* Operative picture showing the fracture and the patella after the removal of the fragment. *D,* Postoperative radiograph after fragment was removed (facetectomy).

Figure 519. This professional baseball player received a sharp blow on the knee with a baseball, had immediate swelling, pain and discomfort. He was treated for contusion. On examination some weeks later, the oblique view shows the fracture, which had been overlooked in the anteroposterior and lateral views. The silhouette view (as in Fig. 517C) would demonstrate this even better.

violent contraction, such as occurs when the knee hits the dashboard in a car accident. The contusion fracture is due to a sharp blow in a relatively localized area, such as is sometimes received by a baseball fielder. As he is squatting down with his knees flexed, the ball caroms to one side and directly hits the patella. This same force may cause chondral damage. A typical example of this fracture is illustrated in Figure 517C. The silhouette view made its diagnosis much easier, since the small fragment is difficult to visualize in the anteroposterior x-ray view unless the x-ray is particularly good

(see Fig. 491). This condition is treated by removal of the fragment and suture of the retinaculum to the patella. Uneventful recovery should be expected. At the time of repair the undersurface of the patella and the cartilage of the patellar groove should be carefully inspected for possible chondral damage.

Care should be taken not to confuse the *bipartite* or *tripartite patella* with acute injury (Fig. 520). The partite patella is usually bilateral and symmetrical and is asymptomatic. Careful examination will demonstrate that the symptoms are not in the area of the anomaly. It should be borne in mind, however, that it is possible for the quadriceps lateralis to avulse or partially avulse the separate piece, in which event the condition will become symptomatic. This condition ordinarily will respond well to rest and protection. If the symptoms persist, one is justified in removing the piece and suturing the tendon to the patella. This condition is quite analogous to avulsion of the accessory navicular in the foot. In both instances there is an underlying congenital anomaly on which an acute injury is superimposed.

Avulsion Fracture

The *avulsion fracture of the upper tibia* (Fig. 521) is basically an avulsion of the anterior cruciate ligament and should be treated as such, the main emphasis being placed on the restoration of the anterior cruciate ligament to its normal length and function. Only in the exceptional case can this be done nonsurgically. I much prefer to expose the knee antero-

Figure 520. Typical bipartite patella. Note the difference in the two sides, but general location is the same. Also note definite rounded-off line between the fragments. This is not an acute fracture. However, this fragment may be avulsed or partially avulsed and become symptomatic.

medially, examine it carefully for other lesions and then carry out whatever measures will best restore the function of the anterior cruciate. The occasional "locking" caused by a displaced fragment obviously demands reduction of the fragment. If there is a large fragment involving a portion of the articular cartilage on either side, it should be replaced and held in its bed by a transfixion screw or by sutures passed through parallel drill holes running from in front of the tibia to the bed of the fragment and then passed through the fragment, using mattress sutures. The sutures must be carefully placed so that the drill holes in the fragment coincide with those in its bed or else the fragment will not be perfectly reduced.

If the fragment is relatively small or comminuted, it should be removed and the cruciate ligament pulled down into the defect and firmly sutured, in which instance it will heal less rapidly than it will if the bone is replaced (Fig. 522). There is little purpose in leaving a small, thin fragment subject to necrosis. On the other hand, when the fragment is large and makes up a substantial portion of the upper tibia, as is frequently the case in young people, it should be preserved in the manner described. Normal function of the knee will not tolerate gross unreduced displacement of the superior surface of the tibia.

In an *avulsion fracture of the distal end of the patella,* the so-called jumper's knee, there is some damage to the tendon attachment at the distal pole of the patella. A similar type of injury is avulsion of a tip of bone from the distal pole of the patella. Sometimes the tendon will be partially avulsed, taking a shell of bone with it, which fills in and makes a prominence at the distal pole of the patella (Fig. 523). Ossification in this area is likely to be diminished by proper immobilization, which permits the area to heal without irritation. Chronic irritation will result in the laying down of a deposit of bone, which may become quite extensive. This is not like the deposit of calcium in the tendon, which is a degenerative change and which will be out in the substance of the tendon. The bone usually forms contiguous to the patella. Occasionally there will actually be a piece of bone pulled off, resulting in fracture. On other occasions the injury will heal without bone formation. Sometimes it does heal with bone formation, making a rather extensive addition to the distal end of the patella, as illustrated in Figure 523C.

If there is fracture of the distal pole of the patella with separation, it is best treated by resection of the bone and repair of the tendon to the patella through drill holes. Actually, even if there is a relatively substantial piece of bone avulsed by the patellar tendon, it is probably better to take the fragment out and sew the tendon to the parent patella, since fracture of the patella is notoriously slow to heal and sometimes will go on to a painful nonunion (see Fig. 523A). Of course if the bone in the tendon is not painful, it requires no treatment. Sometimes there is pain even

Figure 521. Bicycle injury in which the foot was caught in the wheel. The child was thrown off the bicycle. *A,* Illustration of avulsion of the top of the tibia by anterior cruciate. Note the tibial spines are intact, since the cruciate does not attach there. *B,* After replacement and suture. No anteroposterior instability.

Figure 522. This 9 year old female fell from a bicycle, injuring her right knee. The doctor made x-rays and told her she had a "bone sliver" and to keep it at rest for two weeks. No support. No other treatment. *A*, The acute injury showing a large fragment of the upper tibia avulsed by the anterior cruciate. *B*, Four months later, the fragment in the same position. Film made with the knee at its maximum extension. Range of motion, 30 degrees. *C*, Two months after removal of the fragment, some recurrence of the ossification. This knee has had very extensive physical therapy, active and passive motion. Range now (nine months post-injury—five months postoperative) is 20 to 90 degrees. This disability could have been prevented by early adequate treatment.

though there is apparent union, and in some instances, it is justifiable to detach the tendon and take out the exogenous bone. However, this is a pretty major procedure from the standpoint of morbidity and should not be done unless it is definitely necessary.

Avulsion fracture of the patellar tubercle of the tibia may occur. Diagnosis can readily be made by location of pain and tenderness and disturbance of the quadriceps mechanism. It should be confirmed by x-ray. The most important consideration is the function of the tendon rather than the fragment of displaced bone. The tendon should be replaced surgically. If the bone fragment is small or comminuted, it should be removed and the tendon repaired to its bed. If the fragment is large, it may be repositioned and held by internal fixation, preferably using a transfixion screw (Fig. 524). If the epiphyses are open, care must be taken not to close them.

There may also be *avulsion at the superior pole of the patella,* in which instance the quadriceps attachment is pulled away from the patella with or without a shell of the patellar bone. In incomplete avulsion, the mechanism of injury is a powerful contraction of the quadriceps while the leg is being forcibly flexed. This is, in fact, a strain type of injury, and as the forces are arrested, there may be greater or lesser damage to the attachment of the tendon to the upper pole of the patella. This will cause pain on active function of the quadriceps but will not interfere with extension of the knee otherwise. The incomplete injury is treated by protection, local injection and application of heat locally. The degree of protection depends upon the extent of the damage.

If the force is severe enough, the whole quadriceps aponeurosis may be detached from the patella. This is a painful injury. Examination will reveal swelling about the upper end of the patella, with tenderness along its superior margin. The patient will be unable to actively extend the knee completely. When he contracts the quadriceps, a palpable defect may be felt above the patella. The patella will not be displaced downward, since there is no muscular mechanism attaching to the patella from below, and its distance from the tibia will remain constant whether the knee is flexed or extended. X-rays may be of diagnostic value, since often a shell of bone may be avulsed (Figs. 517*A* and 525). Treatment should be surgical repair with snug suture of the aponeurosis to the patella through drill holes. I recall one case in an older man who caught his heel on a step as he descended a stairway. Both of his knees flexed sharply, and in his violent effort to regain his equilibrium, the quadriceps were detached from the patellas on both knees. Uneventful recovery followed surgical repair.

Major fractures about the knee are not particularly frequent as athletic injuries and are readily recognized by the accompanying major disability and by confirmatory x-ray. One should be particularly alert to the *associated ligament injuries*. Avulsion of the collateral ligament with a fragment of bone from the tibial plateau or femoral condyle is in reality a ligament injury and should be treated as such (Figs. 526 and 527). One must be aware that when a small fragment of bone has been pulled off the condyle, the probabilities are that the ligament is attached to it (Fig. 528). One must not assume that it is a chip fracture. For example, if the tip of the fibula is broken, one should suspect avulsion of the biceps (see Fig. 457*B*) or the fibular collateral ligament or both.

If the lateral table of the tibia is compressed, one should examine the leg very carefully to determine the function of the medial collateral ligament, which also was placed under strain by the force that caused the fracture (Fig.

A

B

C

Figure 523. *A,* Interesting case of partial avulsion of the patellar tendon from the patella with marked ossification and painful nonunion. The exogenous bone was removed and the patellar tendon repaired to the patella. *B,* Opposite patella for comparison. This is not a fractured patella but a tendon avulsion. *C,* Another patient who had had previous trouble at the distal pole of the patella, which in the last few months had subsided. Notice he has an old apophysitis with an ossicle in the patellar tendon which is now symptomatic. Following resection of this ossicle from the tendon and a suitable period of rehabilitation, the patient returned to his ordinary activity. This simply illustrates that the deposit of bone, not calcium, at the distal pole of the patella may not be symptomatic if there is union between this exogenous bone and the patella.

Figure 524. Boy injured while high jumping. This leg was not in contact with the ground. *A,* Showing avulsion by violent contraction of the muscle, which pulled off the patellar tubercle and the anterior one third of the upper surface of the tibia. *B,* Two months post-repair showing good healing. He went on to a good and complete recovery.

529). The mechanism of this injury is force applied to the lateral side of the knee, very likely with the knee in extension. The medial collateral ligament and the posterior capsule hold the knee stable in this position, and the relatively sharp edge of the lateral femoral condyle rotates slightly medially and drives into the central portion of the lateral tibial plateau. The force may split the edge of the plateau laterally, may depress the central portion, may cause any type of fracture of the upper tibia or, indeed, may snub off a portion of the femoral condyle. The same force, however, is being applied on the medial side of the knee. These fractures ordinarily occur in older people in whom the ligament is ordinarily stronger than the bone. In a young person there may be ligament damage as well. In the injury which occurs with the knee slightly flexed, the force is accepted mostly on the rounded portion of the condyle. No lateral bony damage occurs, and the ligament tears on the medial side. If the leg is in extension with the support by the posterior capsule, the

Figure 525. Flexion injury of the knee with avulsion of the quadriceps tendon attachment from upper pole of the patella. Surgery revealed the whole quadriceps tendon pulled off the patella.

Figure 526. Acute wrestling injury, with avulsion of the popliteus tendon attachment from the femur with a relatively large fragment of bone. This was the only injury. Uneventful recovery following repair. The osteochondritis dissecans was an incidental finding, was asymptomatic and was not demonstrable surgically.

Figure 527. Medial side injury. This is an avulsion of the femoral attachment of the medial collateral ligament. *Arrow* indicates fragment of bone. Notice the avulsion is definitely below the adductor tubercle. The medial joint space is somewhat wider than the lateral. This is likely to heal with a painful prominence and some redundancy of the ligament. Advise removal of the fragment and repair of the ligament to the fracture bed.

Figure 528. Avulsion of the posterior cruciate ligament, resulting from a motorcycle accident. *A,* X-ray six weeks post-injury. Patient had direct blow to the tibia with the knee flexed, forcing the leg backward. He had four-plus posterior cruciate instability and restriction of extension. Arrow indicates avulsion of the ligament, with a fragment off the tibia. *B,* Postoperative film showing removal of some fragments and repair of the posterior cruciate to the back of the tibia with fragmented bone. Nine weeks postoperative the knee would flex to 120 degrees and was stable in this position.

Figure 529. *A,* Torn medial collateral ligament. Note compression fractures of the lateral tibial plateau. The same force that tears the medial ligament drives the lateral condyle into the tibia. A disappointing result will be obtained if this fragment is not elevated. This is not common in the young athlete. *B,* Postoperative film shows fragment completely elevated and held in place by a strut of bone. Medial collateral ligament was repaired. Good stability.

medial ligament holds for a period long enough so that the bone breaks. If the force is continued on the femoral condyle, further compressing the tibia, the ligament may give way. There are, therefore, injuries on both sides of the knee, either one of which may be easily overlooked.

In checking a case of obvious medial collateral ligament damage, one should inspect the x-ray carefully to see whether there is some compression of the lateral plateau. Similarly, if the lateral plateau is compressed, it is necessary to eliminate the possibility of the presence of medial collateral ligament avulsion. The test of gross instability may be quite misleading because either of these conditions alone will produce instability of the knee, with the leg going into more abduction than normal. In this instance, stress x-rays will be of great value, since they will show whether or not the medial margin of the joint opens up (Fig. 530). It is extremely disappointing to fix the tibial plateau and find an unstable knee resulting from medial ligament damage. It will be equally disappointing to make a skillful repair of the medial collateral ligament, only to find

Figure 530. This patient received a forcible blow on the lateral side of the knee. *A,* Anteroposterior view showing depression of the central portion of the lateral tibial plateau. *B,* The stress picture reveals that his marked instability was due not only to depression of the plateau but to severance of the medial collateral ligament. Note that the femur has moved slightly medially and the edge of the condyle rests on the depression of the tibial plateau. This should be treated by elevation of the plateau but of equal importance is repair of the medial collateral ligament.

that bony damage on the opposite side has impaired the result. The true importance of the treatment of fractures about the knee must be to obtain complete restoration of normal function by whatever method is most effective in a particular case.

Fracture of the Head of the Fibula

Although, strictly speaking, fracture of the head of the fibula is not an injury to the knee, it does sometimes become a diagnostic problem (see Fig. 461). The head of the fibula may be broken by a direct blow in an ordinary comminuted-type fracture without gross displacement. Any fracture below the head of the fibula, actually involving the neck, should cast immediate suspicion on the ankle joint rather than the knee. If the fracture is of the head of the bone, one should determine particularly whether or not there is any displacement and check for involvement of the peroneal nerve as well as the biceps tendon and external collateral ligament. If the fracture involves the ligament and tendon attachments, treatment must be much more extensive than if the injury was simply a direct trauma-type fracture of the bone.

There may occasionally be a *dislocation of the fibula from the tibia* (Fig. 531). Here, again, one should immediately suspect a twisting force, resulting in damage to the ankle joint. The condition, however, may be localized at the knee and have been caused by direct trauma against the fibular head, knocking it away by tearing the relatively weak superior tibiofibular ligaments. In such an instance, replacement should be accurate, and if there is any tendency whatever toward instability of the fibula, it may be fixed by internal fixation with a transfixion screw through the fibula into the upper end of the tibia. This screw should be removed as soon as ligament healing is complete. Use of internal fixation will expedite rehabilitation. Careful attention should be paid to possible involvement of the peroneal nerve, since it is in a very vulnerable location as it crosses around the fibular neck.

Epiphyseal Fractures

A word should be said about epiphyseal fractures about the knee, since they do happen, particularly in children of secondary school age. These fractures are usually readily recognized by careful study of the x-ray. The incomplete fracture of the epiphysis may be overlooked and diagnosed as sprain (Figs. 532 to 536). A careful, detailed examination will ordinarily result in an accurate diagnosis, since the tenderness and pain will be completely around the epiphyseal plate, and strain in any

Figure 531. Gymnast vaulted over a horse and landed off balance, with his knees stiff and with considerable force. The left knee snapped and hyperextended. He had severe pain posteriorly and to the outer side of his knee over the head of the fibula. The injury was treated with heat for ten days and then put in a cast. While in a cast it was still painful. The patient was seen here two weeks post-injury. Examination revealed a very tender, painful fibula, which was quite prominent on the left side compared with the right. Flexion of the leg against resistance was painful in this area. X-ray was interpreted as suggestive but nonconclusive. Surgery revealed that there was a tear of the ligament (proximal tibiofibular ligament), which permitted the fibula to displace away from the tibia. This was held with a transfixion screw, and the fascia was repaired. The screw was removed three months later. Six months later there was a little prominence of the fibular head. Patient was otherwise asymptomatic. X-ray was interpreted as negative. *A,* Preoperative x-ray. Note evident widening of fibula from tibia. *B,* Internal fixation. *C,* Six months post-injury, patient asymptomatic.

Figure 532. Epiphyseal fracture of upper tibia. Note slight separation of medial half of epiphysis, with it split down the shaft. As a result of the injury the fractured part of the epiphysis closed, necessitating surgical closure of lateral tibia and fibula.

direction will tend to cause pain, whereas ligament injury is quite unusual on both sides of the knee at once.

If no displacement is present, *treatment* generally given to injury about the knee will suffice, that is, local measures, use of a compression bandage, and application of ice followed by protection. It should be emphasized that the apparatus applied to protect the knee should result in elimination of pain on stress; otherwise it is not truly protective. When effective it will be adequate for the ordinary incomplete epiphyseal fracture. Any displacement, even of a mild degree, should be corrected (Figs. 537 to 539). Correction becomes increasingly difficult with the passage of time, so that in any doubtful situation, x-rays should be made promptly and treatment carried out as soon as possible, with the patient under general anesthesia. Epiphyseal fractures do not necessarily affect the growth of the bone, and they are much less likely to do so if reduction is anatomical and with a minimum amount of trauma. One should be able to reduce these fractures by closed manipulation, but they may require internal fixation, preferably not crossing the epiphyseal plate, to prevent recurrence of the displacement. If open reduction is decided upon, one must be partic-

ularly careful in handling the epiphyseal cartilage. Prying against the cartilage or levering the fragments into place with instruments may well do more damage than the injury itself. The epiphyseal cartilage as a rule remains with the epiphysis, the diaphyseal portion of bone being denuded, hence one must be particularly careful in handling the smaller fragment.

Fabella

The fabella (see Fig. 442) is a sesamoid bone frequently found in the tendon of the lateral head of the gastrocnemius muscle as it passes under the femoral condyle. Fracture of the fabella is extremely uncommon but is of quite serious consequence when it occurs. One should be aware of the fabella and not mistake it for a foreign body or a loose fragment in the joint. If it is in two or more pieces, the opposite knee should be carefully checked since as a rule the bipartite fabella will be bilateral. The location of the tenderness and pain on function of the gastrocnemius are diagnostic signs. The x-ray may be quite deceptive. If the fabella is actually involved, either by a fracture, osteo-

Figure 533. Illustration of a case of slight epiphyseal subluxation of lower femur. Note the callus formation where the periosteum was stripped up laterally. This is the same mechanism as sprain of the medial collateral ligament and in fact was diagnosed as such until careful examination localized the tenderness on both sides of the lower femoral epiphysis and x-ray showed the fracture across the lateral corner of the metaphysis.

Figure 534. This and the next case (Figure 535) represent a diagnostic problem. Both patients had what appeared to be medial instability of the knee joint. *A,* The original picture showed suggestion of separation of the medial upper tibial epiphysis. *B,* Confirmed by stress x-ray under anesthesia. The apparent widening of the medial joint space is normal for this individual when compared with the opposite knee. This was treated by closed manipulation and repair of the long fibers of the medial collateral ligament. See also Figures 537, 538 and 539.

Figure 535. Another medial side injury (see Figure 534) showing apparently normal upper tibial epiphysis but suspicious buckling of the lateral cortex. *A,* The normal side. *B,* The involved side. *C,* Oblique view confirms the true pathological condition: separation of the medial upper tibial epiphysis with compression of the lateral plateau. Closed manipulation corrected the deformity.

Growth disturbance may become a factor here as well as in the case presented in Figure 534.

Figure 536. Patient injured by collision with another player. He experienced severe excruciating pain down the lateral side of his leg, which was attributable to "nerve." He continued to have trouble and finally developed an effusion in his right knee with ecchymosis in the calf. Careful restudy of his x-rays revealed the fracture line running from across the lateral quadrant of the tibia, beginning just at the head of the fibula and crossing obliquely up through the interspinous area. A, Arrow indicates the fracture line at the time of the injury. B, Three months later the line of the fracture is still apparent.

Figure 537. This 17 year old boy was sent in with diagnosis of acute rupture of the medial collateral ligament and instability of the knee. A, The picture sent in was interpreted as normal, but note the suspicious vertical line extending upward from the intercondylar notch. B, X-ray made with lateral stress under anesthesia revealed the true pathological condition, an epiphyseal fracture across the medial condyle split down into the intercondylar notch. This was treated by transfixion screw in order to permit more rapid mobilization.

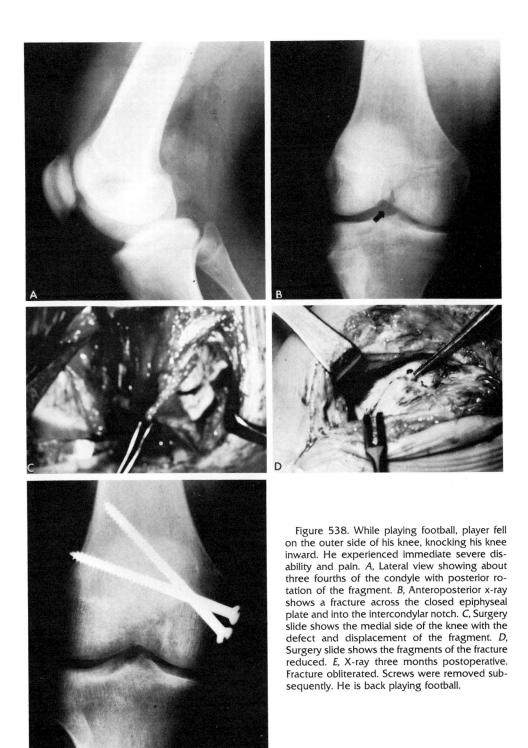

Figure 538. While playing football, player fell on the outer side of his knee, knocking his knee inward. He experienced immediate severe disability and pain. *A*, Lateral view showing about three fourths of the condyle with posterior rotation of the fragment. *B*, Anteroposterior x-ray shows a fracture across the closed epiphyseal plate and into the intercondylar notch. *C*, Surgery slide shows the medial side of the knee with the defect and displacement of the fragment. *D*, Surgery slide shows the fragments of the fracture reduced. *E*, X-ray three months postoperative. Fracture obliterated. Screws were removed subsequently. He is back playing football.

Figure 539. Patient fell about three meters, landing on the flexed knee. He had immediate instability and disability. *A*, X-ray revealed splitting off of the medial femoral condyle and displacement of the patella with the fragment, and avulsion of part of the medial collateral ligament from the tibia. *B*, Twelve weeks postinjury showing repair of the fracture prior to removal of the screws. *C*, Surgical film when screws were removed showing that in spite of the fracture being well healed, there is still a definite fissure in the articular cartilage.

chondritis or chondromalacia, it should be removed. The approach is a lateral one behind the fibular collateral ligament and the iliotibial band—the same approach utilized to expose the posterior horn of the lateral meniscus.

CHRONIC SYNOVITIS WITH EFFUSION
("Water on the Knee")

To be complete, any discussion of injuries to the knee in athletes requires comment on joint effusion. It must be recognized that this is not a specific diagnosis but a finding. In normal circumstances the fluid balance within the knee is finely adjusted, with the fluid formed and absorbed in an equal ratio in order to keep the joint lubricated. There are many and varied causes for irritation of the synovia

and recurrent effusion. I want to emphasize that there is no such thing as "water on the knee" as a disease or an injury. This excess fluid formation results from a pathological condition within the knee. To examine the knee and say "He has an effusion" is like examining an abdomen and saying "He has rigidity." The effusion must be and ordinarily can be accounted for. If the physician is unable to explain the cause of the effusion, his management of the case must be extremely inadequate. If the effusion followed an injury, one may ordinarily dismiss the systemic and indeed most of the inflammatory causes of effusion. However, a word of caution is necessary: The active young athlete will almost always be able to explain the effusion in the knee on the basis of having injured the knee, since he is bumping his knees constantly. Unless the diagnosis is immediately obvious, measures must be taken to successively rule out the various causes of effusion. Here the routine examination of the knee becomes extremely valuable.

First, the patient's *history* is taken. Is there an immediately determinable cause for the fluid or did it develop insidiously? Has there been a change in the activity habits of the patient? For example, if a person has run ten miles when he was not accustomed to this degree of activity, irritation and effusion may well occur. This cause could easily be overlooked, since to the athlete it might not suggest an injury. Inquire as to his general health. Are there signs of a rheumatic disturbance or an infectious process?

On *examination,* observe the knee carefully. Is it swollen, tense and obviously inflamed, or is the suprapatellar pouch merely filled with fluid? On palpation much can be learned as to the nature of the effusion. The ordinary traumatic effusion, even with hemarthrosis, causes little local heat, whereas an inflamed knee will ordinarily be hot. Careful examination for tenderness around the menisci or over the condyles or around the patella may provide a lead as to the diagnosis. Is there a local area of tenderness?

Careful manipulative examination of the knee will help to determine whether there has been ligament damage or whether there is persistent meniscus reaction. Is motion in the knee painful? After careful evaluation and x-ray study, the knee joint should be aspirated and close attention given to the fluid. Cloudy, turgid, viscous fluid is very suggestive of acute inflammatory reaction, and conversely, clear, straw-colored, thin fluid will pretty well eliminate this possibility. If there is gross blood, one may immediately presume an injury. Careful study of the fluid is necessary to determine whether it is actually blood, bloody fluid or merely blood-tinged fluid. If the fluid is at first clear, and then toward the end of the aspiration becomes bloody, one may assume the presence of an inflamed synovium in which the irritation from genupuncture has caused local bleeding at the site of the puncture. Culture of the fluid for the presence of infection is of undeniable importance. Routine microscopic or laboratory examination of knee joint fluid is of some value in diagnosis and may be a useful aid in eliminating the possibility that systemic causes resulted in the effusion. The blood count is important and urinalysis may provide a lead. The best single laboratory procedure is that which tests the blood sedimentation rate; findings should be negative in cases of trauma.

The *treatment* of an effusion in the knee is the treatment of the underlying cause. This predicates accurate diagnosis. If the diagnosis must be deferred or is not possible, certain local measures are of value in the interim. The extent of treatment will vary considerably according to the symptoms. Certainly the joint should not be permitted to remain grossly distended over a long period of time, since this very distention of the capsule will often perpetuate an effusion long after the causative lesion has been arrested. In general, then, the treatment should consist of aspiration, pressure, and protection. Aspiration is repeated as often as the fluid recurs, even though this may be every few days or, in certain very acute circumstances, daily. Injection of various medicaments into the joint may be indicated. I would not recommend injection of an antibiotic into the knee unless definite infection is demonstrable. In chronic inflammation, the corticoid preparations are of value. In my opinion they should not be repeated more than once a week, even though aspiration may be needed more frequently. Corticoids should not be injected over a long period of time.

One of the most difficult decisions in the presence of chronic or so-called idiopathic effusion concerns the amount of protection necessary. If the condition seems to be relatively minor and there is no pain or other local symptoms, one may be under considerable pressure to permit unrestricted activity, particularly in the athlete. I believe that under certain circumstances the patient with an effusion in the knee may continue athletic activity, but I would feel extremely uneasy about permitting it unless I was sure of the underlying pathological condition. To be more specific, in a patient recovering from a meniscectomy in whom the rest of the knee appears to be in good condition, the physician might permit considerable activity in the presence of definite effusion, since he can readily account for the symptoms. On the other hand, if the effusion is spontaneous, the physician must be very sure of the nature of the pathological condition before permitting activity. This can often mean complete immobilization of the joint until either the diagnosis is determined or the effusion has been eliminated. Although the ordinary wrap-on elastic bandage on the knee is of little value for protection of the ligaments, it is very useful in the presence of an effusion into the joint. Following aspiration of the fluid, if it is not necessary to immobilize the knee for other reasons, a snug pressure bandage should be applied routinely, since it exerts the same restraining influence on intercapsular bleeding or effusion as does the pressure of a capsule full of fluid. I much prefer the wrap-on to the pull-on bandage, since the pull-on bandage inevitably fits very few people. It is either too tight or too loose in its ordinary application. Since the elastic bandage does put pressure on the synovium, pushing the irritated surfaces together, it is not advisable to put on a tight elastic bandage and then encourage activity. In other words, if you are going to permit a player to return to play while he still has effusion, it probably would be better to tape his knee, which does give some restriction of motion but does not put the pressure on the synovium that the elastic bandage does.

Physical therapeutic measures are of considerable value in synovitis, whatever its cause. For this reason, modalities such as diathermy, electric pad, whirlpool, hot packs and analgesic packs are recommended. It will be noted that with all these measures, the whole knee is encompassed by the heat. Such modalities as microtherm and infra-red or other rays are so restricted in their application that they tend to get the knee much too hot in one location and not hot enough in another. If only the bulb or infra-red ray is available, it should be used in the form of a baker so that the knee is exposed to the hot air rather than primarily to the ray.

Rehabilitative exercises would seem to be the antithesis of what is beneficial in effusion, since effusion is encouraged by irritation of the synovium by motion. Obviously a compromise must be reached in a given case to decide what degree of rehabilitation will be compatible with recovery of the irritation. There are some rehabilitative measures, however, that are perfectly consistent with treatment of synovial irritation in the knee. These are exercises for the foot, the hip and the rest of the body. Also the isometric contractions of the quadriceps and hamstrings have been shown to be very effective in rehabilitation and yet do not entail any degree of motion of the knee and may be carried out with the knee straight. Since rehabilitation of the quadriceps is extremely important, I routinely encourage straight leg raising, with a progressive weight program. This does not cause the synovium to slide and so should not increase irritation. We ask the player to discontinue weight-lifting exercises that cause flexion of the knee, such as sitting with the foot hanging down and bringing it up to the horizontal level. He can build the same mass by isometric straight leg raising and by resistive extension exercises. (See Chapter 22.) If effusion persists, synovectomy may occasionally be indicated.

APOPHYSITIS OF THE PATELLAR TUBERCLE
(Osgood-Schlatter "Disease")

Apophysitis of the tibial tubercle is a particular type of involvement that is commonly called Osgood-Schlatter disease. The word disease is a misnomer, since the condition is not a disease. Actually, there are three manifestations of Osgood-Schlatter disease. One is *bursitis of the infrapatellar tendon bursa* (see Fig. 438). This bursa lies between the infrapatellar fat pad and the patellar tendon, just proximal to the patellar tubercle of the tibia. In this condition, tenderness is elicited at a point slightly higher than the tubercle. The condition should be treated as a bursitis (see page 466).

The second type of Osgood-Schlatter disease is an *aseptic necrosis of the tip of the epiphysis* of the patellar tubercle of the tibia (Fig. 540). The necrosis occurs in the patellar tendon attachment and is probably traumatic in origin, initiated by a fracture or by an avulsion of the tip of the patellar tubercle. Because of poor circulation, the fragment fails to heal, and the constant irritation or traction of the patellar tendon makes it symptomatic. The mass tends to enlarge with reactive inflammation, so that a rather large tumor may result. The tumor is tender to touch, and there is pain on active extension of the quadriceps against resistance.

The third type of Osgood-Schlatter disease is a *true epiphysitis involving the whole epiphysis* (Fig. 541). This type is not particularly frequent but generally is more severe than the others when it occurs.

The *symptoms* of the latter two conditions are pain on direct pressure and pain on active use of the quadriceps. Rather sharp limitation of the activity of the patient may result. As is true of epiphysitis in other areas, the reaction itself is self-limited, but there may be considerable residue, usually in the form of a large patellar tubercle with separate fragments lying within the patellar tendon attachment (Fig. 542). This may or may not remain symptomatic after the active condition subsides.

Treatment varies with the type of pathological condition and, until recently, has usually been nonsurgical, an attempt being made to relieve the tension in the mass by measures reducing the activity of the knee. They may range from cutting down the patient's activity to putting the leg in a cast. However, following arrest of symptoms, there is a strong tendency for them to recur, so that until the epiphysis closes, it remains a constant source of irritation. Even after the growth period, local symptoms may persist. Surgical treatment will result in much more prompt and complete recovery in the first two conditions, once frank involvement has occurred.

At operation the patellar tendon is split over the area of the involvement, and in the second type, the sequestrated fragment is carefully removed and the area thoroughly curetted down to normal bone. The epiphyseal plate between the tubercle and the tibia is not disturbed. The split tendon is resutured over the area and the knee protected for about four weeks with a cotton cast. If a large mass of bone and cartilage has developed, it should be trimmed down with an osteotome to leave a fairly flat area. Following four weeks of immobilization and a few weeks of rehabilitation,

recovery should be complete. In the actively growing person, great care must be taken that the epiphysis is not surgically closed. If the epiphysis is continuous with the proximal tibial epiphysis, backknee may develop owing to arrest of growth in front while growth persists in the posterior one half of the plate. It should be emphasized to the parents that the condition is self-limited and will not develop into a malignant tumor, and if adequately treated, it will not limit physical activity. Most parents and patients will accept surgical treatment if the alternatives are carefully explained. The recurrence rate is extremely low after surgical treatment and quite high after nonsurgical treatment. Acute fracture of the patellar tubercle is discussed on page 457.

Figure 540. *A,* Normal tibial tubercle epiphysis. *B,* The excavated necrotic area with fragmentation which requires curettement. *C* and *D,* A similar case. Patient had persistent trouble in the knee with a large mass distal to the patella, which had bothered him since adolescence and had gradually increased in severity. Surgical excision was essential. This outcome from untreated apophysitis of the patellar tubercle is not unusual, although the size of the mass is.

Figure 541. Osgood-Schlatter "disease," showing epiphysitis of the entire epiphysis, with irregularity of the epiphyseal line. Since this epiphyseal cartilage is continuous with that of the upper tibia, it should not be disturbed. If surgery is utilized, exposure should be superficial to the epiphyseal cartilage.

OSTEOCHONDRITIS DISSECANS
(Osteochondral Fracture)

Over three fourths of recognized cases of osteochondritis dissecans occur at the knee and usually on the lateral margin of the medial condyle. They extend from the articular margin at the notch toward the medial side of the knee, a position coinciding almost exactly with the femoral attachment of the posterior cruciate ligament. The reader is strongly urged to refer to Chapter 4, page 85, for a more complete discussion of this condition.

Etiology. It cannot be doubted that some of these cases are caused by excessive traction on the attachment of the posterior cruciate ligament, resulting, in fact, in an avulsion or at least a partial avulsion of a fragment of bone by the ligament. I have seen many cases in which the osteochondritic fragment contained a major portion of the attachment of the posterior cruciate ligament (Fig. 543). It is not my contention that all these cases are caused by trauma but simply that many of them are. Trauma would seem to account more plausibly for the frequent occurrence of the lesion in this location that any of the other stated explanations. The theory of spontaneous ischemia

is not wholly tenable. This theory implies that ischemia is more marked in this particular location on the femoral condyle than elsewhere, but actually circulation should be somewhat better here because the posterior cruciate ligament attaches at this point. However, osteochondritis dissecans occurs occasionally in other areas in the knee and also in this same general area without actually including the attachment of the posterior cruciate, so that avulsion by the posterior cruciate cannot be the universal cause.

The lesion is most common at the extreme distal arch of the condyle, an area that is obviously quite subject to trauma, particularly in a fall on the flexed knee. With the knee flexed, the patella rides directly over this area of the femoral condyle, and the transmitted force strikes directly here. The principal argument against direct trauma as the occasional cause is that one would expect the lateral condyle to have received at least equal trauma, whereas actually osteochondritis dissecans is quite unusual in the lateral condyle of the femur. The explanation may lie in the fact that the patella is so much thicker in its medial portion and so transmits the trauma more directly.

In summary, the cause of osteochondritis

Figure 542. Old apophysitis of the patellar tubercle, with fragmentation and painful, unsightly tumor. Treated by excision of the fragments, flattening of the tubercle and reattachment of the patellar tendon, which has been split longitudinally and has become partially detached.

dissecans at the knee may be said to be (1) ischemia with loss of circulation to the bone of the epiphysis, (2) avulsion of the posterior cruciate ligament attachment or (3) direct trauma transmitted through the patella directly against the condyle.

Diagnosis. Some cases give no positive clinical findings and are discovered incidentally in an x-ray examination for other conditions (see Fig. 526). It should be recognized that x-ray has been made for *some* reason, and most frequently the reason is chronic complaint in the joint, which is nonspecific in character and does not suggest internal derangement, ligament injury or chronic synovitis. In such a case, x-ray may show a well-defined lesion of the medial femoral condyle on its articular surface, and one may presume that the lesion may well be the cause of the slight complaint (Fig. 544). As symptoms develop the condition becomes more acute, with chronic synovitis and often mild effusion. Pain occurs after forced exertion. Examination at this time will reveal no specific findings. Results of tests for ligament injury are negative. Meniscus test findings are negative. Occasionally percussion on the patella with the knee flexed to beyond 90 degrees will elicit discomfort. X-ray examination reveals the lesion. As the condition progresses, the bony sequestrum separates from its bed, the cartilage fissures and the fragment may become detached (Fig. 545). The symptoms then become the same as those caused by a foreign body in the joint; occasionally there is a palpable foreign body, with locking, increased synovitis, pain and loss of rhythmic motion of the knee (Fig. 546).

Treatment. If osteochondritis dissecans is seen incidentally without pre-existing symptoms, the degree of needed protection will depend upon the size of the fragment and the extent of the necrosis. If the fragment is large, involves a considerable portion of the weight-bearing surface and necrosis seems quite extensive, the treatment will vary according to the age of the patient. In a patient under 12, prevention of weight-bearing and immobilization of the knee may well permit spontaneous healing. This will require a period of eight to 18 months, which becomes quite disheartening to an active youth. In most cases immobilization in a cast with the knee flexed will be necessary, since the youngster can hardly be expected constantly to remember not to bear weight. In an older patient it is quite unlikely that complete resolution will occur. If it does, it will be so slow as to justify operative treatment to expedite recovery, if for no other reason. Surgery under these circumstances begins with arthrotomy of the knee and careful exploration of the area. If the fragment is completely detached, it should be removed. If the cartilage appears to be intact without separation or depression, one may be justified in drilling multiple 0.3 mm. drill holes through the fragment into its bed in order to increase its circulation and encourage revascularization. It is difficult to assess this method because one can never be certain that healing would not have taken place without operative interference. If there appears to be a defect in the cartilage with any undermining at all, the case should be treated as if the fragment had been completely detached, and the fragment should

Figure 543. *A*, Osteochondritis dissecans. Actually an osteochondral fracture of the femoral condyle, with almost the entire femoral attachment of the posterior cruciate ligament remaining attached to the fragment. *B*, Three months following repair of posterior cruciate to femur. Excellent function. One probably cannot expect complete filling in of this defect at this age.

Figure 544. Patient was injured eight months before and experienced lateral meniscus symptoms. X-rays revealed large chondral defect in the lateral femoral condyle. At surgery, condyle was filling in, and the lateral meniscus was indeed torn and was removed. Inspection of the condyle revealed (as suggested in x-ray *A*) that the defect was apparently beginning to fill in. Thus it was not disturbed. *B,* Same view three years later. Knee is basically asymptomatic. Note the uniformity of the bone and the normal contour in spite of some marginal irregularity.

be removed. I have had little experience with replacement of the fragment and fixation by pins or screws. This method does not appeal to me unless the fragment is large and vital to joint function.

If the condition is symptomatic, operative treatment is the treatment of choice. The knee is exposed by a medial parapatellar incision, with the knee flexed over the end of the table. The medial compartment is carefully explored, special attention being paid to the medial me-

niscus, to the fat pad and to the cruciate ligaments. The femoral attachment of the posterior cruciate ligament is carefully examined and then the condyle and the defect are inspected. If the fragment is completely loose, the knee should be searched until it is found and removed. At this stage it is important to examine the undersurface of the patella, since frequently patellar malacia will be present, particularly if the osteochondritis dissecans has been present for a very long time. Following

Figure 545. Large osteochondritic fragment lodged in the posterior pouch. No source of the cartilage was demonstrated at surgery.

Figure 546. Old neglected case of osteochondritis dissecans with multiple fragments and diffuse arthritis. Note calcareous layers surrounding the original piece.

careful exploration with the knee in this position, the end of the table is raised again to a position that directly presents the lesion itself in the wound (30 to 0 degrees). Again proper aseptic precautions are taken. If the fragment is still in place, it is carefully removed by sharp dissection. If it includes the attachment of the posterior cruciate ligament, this should be detached from the fragment, care being taken to preserve as much ligament as possible. The posterior cruciate ligament is carefully inspected and this detached portion sutured down to the remaining portion of the ligament. However, if as much as one half of the attachment is torn, it is advisable to make two parallel drill holes from the medial femoral epicondyle into the bed of the defect, which is in the intercondylar notch at the articular margin (see Fig. 543B). The suture is passed through one of the drill holes, plicated through the loose end of the torn section of the posterior cruciate and passed out through the other drill hole to emerge on the medial epicondyle. Proper tension will permit close apposition of the cruciate ligament to the bone. Before this fixation is carried out, the crater remaining following removal of the fragment is inspected and curetted down to fresh bleeding bone. The surrounding margins of the articular cartilage are trephined so that there is a vertical margin rather than a beveled edge. Great care is taken to remove any cartilage that is undermined. If

the bone in the bed of the crater appears to be eburnated, multiple 0.35 mm. drill holes are made through to fresh cancellous bone. The knee is now carefully lavaged with warm saline to wash out any fragments or debris. If the patella has been found to be irregular and malacic, the knee is then extended completely, the patella elevated by grasping its margins with tenacula and a chondroplasty carried out designed to leave firm, smooth cartilage. This is similar to the procedure done to repair primary patellar malacia (see page 580). The knee is then closed in layers in the usual manner, and a cotton cast is applied, followed by the usual postoperative care for arthrotomy of the knee.

In postoperative management, active use and active motion should be encouraged. It has been shown conclusively that articular cartilage regenerates better with active use. Hence the belief that trephining, which leaves a smaller defect with vertical margins, is better than shaving, which leaves a larger defect. With a well-defined hole in the cartilage, no actual weight will be borne on the regenerating cartilage until the defect is filled. So active use with full weight-bearing is recommended as soon as operative reaction has subsided.

With a larger lesion on the femoral condyle, I recommend full activity but not full weight-bearing. This may be hard to accomplish in the young active athlete. I would prefer him to have full weight-bearing than to immobilize him completely just to prevent weight-bearing.

PATELLAR MALACIA

The term "patellar malacia" has been used as a catch-all to include the many processes that involve the undersurface of the patella. Many of these conditions are not particularly pertinent to sports. True malacia is a softening or breaking down of a part or tissue. When chronic synovitis of the knee causes the patellar cartilage to break down and the bed to eburnate so that denuded bone is exposed, the condition is called malacia. So also is fragmentation of the patellar cartilage in the young individual with no signs of arthritis. The previous discussion (see page 554) of chondral fractures and their treatment applied particularly to the patella.

Etiologically, patellar malacia falls naturally into three groups:

Group I. In the athlete, a relatively young individual, *trauma* may be the cause. This may be a chondral fracture or infraction either by acute trauma or by repeated lesser trauma to the patella. Infraction of the patellar cartilage subsequently causes irritation of the patellar groove on the femur, and gradual changes supervene with fissuring, absorption and fragmentation of the cartilage. The findings at operation will depend upon the duration of symptoms. I once operated upon a female who was injured while horseback riding. The horse got a little eager to turn into the barnyard and made a sharp turn that drove the patient's patella forcibly into the gate post. She had an immediate severe reaction in the knee joint. The x-ray findings were consistently negative. At operation some four weeks later after diagnosis of chondral fracture of the patella, there was, indeed, a fracture of the cartilage of the patella, which was already undergoing degenerative change. It was early enough, however, that there was still injection of cartilage with hemorrhage into the crater of the fragments, so that there could be no question as to the cause. Similar changes were present in the contiguous portion of the patellar groove. Had operation in this case been postponed for several months, as in the ordinary case, typical chondromalacia of the patella would have been present. In my opinion trauma accounts for many of the cases of isolated patellar involvement in the young athlete (see Fig. 493).

Group II. Another etiological factor in involvement of the undersurface of the patella is *disturbance of the rhythm of the patellar function.* This type of malacia accompanies intrinsic injury to the knee (Fig. 547). Any condition that causes a disturbance in the rhythm of the knee action frequently results in involvement of the undersurface of the patella. The knee is checked abruptly and motion is reversed. The patella is driven against the femur. In fact, in an analysis of 350 cases* of intrinsic injury to the knee, some degree of patellar involvement was demonstrated in 65 per cent of the cases treated by operation, and in 15 per cent of these, the involvement was Grade 4. It was possible to show a direct relationship between the number of lockings of the knee and the degree of malacia (Fig. 548) and, further, that the duration of symptoms and the degree of malacia (Fig. 549) also correlate. These two factors were much more important in indicating the amount of malacia present than was the age of the patient. This seemed so definite that I make a positive

---

*Bulletin of Hospital for Joint Diseases, Vol. 17, No. 1, April, 1956.

Figure 547. Severe chondromalacia of the patella following neglected ligament injury.

recommendation that surgical intervention should be prompt in intrinsic injury of the knee if for no other reason than to prevent damage to the undersurface of the patella. The exact mechanism of this breakdown of the patella has never been wholly explained. This condition also probably occurs as a result of various other causes, including direct trauma, synovitis of the joint and general chondrolytic changes. The particular pathological changes

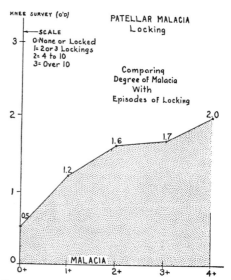

Figure 548. It should be noted in the above graph that there is direct correlation in the number of times the knee locked prior to operative treatment and the degree of malacia. The knee, which locked as many as ten times (category 2), showed 4 + malacia. (Hosp. for Joint Dis. Bull. *17*:5.)

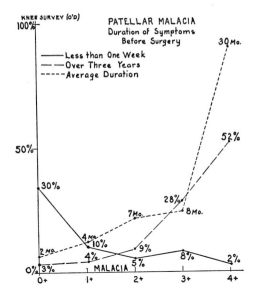

Figure 549. The above chart shows that the great majority with symptoms of less than one week in duration showed no symptoms of patellar malacia; whereas only 2 per cent of those patients with symptoms of less than one week had 4+ malacia, 52 per cent of those with symptoms over three years showed 4+ patellar malacia. (Hosp. for Joint Dis. Bull. *17*:10.)

described usually accompany other intrinsic conditions of the knee.

Group III. A third classification is *primary malacia of the patella*, which is usually bilateral and without any demonstrable etiological factor. These cases are truly puzzling. One cannot rule out the effect of repeated trauma, since the young patients are usually very active physically. They could be expected to traumatize their knee caps repeatedly. However, the simultaneous involvement of both knees with relative lack of involvement of other chondral surfaces equally susceptible to trauma prompts us to seek a cause other than simple contusion.

Careful evaluation of the anatomical development of the knee may give a definite lead to the cause of so-called idiopathic malacia. Patellar alta (see Fig. 481) is very prone to alter the mechanism of the gliding surface of the patella on the trochlear groove and so contribute to malacia. Lateral subluxation of the patella as the knee comes into complete extension may cause malacia of the patella without actually providing any gross evidence of displacement. This may be documented further by the silhouette x-ray view of the patella, which shows the patella displaced somewhat laterally (Fig. 550). A negative finding is not very significant, however, because the silhouette x-ray view is made with the knee flexed somewhere between 30 and 45 degrees, and in this position, the patella may well have slipped back into the patellar groove and may appear to be entirely normal. A significant examination is made by having the patient sit with the leg hanging pendant off the edge of the table at 90 degrees. As he brings the knee up into extension, it will be noticed that the patella slips sharply laterally in this position, and as the knee is bent, it slips back into the groove. In this instance, treatment of the malacia will basically be the same as treatment of the subluxing patella. Obviously, the prognosis for patellar malacia is sharply improved if the underlying cause can be well defined.

Diagnosis. Group I caused by a single severe trauma is usually found in the knee that has been seriously contused to the point that a fractured patella is suspected. The findings remain localized about the patella: pain on

Figure 550. This 35 year old male had a long history (15 years) of trouble with his knees. He has obvious malacia of the patellae with crepitation, pain and disability. Silhouette view reveals lateral slipping of the patella on the left with definite, rather marked narrowing of the patellofemoral space on the lateral side. At surgery the patella was very seriously involved, the central facet being down to bare bone. There was also a chondromalacic area on the trochlear groove of the femoral condyle opposing the area on the patella, which was severe. The patella was removed. (For x-ray positioning of the silhouette view, see Fig. 491.)

pressure of the patella into the groove, pain on active extension of the knee, particularly against resistance and pain on patellar ballottement. The severity of the symptoms will be increased by continued activity of the individual.

Group II occurs coincidentally with other intrinsic conditions of the knee, therefore, the patellar symptoms may well be completely masked by these other conditions, so that the patient may present with the knee locked and swollen with effusion but with no demonstrable patellar symptoms. At arthrotomy one may be surprised to find extensive involvement of the undersurface of the patella. More frequently, however, careful examination prior to operation will reveal subpatellar crepitation and pain on pressure over the patella, provided the condition is fairly severe.

In Group III, with spontaneous degenerative changes, the joint is asymptomatic except for the patella. There will have been gradually increasing discomfort and disability in the knee centering around the patella but without a history of previous trauma. The signs of involvement of the patella are quite obvious. If the undersurface of the patella is rough and irregular, the patella will not glide smoothly in the patellar groove, and gross subpatellar crepitation is usually the first symptom. This is more severe on extension against resistance or on extension of the knee while the patella is held firmly against the patellar groove. There is also pain when going up or down stairs, squatting or doing anything that forces the patella against the patellar groove. This pain may become so severe that it is grossly disabling.

Treatment of the knee having these conditions of the patella is surgical. True enough, the symptoms may be ameliorated somewhat by nonsurgical treatment, such as aspiration, injection of a corticoid, splinting and prevention of weight-bearing. Nonetheless, the future is bleak indeed, since the defect in the patella remains and the symptoms will promptly recur with resumption of activity. Surgery may be directed primarily toward the patella or may be incidental to other operations. After arthrotomy by medial parapatellar incision, the patella is carefully inspected with the examining finger, and the extent of the pathological involvement is determined by palpation and observation. If the diagnosis is confirmed, the incision is enlarged sufficiently to permit the patella to be turned up on edge for thorough inspection of the undersurface. At this time a decision must be made on definitive treatment. This decision will be affected a great deal by the circumstances of each particular case, and treatment will vary from chondral shaving to patellectomy.

Chondral Shaving. In the young athlete it is quite important to retain the patella if this is possible. With an extremely sharp knife blade, the patellar cartilage is shaved down in an attempt to reach firm, uninvolved cartilage. This is frequently possible in the young athlete, since the patellar cartilage is relatively thick at this age. The degenerative changes may be found to be quite superficial. Care must be taken to remove all pathological cartilage, even if this leaves denuded bone. After this step has been completed, the patellar groove is carefully inspected, and if necessary, chondroplasty is also done to eliminate all abnormal cartilage. At the conclusion of the chondroplasty, the patella should slide smoothly in the patellar groove, with minimal irregularity either of the patella or of the groove.

At this stage considerable surgical judgment is required to determine whether or not the patella should be retained. If the patient is young and otherwise has an excellent knee, one may be justified in leaving in a somewhat defective patella. On the other hand, if there are degenerative changes throughout the joint, with marginal osteophytes and rather poor femoral cartilage, the patella probably should be sacrificed.

Trephining and Drilling. The cartilage of a young person has a great deal more regenerative power than the cartilage of an older individual and in a young person, a crater such as that left following removal of an osteochondritis dissecans fragment may readily fill in if it is curetted down to raw bone and no degenerated cartilage is left behind. In the older individual with very thin cartilage, this regeneration does not occur. Localized lesions in the patella in young people are probably traumatic. It is not advisable to shave all the patellar cartilage in order to smooth out such a defect. The area should be trephined and all involved cartilage removed down to the underlying bone, leaving sharp vertical margins. If sclerotic, the bed should be drilled with a very fine Kirschner wire (0.3 mm.). Sometimes with more extensive involvement of the patellar cartilage, a substantial portion of this may be shaved down, leaving a smaller area in the center in which the involvement extends to the bone. In this instance preliminary shaving down to the normal cartilage over the major defect may be followed by trephining the small defect in the center of the area for the reasons indicated.

The exact technique of trephining and drilling is quite important. The major aim is to retain as much normal cartilage as possible; therefore the margin of the pathologic cartilage is definitely defined with a degree of conservatism. In other words, if there is any doubt about it, leave it on the first cut. Using a No. 15 blade with a short tip, simply cut around the defect with the incision in a vertical direction, much as you would take out a defect with a cookie cutter. After this first area has been cut clear around and the center curetted down to subchondral bone, the margins are very carefully inspected to make sure that there are no loose fragments or undermined edges left. This margin should be exactly vertical to the underlying bone if the major part of normal cartilage is to be preserved. If, on the contrary, the margins are beveled off or smoothed off, this simply enlarges the hole and does not add

anything. In fact, it detracts because the fibro-cartilage or hyaline cartilage, whichever replaces this pathological cartilage, will appose better to a vertical edge than it will to a sloping one, whether the bone grows up from the bone below or from the periphery. Each process has been described as the way cartilage regenerates. As this hole is rather small, approximately 1 cm. in diameter, the patella will glide perfectly smoothly in the patellar groove (Figs. 551 and 552).

Facetectomy. Often the malacia will involve either the medial or lateral facet of the patella, whereas the rest of the cartilage is relatively normal. In these cases, facetectomy is a gratifying procedure. One may safely remove up to one third of the patella, either medially or laterally, without appreciable dysfunction or noticeable deformity (Fig. 553). I find that this procedure is indicated much more frequently now than previously. It eliminates all the portion of the patella which is pathological and yet leaves essentially normal function of the

Figure 551. This is a typical case for trephining and drilling. Notice the localized area of the malacic cartilage with essentially normal cartilage surrounding it. The patient had a history of falling directly on his knee cap a year before, with definite symptoms here. Notice the postoperative crater. This is a large defect—larger than is ideal. The drill holes are evenly spaced around the lesion but not enough to destroy the structure of the bone. The shape of the hole is pertinent. It should be shaped exactly to fit the defect rather than to be square, round or oval. A, Preoperative view. B, At surgery.

Figure 552. This boy had a history of serious trouble with both knees. The left knee sustained injury when he fell on the flexed knee. He had pain laterally and a cast was applied. One month later an arthrogram showed a torn lateral meniscus. X-ray showed a very localized area of malacia. The patella was treated by trephining and drilling. This particular patient did not do well. The hole actually filled up with bone, as visualized in the lateral view of the patella. The knee was quite symptomatic.

bone. In the course of treating marginal fractures of the patella, it has long been my practice to remove the fragments rather than to repair them. Results have been so gratifying that the same thing has been done in other defects of the articular cartilage with equally good results when the remainder of the patella is normal.

The technique for facetectomy is relatively simple, particularly when it is done in conjunction with exploration of the patella. For such an exploration, either a medial or a lateral parapatellar incision is made in order to visualize the involved area. Now if it is decided that the pathological condition is largely confined to either the medial or lateral facet, a careful dissection is made to detach the tendon covering the damaged portion of the patella, as one would do for a patellectomy. This dissection should be carried back as far as it is felt to be necessary in order to remove a sufficient amount of bone to eliminate all of the pathological condition. Approximately one third of the bone can be removed without any appreciable loss of function. After this tendon,

which passes over the patella, is reflected, the facetectomy can be carried out either with an osteotome or with an oscillating saw. I prefer the oscillating saw. The patella should be carefully immobilized with a forceps and a vertical cut should be made, with the saw extending completely through the bone and cartilage. There seems to be no particular advantage in making this section of the facet exactly vertical as shown in Figure 553. I have more recently been making it at an angle so as to remove less of the anterior surface of the patella and so disturb less of the patellar tendon traversing it. This angle should not be so flat that there is no possibility of the bony surface articulating with the trochlear groove. The damaged segment is then removed, leaving a clean, smooth cut. This area is carefully smoothed off and covered with a very thin layer of bone wax. Then the retinaculum is closed as it would be had the patellar segment not been removed. In other words, it is not desirable in the ordinary case to tighten the retinaculum by overlapping unless there is some specific reason for doing so that is not related to the facetectomy.

The aftercare of this patient is not altered by the facetectomy. If the wound is to be immobilized for two weeks, there is no reason to add more time than this because of the procedure described. The follow-up care proceeds as indicated for any other pathological condition encountered in this particular case. If the facetectomy is the only procedure carried out, it is advisable to immobilize the knee for two weeks, during which time the usual patellar setting, straight leg raising and so forth may be carried out, since the major tendinous attachments of the patella have not been disturbed.

Patellectomy. If one decides to remove the patella because of defective articular cartilage, the technique of removal is extremely important. The patella should be removed by sharp dissection, care being taken to remove all fragments of bone. The knee is then thoroughly lavaged, and the quadriceps tendon and patellar tendon are inspected. At this stage it is important to remove the superolateral and superomedial margins of the anterior articular surface of the femur with an osteotome, since these margins stand up as a bony prominence upon which, later, the edge of the quadriceps lateralis tendon may catch with a painful snap. This is particularly important on the lateral side, since the patellar tendon does tend to slide laterally. After this articular surface has been carefully taken off and the raw bone covered with bone wax, the adjacent tendons are inspected for roughness or any undue thickening. If either is present the area is smoothed down. Using No. 1 cotton suture and a relatively long curved needle, sutures are placed beginning at the lateral edge of the quadriceps tendon, going from an anterior to a posterior direction through the edge of the quadriceps tendon to emerge anteriorly through the portion of the tendon which had been lying over the patella about two thirds of the way toward the patellar tendon. This suture passes back through the portion of the tendon over the patella again to pass through the patellar tendon from back to front. This tends to loop up and invaginate the thin tendon between the patellar tendon and the quadriceps tendon. About eight of these sutures are placed across the knee. As each suture is placed, the palpating finger determines that the undersurface is smooth. With this invagination of the thin part of the tendon, two things are accomplished: the quadriceps apparatus is shortened by about two thirds of the length of the patella, and the relatively thicker portion of the tendon occupies the previous position of the patella.

The repair is then continued in the retinaculum by direct over and over suture. The previously placed sutures are then tied with the knee in complete extension, closely approximating the quadriceps tendon to the patellar tendon and obliterating the patellar fossa in the tendon entirely. A finger is passed underneath the suture line to make sure that the imbrication is smooth. After all these sutures are tied, it should be possible to flex the knee to 90 degrees and determine whether or not the repaired tendon has a smooth gliding surface. By careful attention to this shortening of the quadriceps tendon mechanism, one will avoid the extremely disabling effect of loss of complete active extension of the knee which so frequently follows patellectomy. One can readily sacrifice some degree of flexion in order to obtain complete active extension of the knee. Usually full motion is regained. If the suture line appears to be very secure and there is no undue tension on the sutures, immobilization may be carried out in a cotton cast (see Fig. 441), although I really prefer a little longer dressing. Therefore, instead of using the basswood or yucca board splints, I use plaster strips extending from just above the ankle to the upper thigh. Weight-bearing is permitted as soon as it is comfortable, which may be the first day postoperative. If your clinical judgment indicates that the suture is secure in good healthy tendon (which is very likely to be the case in athletes), the patient can probably begin motion as early as the second week, providing there is no severe reaction within the knee itself. If there is no synovitis with effusion and if there is no swelling or edema at the end of two weeks, a long leg brace may be applied with a caliper heel and a dial knee. The dial knee may be set just beyond the degree of flexion which is present and the angle steadily increased as range of motion increases. With this mechanism, one may permit free weight-bearing, utilizing what motion is present in the knee and yet protecting the knee against undue force, such as that caused by the patient accidentally stumbling and

Figure 553. This 25 year old athlete had internal derangement of the knee for about three years, with increasing trouble in the patella. Involvement of the medial facet of the patella was noted when medial meniscectomy was done. A, Denuded bone along the medial facet. B, The line of the saw cut. C, The fragment, showing the square edges. Note the remaining normal-looking cartilage of the patella. D and E, Silhouette views of the right and left patellae. The pencil mark shows the line of the facetectomy. F, Five months postoperative. Excellent functional result.

KNEE SERIES

Figure 554. The diagrams above depict the series of exercises utilized by West Point cadets following knee injury or knee surgery. These exercises are instituted following the acute phase of medical care and initial physical therapy. In general they are instituted about the time a patient is ready for brisk walking or light jogging.

Specific notation should be made of the total lower body reconditioning program. All major muscle groups of both thigh and lower leg are challenged. The cadet is started with a low weight, low repetition work-out and is progressed as tolerated until he is ready for competitive athletics.

In conjunction with the above exercises, a program of guided running and jump rope exercise is employed. Running begins with a slow ½ mile and progresses to a 2 mile run in 13 to 16 minutes. Rope jumping begins with jumping on both legs and progresses to three sets of *one* legged jumping (injured extremity), 90 to 120 times in 60 seconds.

It is felt that by employing the above program, re-injury of the involved part or new injury to an adjacent part has been minimized. The above work-out should take at least 30 minutes even if done by the most aggressive athlete. The cadet is returned to full unrestricted activity when lower body performance is approximately symmetrical.

The exercises contained in the diagrams of the West Point knee reconditioning program represent the evolution of rehabilitation spanning many years and many individuals. The West Point Orthopaedic Service, Physical Therapy Department and Office of Physical Education have all contributed to the program now in use.

overflexing the knee. It will require a considerable degree of judgment to decide which patient should be trusted with a brace, since it can be taken off by the patient. If there is any question concerning this or if the patient seems to be unusually active, it probably would be better to put him in a long leg walking cylinder or a long leg walking cast. I think the brace is very effective, particularly in older people, who have a real problem regaining motion. Regaining motion is not a serious problem in the young person. Rehabilitation begins on the first postoperative day. (See Chapter 22.)

The *prognosis* in patellar malacia depends largely on the etiology. If the cause was a chondral fracture, the prognosis should be very good, with no fear of recurrence provided a good patella was left. If the condition resulted from an intrinsic pathological condition in the knee and this is corrected, the prognosis is also good. If the patellar malacia is a component of a generalized degenerative change in the knee or if it is a spontaneous type of degenerative change, the prognosis is much less favorable, since the etiological factor probably has not been eliminated.

The question of athletic participation following involvement of the patella will inevitably arise. If the physician can be reasonably sure that he has left a relatively normal patella, there should be no reason to forbid participation. Such would be the case in chondral fracture or malacia following rupture of the medial meniscus, for example. In the more chronic type of involvement, one would hesitate to permit active competitive sports which cause overuse of the patella. If it is already questionable that the patella will withstand the rigors of ordinary use, one is not justified in encouraging athletic participation, which would only precipitate the trouble. The decision rests on the same considerations as those following any other pathological condition and must remain a matter of personal judgment.

Particularly to be considered is the importance of athletic competition to the individual. If his livelihood or his education depends upon it, greater effort should be made to permit him to participate. If, on the other hand, it is a casual thing and his interest can be diverted into less strenuous pursuits, this should be encouraged. Once again, it should be emphasized that treatment should be definitive and prompt in order that the proportion of patients with good recovery may be increased.

REHABILITATION

For the athlete the rehabilitative period is as important as the actual treatment of the local lesion. The athlete should return to full activity as soon as he can safely do so. Therefore, rehabilitation should be planned and initiated on the day of the injury, with particular effort made not only to restore the injured member to normal strength and activity but also to prevent deterioration of the athlete's physique as a whole. This cannot be done casually. It may be quite difficult to persuade the young high school athlete that he should be doing rather rudimentary exercises when he has pretty largely taken his physique for granted, except when training for some particular activity. Dr. Fred Allman, a nationally known authority on the subject of rehabilitation of the athlete, has kindly provided a chapter on this subject for this book. I urge the reader of this material on the knee to study his recommendations in Chapter 22 carefully.

The West Point Military Academy also has long had an excellent rehabilitation program and has given me permission to reproduce their exercise schedule for rehabilitation following injury of the knee. I gratefully acknowledge their contribution to this problem. These exercises are listed in Figure 554.

Injuries of
the Leg

19

For the purposes of this discussion, the leg will be considered the area between the knee and the ankle and not immediately concerned with the two joints themselves.

ANATOMICAL CONSIDERATIONS

The upper portion of the leg receives the muscles from the thigh, and involvement of these attachments has been discussed elsewhere (page 457). Likewise, the lower portion of the leg is intimately involved with the function of the ankle joint, which also will be discussed in detail elsewhere (page 603). The shafts of the tibia and fibula serve as the origin of the muscles that move the ankle and foot. The tibia is the only weight-bearing bone, since the fibula does not have a weight-bearing component. The fibula situated posterolaterally is not directly involved in the knee joint but forms a vital part of the ankle.

Throughout its length the fibula is bound to the tibia by the interosseous membrane. The interosseous membrane forms a "Y" above to surround the upper tibiofibular joint, the anterior division being called the anterosuperior tibiofibular ligament and the posterior division the posterosuperior tibiofibular ligament. A similar arrangement is formed below, the interosseous membrane thickening and dividing to surround the inferior tibiofibular syndesmosis, and the two components being called the anterior and posterior inferior tibiofibular ligaments. Although the upper portion of the fibula is largely for muscle attachments and may serve to some extent as a brace, it has no vital function and in fact may be sacrificed without material loss of function as long as proper security is provided for the structures attaching at the top of the fibula. The lower one third, as mentioned, is extremely important because it is vital in the formation of the ankle mortice.

The interosseous membrane serves as the floor of the anterior compartment of the leg (see Fig. 557). This is a closed space, the boundaries being the anterior fascia of the leg in front, the interosseous membrane behind, the fibula laterally and the tibia medially. This space permits little, if any, expansion of the structures contained within, whereas the posterior compartment is a loosely contained space with a relaxed and redundant fascia. This space is not subject to constriction to the same degree as the anterior compartment.

The tibia, the main weight-bearing bone, is roughly triangular in cross-section and has muscle attachments at the posterolateral and posterior surfaces. The anterior border, the anteromedial surface and the posteromedial border are all subcutaneous.

CONTUSION

Contusion is extremely common in the lower leg, since this part, particularly in athletics, is very much exposed to direct blows. The nature of the contusion will vary according to the location of the blow. If the blow is over the subcutaneous portion of the tibia, the contusion is much more likely to be severe, since the integument and periosteum are caught between the external force and extremely hard bone. This may result in a simple bruise with extravasation of blood in a localized area, or the periosteal damage may result in severe traumatic periostitis, also usually localized. It is also possible to have contusion over the muscles of the anterior compartment; the resulting swelling within the compartment may be extremely uncomfortable owing to the closed nature of the space. Contusion of the muscles of the calf is also common, but circulatory embarrassment is not usual here. An unusual type of contusion is of the peroneal nerve as it winds around the upper portion of the fibula (Fig. 555). This may result in a painful neuritis or even in transient paralysis

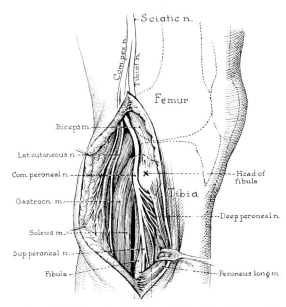

Figure 555. Drawing showing relationship of peroneal nerve to the head of the fibula.

of the peroneals with drop foot, which may be very distressing to the athlete.

Contusion and Hematoma

Implicit in the pathology of a contusion is some degree of hematoma. In the lower leg this may be extremely disabling. A severe hematoma in the anterior enclosed space may become a surgical emergency, since it may go on to actual ischemia and necrosis of the muscle (see Anterior Compartment Syndrome, page 590). A subperiosteal hematoma complicating a contusion of the skin may also be painful and actually disabling if it is severe. Hematoma within the muscle is not as common in the calf as in other areas in the body.

Diagnosis. Following injury of the lower leg, careful analysis should be made of the patient's history to determine, if possible, the type of blow and the type of instrument. A large blunt object such as player's helmet will usually cause a different type of injury than a relatively sharp object such as a cleat or the hard toe of a shoe. The leg should be carefully examined to determine the degree of swelling and whether a hematoma is present. Function should be carefully checked, since this may well give some indication as to whether the muscle or a nerve is involved. The leg should be carefully examined for a possible fracture from a direct blow on the tibia or fibula. The tibia is readily palpable, but it may be more difficult to examine the fibula, since it is well

surrounded by muscle. If there is any question as to the degree of localized injury in either bone, x-ray studies should be done.

Treatment. If a diagnosis of contusion or hematoma is made, treatment will depend upon the degree of involvement. If hematoma is present, it should be aspirated under aseptic technique and injected with anesthetic. These measures should immediately be followed by the application of a pressure bandage and a cold pack for six to eight hours. Further analysis can then be made as to the severity of the injury. If fluid or blood has recurred, it should be re-aspirated. At the end of 24 to 48 hours, depending upon the degree of injury, heat therapy should be substituted for cold. The degree of protection of necessity will depend upon the location of the injury. If the injury involves the bone and periosteum and is not severe, treatment should be by wearing a protective pad, and function need not be interfered with unless it is a major injury. If, on the other hand, the blow involves the muscle, the muscle should be kept at rest by proper strapping or splinting until it is determined that there is no major bleeding or laceration within it. Protective strapping should be used until such time as the part is symptom-free.

Contusion of the Peroneal Nerve

As the peroneal nerve continues downward after leaving the popliteal space and passes laterally, it crosses directly behind the neck of the fibula (Fig. 555) and winds around the lateral surface of the fibular neck to pass into the extensor muscles anteriorly. It is extremely vulnerable to injury either posteriorly or laterally, since it lies directly between the skin and the bone. An ideal situation is present for contusion of the nerve, since the nerve will be caught between the hard contusing object and the underlying bone. A relatively minor blow may cause serious nerve injury.

The *pathology* will vary greatly according to the severity of injury, since the nerve may be only slightly shocked or may be crushed in two. The usual effects of contusion are congestion and edema, with local swelling. Since the nerve is contained within a sheath, this swelling will cause pressure on the nerve fibers with resulting symptoms of pain, numbness and paresthesia. If there is actual hemorrhage into the sheath, the increased tension may proceed to actual paralysis caused by intrinsic pressure. Indeed, this may result in necrosis of the nerve fibers with permanent functional loss. As a rule, the congestion diminishes, the swelling subsides and the nerve slowly returns to normal. If there has been actual damage to the nerve fibers themselves, they may be replaced by fibrous scar and greater or lesser loss of function results, depending upon how many nerve filaments remain undamaged.

Contusion may cause hemorrhage in the surrounding tissues, and this may cause secondary pressure on the nerve. However, this is not likely in this particular area.

The *symptoms* will be those caused by the local blow plus the effect on the nerve itself. The immediate symptom is almost always a "shocking feeling," with pain shooting throughout the distribution of the nerve to the lateral side of the leg and foot. Acute tingling and numbness remain after the pain subsides. These may be transient and may disappear within seconds or minutes if actual damage to the nerve has not resulted. In such a case the patient may completely recover before he is ever examined by the doctor.

If the injury is more severe, a different pattern of symptoms will emerge. The initial symptoms may be as indicated, but they are followed by a completely asymptomatic period, which is followed in turn by symptoms of pressure within the nerve. The pain and paresthesia return and increase in severity. As the pressure continues, signs of loss of function develop. This is evidenced by hypesthesia throughout the distribution and by weakness on dorsal flexion of the foot. This may progress to complete paralysis of the nerve, with sensory loss and muscular nonfunction. There follows a longer or shorter period during which the only symptom is loss of nerve function, namely, sensory and motor loss with no pain. This may develop within days or it may be several weeks before the painful stimuli have ceased. After a variable lapse of time, function will begin to return, usually in the sensory distribution first. One may be able to elicit a Tinel sign by tapping along the nerve distal to the injury and so get some idea as to the progression of recovery. This is rather difficult, since the peroneal nerve becomes deep-seated a short distance below the knee. Recovery may be complete or may be only partial.

This whole train of symptoms may be interrupted at any time by the recovery process. The earlier the recovery begins, the more rapid and complete it will be. Very careful examination of the leg and foot in a case involving the peroneal nerve will be extremely rewarding, since it is quite important to be able to follow accurately the succession of events. If the paralysis is immediate and complete, one may assume a major injury and govern treatment accordingly. Rapidly progressing development of signs of nerve pressure indicate increasing swelling within the sheath. The rate of its development is of considerable importance in determining the proper treatment. One should carefully outline the area of sensory involvement and determine not only touch but also sharp and dull and hot and cold sensitivities, although this is not as important here as it is in central nervous system lesions. A good practice is to outline in ink on the skin the area of involvement or to record it faithfully in notes. On re-examination of such a patient it is very gratifying to find that the area of involvement has decreased and to be able to give the patient a favorable prognosis. Conversely, if the area increases one can be prepared to modify the treatment accordingly.

When one is faced with involvement along the peroneal distribution without definite history of an injury, by careful palpation around the fibular head it may be possible to locate areas of local tenderness that give some clue as to the possibility of a direct blow on the nerve. In the heat of an athletic contest, such a blow may be readily overlooked and the patient may have no knowledge of an injury.

Treatment. The vast majority of these patients with contusion of the peroneal nerve will require no specific treatment. If the blow is severe enough that the soft tissue contusion requires care, the customary treatment is in order—application of ice packs early, followed by local heat. However, as the nerve symptoms develop and there is motor paralysis or specific weakness, the muscles will require protection. Support of the ankle and foot must be provided by cast, splint or brace. A carefully applied drop-foot brace holding the foot at a right angle by a mechanical spring will permit ambulation without disconcerting drop foot. This will make walking easier and will prevent overstretching of the paralyzed muscles. Some such apparatus is also important in rehabilitation as the muscle strength returns. During the early phase of such a condition, we would recommend wearing the brace and shoe during sleeping hours to prevent contracture of the calf. Once the acute symptoms have subsided, there is no particular need to proscribe athletic activities. The presence of a drop foot is a real handicap in running, however, particularly in cutting and turning, and the player's efficiency will be sharply reduced until the drop foot recovers. Overfatigue of any weakened muscle should be avoided and strength should be

Figure 556. Reconstructive exercises for the foot and leg. See explanation on this page.

In other instances, the quiescent period may be much longer only to be followed by the same pattern of progressively increasing nerve symptoms. This is due to scar formation with gradual constriction of some of the fibers of the nerve by the maturing scar. In such an instance, if the condition is steadily progressive, there is no advantage in undue delay and early neurolysis should be done.

Another indication for surgery is the case in which there is intractable pain along the nerve that persists for several weeks. These patients should be treated by exploration of the nerve. The nerve should be carefully dissected free of all adhesions and appropriate neurolysis carried out, either surgically or by saline injection, in order to expand the sheath.

Some typical sets of exercises follow (Fig. 556). (See also Fig. 610.)

1. First Stage (check range of motion):
   A. Flexion—flex foot as far as possible (point toes upward (see Fig. 556A).
   B. Extension—extend foot as far as possible (point toes downward) (see Fig. 556A).
   C. Inversion—turn soles of feet inward.
   D. Eversion—turn soles of feet outward.
2. If the preceding exercises can be done in full range of motion and without pain, do the following exercises:
   A. Foot circles—foot circumscribes a small circle. Ball of foot down first, then in, up and finally out (see Fig. 556B).
   B. Alphabet—sitting on table with knee straight and only ankle extended over the end of the table, print the entire alphabet in capital letters with your foot.
3. If the preceding exercises can be done in full range of motion and without pain, do the following exercises:
   A. Towel exercise—sitting on a chair with your foot on a towel, pull the towel up under the foot with your toes. After completing this part successfully, place a weight on the other end of the towel to offer resistance (see Fig. 556C).
   B. Pick-up exercise—with the toes pick up marbles or a small piece of sponge rubber. Alternate placing the object in the hand in front of and behind the opposite leg (see Fig. 556D).
   C. Toe rises—stand with feet one foot apart and toeing in. Rise on toes as high as possible without pain. Also repeat this exercise with toes pointed straight ahead and pointed out.

painstakingly restored by graduated exercises. An example of the type of exercise we use is included at the end of this section (Fig. 556) and also shown in Figure 610.

Should a blow be followed by a quiescent period and then by a rapidly developing paralysis, one is justified in exploring the peroneal nerve and performing neurolysis to be sure that the tight sheath is not constricting the nerve beyond the point of its tolerance. This procedure is not often indicated. Even if the paralysis is immediate and complete, one is justified in a period of watchful waiting to give the nerve a chance to recover spontaneously. If there are no definite signs of recovery within three months, I would recommend surgical exploration of the nerve with neurolysis or nerve suture, as indicated.

STRAIN

Strain of the muscles and tendons about the ankle and foot will be discussed elsewhere (page 603). Here, in addition to the well-delineated entities of strain involving the leg proper, some rather unusual conditions will be covered, although there may be some question as to whether strain is actually the cause.

Anterior Compartment Syndrome

It will be recalled that in the anterior compartment of the leg the anterior tibial, the extensor hallucis and the extensor digitorum longus muscles arise from the sides of the tibia, fibula and interosseous membrane, completely filling the anterior compartment. This compartment is tightly roofed by the anterior fascia of the leg (Fig. 557). In the anterior tibial syndrome, for various reasons there is a rapid swelling of the muscle within this compartment. This may come on following active exercise alone and in theory is due to the fact that muscles which have not been previously conditioned are overused and respond by swelling and edema. It may also occur following direct injury in which there is excessive swelling and hemorrhage into the space. The condition can also be caused by localized infection within the space. In fact, anything that causes intractable swelling may cause this syndrome.

At onset there is severe pain over the involved area and loss of function, so that contraction of the muscles contained in the space rapidly becomes impossible and a drop foot ensues (Fig. 558). Very soon even passive stretching of the muscles becomes quite painful. This is not ordinarily preceded by the symptoms of tenosynovitis however. The skin over the area becomes red, glossy, warm and markedly tender, with a feeling of woody tension even to the point of real hardness of the fascia over the space. There may occasionally be involvement of the peroneal nerve with sensory loss, but the loss of muscle function is usually not due to nerve involvement but to pathological change within the muscle itself. The muscles go on to ischemic necrosis, often called "Volkmann's ischemia of the leg," with swelling, edema, extravasation of red blood cells, destruction of blood cells and replacement of muscle tissue by fibrous scar. The result is a firm, inelastic, noncontractile muscle group. This can be extremely disabling and defies reconstructive treatment.

Treatment depends upon the extent of involvement. Any delay is disastrous. Early treatment should be prompt application of ice without pressure dressing. If the symptoms do not respond within a few hours, treatment must be surgical. If the anterior fascia of the leg is promptly sectioned, complete relief is obtained from pain and the other symptoms. If the operation is postponed until necrosis of the muscles has already occurred, fibrous replacement will still leave irreparable scarring.

This condition is not common but when it occurs it is an extreme emergency. The danger lies in the similarity of the early symptoms to so-called cramping, muscle spasm, "shin splints" or contusion. Any of these conditions that do not respond promptly to treatment should be carefully investigated. Of particular

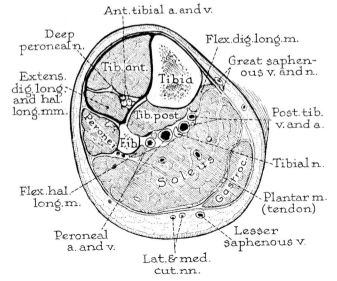

Figure 557. Cross section of leg showing its anterior compartment, outlined by heavy line, indicating muscles and vascular bundle within the compartment.

Figure 558. Anterior compartment syndrome, late. This is an intractable deformity of the foot due to pressure of the vessels in the anterior compartment of the leg. Triple arthrodesis was necessary.

importance is the patient's complaint of constant, boring, aching pain, made more severe by function but not disappearing at rest. The anterior compartment syndrome may spell the end of athletic competition for the affected individual. Because of the extreme urgency of this situation, any time there is intractable pain in the front of the leg, accompanied by some loss of function of the toes which is not relieved by ordinary sedation, it must be assumed to be anterior compartment syndrome, and preparation must be made for surgical release of the fascia of the leg. If one waits until this condition is completely defined, necrosis of the muscle has occurred and surgery is of little value. This often results in complete drop foot as well as symptoms of ischemia of the leg.

Shin Splints

Another condition unique to the leg is so-called "shin splints." As with many names in common use, there is considerable and often heated argument as to what is actually meant by the term. As is usual in these circumstances,

the term "shin splints" is a wastebasket one including many different conditions. The authors of various articles on the subject are inclined to state very definitely that it is caused by one particular thing to the exclusion of all others, which causes great confusion.

Shin splints ordinarily occurs early in the training period, frequently in training on hard floors such as an indoor track. It also may occur as a result of training on the hard ground in the early fall or on the basketball court. One of the conditions sometimes called "shin splints" is irritation of the attachment of the posterior tibial muscle along the posterior face of the tibia, with resulting periostitis. Here the tenderness will be along the posterior medial angle of the tibia and pain will be on function of the posterior tibial muscle. Another cause is an actual tearing of the attachment of the posterior tibial muscle along the tibia. "Shin splints" may also be caused by irritation at the interosseous membrane, in which case the symptoms are somewhat more posterior and seem to be deeper in the muscles of the calf. An ordinary periostitis along the posteromedial angle of the tibia may also be called "shin splints." Indeed, the involvement of the anterior tibial muscle at the anterior border of the tibia and onto its anterolateral face is called "shin splints" by some. The last-named condition may go on to serious involvement of the anterior compartment. A stress fracture of the tibia may also be misdiagnosed as "shin splints" by the unwary.

Treatment. A condition having so many etiological factors must of necessity require varying types of treatment. However, certain basic measures are of importance regardless of the etiology, the primary ones being rest and use of heat locally. A word of caution is nevertheless needed about use of heat in involvement of the anterior compartment, since heat may only aggravate the tension within the space. In the ordinary case of "shin splints" local heat, rest of the affected part, and strapping to prevent stress of the posterior tibial muscle will give marked improvement. The outcome may be disappointing, however, since the condition has a great tendency to recur and may indeed keep a track man off the boards for a whole season. A longer initial period of rest and protection will pay dividends in a more complete recovery. Various measures have been recommended, such as binding of the leg with elastic or adhesive over foam rubber or various other types of padding. This has but little effect upon a condition that is basically due to overuse of the muscles. Physical therapeutic measures should be continued until the leg is symptom-free. Resumption of activity should be on a very carefully supervised basis and function should always be kept below the level that causes pain.

There has recently been a great deal in the literature and at various meetings about treatment of shin splints by support under the arch of the foot. I call your attention again to the fact that the cause of the shin splint should be determined before treatment is planned. If the patient has a tendency to pronate the foot, he may well be susceptible to chronic stress of the muscles of the leg. If the deficiency of the arch is corrected by overtension on the posterior tibial, or even occasionally on the anterior tibial muscle, this can cause extreme overfatigue of these muscles with resulting muscle spasm and that condition which we, for lack of a better word, call shin splints. Certainly careful analysis of the arch should be carried out. If there is any tendency toward pronation, appropriate support should be put under the arch of the foot. This is particularly pertinent because most athletic shoes have no support to the arch. Many of them do not even have a heel of any sort. Possibly simply elevating the heel with a ½ in. felt pad inside the shoe and/ or inserting a cork and leather arch support flexible enough to permit the foot to flex but that will still give some support to the inner arch may solve what has seemed to be an insoluble problem. Again, the emphasis must be on accurate diagnosis of the actual trouble so that you are not treating "shin splints" but the cause of the pain and disability in the patient's leg.

Rupture of the Plantaris Muscle

Another condition unique to the leg is rupture of the plantaris muscle. This is a pencil-sized muscle arising from the lateral condyle of the femur, passing beneath the gastrocnemius and soleus muscles to attach to the tendo Achilles or the tubercle of the calcaneus on the medial side. The tendon is no larger than a piece of twine and is easily broken. To the freshman anatomy student, it is the "fool's nerve." This muscle itself is sometimes completely ruptured, in which case pain will be deep in the calf and may be quite disabling. Actually, function of the muscle is of little importance in the human and there is no necessity for repair. A relatively short period of protection will result in complete recovery.

One must carefully distinguish between rup-

ture of the plantaris muscle and *rupture of a portion of the calf;* in the latter case the symptoms will be much more severe and much longer lasting. Because of the extremely explosive action of the calf muscle, a vessel in the muscle or in the subcutaneous or fascial area will frequently be ruptured. This also gives a sharp stinging pain without serious disability but with development of ecchymosis, which may be disquieting. This ruptured vessel requires no treatment other than of the symptoms, but the condition must be distinguished from rupture of the plantaris. The ruptured vessel may be somewhat more disabling.

Muscular Strain

The muscles of the lower leg are particularly subject to strain, and this will be discussed at greater length elsewhere (see Ankle Strain, page 603). One of the most common locations for strain is at the musculotendinous junction of the calf. Much of the accustomed activity of the athlete involves forcible contraction of the calf, so that the whole body weight is abruptly thrown on the calf mechanism. Strain here may be caused either by chronic overuse in the poorly conditioned calf or by a single violent stress. Strain in the calf mechanism may be extremely disabling.

Treatment. Ordinarily strapping or taping is of little benefit except to prevent overstretching of the strained area. The athlete must be withdrawn from competition and instructed to do nothing that causes pain. The condition will frequently progress to chronic strain. Early treatment consists of rest, application of local heat and immobilization, followed by protective strapping and very gradual return to activity. In the early period the most efficient means of immobilization is a walking boot cast that will permit the patient to have fairly good activity and still prevent any strain on the calf. If the strain is less severe, primary elastic adhesive strapping will be adequate. Strapping is also used subsequent to removal of the cast (Fig. 559). This strapping is of the type designed to prevent dorsal flexion of the foot. The foot should be placed in equinus and the major anchor strap should begin above the bulge of the calf and pass directly down the back of the leg, over the heel and along the sole of the foot to the toes. The cross-stretch adhesive that stretches laterally rather than longitudinally serves well for this purpose. It has the advantage of rigidity in its long axis, while the lateral stretch permits it to be molded well around the ankle and heel without wrinkling (see Fig. 559). This can be placed to limit dorsal flexion to any desired degree, and the foot may actually be held in plantar flexion. If the foot is held in plantar flexion by the strapping, the shoe heel must be built up a proportionate amount. Even after recovery, it is advisable to elevate the heel of the street shoe and put a ½ in. pad in the heel of the athletic shoe to give some degree of relaxation to the calf. Once a strain has occurred, it is advisable to strap the foot at each practice session or game so that it cannot be dorsiflexed beyond the point where it becomes painful or sensitive. By this means one may at least prevent the strain from excessive dorsal flexion, although the strain caused by violent muscle contraction cannot be limited by taping.

In a similar manner there may be strain to the anteromedial muscles of the foot, most often the anterior tibial and less frequently the posterior tibial, except in relation to the muscle origins (see Shin Splints, page 591). In these instances the strapping should be applied so as to relieve the tension on the muscle involved. The peroneal group is not frequently involved, since athletic activity does not ordinarily subject these muscles to the same tensions received by the posterior and medial groups.

Severe (Third Degree) Rupture

The calf muscle may be ruptured partially or completely any place from its origin on the posterior part of the femoral condyles and back of the tibia to its attachment to the calcaneus. The tear may be in the muscle belly itself, but more frequently it occurs in the musculotendinous junction between the gastrocnemius and the conjoined tendon with the soleus. The unit may rupture through the tendon itself or at the attachment to the heel, sometimes avulsing a fragment of bone. As in a muscle rupture anywhere, determination of the location and extent of the injury is extremely important. The location is usually readily determined when the injury is examined early, since the tenderness will be found to be quite localized. After several hours, swelling, edema and inflammation become diffuse and the exact location of the injury may be in doubt. Both active contraction of the muscle and passive stretching will cause pain. If there is complete severance of the whole muscle-tendon unit such as (1) the head of the gastrocnemius, (2) the entire gastrocnemius from the conjoined tendon, or (3) rupture of the tendon, loss of function will be noted so that on contraction the muscle will bunch up rather than flatten down as it normally does. If the rupture is in the tendon or musculotendinous junction, a palpable defect can often be felt. The condition is quite disabling even with a relatively minor degree of tearing. It does not permit running or any activity that causes the athlete to be on his toes. This loss of function may be due to actual loss of continuity of the tendon, but it is more frequently due to muscle spasm and

Figure 559. A 3 inch strip of cross-stretch elastic adhesive is run down the back of the calf and over the sole of the foot to the metatarsals. It is anchored in place by a Gibney-type of basket weave, as shown on the right.

Figure 560. A 27 year old male playing handball felt a sharp pain in the back of his leg above his ankle. He tried to continue playing but his ankle swelled up and he had to quit. The ankle stayed sore, and he noticed he could not go up on the tip of his toes. Four weeks later an examination revealed a definite defect about 2 in. above the attachment of the tendo Achilles with almost complete loss of function of the calf. A, View showing the rather stumpy end of the tendon attachment of the calcaneus *(right)* and the badly frayed-out tendon above, near the muscle-tendon junction *(left)*. B, The difficulty in getting the ends together is shown. C, The final imbrication of the stumpy distal end into the more frayed-out proximal end with marked plantar flexion of the foot is shown. Result equivocal, even though reconstructive support by the peroneus brevis was added.

pain. If the rupture is complete and seen early, repair is quite feasible even in the muscle belly.

Treatment. Surgical repair of the tendon is mandatory even if the patient is seen late (Fig. 560). In the early case incision is made directly over the involved area, the underlying muscles are inspected, the clot is evacuated and the muscle ends are apposed by mattress sutures placed with the knee flexed and the foot in plantar flexion. The extremity must be kept in this position for about four weeks if the repair is in the muscle itself. If the repair is in the tendon or tendon to bone, a much firmer internal fixation may be obtained and the extreme flexion position may not be necessary. In any instance, it is advisable to hold the foot in equinus for a period of time. When a fragment of bone is avulsed, this fragment should be excised unless it is so large as to be vital to calcaneal function. One of the major sources for tension on the suture following repair of any part of the gastrocnemius-soleus complex is a spasm in the calf muscles. If the rupture is actually in the muscle, this is not quite so pertinent, since the lesion in the muscle will tend to prevent overcontraction. However, if the lesion is in the tendo Achilles or at its attachment, it is necessary to undertake some measure to prevent overstress of

the calf during the convalescent period. For this reason a mattress suture holding the calf muscle down, with a pull-out wire to take out the wire suture later, is extremely important. Technically, the wire is woven back and forth through the muscle above the level of the lesion, terminating with one wire on either side of the tendon. These wires are led down along the side of the calcaneus and through the sole of the heel, where they are tied over a suitable block or button to securely accept the tension of the calf muscle. The pull-out element is a wire loop passed through the proximal portion of the mattress holding the calf. This exits through the skin on the calf above the level of the wire suture holding the muscle. With such a measure it is not necessary to hold the foot in such extreme equinus for a long period of time, which often results in equinus contracture. At eight weeks or so the wire can be cut on the button at the sole of the heel, and, using the pull-out wire, can be pulled out. This aids materially in the general management of rupture of the tendon below the level of the muscle-tendon junction. It is important to be sure that the mattress wire will slide freely through the muscle with no kinks, so that it is not difficult to remove with the pull-out loop.

Good surgical judgment is required to determine just how long the foot must be kept in equinus after the repair. If it is held too long it may be difficult to get the calf muscle stretched out to its normal length. If the injury is fresh, the tissues strong and the suture material well placed, it may be possible to put the foot at right angles immediately after suture. If the strength of the fixation is questionable because of shredding of the tendon, the equinus position must be maintained longer. It should be borne in mind that at least four weeks are needed for the tendon to start to heal, and even then union is quite insecure. In order to minimize morbidity, a walking cast may be utilized after a week or ten days so that disability is not unduly prolonged. One should not anticipate return to competition in the same season in which the injury occurs. A little more time spent to get a complete recovery is well rewarded by the completeness of the recovery. A tendon as large as the tendo Achilles could not be expected to resume anything like its normal strength under three or four months, although some function may be permitted as early as eight weeks.

SPRAIN

Sprain occurs in the leg proper only at the upper end of the fibula. The upper end of the fibula does not participate primarily in the knee joint but may be involved in a knee injury. This is especially likely in relation to the fibular collateral ligament attachment (see page 475). There may be damage to the upper tibiofibular ligaments, to the extent of an actual dislocation of the upper end of the fibula. The exact mechanism of isolated strain of this area is difficult to determine. It may be that some of the lesser sprains are caused by forcible traction of the biceps tendon with the knee in flexion (Fig. 561). The type of injury that damages the fibular collateral ligament of the knee would not ordinarily damage the tibiofibular ligament, since its force tends to pull the fibula toward the tibia. If, however, the distracting force occurs with the knee flexed, the lateral collateral ligament may possibly pull the fibula backward in relation to the tibia. It is certain that sprain to the extent of complete dislocation may occur from a direct blow to the upper end of the fibula, driving it away from its tibial attachment.

It may actually be possible to manually subluxate the head of the fibula back and forth or to dislocate it from the tibia if the ligament tear is severe, since the bone is subcutaneous and can be readily manipulated. Distinguishing symptoms are pain and tenderness around the anterior and posterior tibiofibular sulci at the superior end.

Treatment. If the fibula has dislocated and spontaneously replaced, it may be difficult to determine that there has actually been a rupture of the ligaments. Occasionally the dislocation remains unreduced (see Fig. 531, page 565). If it is seen early it may be readily reduced by manipulation. It may be held in place by simple splint fixation protecting the knee. The splint should extend from above the

Figure 561. Drawing showing flexed knee, the biceps tendon pulling the fibula back.

ankle to the groin. One must be extremely wary of trying to hold the fibula to the tibia by a constricting circumferential bandage because of the extreme vulnerability of the peroneal nerve. There may be a chronic dislocation of the upper end of the fibula, and in many instances this will not be troublesome. However, the fact that the biceps and fibular collateral ligament attach to the fibula may cause this condition to become symptomatic. If it is symptomatic to the degree that it causes disability, surgical repair should be carried out by screw fixation across the upper end of the fibula into the tibia. This is rarely necessary.

FASCIAL HERNIA

Fascial hernia occurs in various areas of the body. One of the most common hernias of this type and one of the most likely to be symptomatic occurs in the anterior fascia of the leg. This rent usually takes place at the attachment of the anterior fascia to the anterior border of the tibia. The early symptoms will be those ordinarily connected with "shin splints," periostitis, or, in fact, simple contusion. As acute symptoms subside, the patient will complain of a sharply localized mass that appears just lateral to the tibial crest but is not constant. It may or may not be tender. He may notice aching pain in the leg after continued use, but at other times the condition may be almost wholly asymptomatic. Careful examination reveals a palpable defect in the fascia through which a tumor mass bulges that is particularly noticeable when the muscle is relaxed. When the anterior tibial muscle is contracted the mass will disappear, since on contraction the tension in the muscle prevents it from bulging through the defect. The rim of the defect may readily be palpated.

Treatment. Ordinarily a careful, detailed explanation to the patient of the nature of his defect will suffice to reassure him and permit him to go on without further management. Occasionally, however, the condition is symptomatic enough that it causes disability in the form of chronic pain involving the anterior tibial muscle. In these cases the defect is usually relatively small and there may be impingement of a portion of the muscle or soft tissue between the sharp edge of the fascia and edge of the bone. Here surgical interference is justified and consists of suture of the fascia to the tibia. This is successful if the sutured edge of fascial tissue is firm. Frequently, however, the edge of the fascia will be torn and efforts to draw it to the tibia simply result in splitting it further. In this instance, extending the rent to a distance of 2 to 3 in. will give symptomatic relief so far as pain is concerned. The bulging will persist, but its discrete character has been lost so that it no longer resembles a tumor mass.

EXOSTOSIS

There is no particular propensity toward traumatic exostoses in the leg. Although they frequently occur at the upper and lower ends of the tibia (Fig. 562), they are not frequent in its shaft. If they do occur they are managed as exostosis anywhere, except that a much smaller exostosis will be symptomatic in a subcutaneous bone than in one surrounded completely by muscle. If the condition is symptomatic and cannot be handled by a simple protective pad, surgical excision should be entirely successful. Occasionally a small exostosis at the upper end of the tibia will lie directly under the pes anserinus. While a player is running, or more particularly, cutting, one of the tendons of the pes may snap over the exostosis and in fact may even catch on it and simulate locking or catching of the knee. Careful attention to the location of the tenderness and to the absence of knee symptoms will prevent an embarrassing error in diagnosis. The condition is readily relieved by removing the exostosis surgically.

FRACTURE

It is not our intention to relate in detail the treatment of fracture of the bones of the leg. The tibia and fibula are both very subject to fracture from unusual forces.

Tibial Fracture

Fracture of the tibia is not common as an athletic injury but does occur. A complete fracture of the tibia will be symptomatic enough to warrant x-ray studies that will readily diagnose the condition. Needless to say, treatment should be prompt and definitive. Competition within a season would not be expected following a fracture of the tibia, even if it were an incomplete one.

Fibular Fracture

Whereas fracture of the tibia is relatively infrequent in athletic injury, fracture of the fibula is relatively common. In any fracture of the fibula, one is obligated to rule out associated injury to the ankle joint, and I shall categorically state that any time there is a complete fracture of the fibula (see Ankle, page 606) above the level of the lower tibiofibular syndesmosis, one is obligated to rule out accompanying complete rupture of the inferior tibiofibular ligaments. This is without doubt the most serious and most important consideration in the fracture of the fibula. The actual fracture of the fibula is usually quite inconsequential, except that it does require a certain period of healing. But if the fracture is accompanied by a rupture of the tibiofibular ligament with resulting instability in or separation of the ankle mortice (see Fig. 578), the outcome is a serious permanent disability. The condition is readily managed if it is recognized early and treated promptly. It is very difficult to handle as a reconstructive measure. So the first step in considering the fracture of the fibula is to determine the integrity of the ankle joint.

The fibula is subject to fracture by direct blow. This is usually in the lower one third and may be caused by contact with a shoe or other hard object. There is immediate severe pain but not necessarily severe disability. Upon examination, local tenderness will be present at the site of the injury. There may or may not be local crepitation. There is prompt swelling with localized hematoma formation. The individual can usually walk quite well, and in fact may complete the game, since in a fracture of the fibula by direct blow the integrity of the ankle is not involved and disability is due to contraction of the muscle attachments on the fibular shaft. Diagnosis is confirmed by x-ray study, which should always be carried out in a case of localized tenderness over any bone.

Treatment consists of management of the localized area and protection of the part. If there is definite hematoma with localized swelling, aspiration by surgically aseptic technique and injection of hyaluronidase are of some value. These measures are ordinarily not necessary. After a short period of packing in ice or wearing a compression bandage, the extremity should be placed in a walking boot, which should be worn for about three weeks. Union will not then be complete, but by this time it is usually possible to strap the extremity so that some degree of function may be resumed. At least activity may be permitted to the point of starting rehabilitation, but nonparticipation in contact sports probably is advisable for as long as six to eight weeks. One has a quite effective indicator in the degree of the patient's discomfort.

Stress Fracture (Fatigue Fracture)
(See Page 69)

The fibula is particularly prone to stress fracture (Fig. 563), being second only to the

Figure 562. Exostosis of tibia. Note that the lateral view *(A)* is negative. The anteroposterior view *(B)* is inconclusive as to the nature of the mass, whereas the oblique view *(C)* reveals the tumor very distinctly.

Figure 563. This boy was examined by a physician because of persistent pain in the lower fibula. X-ray was made *(A, B)* and he was advised that he had a malignant tumor and operation was scheduled. On seeing him in consultation a careful history elicited the fact that three weeks before he had sprinted off the curve of a track and up an incline and pulled up lame in his left leg. Two days later he ran in a race and had increased pain, particularly after the race. The pain and tenderness persisted but actually had seemed somewhat less in the past several days. He was advised that he probably had a stress fracture. The subsequent pictures *(C, D)* three weeks later show some increase in the extraperiosteal shadow but also some increased modeling. Meantime, the clinical symptoms had materially improved. Eight months later *(E, F)* the films show almost complete resolution. The patient had long been asymptomatic.

Figure 564. Blown-up view of "fatigue" fracture of the tibia. Differential diagnosis here was of tumor because of no injury and the presence of severe aching pain. Time gave complete relief.

Figure 565. *A,* Anteroposterior view showing periosteal proliferation indicated by arrow, four months after onset of pain. Patient had no specific injury. *B* and *C,* One month later, anteroposterior and lateral views show definite callus solidification at the fracture line.

Figure 566. *A*, Four weeks following the onset of pain, radiograph shows callus (indicated by arrow) with an indefinite line. *B*, Four weeks later radiograph shows the solidification of callus and obliteration of fracture line. This is a typical stress fracture and should not be confused with a tumor.

metatarsals in this respect. This condition arises early in the training period and appears as aching pain, soreness and some distress on function, usually localized near the neck of the fibula. There is no history of injury. Examination will reveal localized tenderness over the bone. Early x-ray findings will usually be negative. The patient will be treated for contusion or sprain, but the complaint persists and remains quite localized. After 10 to 14 days x-rays will often reveal a transverse crack across the bone. Possibly callus formation will appear with no fracture line visible. The significance of stress fracture of the fibula is not as great as that in the foot, since the fibula is a non-weight-bearing bone, but the patient should be carefully rehabilitated so that he does not develop chronic muscular disability in the leg. Frequently by the time the fracture is found the time for immobilization will be past, and treatment will be by careful muscular rehabilitation and other physical therapeutic measures such as application of heat locally and muscular massage. Stress fracture of the tibia is not as frequent as that of the fibula, but it does occur, principally in athletes (Figs. 564 to 566). It is of necessity more disabling than in the fibula, since the tibia is a weight-bearing bone. When the fracture is recognized, a protective cast should be applied until union has progressed to the point of good stability with no pain.

20

Injuries of the Ankle

ANATOMICAL CONSIDERATIONS

Injuries to the ankle joint are the most common conditions encountered in the treatment of injuries to the athlete. There is no doubt that many ankle injuries are treated overcasually, which may account for the expression "Once a sprain, always a sprain." Often insufficent consideration is given to the exact nature of the damage in the individual case. In order to be able to treat any injury of the ankle joint intelligently, a definitive diagnosis must be made. This predicates a working knowledge of the anatomy of the region involved.

Let us consider those anatomical characteristics of the ankle joint that have a direct bearing on the type of injury that occurs in response to various forces applied (Figs. 567 to 569). The ankle joint is functionally a hinge joint, having motion in only one plane—flexion and extension. The bony structure is designed as a mortice and tenon, with considerable inherent stability (see Fig. 568). The mortice is formed by the lateral malleolus, the undersurface of the tibia and the medial malleolus. The tenon is the body of the talus, which is shaped to fit snugly into the mortice. It should be noted that the lateral malleolus is longer than the medial malleolus. Its distal tip extends to the bottom of the talus at the level of the talocalcaneal joint. It is roughly rectangular in outline but actually somewhat narrower at the level of the lower end of the tibia. The medial malleolus, on the other hand, is short and thick, being roughly pyramidal in shape with its base upward. Its distal tip extends only halfway down on the body of the talus.

The distal tibia and fibula are bound together by the anterior and posterior tibiofibular ligaments, which are really thickened expansions of the interosseous membrane that fastens the two bones together throughout their length. Although some motion is present in the syndesmosis between the tibia and fibula at the lower end, there is to all practical purposes complete stability between the two bones. Definite motion has been demonstrated in the distal tibiofibular syndesmosis, so that a certain amount of disability occurs from ankylosis between the tibia and fibula at the ankle joint. Thus, the ankle joint has stability from two sources: first, the mortice and tenon bony structure, and second, the extensive investiture of ligaments that surround the joint.

The ligaments are thin fore and aft (capsule) to permit flexion and extension of the joint, but on each side they become heavier and stronger as the tibial and fibular collateral ligaments. The medial collateral, or deltoid, ligament is particularly strong, has a very broad attachment to the internal malleolus and extends downward in many bands to become intimately connected to the ligaments supporting the arch of the foot. In addition to stabilizing the ankle joint on the medial side, the medial collateral ligament serves to support the arch and hence is a doubly vital structure.

It is possible to dissect the lateral collateral ligament into many separate ligaments, but there are three primary fasciculi: (1) one running forward to attach to the talus anteriorly (anterior talofibular), on the lateral margin of the nonarticular portion of the body of the talus just in front of the articular surface; (2) another running backward to attach to the posterior portion of the talus (posterior talofibular), again just adjacent to the articular surface on the nonarticular portion near the top of the bone; and (3) one extending directly downward to attach to the calcaneus (calcaneofibular), bypassing the talus, the second and stronger branch passing from the talus directly to the fibula. These ligaments also blend into the lateral ligaments of the foot, extending forward onto the cuboid and to the base of the fifth metatarsal. Together the me-

Figure 567. Anatomical drawing of ankle, posterior view, showing the tibiofibular ligament, which is heavy distally, thinning out to become the interosseous membrane proximally. The posterior and lateral fasciculi of the lateral collateral ligament and the posterior and medial fasciculi of the medial collateral ligament are shown. Note the different lengths of the two malleoli. The guideline indicates top of dome of talus.

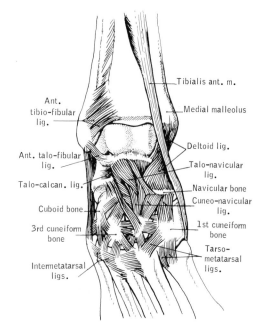

Figure 568. Anatomical drawing of ankle, anterior view. Note massive deltoid ligament and very weak anterior talofibular ligament. Note no ligament from front of tibia to top of talus. The joint capsule has been removed.

dial and lateral ligaments, acting in conjunction with the two malleoli, serve to prevent lateral instability at the ankle joint.

The long lateral malleolus, acting with the medial ligament, prevents excess motion to the outer side. The length of the lateral malleolus firmly holds the body of the talus so that lateral motion in the tarsus is more restricted than medial motion. A normal range of flexion-extension is permitted with its axis at the tip of the medial malleolus.

The body of the talus is not rectangular in its general shape. The anterior portion of the body is distinctly wider than the posterior portion so that, as the foot goes into dorsiflexion, the wider part of the talus is forced between the two malleoli and the ankle is very stable in this position. As the foot goes into plantar flexion, the narrower part of the body of the talus moves into the mortice and some lateral instability results in this position, predisposing to injury. It also adds distinctly to the mobility of the foot, so that with the foot in equinus there is definite lateral motion in the ankle joint, whereas with the foot in dorsiflexion there is no lateral motion. On forced dorsiflexion of the foot, the fibula is forced away from the tibia and injury may result. On forcible dorsiflexion of the foot, the anterior edge of the tibia nestles into the sulcus between the head and body of the talus. The anterior inferior angle of the tibia inclines slightly backward in order to prevent direct impingement of the talus on the tibia. As the foot dorsiflexes and everts, the talus is driven forcibly against

the lateral malleolus. These factors are of considerable importance in the study of injuries to the ankle.

The two malleoli are subcutaneous and as such are subject to direct injury. The posterior tibial and flexor hallucis tendons medially and the peroneal tendons laterally lie in very intimate association with the back of the medial and the lateral malleolus, respectively, whereas the dorsiflexors of the foot have a much less intimate relationship with the osseous structures in front of the ankle.

CONTUSION

There is nothing particularly significant about contusion of the ankle. The contusion is usually to one of the malleoli. The most critical factor is accurate diagnosis of the injury. Once it has been confirmed that a contusion, and not a fracture or a sprain, is present, the treatment is simple. A few words of caution: in many sprains the maximum tenderness will be on the malleolus itself. A negative x-ray finding does not necessarily mean that the injury is a contusion only. An incomplete or fissure-type fracture may simulate a contusion, and one should be suspicious of the condition that is particularly slow to heal or causes pain on function. In an ordinary contusion of the

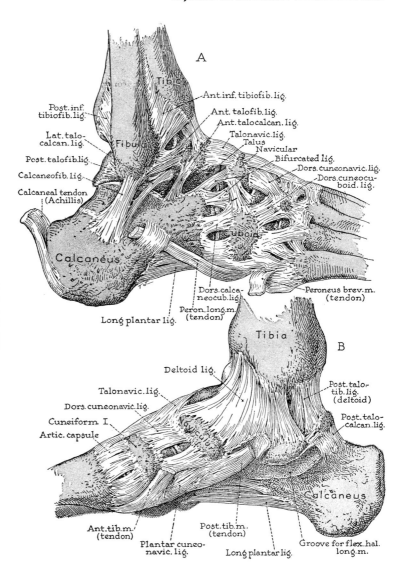

Figure 569. Ligaments of the ankle and foot. *A*, Lateral side. Note very weak lateral ligaments. Distal end of fibula is at level of talocalcaneal joint. *B*, Medial side. Note massive deltoid ligament and short medial malleolus. Deltoid ligament extends down over medial side to support arch. The calcaneal tendon has been removed in *B*. (From Jones and Shepard, *A Manual of Surgical Anatomy*, p. 116.)

ankle, ankle function is disturbed very little unless there has been a severe crushing injury of the soft tissues. A blow over the tendo Achilles may lead to tenosynovitis, complicating a contusion. A blow over the peroneal tendons may actually dislocate them from the groove—an injury very much more serious than simple contusion. These facts suggest that a careful examination should be done to eliminate other possible injuries before treatment for contusion is initiated.

Treatment is the same as for contusion elsewhere: aspiration of the hematoma, local injection (hyaluronidase), compression, and application of cold packs to be followed in a few hours by heat. Immobilization and support per se are not necessary. Protective appliances such as sponge rubber or felt doughnuts are useful. Rehabilitation should be rapid, and

athletic participation is not unduly interfered with.

STRAIN

The area of the ankle joint is subject to strain perhaps more than any other area in the body. This is attributable to several factors. The ankle is a weight-bearing joint and in the athlete is subject to very dynamic forces as a result of the explosive character of its motion under certain circumstances. The broad jumper, for example, takes off with a terrific drive and on landing forces both feet into extreme dorsiflexion, with resultant strain on the tendo Achilles. This strain may occur either at the attachment of the tendon to the calcaneus or frequently at the musculotendinous junction, occasionally along the course of the tendon. It is frequently complicated by tenosynovitis. Another tendon particularly subject to strain is the anterior tibial. A most annoying disability can arise from strain of this tendon at its attachment to the medial side of the foot. The posterior tibial tendon is unusually vulnerable because of its dual role in supporting the arch of the foot and in supplying plantar flexion and inversion. A frequent problem is a tendinitis at its attachment to the tuberosity of the navicular bone, or under the navicular in the arch of the foot. Switching from street shoes, which have a heel and a firm medial support with a strong counter, to athletic shoes, which, as a rule, have no heels, minimal support and very little counter, can cause a static strain which is very difficult to handle. The tenderness occurs at the medial border of the arch. Pain and aching may spread around under the arch of the foot and behind the medial malleolus. The peroneal tendons are much less frequently strained, since the nature of the activity of the ankle does not require such forcible use of the everters as of the other muscles of the ankle. So it can be seen that strain does not involve the ankle joint proper. It involves the many dynamic forces through the muscle tendon units which encompass the lower leg and foot.

Treatment of the acute condition is rest of the muscle involved, use of heat locally, injection with a local anesthetic, and protection against further injury. The proper degree of protection may be very difficult to decide.

Since the condition involves the integrity of the muscle, it is obvious that the strain cannot be well protected while activity of the muscle is permitted. An attempt to shorten the treatment period often results in prompt recurrence of the disability, and the situation may become quite frustrating to the physician and doubly so to the athlete. Certain protective measures can be used, however, the general rule being that no function should be allowed that causes pain. In strain of the tendo Achilles, for example, the pain may be caused mainly by overstretching of the tendon, and this can be prevented by adequate strapping to prevent hyperdorsiflexion of the foot (see Fig. 559). With such protection the athlete may be able to jog or even run at a relatively steady pace, but he should not be allowed to charge out of the blocks or to jump or to hurdle. In short, he should do nothing that requires explosive activity of the muscle. Ordinarily treatment of the condition will require at least ten days of relative inactivity and sometimes much more than this. Unrestricted activity should be permitted only when it is entirely pain-free. Since pain is a relative thing, it may be very difficult in a given case to decide just when unrestricted activity will be safe. If the strain involves the posterior tibial tendon, a well-fitted arch support may be a useful adjunct. After a period of taping (Fig. 570) to slightly invert the foot and support the arch, a flexible arch support should be used for the rest of the season, particularly when the athlete is wearing athletic shoes.

Figure 570. Drawing shows a classic arch strapping on an adult. Several strips of 2.5 cm. adhesive tape will be necessary. Strip 1 starts at just above the lateral malleolus and passes under the heel and up the inner side of the foot to above the bulge of the calf. Strips 2, 3 and 4 pass up the leg in a similar course; the number of strips used depends somewhat on the size of the leg. As the strip reaches the front of the ankle it is then twisted across the front of the leg to the lateral side. Five or six strips are utilized, with the arch strapping extending clear up and forward to the base of the head of the metatarsals. Strips are anchored at the calf and above the ankle with one or more circumferential strips. If the injured arch is high, a felt pad should be inserted under the arch and held in place by short strips of tape, particularly if a flat support shoe is worn. This felt pad is probably not necessary in a shoe having a heel and a good support.

TENOSYNOVITIS

Tenosynovitis is quite frequent about the ankle and, as indicated in the preceding section, frequently follows strain. Tenosynovitis can result from contusion or infection, but at the ankle the most common cause is overuse of the tendon. This causes irritation between the tendon and surrounding tissues, with resulting loss of the smooth gliding pattern. The significant findings are pain on motion of the tendon, particularly under tension, "snowball crepitation" on motion, tenderness along the involved area, local heat and redness and other signs of inflammatory reaction. Differentiation between tenosynvovitis and strain may be extremely difficult, but since their treatment is quite similar this is not a vital problem. In fact, the two often coexist. When they do the condition becomes more resistant to treatment.

Treatment should be prompt. Complete rest of the involved tendon, together with the use of a long-acting local anesthetic, is indicated. Extreme care should be taken that this is injected around the tendon and not into it. If it is impossible to be sure you are in the tendon sheath, no injection should be given. There is a certain resistance to injection into a tendon which is quite different from that felt when entering the sheath, so if you encounter any resistance at all the injection should be discontinued. Local injection of anesthetic agents should not lead one to the false conclusion that the inflammation has subsided, since return to function under these circumstances will result in prompt exacerbation of the condition. Local injection is of value as a measure of active treatment, not as a means of rehabilitation. Athletic participation is extremely difficult in cases of tenosynovitis of the ankle, since the only real way to prevent motion of the tendons of the ankle is to immobilize the ankle, and this is not consistent with ordinary athletic endeavor. As rehabilitation progresses, protective measures should be designed to prevent extremes of motion in the involved tendon. If the heel cord is involved, strapping to prevent dorsiflexion will help (see Fig. 559). If the anterior tibial or posterior tibial tendon is involved, strapping in inversion in the early stage (see Fig. 570) and later a properly fitted arch support or wedging the shoe on the medial border of the sole and heel will serve to eliminate some of the static stress of this condition.

Tenosynovitis is more likely to be disastrous to a season's play than strain, but for the same reason, namely, a marked tendency toward recurrence. The track man who develops a tenosynovitis running on the boards in the winter will frequently have a very ineffectual season since, when he puts out his maximum effort, he is likely to be pulled up short by recurrence of his tenosynovitis. As in so many other instances, early adequate treatment is the very best insurance of success. A period of complete nonparticipation may well be followed by a highly successful season, whereas an attempt to continue athletics in spite of pain and discomfort can result only in continued ineffectual activity.

My best recommendation for treatment of severe acute tenosynovitis in the tendo Achilles or anterior tibial tendon is a period of elevation of the foot and application of hot packs until the acute tenderness has disappeared, followed by the wearing of a walking boot cast for 10 to 14 days. By this time the symptoms will have largely subsided and adequate strapping can be applied to permit gradual return to function. Protective strapping should be continued for several weeks until one is sure there is no real likelihood of recurrence. The strapping must be specifically designed to protect the tendon involved. Great care must be taken that the adhesive straps do not actually constrict the tendon and so make the condition worse. For anterior or posterior tibial strain, the strips should start on the lateral border of the dorsum of the foot, pass under the sole of the foot and swing under the arch and up the medial aspect of the leg (see Fig. 570). They are applied with the foot in neutral flexion and slightly inverted.

To support the tendo Achilles the foot should be strapped in plantar flexion (see Fig. 559).

DISLOCATION OR SUBLUXATION OF THE PERONEAL TENDONS

A condition unique to the ankle area is dislocation or subluxation of the peroneal tendons. This condition may be acute or chronic.

Acute

In the acute condition the history usually is of a blow at the back of the lateral malleolus while the peroneal tendons are taut in dorsiflexion and eversion of the foot. The peroneal retinaculum gives way. One or both of the tendons pop out of the groove onto the lateral side of the malleolus. They usually reduce spontaneously. One may confuse this condition with an ankle sprain. Careful history and physical examination will eliminate the confusion, however. Tenderness is directly over the peroneal tendons, and it may be confused with tenosynovitis. Indeed, tenosynovitis may be a sequel. In the acute case, it is usually not possible to displace the tendons at examination.

If the diagnosis of an acute dislocation is made, the *treatment* is surgical. Incision is made posteriorly along the peroneal groove; replacement of the tendons with resuture of the torn or redundant retinaculum may be effective. In many cases there will be a shallow peroneal groove, which predisposes to this condition. In this instance, repair should be accompanied by deepening of the groove in order to make the tendons more secure. If the groove is to be deepened, the tendons are displaced forward in order to expose the furrow behind the fibula. With a very sharp osteotome, a thin, flexible layer of bone is elevated from the posterior fibula beginning on the lateral margin and extending to the medial edge. Care should be taken not to detach the medial margin of the cut. It is important that this thin strip of bone, including the fibrocartilage of the peroneal groove, remain attached on the medial side. This may be retracted medially while the furrow is deepened beneath it. This flap includes the smooth membrane which overlies the fibula and forms the floor of the peroneal groove. After this layer is carefully reflected from a lateral to medial direction, the underlying bed is scooped out with a sharp gouge until a smooth deep furrow large enough to contain the tendons is formed. The reflected flap is placed back over the raw bone and sutured down through drill holes in the fibula if necessary, in order to make a smooth bed for the peroneal tendon. The redundant sheath is plicated over the tendons in order to make a strong roof. If the tissue seems too redundant or too inadequate, a strip of periosteum can be resected up from the tibia and pulled back over to help support the roof of the groove. This completes the tunnel. Following surgery, fixation in a stirrup splint for two weeks, then wearing a walking cast for four weeks, will give adequate protection. Active athletics should not be permitted before eight weeks, however.

Chronic

Chronic or recurrent subluxation of the peroneal tendons may be congenital or it may follow an acute episode that was untreated. In the latter instance there will be a history of acute injury with considerable soreness for many weeks, followed by recurrent episodes of feeling something slipping out of place at the back of the ankle, with or without sharp pain. These episodes occur as the athlete everts the foot with the tendons tight. They are quite distressing. The tendons slip back into position and all is well until the next episode. A careful history will usually disclose the original accident, and the patient can describe the recurrent episodes quite graphically. Physical examination will usually demonstrate the shallow groove, with thickening of the retinaculum. The tendons often can be slipped completely or partially out of the groove on manual manipulation.

This condition should be treated by surgical reconstruction of the groove and repair of the retinaculum, suitably reinforced by adjacent tissue. The groove should be reconstructed, as indicated in the discussion on Acute Dislocation, taking particular care to obtain further soft tissue from the tibial periosteum or even a strip of tendo Achilles in order to get a very substantial roof over the groove. This is a very successful type of reconstruction. This should give prompt relief, but eight weeks of immobilization of the ankle will be needed to insure stability.

SYNOVIAL HERNIA

Synovial hernia about the ankle will be discussed in the section dealing with this condition in the foot (page 650).

SPRAIN-DISLOCATION-FRACTURE

In injuries to the ankle there is such a close association of these conditions, namely, sprain-dislocation-fracture, that it is unwise to place them in separate categories. This is particularly true in the athlete, since the same forces may well cause a combination of injuries. Resultant pathology may be determined more by the strength and duration of the forces causing the injury than by the exact type of stress. In the athlete the injury is usually caused by stress forces which may result in either a sprain, a dislocation, a fracture, or all three at the same time.

Mechanics of Injury

Since the ankle is functionally a hinge joint normally permitting only dorsal and plantar flexion, it follows that injuries to the ankle are primarily caused by lateral stresses that force the ankle through an arc of motion which it does not normally possess. Less frequently they are due to hyperflexion or hyperextension. The injuries produced by lateral stresses may readily be divided into two categories, namely, inversion injuries and eversion injuries.

Inversion Injury

Inversion injuries to the ankle (Fig. 571) are as a rule not due to pure inversion. The force usually consists of inversion, internal rotation and plantar flexion of the foot in relation to the leg, so that the foot is inverted and the ankle and leg are thrown to the outer side. The push is against the medial malleolus and the pull is away from the lateral malleolus. As the foot inverts in relation to the leg, strain is put upon the lateral collateral ligament, which is the ligament primarily constructed to restrict this motion. As a result of this overinversion, the ligament will tear slightly, partially or completely, according to the severity of the force. If the inverting force continues as the lateral ligament gives way, the ankle "opens

Figure 571. *A,* Mechanics of inversion injury of the ankle. Drawing showing talus rolling over medial malleolus. *B,* Inversion injury showing complete severance of the lateral collateral ligament, permitting the talus to roll over the medial malleolus. There is no fracture. The ossicle on the medial side is the os trigonum. Drawing in insert shows the wide space between the top of the talus and the bottom of the tibia. *C,* The same stress on a normal ankle.

Figure 572. Inversion injury of the ankle. *A,* Drawing showing vertical fracture of the medial malleolus, with a split up the shaft and complete tear of the lateral ligament with no fibular fracture. *B,* Another inversion injury. The talus pushed the medial malleolus off instead of rolling over it, and the fibula was fractured. This should be treated by reduction and internal fixation.

up" on the lateral side and the talus is forcibly thrust against the medial malleolus. The medial malleolus, being short and stubby and extending no more than halfway down the vertical height of the body of the talus, will act as a fulcrum, with its tip impinging against the central portion of the medial face of the talus. The talus thus rotates over the malleolus rather than pushes it off. In such a case the injury will probably be confined to the lateral side, and there will be more or less complete laceration of the lateral collateral ligaments. It is unusual for this type of force to break off the lateral malleolus in the athlete. In the elderly person in whom the bone is brittle and fragile, the lateral malleolus may break rather than the ligament tear. If this same inversion force is continued as the talus is driven against the medial malleolus, the latter may break off. In this instance the fracture line will ordinarily extend more or less vertically up the shaft of the tibia beginning at the lateral margin of the medial malleolus (Fig. 572*A*). There is injury on both sides of the ankle. This may be a bimalleolar fracture or perhaps a fracture of the medial malleolus plus an avulsion of the lateral collateral ligament (see Fig. 572). If the x-ray shows a vertical fracture of the medial malleolus as in Figure 572*B,* one must presume that the lateral components are torn until proved otherwise. Open repair of the torn

lateral ligaments with screw fixation of the medial malleolus is recommended.

Approximately 85 per cent of all injuries to the ankle are inversion injuries and are confined to ligament injury, so-called sprain or "sprain-fracture" of the ankle (Fig. 573). The vast majority of these may be classified as mild (first degree) sprains without any particular loss of function of the ligament. If the force is violent, other fractures may occur such as fracture of the superomedial portion of the talus and fracture of the back of the articular surface of the tibia, but as a rule injury is confined to the ligament on the lateral side, with occasional instances of avulsion fracture of the tip of the fibula (Fig. 574) or "push-off" fracture of the medial malleolus.

Eversion Injury

If the opposite force is applied and the foot is carried outward in relationship to the leg, the talus is forced laterally and into dorsiflexion (Fig. 575). The anatomical difference between the two malleoli becomes doubly significant here. Whereas on the medial side the malleolus is short and the talus may rotate over it, on the lateral side the malleolus is at least as long as the height of the talus, so that it is extremely difficult for the talus to rotate over the lateral malleolus with the malleolar

Figure 573. *A,* Drawing showing avulsion of lateral malleolus. *B,* Avulsion fracture of the tip of the lateral malleolus by inversion injury, so-called sprain fracture. The fragment will usually be smaller than is shown in the drawing.

tip as the fulcrum. In eversion force, since the push is toward the lateral side, the talus is driven forcibly against the lateral malleolus, and severe pressure is applied to the malleolus before overstress of the short medial collateral ligament occurs, since it can permit some degree of lateral tilting of the talus. When applied to the lateral malleolus this stress may cause several types of injuries, but all are due to the same forces. Perhaps the most common injury is fracture of the fibula somewhere below the level of the lower end of the tibia, resulting in a single malleolar fracture (Figs. 576 and 577). This may occur without significant damage to the deltoid ligament, but it is more often accompanied by a rupture of this ligament. This same force may actually drive the fibula away from the tibia after rupturing the tibiofibular ligament and so permit separation of the ankle mortice (Fig. 578). As the force continues, the medial collateral ligament gives way, the tibiofibular ligament tears, the fibula is driven further away from the tibia, and the fibula may break anywhere along its length. The most common location of the break is somewhere on its lower third. If a fibular fracture appears above the level of the ankle joint, one must assume that the tibiofibular ligament has been torn and that the integrity of the ankle mortice has been lost until proved otherwise. This is an extremely important point from the standpoint of treatment. Before this lateral stress is sufficient to push the fibula

Figure 574. This ten year old female twisted her right ankle broad jumping. No treatment. Persistant pain three years later at the tip of the lateral malleolus. X-ray shows avulsion of the tip of the lateral malleolus. This fragment was removed and two months later the patient was allowed full activity, except for basketball for another six weeks. Four months postoperative she returned because she hurt her wrist. At that time her ankle was asymptomatic.

Figure 575. *A,* Drawing of eversion injury of the ankle. The talus pushes the fibula laterally, rupturing the tibiofibular ligament. The fibula may break at any level above the tibiofibular ligament. The medial collateral ligament is torn. *B,* X-ray showing normal ankle. *C,* Eversion injury. Eversion stress would displace the talus further. Severe example of this same injury is shown in Figure 583. There may be no fracture or the fibula may break anywhere in its distal half — usually just above the tibiofibular ligament.

away from the tibia, something must give way on the medial side of the foot. This may consist of laceration of the medial collateral (deltoid) ligament or an avulsion of the medial malleolus.

Another common injury is the *bimalleolar fracture* (Figs. 579 and 580), namely, fracture of both malleoli at or below the level of the lower end of the tibia. This is also an eversion injury. If a fracture of the lower end of the fibula is observed at the level of the lower end of the tibia, one should very carefully check the integrity of the deltoid ligament. While the great majority of injuries of the ankle joint are sprains and are the result of inversion injury, most fractures of the ankle are of the lateral malleolus and are caused by lateral angulation, eversion and external rotation.

Figure 576. *A,* Eversion injury, showing fractured fibula without separation of ankle mortice. Note rupture of the deltoid ligament. Tibiofibular ligament is intact. *B,* X-ray of injury shown in drawing. Note the vertical direction of the fracture line of the fibula, typical of the push-off injury. The deltoid ligament must be repaired and internal fixation of the fibula done. In this instance, with the tibiofibular ligament intact, pin or rod fixation in the fibula will suffice.

Figure 577. *A*, "As is" picture without stress showing oblique fracture of the fibula and widening of the ankle mortice. *B*, Carefully positioned anteroposterior view shows no pathological change. *C*, Lateral stress reproducing displacement which occurred at the time of the injury. Note the tibiofibular ligament is intact. *D*, Repair of the deltoid ligament and fixation of the fibula by transfixion screws, which should be extended to engage the opposite cortex of the tibia. Note in this picture the fracture line has again disappeared.

Figure 578. This injury differs from that in Figure 577 in that the fracture is higher in the fibula and the tibiofibular ligament is ruptured. *A*, Eversion injury. Fracture of fibula in which fibula is actually pushed off with separation of ankle mortice and rupture of the tibiofibular ligament. *B*, X-ray of same injury. Rupture of the medial ligament, separation of the tibiofibular ligament, lateral displacement of the talus, fracture of the fibula above the level of the joint. This fracture cannot occur without rupture of the medial ligament and almost always of the tibiofibular ligament. *C*, After repair of the medial ligament and fixation of the fibula to the tibia.

Figure 579. Bimalleolar fracture. All ligaments intact. This should be treated by replacement of the medial malleolus and internal fixation. In this case no treatment was necessary on the lateral side of the ankle, since the fibula is relatively stable by virtue of its intact periosteum. In many cases fibular fixation is advisable (see Fig. 589).

From the description of the mechanics of injury it becomes quite apparent that it is of great importance in any individual case to try to determine the type of forces involved and so be able to forecast to some extent the area upon which the strain is to be expected.

Dorsiflexion Injury

Characteristically, the eversion injury is some combination of eversion, external rotation and dorsiflexion. Thus, strictly speaking, the dorsiflexion injury is a type of eversion injury, but it is so frequent that it merits individual description. As was indicated in the description of the anatomy of the ankle, the talus is broad in front and narrow behind. As the foot is pushed into dorsiflexion, the broad part of the talus seats firmly between the two malleoli, and this stress is readily supported by the distal tibiofibular ligament. If the force continues or if some eversion component thrusts the talus more forcibly against the fibula, the result is unusual strain against this ligament, which binds the two bones together. This same force puts tension against the musculotendinous unit of the calf and may result in strain or actual rupture of this mechanism. Far more frequently the dorsiflexion simply

Figure 580. Classic bimalleolar fracture with eversion type of injury. Note (A) the complete fracture of the medial malleolus, which is displaced laterally. Note the oblique fracture of the lateral malleolus, a little higher than usual but still quite typical. Note also that the tibiofibular ligament, although partially torn where it attaches to the distal fragment of the fibula, has remained intact to the proximal fragment of the fibula and the interosseous membrane, so that there is complete stability of the fibula. This is properly treated as a bimalleolar fracture (B) by reduction of the malleolar fracture, by internal malleolar fracture fixation with a long screw and by immobilization of the distal fragment of the fibula by a transfixion screw through the tibia. It is better for each of these screws to transverse the opposite cortex. View B was made the day after the injury. Note the complete disappearance of the fracture line because of the obliquity of the fracture of the tibia.

springs the tibia and fibula apart, the force is resolved, the two bones fall back together and the disability does not seem to be severe. Simple dorsiflexion probably will not avulse the ligament completely.

Symptoms. The patient usually presents with a rather indefinite history. He may say that his foot was pushed too far in dorsiflexion but usually he cannot be sure. He may have noticed that he experienced pain at the ankle and this subsided as the foot came down into the normal position. Contrary to the ordinary sprain of the ankle, local swelling is not manifested because the hemorrhage occurs deep in the leg and is not readily detectable under the skin. This is the patient who continues to play, tries to run, and who has increasing pain and discomfort as he increases his activities. He may be able to run well at a normal pace, but if he puts the pressure on, he will notice pain in the ankle. He will often be able to associate this pain with dorsiflexion of the foot.

Examination reveals a moderate degree of swelling with some fullness in the area back of the lateral malleolus, between it and the tendo Achilles. Palpation directly along the sulcus between the tibia and fibula will demonstrate tenderness posteriorly and anteriorly. The findings at this stage are ordinarily not marked, however, unless the injury has been a severe one. On manipulation of the foot ordinary motion is free and pain-free. Inversion and eversion do not cause pain. Pain will be elicited on complete dorsiflexion of the foot, particularly with the knee flexed to relax the calf. These symptoms are very similar to those of talotibial exostosis, the distinction being that, in the sprain, pain is usually tibiofibular, whereas in the exostosis it is ordinarily in front of the ankle. The two conditions may coexist. If the injury seems severe, an x-ray should be taken with the foot sharply dorsiflexed and slightly everted. If this now shows any tibiofibular displacement, as compared with a similar view of the opposite ankle, it indicates that there has been a complete tear of the tibiofibular ligament.

Treatment. Early attention to this injury will result in prompt recovery in the moderate (first or second degree) sprain, since it is relatively easy to protect the injured part and even permit a fairly high degree of activity. Measures designed to prevent dorsiflexion, such as strapping of the foot (see Fig. 559) and the use of an elevated heel on the shoe, will be effective. The foot should be strapped so that dorsiflexion cannot take place even under very

severe stress. In too many instances the condition is minimized by both player and physician, and the true nature of the injury is recognized only after weeks of frustration.

If the injury is third degree (severe), treatment must be much more comprehensive. In this case if an x-ray of an anteroposterior view of the ankle, made when the patient is standing, does not show separation at the tibiofibular synchondrosis, as compared with the opposite side, one may treat this condition by immobilization with a plaster cast. Posterior and lateral boot stirrup splints should be used, with no weight-bearing permitted until the swelling is well controlled. Then a boot cast with a walking heel should be worn for at least four weeks post-injury. At this time if the symptoms seem to be minimal, a very adequate strapping may be substituted. This treatment must be continued for at least another four weeks or longer if active participation of athletics is initiated at that time.

If there is any question about the separation, an oblique x-ray view should be made of each ankle in addition to views in sharp dorsiflexion. If any of these views show a separation between the tibia and fibula, surgical treatment will be much more effective. It is relatively simple to place a transfixion screw through the fibula and across both cortices of the tibia just above the level of the tibiofibular joint through a small lateral incision over the shaft of the fibula. This will maintain continuity of the ankle mortice and so prevent instability of this joint. It goes without saying that the reduction must be complete at the time the screw is placed. This screw should be removed later (eight weeks) in order to permit motion in the tibiofibular joint.

If reduction cannot be carried out under anesthesia, an incision must be made in order to free the space between the tibia and fibula before the fixation is inserted. Although the fibula is situated somewhat posteriorly, visualization is more easily and completely obtained by an anterior approach, since this will not disturb the peroneal tendons. A vertical incision, right over the syndesmosis, just lateral to the peroneus tertius tendon, permits ready access to the area with no vital structures involved. It is extremely important that all the soft tissue debris be trimmed away with minimum disturbance of the bone, since a fusion across this syndesmosis is not desirable.

The dorsiflexion injury accounts for the relatively high incidence of ossification noted between the tibia and fibula in x-rays of the

Figure 581. College athlete who had a dorsiflexion injury apparently resulting in a mild sprain. Inadequate treatment, which did not prevent dorsiflexion, resulted in persistent pain. Patient made repeated, unsatisfactory efforts to return to football. The player could not run all out. At the season's end, more thorough study revealed the true nature of the condition, with ossification of the tibiofibular ligament over a considerable space. There was mild diastasis. Removal of the bone and screw fixation for eight weeks resulted in improvement, but some symptoms persisted. A, Anteroposterior view showing slight tibiofibular diastasis with ossification. B, Oblique view revealing the extent of the bone deposit and diastasis. C, Postoperative view showing reduction of the diastasis and fixation.

ankle, since ossification is prone to occur where chronic irritation takes place (Figs. 581 and 582). The late manifestation of this chronic condition may be quite discouraging. I do not believe there is real justification for removing the ossification, unless there is separation between the tibia and fibula or intractable pain on function, making it advisable to restore the ankle mortice. Probably conservative treatment is better in the ordinary case of ossification. The foot should be carefully strapped to prevent the motion causing the pain.

Diagnosis

History. Since the forces that cause ankle injuries are of such significance in the resulting damage, one must determine, if possible, the exact mechanics of the injury. Was the foot inverted or everted? How did the accident occur? Was disability immediate? Is disability the result of swelling and edema? Was there a primary deformity which was corrected by the patient, a friend or the x-ray technician before making the picture? How long ago did the injury occur? What was the treatment? Has heat or cold been applied? All these factors give important leads not only as to the type and location of injury but also as to its severity.

They may be invaluable guides to the treatment indicated.

Examination. Examination of the injured ankle should be preceded by careful examination of the opposite leg in order that a normal standard may be obtained for comparison. One then proceeds with a meticulous but extremely gentle examination of the involved extremity. If one begins by simple observation, the confidence of the apprehensive patient can be obtained and with it more detailed information. Observation will reveal deformity, the location and amount of swelling, the degree of tension in the skin, and the extent of circulatory impairment. Following observation, by careful palpation one can determine the tension and the degree of swelling. There may be obvious bony crepitation on careful palpation through the skin. Then, by gentle manipulation the pain-free range of motion is determined and a test is made for increased lateral motion. If abnormal lateral motion is elicited, note is made as to whether there is pain on attempting to force lateral motion or dorsiflexion. Any abnormal motion indicates serious ligament or bone injury.

X-ray Examination. Examination by x-rays should be done only after careful clinical examination by the surgeon. If possible, he should examine the foot before the x-ray is

Figure 582. The findings at the time this 20 year old male was first seen were rather nonspecific, except for some swelling of the ankle. The lateral ligament seemed to be entirely intact. He continued to play for the rest of the season, although he could not cut well. X-rays findings were negative. Three months later, (A), x-ray revealed ossification between the tibia and fibula. Relatively immature at this time. He was advised to leave it alone until this became more mature. Examination six months post-injury revealed pain on forced motion, such as sprinting; tenderness along the front of the fibula from about 5 cm. above the ankle upward for about 8 cm. There seemed to be a hard, firm, bony mass here. B, X-ray at this time showed ossification very much more mature, the bone uniting the tibia and the fibula. C, At surgery, revealing the plowshare-shaped mass of bone extending directly forward from the fibula and fastening over to the tibia. Note there is synostosis between the two bones. This mass was completely excised. D, Although four months later he had some x-ray evidence of recurrence of ossification, he was asymptomatic. Since that time he has gone on with good function and is able to play football. It should be pointed out that these exogenous bony masses should be left alone until they mature. If they are, there is a good chance that significant recurrence will not take place.

Figure 583. *A,* The "as is" view. Original film of severe sprain, which illustrates dramatically the nature of this injury, namely ruptured medial collateral ligament and ruptured tibiofibular ligament. Repair of medial ligament and fixation of fibula to tibia by long screw resulted in normal ankle. *B,* After reduction the positioned anteroposterior view showed no pathological changes.

made. X-ray technicians are trained to position extremities in certain standard ways, and often manipulation of the part to get proper position will reduce deformities or screen injuries that might otherwise be obvious. The x-ray technician should be instructed to make the original picture without correction of the position of the foot, the "as is" view, since this may provide an invaluable guide to the degree of injury (Fig. 583). Following this original picture, the foot can be positioned to obtain the standard views. At least three views should be obtained: an anteroposterior of the foot, an anteroposterior of the ankle and a lateral of the ankle and foot. Oblique views are invaluable and may reveal fractures not seen on conventional views (Fig. 584). If abnormal motion can be elicited, an x-ray made with the foot in the abnormal position is of considerable value. If the x-ray examination does not appear to be consistent with the clinical findings, a careful review of all findings must be made. Further x-ray views may be needed to clarify the situation, such as an anteroposterior view in forced dorsiflexion.

Careful attention to all these details of history, physical examination and x-ray visualization will usually permit early diagnosis of a serious injury. Definitive treatment may then be carried out promptly rather than after a period of time pending determination that the

injury is more serious than it was first considered to be. Although the majority of injuries to the ankle are sprains without bone involvement, it is extremely embarrassing to discover after several weeks that treatment was woefully inadequate because of more extensive damage than was recognized at the time.

Here is a useful checklist indicating the common association of injuries. Given certain x-ray findings as indicated, one might expect the corresponding injury to be as follows:

I. Fracture of the fibula above the tibiofibular joint
   A. Lateral side:
      1. Ruptured tibiofibular ligament.
   B. Medial side:
      1. Ruptured medial collateral ligament, or
      2. Fractured medial malleolus.
II. Fracture of the fibula below the joint line
   A. Lateral side:
      1. Fractured lateral malleolus.
   B. Medial side:
      1. Fractured medial malleolus, or
      2. Ruptured deltoid ligament.
III. Fractured medial malleolus
   A. Lateral side:
      1. Ruptured lateral collateral ligament, or
      2. Fractured lateral malleolus.
      3. Ruptured tibiofibular ligament.
         a. Separation between tibia and fibula.
         b. Fractured fibula above the joint line.

Figure 584. Routine anteroposterior (A) and lateral (B) x-rays are apparently negative. Oblique view (C) reveals true condition, namely fracture of medial malleolus and rupture of tibiofibular ligament. In this instance the x-ray examination did not agree with the clinical findings, so further x-ray study was made. This should be treated by reduction and fixation of the fibula to the tibia with a screw. Exact reduction and fixation of the medial malleolus by a screw is vital in this injury.

IV. Separation between tibia and fibula
    A. Lateral side:
        1. Ruptured tibiofibular ligament.
        2. Fractured fibula above tibiofibular syndesmosis.
    B. Medial side:
        1. Ruptured deltoid ligament, or
        2. Fractured medial malleolus.
V. Negative x-ray findings may not indicate serious pathology, but there may be:
    A. Lateral side:
        1. Ruptured lateral collateral ligaments.
        2. Ruptured tibiofibular ligament.
    B. Medial side:
        1. Ruptured deltoid ligament.

Treatment

Before treatment can be properly initiated in any individual case, it is important to classify the injury not only as to type and structures damaged but also as to severity. It is axiomatic that the closer an injury approaches the joint, the more necessary it is to get completely accurate repositioning of the injured structures. One must not be satisfied with incomplete reduction or partial replacement of fractures or dislocations about the ankle any more than about any other joint. Indeed, it is more important to get accurate repositioning in a weight-bearing joint than in the nonweight-bearing joints in the upper extremity.

Complete reduction must be accomplished by the method that will insure the best result, not by the method that at the time seems the most convenient. A little extra care at the time of injury will save a great deal of time and trouble at a later date. It is well known that surgery will be required in a certain percentage of injuries about the ankle joint. Recognizing this fact, it is extremely important that surgery be considered as a method of treatment per primam. If it is going to be necessary for best results, it should be carried out promptly at the time of injury rather than backed into after nonsurgical treatment has failed.

Sprains

Sprains, which constitute the majority of injuries about the ankle, can conveniently be classified into three groups—mild (first degree), moderate (second degree) and severe (third degree). This arbitrary division is subject to a good deal of variation according to the views of the individual physician. The groups will, of necessity, overlap.

Mild (First Degree) Sprain. There is no functional loss and treatment is symptomatic. A mild sprain (Fig. 585A) is one in which there

Figure 585. Drawings showing *A*, partial tear of ligament, mild (first degree) sprain; *B*, moderate (second degree) sprain, with more complete tear but still integrity of ligament; *C*, severe sprain with (third degree) tear and loss of integrity.

has been a partial tear of elements of one of the ligaments at the ankle joint but without any actual functional weakening of the ligament as a whole. In such a case, one would expect to find minimal symptoms: local tenderness, local swelling and mild disability. Indeed, the disability may be so mild that the patient does not even seek advice from a physician.

Examination will reveal no pain on normal motion, no abnormal motion and only a moderate degree of pain on applying the stress that caused the original injury. X-ray examination is normal. This condition requires no extensive treatment and responds dramatically to the local treatment that was so popular a few years ago. Unfortunately, these local methods have been applied in many cases in which they were woefully inadequate.

Local application of ethyl chloride spray tends to break down the cycle of vessel spasm and reduce the local swelling and edema. It has no effect on the strength of the ligament itself or on its healing. This should be kept in mind since, although it does tend to relieve the symptoms, it does not protect the joint against further damage. However, in the mild case, local injection of procaine and hyaluronidase will tend to permit more rapid absorption of the hematoma and to reduce pain. In this sense it is valuable in treatment.

In this group of injuries ideal treatment would be rest with application of ice followed by heat. However, in a mild (first degree) sprain this is usually not necessary. It is not justified if it interferes unnecessarily with the patient's occupation. Local injection followed by adequate strapping (Fig. 586) and a well-fitted shoe are the only treatment measures necessary, since there is no actual weakness of the ankle joint. It should be pointed out again, however, that if one is to permit activity, one must be extremely sure of the diagnosis. It is unwise in any case to use local treatment that relieves the symptoms and then permit the injured person to participate in active sports immediately. A lapse of several hours will help to determine the extent of injury more accurately.

Moderate (Second Degree) Sprain. There is definite loss of strength in the ligament, and treatment is protective. A moderate sprain consists of one in which there has been an actual tear of a portion of the ligament but in which the integrity of the ligament has not been entirely lost (Fig. 585*B*). There is some weakness of the ligament, but no abnormal motion is elicited. Ordinarily, the history is of sharp inversion of the foot followed by a fall with immediate severe pain. The patient is not necessarily wholly incapacitated for walking, since direct weight-bearing does not put a strain on the injured ligament.

Symptoms are usually so severe that medical aid is sought. On examination there is severe pain in the ankle, diffuse swelling throughout the ankle and foot and tenderness over the lateral side of the foot and ankle, usually sharply increased at the area of the damaged ligament. This may be at the attachment of the ligament to the foot, or at the malleolus, or it may be in the substance of the ligament. The patient may tend to hold the foot in an everted position and any attempt to invert the foot beyond this point will cause severe pain. Even normal motion may be painful. An attempt to reproduce the forces that caused the injury will produce severe pain. However, there is no abnormal motion, since some portion of the ligament is still intact. X-ray findings are negative except that they may show a sprain-fracture at one or the other attachments of the ligament (see Fig. 573).

In choosing treatment it should be borne in mind that whereas in the mild sprain there is no weakness and protection is not vital, in the moderate sprain there is definite weakness of the ligament and treatment should be protective. The first aim of treatment is to protect the ankle against further injury until healing occurs, the second to promote repair of the damage already present. Rather mild stresses superimposed on the already weakened ligament may cause complete avulsion.

Treatment consists of local injection of the area with hyaluronidase and procaine, followed by application of a compression bandage and an ice pack for several hours. Relief of symptoms by local injection should not lead to early ambulation or early function of the part, since this will have a detrimental effect upon healing. The patient should stay in bed with a pressure bandage and an ice pack for 10 to 24 hours. At the end of this time, further analysis should be made as to the extent of the injury.

Following the period of ice packing, a posterior and a lateral stirrup boot splint is applied from below the knee to the toes in order to maintain the part in the normal weight-bearing position. The patient is then allowed to get up on crutches but should be advised not to bear weight on the extremity. Several days later, after the swelling subsides, this splint should be replaced by a walking boot cast which may be worn for ten days to three weeks, depending upon the extent of the damage. Active weight-bearing is encouraged as soon as this cast has dried.

It may be argued that a cast handicaps the patient needlessly. Usually, it will be found that in a ligament injury of this degree, the patient will be substantially disabled in any event. He will actually get around more efficiently and with less pain in the walking cast than he will with ordinary wrapping or strapping. Some liberties with this regimen may be permitted in a well-organized training program. For instance, during the early period of protective splinting, the splints may be removed daily for utilization of physical therapy. Whirlpool therapy is not indicated under these circumstances because it allows the foot to be

Figure 586. Typical Gibney strapping. *A*, Shows the patient holding the foot with a loop of muslin to keep it at the right angle and inverted or everted as the case may be, depending on the location of the sprain. *B*, Shows the first strip of 1 inch adhesive tape, which begins well back on the calf, at the bulge of the calf, extending down under the heel and up the opposite side. If the sprain is a lateral sprain the strip should start on the medial side and come to the lateral side. *C*, Shows the other portion of the weave, a strip running from the base of the first toe behind the heel and back to the base of the fifth toe. *D*, Shows application of successive strips, as many as necessary to reach the front of the foot. In the acute case these transverse strips should not overlap in front because of danger of impairment of circulation. If the strapping is for a chronic case in which swelling is not a factor, it would be more secure to overlap the strips in front. The whole is secured by a circumferential strip around the top of the dressing and then further secured by a gauze bandage. It should be emphasized again that in an acute case there should be no circumferential wrapping overlapping on the front of the foot or on the front of the ankle. NOTE: The foot is held at a right angle to the leg and inverted or everted, depending upon the location of the sprain.

A

B

C

D

pendant and so may increase the local swelling. It is not very feasible to remove the walking cast daily, since it is difficult to replace it with sufficient security to permit pain-free weight-bearing. Sometimes in the exceptional case, under ideally controlled circumstances, a very thorough strapping is utilized in place of a walking cast, and this is removed each day for physical therapy and conscientiously replaced when treatment is finished. This should not be accepted for routine treatment. It should be emphasized again that in ordinary practice it is not feasible to remove the splints and cast daily for exercise. Certainly this is not acceptable in the high school program. In those cases the cast should be left intact. There will be no particular trouble with limitation of motion in the high school person. It is unwise to assume that the motion of the ankle will be confined to normal motion unless it is in a very well-controlled, adequately supervised training program which is available in very few high schools.

Following removal of the cast after 10 to 20 days, it is advisable to apply well-fitted adhesive strapping of the Gibney type (see Fig. 586) to protect the ligament against further injury. This strapping should be worn until symptoms are minimal, ordinarily for at least six weeks from the time of injury. If the original injury is treated adequately in this manner, there is little reason to expect recurrent injuries, since the ligament may heal at its normal length and strength. I would like to emphasize again that the ligament injury will heal completely if given adequate opportunity. It takes as long for a ligament to heal as it does a bone. If this is borne in mind and protection is continued for an adequate period, the ligament injury should heal completely and leave no permanent disability.

Severe (Third Degree) Sprain. In a severe, or third degree, sprain there has been a complete rupture of one or more of the ligaments of the ankle so that its function has been completely lost (see Fig. 585C). Treatment here must be restorative to restore the integrity of the ligament and permit it to heal. Either the ligament is torn completely or one or the other of its attachments has pulled loose from the bone. The history will be essentially the same as for moderate sprain, but all complaints will be more severe. The patient will frequently volunteer the information that the foot had been out of place but was reduced by manipulation, and that pain was relieved by the reduction.

Examination will reveal more serious and extensive findings than in the other groups of sprains. The swelling is more extreme. The pain is more severe. The patient resists any attempt to move the foot and is extremely apprehensive. If the foot is examined very early, abnormal motion may be elicited without undue pain. It is justifiable, in certain cases, to inject procaine into the painful area or even to induce short general anesthesia in order to determine whether or not there is complete disruption of one of the ligaments of the ankle joint. An x-ray should be made in the abnormal position if possible (see Fig. 583A). These cases are relatively infrequent, but when they occur the consequences may be extremely disastrous if the true condition is not recognized and appropriate treatment instituted. Many of the most disabling injuries reveal no demonstrable fracture but are caused by dislocation. Ligament injury may be extremely severe.

An example of these serious injuries to the ankle is disruption of the medial collateral and tibiofibular ligaments, in which case the x-ray findings may be completely negative (see Fig. 583B). Also the external collateral ligament may be completely torn and yet the x-ray picture may appear normal. One must recognize the exact condition present in order to plan the best treatment, which obviously must be far more comprehensive than that for an ordinary sprain of the ankle. For this reason the diagnosis must be made at the earliest possible moment. If surgical repair of the ligament is to be carried out, it must be done promptly in order to secure the best results. If there is a complete severance of the medial collateral or tibiofibular ligament, or both, surgical treatment is certainly the treatment of choice.

Complete avulsion of the external collateral ligament has customarily been treated by simple immobilization, since it is relatively easy to protect the foot against inversion by splints in an everted position. However, there is no more reason to expect these completely torn ligament ends to fall together on the lateral side of the foot than there is elsewhere. The typical patient in whom the injury is treated nonsurgically goes on to have repeated sprains caused by the overlength of the ligament. He can tolerate this to some extent, since this ligament does not support the weight of the body, but it is extremely distressing to someone who wants to play tennis, handball or any other active sport to have recurrent, relatively minor injuries. If it can be determined that a complete tear of this ligament is present, surgical repair not only will speed recovery but also will improve the probability of obtaining a perfect functional result.

The warning is explicit that in these serious injuries one must not temporize but must decide quickly whether or not surgery is indicated. The time to carry out an operation is at the earliest possible moment after the need for one is determined. While late surgery is not nearly as favorable as early operation, it should not be refused simply because the diagnosis was not made at the time of the injury (Fig. 587). However, we have found that if surgery is postponed, after two or three weeks it is impossible to define the ligament ends and under these circumstances reconstruction is necessary to obtain support for the collateral ligaments from some other source. Late repair

is usually not successful, but reconstruction may be (Fig. 588).

If nonsurgical treatment is chosen, then the same treatment is indicated as for a moderate sprain, namely, local injection, compression, ice packs, splints, a walking cast and adhesive strapping. All these treatment phases must be somewhat more extensive and protection must be continued for eight to ten weeks, since there is marked functional loss in the ligament. If such a long period of immobilization is required, formal rehabilitation becomes necessary. Usually rehabilitation is required in direct proportion to the length of time it was necessary to immobilize the joint.

Following operative repair, posterior and lateral below-knee stirrup splints are applied for about two weeks. Then stitches are removed and a walking boot cast is applied, which the patient wears for an additional four

Figure 587. Fracture of tip of lateral malleolus with nonunion, resulting pain and disability from involvement of peroneal tendons as well as the lateral collateral ligament. This patient was treated without immobilization. This is in reality a sprain-fracture, the tip having been avulsed by the lateral collateral ligament. Surgical removal of the fragment resulted in marked improvement. Early surgery should have given complete recovery. A, Illustration of the value of the oblique view. Drawing in insert shows the pathological condition clearly. Note the avulsion is not of the extreme tip of the fibula, which is where the ligament attaches. B, Stress film demonstrating no instability.

weeks. Even six weeks is an inadequate time for healing to occur, but after six weeks careful adhesive strapping should give enough support so that rehabilitation can commence. Actually, rehabilitation will be far less necessary if a walking cast has been used, since the muscles in the extremity that are not immobilized by the cast will be in good condition. I do not believe the oft-repeated statement that "ligament injuries are worse than fractures." This aphorism has arisen from the fact that serious ligament injuries have been undertreated and so the consequences have been more severe than those from an adequately treated fracture. Careful investigation of the patient having painful recurrent sprains of the ankle will probably uncover an initial injury that was treated inadequately (see Fig. 588).

Fractures

I have noted earlier that while the most common injury to the ankle is sprain and is an inversion injury, the most common eversion injury to the ankle is actually a fracture. The two most important factors in the treatment of fractures about the ankle are: (1) maintenance of the integrity of the ankle mortice, and (2) complete re-establishment of the weight-bearing surfaces of the talus and tibia.

Uncorrected separation between the tibia and fibula with corresponding widening of the ankle mortice is not compatible with normal ankle function. While irregularity of the weight-bearing surface is usually quite obvious on x-ray examination, separation of the ankle mortice may not be so readily apparent. It is extremely important that one carefully analyze the relationship between the tibia and fibula in order to determine whether there is separation between the two with widening of the mortice. Actually, the vast majority of fractures around the ankle are malleolar fractures. If they are complete, they have been accompanied by some dislocation of the ankle.

If there is a fracture of the lateral malleolus with displacement and with no fracture of the medial malleolus, there is usually avulsion of the medial collateral ligament. If there is a fracture of the medial malleolus by an inversion force, an avulsion of the lateral ligament must be present. If there has been a fracture of the medial malleolus because of an eversion force, either the lateral malleolus must be broken or the tibiofibular ligament must be ruptured. The same force that causes a bimalleolar fracture may cause fracture of the medial malleolus with a ruptured tibiofibular ligament, or it may cause rupture of the medial and the tibiofibular ligaments with no fracture at all (Fig. 589A). Thus, it can be seen that the treatment of ligament injuries and fractures of the ankle cannot be separated. If the two basic goals are borne in mind, namely, the integrity of the ankle mortice and the restoration of normal weight-bearing surfaces, the type of treatment indicated is clear. Actually, it is not common for the weight-bearing surfaces to be involved. Ordinarily the lower end of the tibia and the upper surface of the talus

Figure 588. This 19 year old received an injury to his right ankle two years ago, which was seen here four months post-injury with complete instability of the lateral collateral ligament. A Watson-Jones reconstruction was done four months after the injury, resulting in good stability. The opposite (*left*) ankle then had an identical situation. He hurt his left ankle one year ago and received the same casual treatment which he had received on the first injury and again had complete loss of the lateral collateral ligament. *A*, Anteroposterior view of both ankles. Note hole for the reconstruction in right fibula. *B*, Stress film on both sides. Right shows good stability with tilt within the acceptable range. Left shows complete dislocation of the talus out of the mortice. The stress film on the right originally looked exactly like the present film on the left. More thorough treatment of the original injury might have prevented this chronic instability. The left ankle has now received a similar type of reconstruction of the lateral collateral ligaments with good stability.

Figure 589, Case A. This 20 year old male received an injury playing football when his foot was forced out and his leg forced in. He had immediate swelling, diagnosed as sprain. A, Eight hours after the injury he had tremendous swelling of the calf, foot and thigh, with definite lateral instability of the ankle. B, X-ray shows lateral displacement of the talus on the tibia, with separation of the distal tibiofibular ligaments and ruptured deltoid ligament. At surgery the posterior tibial tendon was lying between the talus and the malleolus, preventing reduction. The deltoid ligament was completely torn and was treated by direct suture. C, Since it was completely dislocated, I thought it would be more secure to have two screws across the tibia and fibula rather than the ordinary one screw fixation. His postoperative course was satisfactory. Three months postoperative he had no complaint except soreness over the end of the screws. The screws were removed five months postoperative. He returned to full activity, including football.

(Continued on the following page)

Figure 589, Case B. Bimalleolar fracture with adequate internal fixation. In this instance the lateral screw transfixes the fibular fracture site and enters the tibia, coming through medially far enough that it can be removed from the opposite side if it breaks. In other instances an intramedullary pin may be placed in the fibula if the tibiofibular ligament is intact.

are not fractured in ankle injuries, so that the fracture that is actually being discussed here is the malleolar fracture. This is caused by the same forces that cause sprains.

In bimalleolar fractures, it is virtually impossible to obtain and maintain accurate reposition of both malleoli without internal fixation in at least one of them. In these cases, internal fixation has long been the rule. The excellent results obtained by this method have encouraged me to apply it to injuries that are apparently less severe. With fracture of the medial malleolus accompanied by a tibiofibular separation, I feel that open reduction should be carried out, and the internal malleolus accurately replaced and held by screw or some other method of fixation (see Fig. 589*B*). At the same time, the tibia and fibula should be held together by a long metal screw transfixing the lower fibula and crossing both cortices of the tibia. Since it has been demonstrated that under normal usage there is definite motion in the distal tibiofibular joint, I consider it advisable to remove the screw that holds the tibia and fibula together after a suitable interval for healing of the tibiofibular ligament. This period is usually between 8 and 12 weeks. It is not unusual for the screw to break when normal activity is resumed earlier. If this happens it is extremely difficult to remove the tibial

Figure 590. *A*, Fracture-dislocation of the ankle, treated by two transfixion screws. Note that the upper screw is broken whereas the one which is slightly bent is intact. *B*, The screws were later removed, but the broken screw was inaccessible. Note that it has freed itself from the fibula by forming a cul-de-sac in the bone around the screw, thus permitting normal tibiofibular motion. (This was visualized even better in the lateral view.)

section of the screw (Fig. 590). This is of little consequence unless the metal is reactive, since once the screw breaks normal motion is permitted and it is usually not necessary to remove either part of the broken screw. If the injury is a fracture of both malleoli, it is better to use internal fixation on both sides.

Surgical treatment should be carried out only by one well versed in the anatomy of the ankle. The proper surgical environment is a *sine qua non* to success. Although the techniques of these various surgical procedures are available elsewhere, a brief description may be useful in order to emphasize some of the vital factors involved in the different situations.

Medial Side. If the injury is a fracture of the medial malleolus, I prefer to make a linear incision beginning 2 in. above the tip of the medial malleolus, extending downward along the posterior medial border of the tibia to the tip of the medial malleolus. The incision then should swing forward and downward directly along the line of the posterior tibial tendon as far as the tubercle of the navicular. Once this flap is reflected forward, taking care to include all the subcutaneous tissue in the flap, the whole malleolus will be exposed. One must not bring the incision forward beneath the medial malleolus but should extend it downward parallel to the posterior tibial tendon toward the navicular tubercle. Otherwise, great difficulty may be encountered in exposing enough of the area below the malleolus to permit the insertion of the internal fixation. It is necessary to sacrifice the posterior branch of the saphenous vein in this incision.

After the flap is reflected, the fracture is defined and the fracture line is exposed. Great care must be taken to remove all soft tissue which is frequently found interposed into the fracture site. By displacing the malleolar fragment it is possible to visualize the medial portion of the talus, including its neck. By retracting the capsular incision forward it is possible to expose a good portion of the dome of the talus, and by plantar flexing the foot one can make an even more extensive examination, including the leading edge of the distal end of the tibia. Careful search here may well reveal osteochondral fractures of the talus or of the tibia which are not demonstrated on the x-ray.

When one is satisfied that the joint does not contain any foreign bodies or any other fracture line, the wound should be copiously lavaged with saline. The malleolus then should be fitted meticulously into position. This must be done with hairline accuracy. The articular cartilage extending from the malleolus onto the tibia should be exposed to be sure that ıt is in direct continuity. The fragment may then be held in this position with a Bishop clamp or some similar type of tenaculum; it is very difficult to hold manually. Fixation is then inserted.

If the fragment permits, it is desirable to use two screws at slightly divergent angles. Each must pass through the medial malleolus, across the fracture line, traverse the tibia and penetrate its opposite cortex (see Fig. 589, Case B). This requires a relatively long screw but does give much better fixation, particularly in older people in whom the cancellous bone may seem quite inadequate for fixation. If one uses a single screw, the fragment will often rock or rotate and the exact repositioning may be lost. After one is certain that the fragment is securely held in position and will stand a considerable degree of manipulation of the foot, the wound is closed in layers. It is possible to use various other appliances to fix the medial malleolus, but I prefer the long screw. On occasion the malleolus fragment may be very small and include the articular portion only. This makes it very difficult to screw from below. In this instance retrograde screws can be placed from the tibia into the fragment with less disruption of the fragment and the deltoid ligament.

Medial Approach—Repair of the Deltoid Ligament. This incision is similar to that for the medial malleolus except that it is carried somewhat more distally before it is brought forward across to the tubercle of the navicular. If the incision is extended a little bit further distally before it is extended forward, the deltoid ligament is more readily available, particularly if it happens to be torn beneath and behind the tendons. The pathology is carefully defined by meticulous dissection with minimal damage to any of the ligament fibers. If the ligament is pulled off the malleolus, as it frequently is, it is best replaced by mattress sutures, imbricated through the ligament so as to get firm security, and then passed through multiple drill holes placed in the blunt end of the medial malleolus. My preference here is to use No. 0 cotton and to have at least three and possibly four mattress loops. If the deepest, most lateral portion of the ligament is damaged beneath the tendon bed, this should be carefully sutured by inverted sutures, leaving the knot buried in the ligament. When all the sutures are placed, the tendon sheath is closed. It is extremely important to repair all the components of the ligament so that the edges accurately appose. Occasionally the fracture in the medial malleolus may be such that it is difficult or impossible to get fixation screws from the malleolus upward into the tibia.

Lateral Approach. The preferable incision for exposing the lateral malleolus and the lateral collateral ligament parallels the posterior border of the fibula and extends down across the tip of the fibula to swing along the line of the peroneal tendons toward the base of the fifth metatarsal bone. Reflecting this flap forward, together with all the subcutaneous tissue, exposes the various components of the fibular collateral ligament. The ligament then should be carefully defined and replaced with as many stitches as are necessary to appose the various fibers. Actually, the ligament is such that No. 0 cotton is probably adequate. Stronger suture tends to necrose the ligament if it is tied too tightly. After all the components are carefully sutured, the wound is closed in the usual manner.

Lateral Malleolar Fracture. The same incision may be used for fixation of the lateral malleolus. It may need to be extended proximally if the fracture is higher up the shaft. It may not be necessary to use the distal curved portion in this instance. There are various ways to fix the fracture of the malleolus. These vary according to circumstances. If the fracture is transverse at the level of the line of the joint, some sort of intramedullary fixation is preferable, either with a long screw, a threaded pin or even a smooth type Steinman pin drilled up the fibula from the distal end. In this instance the tibiofibular ligament is not involved and good stability can be obtained in the malleolar fragment by intramedullary fixation.

If the fracture is oblique and through the tibiofibular joint, as it often is, with the fracture line oblique from above downward and inward, it is probably better fixed by a long screw through the distal fragment crossing the tibiofibular synchondrosis and tibia to engage the opposite cortex of the tibia (see Fig. 589, Case B).

If the fracture is above the tibiofibular joint and there is tibiofibular separation, it is not adequate to use simple intramedullary fixation. In this case, the most important consideration is to get fixation between the tibia and the fibula. This is best obtained by placing a long screw just above this synchondrosis. It should traverse the fibula and both cortices of the tibia, taking care not to overcorrect the fibula

at this level (see Fig. 590). If the screw happens to be a little high, it may pull the fibula too close to the tibia and so tilt the tip of the malleolus outward and defeat the purpose of making a stable mortice.

If it is a gross fracture-dislocation with major instability, it may be advisable to put a plate on the fibular fracture above to obtain stability of the fibula. This is not often the case in athletic injuries.

Of primary importance in open reduction for a fractured fibula with separation between the tibia and fibula is to be sure that there is no foreign material between the two bones. If the two bones do not completely appose, as checked by x-ray on the operating table, the fracture line and the syndesmosis should be explored and all intervening tissue removed. As indicated on the medial side, if the joint is involved it should be inspected as far as possible by displacing the fragment and determining whether or not there is damage to the articular cartilage of the talus, lateral tibia or lateral malleolus.

Following surgical repair, postoperative fixation should be by posterior and lateral stirrup splints (see Fig. 452). Under ordinary circumstances it is better to extend these splints above the knee for at least two weeks while the wound is healing. At the end of that time a cast is applied. A decision must be made whether or not to put on a walking heel and whether or not the cast needs to extend above the knee (see Fig. 454). This depends on the stability of the internal fixation. If there is any danger of displacement of any of the fragments or stress on any of the repaired ligaments by rotation of the foot and leg at the knee, the cast fixation must extend above the knee. For example, an injury involving a ruptured deltoid ligament and tibiofibular ligament should not be subjected to weight-bearing this soon. Weight-bearing in a walking cast should not be permitted if any weight-bearing bone is involved. Some judgment is required in the utilization of a walking cast to be sure that the cast gives proper fixation. This is much more easily done with a patient who is long-legged and slender than it is with one who is short and fat. It is always better to err on the side of adequate protection if there is any question about whether or not protection should be extended above the knee. If you bear in mind that it requires 10 to 12 weeks for a ligament to heal, even with partial strength, and that simple subsidence of symptoms is not an indication that healing is complete, the importance of adequate protection is clear. We have a guide for healing in fractures, and they should be carefully checked by x-ray for degree of union. Following removal of the plaster fixation, the ankle must be protected against unusual stress by either taping, elastic bandaging or wrapping.

Since in many instances open surgery may be simpler to carry out and easier to manage postoperatively than manipulative treatment, it follows that adequate training is essential before any physician should attempt to manage a serious fracture or dislocation about a joint.

Only by extreme care in examination, conscientious selection of the best method of treatment and thorough preparation in technique can one expect to obtain optimum results in treatment of injuries about the ankle.

EXOSTOSES

Exostosis in its various manifestations appears quite frequently about the ankle and foot; in fact, it is seen so frequently on the top of the talus and the front of the tibia that it has been described as a separate entity, namely, *talotibial exostosis.* An exostosis should be distinguished from a marginal osteophyte. An exostosis is an actual piling up of bone at the site of the irritative lesion, whereas the marginal osteophyte is an osteochondral ridge developing at the joint margin as a result of a chronic synovitis or chronic arthritic change. An exostosis will characteristically develop as a response to direct trauma so that it may be seen on the back or front of the lower margin of the tibia, or less frequently in front of the medial malleolus or of the lateral mal-

Figure 591. *A,* X-ray showing talotibial spurs, 3 plus. *B,* X-ray showing impingement occurring when the foot is dorsiflexed.

Figure 592. Roentgenograms showing the area of opposition between the tibia and the talus. *A*, The foot in a neutral position. *B*, The foot in dorsiflexion. *C*, The foot in hyperdorsiflexion.

leolus as the result of impingement of the talus. On the talus the exostosis forms just back of the head superiorly (Fig. 591). Here the trauma results from repeated overflexion or overextension, overinversion or overeversion of the ankle joint beyond its ordinary range. For example, when the foot is driven into dorsiflexion, the leading edge of the tibia impinges against the concavity of the neck of the

talus. The resulting irritation causes a piling up of bone that simply serves to aggravate the condition.

It will be recalled that in extreme dorsiflexion of the foot, the anterior lip of the tibia nestles into the sulcus, which is located on top of the talus between its body and head. It should be noted that the leading edge of the lower end of the tibia normally inclines back-

Figure 593. Avulsion of the capsular attachment on top of the talus, together with fragment of bone 18 months after injury. This probably was a relatively big fragment to start with. The patient's complaint now is on forceful running, which impinges the fragment against the lower end of the tibia, similar to a talotibial spur. This is not the typical impinging exostosis in the athlete.

ward in order to prevent impingement against the talus during dorsiflexion (Fig. 592). There actually is no true ligamentous attachment at either of these locations. The anterior capsule of the joint attaches slightly higher on the tibia and runs forward to the navicular bone, with little attachment to the superior surface of the neck of the talus. Spur formation in this region is the result of direct trauma during forcible dorsiflexion of the foot on the leg. It is not the late result of a ligament injury caused by extreme plantar flexion at the ankle, so-called traction sprain. The injury occurs not during ordinary running but during the "drive" of the athlete when his cleats are fixed to the ground with the foot forcibly dorsiflexed and the neck of the talus in direct apposition of the tibia (Figs. 591 to 593).

In many instances, much more often than is usually noted, the reaction to direct trauma during such "driving" running is the formation of bone at the area of impingement. This reaction apparently is similar to the formation of calluses on the skin. This mass has an adverse rather than a protective effect, however, for as more bone is piled up the impingement occurs more easily, and so a vicious cycle begins, resulting in gradually increasing disability.

Characteristically, the player loses his "drive." As a rule, he has rather vague complaints which do not seem sufficient to account for his disability. Ordinary examination reveals little; there is no swelling, no pain on inversion or eversion of the foot, and no tenderness around the malleoli. The impression grows among teammates and coaches that the player is "dogging it." This is especially likely because

he can often run, cut and jump without pain so long as he does not go at full speed. The result may well be disappointment of the coaches, disheartenment of the player, and the ultimate blighting of an otherwise promising athletic career.

Such a patient presents with a history of aching pain in the ankle that is sharply increased by "driving," often to the point that he feels he cannot "go all out." He is unable to explain his failure to get that extra push that differentiates the star from the ordinary athlete. He simply realizes that his previous speed and force have been unaccountably diminished.

Examination will almost uniformly elicit particular findings. One is pain on forcible dorsiflexion of the foot—an impingement type of pain located at the anterior talotibial sulcus. Another is pinpoint tenderness directly over the spur on the talus or tibia. Roentgenographic examination will reveal that the anterior margin of the lower end of the tibia has lost its slanted character and that the edge is sharp, often with an identifiable exostosis extending forward over the articular surface of the talus (see Fig. 591A). The condition may vary from a simple change in contour to a spur a centimeter or more long. This spur extends along the whole width of the bone and is in reality a ledge rather than a spur. In addition, an exostosis of a greater or lesser size may appear on the top of the neck of the talus. Upon dorsiflexion of the foot, the two will be seen to impinge (see Fig. 591B). Either one or both of these exostoses may be present.

These prominences are relatively small in the early stages but may be tremendous in the

Figure 594. Advanced tibiotalar exostoses. Note fragmentation between talus and fibula. The tarsal joints are not degenerative. This is not degenerative arthritis. Note normal tibiotalar joint space.

later stages, at which time the diagnosis becomes obvious. The condition may extend onto the front of the medial malleolus and, rarely, to the anterior edge of the fibula; in severe cases it may also occur in other areas of the foot in which there are impinging bones, such as the posterior part of the ankle. These exostoses appear to be similar to but are not etiologically the same as the spurring that is found on adjacent articular surfaces such as the metatarsal-cuneiform joints. The latter condition is almost always accompanied by degenerative change in the articular cartilage and an actual narrowing of the joint space and falls into the category of chronic arthritic change or so-called marginal osteophytes. This is not the condition to which we are referring when we speak of impingement exostoses of the talus and tibia. The typical impingement exostosis is most common at the anterior edge of the tibia and neck of the talus and is not accompanied by marginal osteophytes, degenerative changes (Fig. 594), or other signs of chronic joint involvement. This is reflected in the prognosis since the result, from an athletic viewpoint, can hardly be classed as excellent if degenerative changes in the foot and ankle or, in fact, any other changes persist. The conditions may coexist, but one is not necessarily the forerunner of the other. When severe, the impingement exostosis may be extremely disabling, precluding athletics or any real activity. In some instances the spur is broken off and is found as a loose body lying on top of the talar neck or elsewhere. As such, it may cause acute disability in an ankle already chronically impaired.

It seems doubtful that the condition is initiated by repeated mild sprain of the very weak anterior capsule. Rather, it would appear that the reaction is initiated by repeated mild trauma caused by direct impingement and is often made severe by acute injury. There seems no question that repeated insult is the definitive factor in this progressive syndrome.

In order to determine the frequency of talotibial exostosis, we checked a long series of students of the same age group and of the same general characteristics. One half of them were scholarship athletes and one half were nonathletes. We found that the presence of talotibial spurring was much more frequent in the athletes (Table 20–1), 45 per cent of whom had some degree of spurring, while only 15 per cent of the nonathletes did. It should be understood that these were all asymptomatic cases.

The mere presence of a spur is not justification for *treatment*, since the great majority of them are completely asymptomatic. Surgical treatment is highly successful in young, healthy adult males provided the proper indications for it are present. The athlete is, of course, the one to whom surgical correction has the most appeal, since if he has to restrict his activity he is no longer an athlete. On the other hand, the casual player may well prefer to give up his athletic activities rather than to submit to surgical correction.

Surgical Treatment

In the ordinary case, an anterolateral approach will suffice to remove both talar and tibial exostoses (Fig. 595). However, in some cases it will be necessary to make both medial and lateral incisions, and occasionally a posterior exposure will be necessary.

Anterolateral Approach. After the usual preparation and the application of a tourniquet, a skin incision is made just lateral and parallel to the peroneus tertius tendon, beginning about 4 cm. proximal to the articular surface of the tibia and extending distally for approximately 7.5 cm (see Fig. 595A). The extensor tendons are retracted medially (see Fig. 595B), and the incision is carried through the very weak anterior capsule of the ankle joint, including the anterior fasciculus of the talofibular ligament. It is not ordinarily necessary to disturb the short extensor muscles, nor is it necessary to clean out the sinus tarsi. After the capsule has been opened, the anterior articular lip of the tibia is readily apparent, and by firm retraction the neck of the talus may be exposed (see Fig. 595C). Using a sharp osteotome, the exostosis along the lower portion of the tibia is carefully removed and the posterior inclination of the surface restored. The front edge of the lateral malleolus is visualized, and any spurring found is removed. The exostosis on the neck of the talus is best removed by means of a gouge shaped to conform to the concavity of the neck; a small osteotome is also useful. The roughened bone is very carefully smoothed and all fragments removed. The area is then thoroughly lavaged and the raw bone surfaces are sealed with bone wax. Following this, the wound, including the divided ligament, is closed in layers.

Medial Approach. The incision on the medial side begins 2.5 cm. above the lower end of the tibia, just medial and parallel to the

Table 20-1. Roentgenographic Findings in a Survey of the Ankles
of 120 Athletes and Non-Athletes

ATHLETES		NON-ATHLETES	
No exostosis	66 (55%)	No exostosis	101 (84.2%)
Exostoses in only one bone		Exostoses in only one bone	
Talar		Talar	
Grade 1 14		Grade 1 8	
Grade 2 3		Grade 2 1	
17 (14.2%)		9 (7.5%)	
Tibial		Tibial	
Grade 1 4 (3.3%)		Grade 1 6 (5%)	
	21 (17.5%)		15 (12.5%)
Exostoses in both bones		Exostoses in both bones	
Grade 1 22		Grade 1 2	
Grade 2 7		Grade 2 2	
Grade 3 4			
	33 (27.5%)		4 (3.3%)
Total	120 (100%)	Total	120 (100%)

(From the Journal of Bone and Joint Surgery. Vol. 39-A, p. 851.)

anterior tibial tendon. The incision extends distally to the posterior edge of the navicular. The saphenous vein may be retracted by cutting either its anterior or its posterior branch, and ready access may be had to the front of the ankle by opening the capsule. The procedures described in the previous section for the removal of the exostoses are then carried out.

The medial malleolus and the medial border of the talus are examined by digital palpation. If spurring is found, a portion of the deltoid ligament may be divided in order to obtain better access to the area involved. The same method of closure is used as on the opposite side.

Following these procedures, posterior and lateral stirrup splints are applied from below the knee to the toes, with the foot in neutral lateral position and in 90 degrees of dorsiflexion. After ten days the stitches are removed and a walking cast is applied, to be worn for another ten days. Following removal of this cast, three weeks after the operation, further support is used only as indicated. An elastic

Figure 595. Anterolateral approach: A, The skin incision. B, The skin has been separated, exposing the lateral edge of the extensor tendons. C, The tendon and muscles have been retracted and the capsule has been opened, exposing the spurs.

bandage may be useful if swelling persists, but it is urged that active use, in fact, unlimited activity, be begun as quickly as possible.

It should be re-emphasized that the condition we are calling talotibial exostosis is not accompanied by degenerative changes in the joint. Frequently, as mentioned previously, the ankle joint will be surrounded by marginal osteophytes resulting from chronic degenerative changes in the articular cartilage. These are characterized by roughened joint space, eburnated articular cartilage, chronic pain in the joint and an altogether different picture than that of exostosis. Prognostically there is a vast difference, since cleaning up of the marginal osteophytes has little effect upon the chronic arthritis that is present and will as a rule prove disappointing. It may be necessary if the osteophyte is large or fragmented, but one should not be misled into believing that the ankle will be wholly cured by removing the loose fragment from a degenerative joint. This condition (marginal osteophytes) is also quite frequent in the joints of the foot and will be discussed in that section.

CHONDRAL FRACTURE (OSTEOCHONDRITIS DISSECANS)

Osteochondral fractures have not been recognized as frequently in the ankle as in the knee. It is probably true that they do not occur as frequently. I am sure, however, that a great many more cases are overlooked than are recognized, since the lesion is readily confused with an ankle sprain followed by traumatic arthritis in the ankle. The most common cause of the condition is trauma. By far the most frequent location for chondral fracture of the ankle is the dome of the talus, where it occurs either on the superolateral margin of the talus, usually in a central location, or on the superomedial margin of the talus, usually posteriorly.

The mechanism of the injury has been described by many authors. It is an inversion type of injury (Fig. 596). Dorsiflexion of the foot forces the broader anterior part of the body of the talus deeper into the tibiofibular mortice, so that there is snug contact between the long lateral malleolus and the lateral sur-

Figure 596. Osteochondritis dissecans showing mechanisms of injury. (Journal of Bone and Joint Surgery, Vol. 41-A, 1959; A. L. Berndt and Michael Hardy.)

Figure 597. Chondral fracture of superolateral border of the talus. This is an inversion injury catching the corner of the talus against the fibula.

face of the talus. If sharp inversion occurs in this position, the superior margin of the talus impinges forcibly against the side of the fibula. The resulting lesion is a snubbing type of fracture in which the cartilage of the superior surface of the talus is "peeled off" the subchondral bone, usually taking a greater or lesser fragment of bone with it. The resulting lesion is a flap of cartilage similar to a piece of linoleum being peeled off the floor. The force may be strong enough to actually dislodge the whole fragment or may simply hinge it upward, leaving the medial portion of the cartilage flap intact (Fig. 597).

As it drives the talus against the side of the fibula, this same inversion force may cause chondral damage to the medial side of the lateral malleolus. The fibular cartilage may be damaged (Fig. 598), but is much less likely to be, because there is no margin or edge to be peeled away. I recall one patient with an extremely resistant ankle injury with symptoms along the anterior talofibular fissure in which surgical exposure revealed a completely loose fragment of articular cartilage with a corresponding defect in the fibular articular surface.

When the lesion of the dome of the talus (Fig. 599) is on the medial side, the cause, strangely enough, also appears to be an inversion injury. Since it is found at the back end of the superior surface of the talus, one must assume that it thus occurs in plantar flexion when the weight of the body is on the narrow posterior portion of the talus. In this position of the ankle joint, the talus may rock to a considerable degree before any tension is placed on the collateral ligaments, since the narrow posterior width of the talus does not provide good bony stability in the too-wide mortice. Landing from a jump may cause direct trauma to a relatively small area, the typical instance being the basketball player who leaps in the air and lands on his toes with his foot slightly inverted. The mechanism in this instance is a compression type which dislodges the talar cartilage, together with some subchondral bone, quite similar to that which occurs at the knee following a direct blow on the patella with the knee flexed. These osteochondral fractures may occur at other places in the ankle or foot (Fig. 600). I do not recall having seen a case involving the head of the talus unless there was an actual fracture of the talar head in which a relatively larger fragment of cartilage and bone was broken off.

Osteochondral fracture occasionally occurs at the superior margin of the posterior articular surface of the navicular bone. The x-ray appearance of the small fragment is characteristic; there is a translucent area between it and the parent bone, giving a scooped-out appearance at the cartilage surface (Fig. 601). One must assume that these same fractures occur on the inferior surface of the talus and on the superior surface of the calcaneus, but if so they are difficult to recognize and must be rare.

The most important single factor in diagnosis of these injuries is an acute awareness that they occur. It is recommended that in any injury to the ankle, x-ray study should be made even though the injury does not appear to be severe. I know of no way to diagnose these conditions in the acute stage except by x-ray examination. We have for many years insisted upon x-ray studies. Perhaps it has not been emphasized enough that the films should be adequately studied after they are made. When these injuries occur they are often seen as emergencies, and the films are frequently taken by a substitute technician. These films may be examined briefly without detailed study for chondral damage. Such casual observation will not reveal these lesions. Injuries to the ankle and foot should be x-rayed in at least three positions, namely, an anteroposterior view of the ankle, an anteroposterior view of

Figure 598. Osteochondral fracture of the articular cartilage of the fibula, old. *A,* The fragment is rounded off and displaced downward. *B,* Following removal.

Figure 599. An 18 year old baseball pitcher with persistent "sprain" of both ankles. He had had extensive treatment for sprain with prompt recurrence of symptoms on resumption of activity. Examination revealed none of the classic symptoms of sprain. In fact, interim examination was essentially negative, except for some discomfort on forced inversion. X-ray revealed chondral fractures of the superomedial angle of the talus of each ankle. Surgery through *A,* an anteromedial incision parallel to the anterior tibial tendon, exposed a normal talar cartilage. *B,* Plantar flexion of the foot revealed a chondral fracture with nonunion. *C,* This was a large fragment with only a very small segment of bone attached. It was removed, leaving a wide gap. *D,* The sclerotic bed after curettement, being drilled with multiple drill holes with a K-wire. This patient resumed baseball pitching after a few months without symptoms. Earlier diagnosis might have saved many disheartening months.

Figure 600. Osteochondral fragment between medial malleolus and talus. This is not in the deltoid ligament. There is also a fragment lying between the fibula and the talus. Removal of these fragments gave substantial relief.

Figure 601. A, Chondral fracture of navicular. B, Patient treated for sprain of the foot for many months primarily by manipulation and physical therapy. Note fracture through the tubercle of the navicular, unrecognized. Also note extreme atrophy in spite of misguided efforts at making him exercise. Removal of the fragment resulted in gradual improvement. Apparently both of these conditions were from the same injury. The talar tubercle fracture is not an accessory navicular bone.

the foot and a lateral view showing foot and ankle. If there is the slightest doubt about complete visualization, oblique views should also be done. In studying the film one should carefully outline each involved bone as a separate entity. Mentally or actually with a pencil, one should follow along the line of the superior dome of the talus, being particularly careful where it superimposes over the tibia. The appearance of a cloudy shadow, any type of irregularity or any extra fissure line demands further study from different angles.

Many of these cases are not suspected until the so-called sprain has not responded well to treatment. Indeed, the majority of them will not be examined by a doctor in the early stages, since the sprain itself may be relatively minor. These fractures, particularly those of the medial surface of the talus, may occur without any actual tearing of the ligaments of the ankle. The usual history is for the patient to present with a painful ankle which has resisted all the usual modalities of treatment. Sometimes the treatment for the original injury was quite inadequate (Fig. 602). At other times completely adequate treatment for a sprain has been carried out. In spite of the measures used, the symptoms persist much longer than they should in a sprain. Careful examination at this time will soon determine that one is not dealing with a "chronic sprain" of the ankle. There is no tenderness along the lateral collateral ligaments. There are no symptoms involv-

ing the tip of the lateral malleolus or along the cuboid or superolateral surface of the foot. The local symptoms, if any, will actually be in the ankle joint, either at the anterolateral confluence of the talus, tibia and fibula or along a similar area on the posteromedial side of the joint. A patient presenting with chronic symptoms that are aggravated by activity and that subside almost completely with rest very frequently is suffering from an osteochondral fracture. By that time the condition which we identify as osteochondritis dissecans (although it is neither dissecting nor an osteochondritis) may be present. Careful x-ray study will reveal the typical appearance, with a crater in the articular surface usually occupied by a line of opacity surrounded by an area of radiolucency (Fig. 603). In many instances only the crater appears, since the fragment may be dislodged from the bone or may not throw enough shadow to show in the film. This is particularly true in cases of some duration. One should not withhold treatment simply because the opacity is not present.

Treatment. It is my opinion that, in the vast majority of cases, treatment is surgical. True enough, we have learned (particularly at the knee and also at some non-weight-bearing joints) that a prolonged period of protection against weight-bearing may permit these conditions to heal, particularly in the young individual. It has been suggested by some that this period should be at least six months and by

Figure 602. Case treated elsewhere for rupture of deltoid and tibiofibular ligament. Patient remained symptomatic. Examination of x-rays revealed chondral fracture of the superomedial surface of the talus. The patient improved after removal of this fragment and removal of the screw. Note incomplete reduction of tibiofibular diastasis.

Figure 603. Osteochondritis dissecans of the superolateral portion of the talus. *Left,* Arrow shows fragment in oblique view. *Right,* Anteroposterior view finding was negative.

others as long as a year. In my experience, the success of conservative treatment has not been great enough to justify denying weight-bearing on the ankle to an active young athlete for a period of a year. On the other hand, surgical treatment has been almost uniformly successful in those cases in which a pure lesion was involved. This qualification is made because a long-standing osteochondritis dissecans may cause irreversible chronic arthritic changes in the joint cartilage and in the capsular structures. In such an instance simple elimination of the primary lesion will not cure the condition, even though it may result in marked improvement. It is my belief, therefore, that early operation is desirable.

In the unusual instance in which the injury is recognized at once, there may seem to be some justification for conservative treatment. One should bear in mind, however, that no weight-bearing can be permitted. Elimination of weight-bearing on the area is not accomplished by the walking cast. In fact, the only way I know for one to be relatively certain of no weight-bearing is to use a long leg cast with the knee flexed to 90 degrees. Since many months of casting are necessary for this treatment, it is not without its hazards and is, to say the least, very difficult for the young and active athlete. It would not be tolerable in an adult. It might conceivably be tolerated by a

youngster under 12. The only justification for such nonsurgical treatment would be the risk of surgery and the belief that surgery will not be highly successful. Neither of these is a tenable presumption. Therefore, treatment of these fractures is surgical at whatever stage they are seen.

In the lateral lesion the area may be approached by an extremely atraumatic incision over the anterolateral ankle parallel to and just lateral to the peroneus tertius tendon (see Fig. 595). The dorsal retinaculum is divided, the anterior fasciculus of the lateral collateral ligament is sectioned transversely and the capsule is exposed. (See page 630, operation for spurs.) Similarly, the medial side may be exposed by an incision medial to and paralleling the anterior tibial tendon. It is necessary to tie off the anterior division of the saphenous vein below the ankle. Both incisions may be made and the whole mass of tendons, vessels and nerves may be elevated forward out of harm's way. These approaches seem much better than the single incision directly anterior, which involves the vascular bundle and the tendons.

In the early case, the capsule will be distended with blood. If the case is of longer duration, a diffuse synovitis will thicken the capsule. (The author operated on a patient in whom there was tremendously thickened synovium, at least ⅜ in. [1 cm.] thick, which presented all the gross characteristics of a xanthomatous synovitis. A classic superolateral talar lesion was found and the other joint changes appeared to be confined to synovitis). On dividing the capsule along the line of the incision, the anterior margin of the lateral malleolus, the leading edge of the lower end of the tibia and the dome of the talus are exposed. On initial examination all the cartilage appears to be intact and without any apparent defect, but as the foot is plantar flexed to expose the central portion of the talus, the defect comes into view. In the majority of instances the defect can readily be seen as a separate piece of cartilage, a depressed area with a cartilaginous wrinkle, or a fissure in the cartilage of the superior surface of the talus. In these cases the fragment can be readily lifted up and removed, using a small, curved hemostat or similar instrument. Since the fragment may be as long as 2 cm. or more, it is frequently necessary to go back under the tibia to complete the removal. This can be more easily accomplished if its anterior portion is removed first, since this allows ample room to explore the area completely. The chondral margin of the defect should be palpated carefully and any loose or undermined cartilage removed. The crater will be seen as an area lined with chronic granulation tissue which can be scraped away with a curette. The underlying bone is extremely sclerotic. The older the lesion, the more sclerotic the bed will be.

At the conclusion of this procedure, there is a dished-out oval of bone including the superior lateral margin of the talus for a major portion of its middle one third. This crater may be as large as 1 cm. wide, 1 cm. deep and 2 to 3 cm. long, but as a rule it is smaller and is quite avascular even after brisk curetting. If this bed is sclerotic and avascular, it should be drilled (see Fig. 599). Using a small size Kirschner wire and a hand drill, my own practice is to drill 8 to 12 holes in the bed deep enough to permit exudation of blood as the wire is removed. Several fresh drill points may be needed if the bone is extremely sclerotic. The area is not plugged with bone wax as in removal of marginal spurs, since in this instance we want to encourage exudation of blood and formation of vascular buds at each of these drill holes. The wound is then closed in layers after thorough inspection and copious lavage of the whole operative area. One will be surprised to discover a considerable amount of debris in the basin after lavaging a joint that appeared quite clean to the naked eye. The lateral collateral ligament and the extensor

retinaculum are carefully repaired. Posterior and lateral stirrup splints are applied to below the knee. At the end of 12 to 14 days the stirrup splints are removed, the stitches are removed and the walking cast is applied. This is worn for an additional two weeks, depending to some extent upon the attendant joint changes, since the ankle joint should be protected longer if there has been long-standing chronic synovitis.

I am convinced that early weight-bearing and active use are better than prolonged protection if the defect in the talus is to become filled. Cartilage replaces much better with active use than with immobilization. If the fragment is left in place, prolonged protection is needed to permit it to unite to the talus; on the other hand, after its removal and curettement of the bed, active use will stimulate formation of granulation tissue followed by scar formation and in many cases by metamorphosis of the scar into fibrocartilage. So, as soon as the operative reaction and attendant arthritic changes have subsided, activity is encouraged. Nor do I see any reason to limit the patient's physical activity, provided that the ankle remains relatively sympton-free. However, in contact sports I think the ankle should be carefully strapped to prevent recurrence of the type of injury that caused the condition in the first place. The prognosis is extremely favorable in young patients and in those cases which have not already progressed to chronic joint changes. Similar lesions occurring elsewhere in the ankle and foot should be treated in a similar fashion.

Some surgeons have recommended that the osteochondral fragment be removed, the bed freshened up and the fragment replaced and pinned to its bed. This seems to me quite unsuitable in the talus. In the first place the lesion is not usually recognized early when the fracture is fresh and union could be expected to occur. In the second place, a major portion of the lesion is pretty well covered by the lower end of the tibia and, while it is available for removal and the bed may be reached for curetting and for drilling, it would be extremely difficult to replace the fragment and pin it adequately without more exposure than seems justified. Exposure can be obtained laterally by transection of the lateral malleolus and medially by transection of the medial malleolus. However, these measures are not without danger of complications and at the very best needlessly prolong convalescence. The success of repinning the fragment would seem to depend upon early recognition and treatment. These are the very cases in which removal of the fragment also gives very good results. Following pinning of the fragment, a prolonged period of nonweight bearing is desirable. As pointed out earlier, this presents difficulties and is not acceptable to many young patients, so that their cooperation is likely to be poor. For these reasons I do not recommend replacement and internal fixation of the fragment.

SYNOVITIS OF THE ANKLE

Although synovitis is much less of a problem at the ankle than at the knee, some degree of synovitis will occur with any injury involving the capsule of the ankle joint. The manifestations of synovitis at the ankle are quite different from those at the knee. The very nature of the ankle joint is not consistent with extensive effusion. There is relatively little synovium in the ankle, the joint space is snug and tight and there is actually no area of the ankle joint where the synovial surfaces are in contact with each other, as they are for example in the suprapatellar pouch. Therefore, one can infrequently make a diagnosis of synovitis with effusion per se, although effusion will occur with injury or with disease. There is no such evident collection of fluid. The condition appears simply as diffuse swelling of the ankle.

As with other joint problems, it is extremely important to make a definitive diagnosis if at all possible. In the acute synovitis which may follow an injury or an infection or a metabolic disturbance such as gout, the ankle is painful, swollen, and hot and has all the appearance of an acute inflammatory reaction. Aspiration ordinarily will not recover much, if any, fluid. The treatment of such an acute condition is systemic and local. Systemic treatment is treatment of the underlying condition: antibiotics should be administered if there is an infection,

and whatever general condition may be present should be corrected. Local treatment is rest, elevation, support and local heat. Although it is difficult to aspirate the fluid from the ankle, the ankle may be readily injected. This is not indicated usually in the acute condition. As the acute symptoms subside, it is important to protect the ankle against stress and strain until healing is complete, since synovitis will have a great tendency to recur.

Chronic Synovitis

A much more distressing condition is a chronic synovitis of the ankle. As previously indicated in this chapter, there are many conditions about the ankle which are difficult to diagnose. There are mild tibiofibular separation, osteochondral fracture of the talus and instability of the lateral collateral ligaments. All of these will cause the symptoms of a chronic synovitis, namely, swelling, pain and disability, yet the synovitis is simply secondary to a primary condition which may well be amenable to treatment. If careful search does not reveal any particular etiology, treatment must be local. Of prime importance is a period of rest for the ankle. Since this is difficult to obtain in the athlete, rest should be carried out by means of immobilization with plaster fixation. Stirrup splints should be used if swelling is marked. As swelling subsides, a walking boot cast may be substituted. It will take several weeks of adequate protection followed by a period of strapping and wrapping in order to permit the condition to heal and athletic endeavor to resume. One of the most distressing situations is to relieve the synovitis only to have it recur because the underlying disease has not been eradicated. A chronic synovitis is not consistent with successful athletic participation.

21

Injuries of the Foot

ANATOMICAL CONSIDERATIONS

The foot is an extremely ingenious mechanism designed to transfer the body weight from the leg to the ground. The arch of the foot provides an elastic, springy connection so that to a large extent the jar of weight-bearing is dissipated before it reaches the long bones of the leg and thigh. The arch also has the function of improving locomotion by adding speed and agility to the gait. Additionally, the foot is capable of rolling from side to side when contacting surface imperfections, permitting the leg to remain vertical while the foot rolls into inversion or eversion.

The leg contacts the foot in its posterior one third, giving the longer lever arm from the heads of the metatarsals to the ankle a marked advantage over the shorter lever arm from the ankle to the back of the calcaneus. Space does not permit a full description of all the many joints of the foot or of its multiplicity of ligaments and tendons, each designed to improve function. A careful study of the anatomy of the foot is extremely interesting and quite rewarding to the surgeon who has to treat injuries to this area.

Basically, the foot is divided into three divisions: the posterior part, consisting of the talus and calcaneus; the central part, consisting of the navicular, cuboid and the three cuneiforms; and the anterior part, consisting of the metatarsals and the phalanges (Figs. 604 to 606). Each of these areas has characteristics that account for distinctive types of injuries. Thus, injuries to the posterior division are usually of the compression type, produced as the forceful drive of the leg into the foot collapses the bone. In the central portion of the foot, the injury is usually an avulsion type as the foot is forced through a range of motion beyond its capacity and either the ligament tears, the bone fractures or both. In the anterior part, the injury is similar to that occurring in long bones anywhere.

The ankle is functionally a hinge joint permitting flexion and extension of the foot on the leg. Lateral motion and circumduction occur largely on the pivot of the talonavicular joint, which is essentially a universal joint. This rotatory motion is permitted by the talocalcaneal and talonavicular joints, which in many motions act as a single unit. There is only slight motion in the remaining joints of the midfoot, particularly the calcaneocuboid, the naviculocuneiform, the intercuneiform and the tarsometatarsal joints. This entire area of the foot is firmly bound together by ligaments from the front of the talus to the metatarsal heads. In dissection of the foot it is difficult to delineate the actual joint lines in the cuneiform-metatarsal areas, so close is the fit. Since there is such intricate apposition of the many bones of the foot, it is very important that the joint surfaces be maintained in the proper position and without undue irregularity. Failure to do so accounts for the severity of the disability following what appears to be a relatively minor injury.

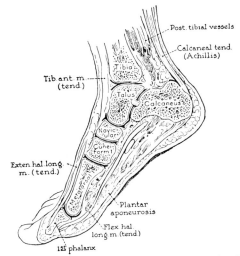

Figure 604. Sagittal section of right foot and ankle, showing bony structure and superficial muscles. (From Jones and Shepard, Manual of Surgical Anatomy).

641

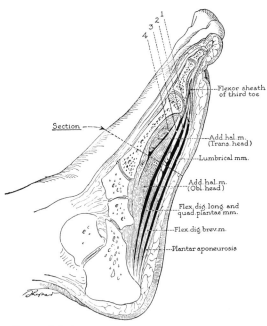

Figure 605. Sagittal section through plantar spaces (1, 2, 3, 4) of right foot. (From Jones and Shepard, Manual of Surgical Anatomy.)

The general contour of the foot is a longitudinal arch resting posteriorly on the bottom of the calcaneus and anteriorly on the metatarsal heads. This arch is supported by the

Figure 606. The bones of the right foot, viewed from below. (From Jones and Shepard, Manual of Surgical Anatomy.)

plantar ligament arising from the calcaneus and extending forward to attach near the metatarsal heads. In the normal foot the lateral portion of this arch rests on the ground, giving additional support to the foot. The plantar ligament is reinforced by the short flexors and other intrinsic muscles and by the ligaments of the foot. Thus, the integrity of the longitudinal arch is preserved by bony architecture, by strong ligaments and by active muscle.

The undersurface of the foot is covered with unusually heavy skin. The underlying fat pad is compartmented by dense, fibrous bands, so that the skin makes a very adherent contact with the deep fascia. The skin of the sole does not slide back and forth as does the skin on top of the foot.

Muscle attachments are arranged to move the foot through its various ranges of active motion and still give static support. The synchronous action of the muscles of the foot is not dissimilar to that of the hand and wrist. The muscle assumes a different function, depending upon the starting position of the foot and the motion involved—in equinus, calcaneus, inversion or eversion. The rapidly reversing motions by the athlete cause excessive strain on the various components of the foot.

CONTUSION

Contusion of the foot is a frequent occurrence and may be caused by any sort of direct trauma, such as a dropped weight or trampling or striking by another player. Contusion of the dorsum of the foot may be quite distressing because of the extremely sensitive nature of this area. Thin integument overlies the tendons, blood vessels and nerves so that they are caught between the underlying bone and the striking object over thin skin.

The complications of contusion may be more important than the contusion itself. The blow may cause damage to a nerve, resulting in intractable pain over the dorsum of the foot, damage to the blood vessels with phlebitis or hemorrhage, damage to the tendons with resulting tenosynovitis, and damage to the periosteum or to the joints. Each of these conditions should be treated appropriately, the important element being recognition of the complication so that one will not continue to reassure the patient that he has a minor condition from which he will promptly recover when the patient is convinced that he has a rather severe condition that definitely is not improving. This is particularly true of tenosynovitis, which has the same tendency to recur here as elsewhere.

The necessity for weight-bearing adds to the seriousness of contusions to the undersurface of the foot. These frequently are caused by a faultily placed spike, a loose cleat, or even a wrinkle in the sock. The subcutaneous tissue lying between the thick plantar skin and underlying bone and muscle becomes ecchymotic and reacts by inflammation, forming the characteristic "stone bruise." This may be very persistent under the heel or under the metatarsal heads.

The anatomical characteristics of a particular foot have a great deal to do with this type of injury. The extremely high-arched foot with a tight heel cord puts unusual stress on the metatarsal heads as they strike the floor or track. The tightness of the calf does not permit the ankle to dorsiflex, and a good deal of the elasticity of the forefoot is lost. To this is added the fact that the weight is borne on the metatarsal heads and on the heel rather than along the lateral margin of the foot. Thus a contusion to the heel or to the metatarsal heads may result because of the excess pressure of weight-bearing. This is particularly pertinent under the first metatarsal head, where the equinus of the forefoot throws excess stress against the two sesamoids lying under the first metatarsal head, possibly resulting in severe contusion of these bones. The same type of foot, with a high arch, often has marginal osteophytes at the junction of the metatarsal bases and the cuneiform bones, so that the bone is quite prominent under the skin and thus much more subject to damage. Under the heel the relatively vertical position of the calcaneus may cause repetitive bruising in the running gait so that a deep-seated hematoma may form and may develop into an adventitious bursa, thus complicating recovery. The remedy is to relieve weight-bearing until the condition has been arrested. This is frequently incompatible with athletic participation. It is particularly distressing to the track man or basketball player, since it seems to him to be a minor condition but it interferes with his competing effectively. Early local injection with a long-acting anesthetic agent, followed by one of the corticoid preparations, is a valuable adjunct in the treatment. Some ingenuity can be utilized to prevent weight-bearing on the tender part and so permit running. Various types of felt pads, combined with strapping of the foot, may give substantial relief. In this instance it is not the pull of the muscle or the motion itself which causes the

distress but the blow against the hard surface. In some instances foam padding will give a good deal of relief. This is much more feasible in football shoes than it is in track or basketball shoes. The usual physical therapeutic measures are of some value in expediting recovery because they serve to improve the local circulation, relieve congestion and promote absorption.

STRAIN

Strain is particularly common in the foot. The complex of intrinsic muscles making up the foot is very extensive and is subjected to very strong forces by athletic activity. Some areas are much more frequently involved than others, one of the most common being the insertion of the **tendo Achilles** to the calcaneus. Strain here may be severely incapacitating because, each time the calf is contracted in walking or running, severe pain occurs at the attachment of the tendon to the heel. Occasionally, chronic strain in the tendo Achilles may result in calcification in the tendon, with distressing recurring pain on function (Fig. 607). Another common location is at the attachment of the **anterior tibial** tendon on the medial side of the foot. Strain is particularly likely to occur here if there is a tendency for the athlete to pronate the heel so that the talus tends to rotate downward and inward in relation to the foot. The anterior tibial is the most active muscle in dorsiflexing the foot and is the opponent of the tendo Achilles. Early in the season, running will frequently cause irritation at either site. Less frequently there will be strain at the attachment of the **peroneals** or of the **posterior tibial** or of the **flexors of the toes** (see page 603).

Treatment of strain has been detailed elsewhere (page 51). Elimination of stress is of prime importance. In the heel, strapping to prevent dorsiflexion of the foot and elevation of the heel by a pad in the shoe or an extra rubber heel will serve to relieve the condition provided that violent activity is avoided. Physical therapy, especially application of heat locally, is of value but protection is the true remedy for the condition. A longer period of inactivity will be rewarded by complete recovery, whereas temporizing measures often result in repeated recurrence. If the patient has had a strain of the attachment of the tendo Achilles, he probably should keep the foot strapped throughout the remainder of the season to prevent forcible dorsiflexion, although

Figure 607. Young skier had persistent pain at the attachment of the tendo Achilles to the calcaneus. *A,* Note calcification in tendon. Pain had become so severe that skiing was impossible. Removal of calcification and scarification of the attachment plus immobilization resulted in complete recovery. *B,* One year postoperative. In this case the prominent superior tubercle at the back of the calcaneus was exicsed.

this will not prevent active traction by the calf muscles. It will reduce passive stretching, which may be an important factor, particularly in contact sports. On the other hand, if the anterior tibial is injured the foot should be strapped to prevent extreme plantar flexion (see Fig. 14). The shoe should be wedged on the inner side of the heel to throw the weight toward the outer side of the foot. An arch support may be helpful.

While discussing strain of the tendo Achilles attachment, one should mention **Apophysitis of the calcaneus** (Fig. 608). This is another of the group of aseptic necroses which occur at various places in the epiphyses of the young athlete. At the calcaneus it is not ordinarily as disabling as at the hip or knee. The calcaneal epiphysis has a wide attachment to the calcaneus and therefore is not particularly subject to extensive irreversible necrosis. Faulty circulation is manifested by sclerosis of the apophysis, frequently accompanied by fragmentation, but the condition is self-limited and usually does not demand drastic treatment. Symptomatically there is pain at the posterior point of the heel, usually somewhat below the actual attachment of the tendo Achilles. Pain is elicited only by forcible activity; therefore the adolescent can usually go about his regular activity without trouble. Pain will recur only if he starts to run or jump or if he violently exercises his foot.

Unlike strain of the tendo Achilles, this condition can usually be completely relieved by restricting dorsiflexion of the foot. Ade-

quate strapping down the back of the leg and over the sole of the foot anchored properly around the ankle, combined with elevation of the shoe heel, is usually all the treatment that

Figure 608. *A,* Typical calcaneal apophysitis, indicated by sclerosis and fragmentation. *B,* Another manifestation of calcaneal apophysitis with irregular and delayed epiphyseal formation.

is necessary. In my experience a few weeks' reduction of activity will usually result in complete relief from symptoms, although the x-ray evidence of apophysitis will persist for many months. The very acute or resistant case may require the patient to wear a walking cast for six to eight weeks. There is no residual except occasionally some prominence of the back of the heel, which may cause symptoms by pressure against the heel of the shoe. During the acute stage, if the tenderness is quite poignant, it may be necessary to cut the counter out of the back of the shoe in order to relieve pressure here and to apply suitable felt padding. Obviously, if the condition is acute, athletics are contraindicated.

SPRAIN

We have defined sprain as a ligament injury and have discussed it particularly from the standpoint of the acute sprain. However, in the foot one must definitely distinguish between static sprain and acute traumatic sprain.

Traumatic Sprain

Traumatic sprain of the foot is similar to sprain elsewhere and may be acute or chronic. It is caused by violent overstretching of a ligament or ligaments by forcing the involved joint through a wider range of motion than the ligaments will normally permit. The same force applied repeatedly may result in a chronic irritative lesion in the ligament itself. It is basically due to abnormal motion.

Treatment is similar to that of sprain anywhere. In the early stage the treatment of choice comprises local injection into the hematoma, compression, and application of ice followed by adequate support and use of heat locally. Usually support can be accomplished by adequate strapping and elimination of weight-bearing. The exact type of support depends upon the ligament involved. Thus, if the sprain involves the calcaneocuboid ligament, it will be treated much like a sprain of the ankle. In the plantar ligament the sprain will be treated by support under the arch to prevent distraction between the heads of the metatarsals and the calcaneus. Acute sprain should be evaluated as to its severity, since to a considerable extent this will determine the degree and duration of immobilization (Fig. 609). If the sprain was caused by inversion or eversion of the foot, suitable strapping of the ankle type (see Fig. 586) is advisable, since it is difficult to immobilize the foot properly without including the lower leg. This is particularly true of sprain of the arch, where it is important to keep the foot inverted (see Fig. 570). Additional support can be provided by placing a wedge on the shoe heel so that, if an arch sprain is present, a medial heel wedge to invert the foot will relieve tension. If the sprain is in

Figure 609. Two day old injury to the foot, with swelling and exquisite tenderness under the heel. Note avulsion of plantar ligament with fragment of bone, so-called sprain fracture. No relationship to calcaneal spur.

the lateral ligaments of the foot, a lateral wedge on the heel or on the sole worn on a temporary basis for a matter of a few weeks will be of considerable value in relieving the stress until healing is complete.

If the injury appears to be quite severe at the time of the initial examination, careful x-ray study must be done to rule out any fracture or dislocation. The proper local treatment should then be instituted, followed by elevation of the foot and use of a compression bandage and an ice pack overnight. Evaluation the next day will permit one to determine the extent of injury somewhat better. In some instances it may be necessary to continue elevation of the foot and application of cold followed by heat until the swelling subsides sufficiently to permit application of a plaster splint for a few days, followed by a plaster boot. This boot should be worn for ten days and followed by adequate strapping, arch support and a wedge on the shoe heel until the foot is symptom-free.

The acute sprain may involve the intermetatarsal ligaments at the distal end of the metatarsal. It is particularly likely to occur in the track athlete who runs in a very light shoe or may run barefooted and receive an injury to the anterior ligaments. This should be treated in the usual manner, but the strapping in this case should be circumferential around the forefoot. This injury must not be confused with chronic sprain of the intermetatarsal ligaments, which may be extremely resistant to treatment. Once the acute sprain occurs, the forefoot should be strapped for the remainder of the season (see Fig. 586).

Static Sprain

Static conditions of the foot can be a very complicated and serious problem but will not be dwelt upon at length here. However, one will be called upon frequently to distinguish between a chronic sprain of the foot and a static sprain of the arch. Whereas the chronic sprain is due to repeated episodes of overmotion, the static sprain is due to the constant stress of superimposed weight on the arch of the foot. This is most frequently manifested by pain along the plantar ligament from the attachment of the calcaneus to its attachment near the metatarsal heads. It is promptly relieved by elimination of weight-bearing. There is no history of any particular injury. The condition is more likely to occur early in the season, when the patient abruptly changes

from his regular shoes which have considerable support in the arch, to the flat shoes of athletic equipment. Additionally, the superimposed weight of his equipment, and more violent exercise plus long hours on his feet, may combine to cause a sprain of the arch. The diagnosis is often suggested by the fact that the player has had foot trouble before and frequently he may be wearing arch support shoes or arch supports in his street shoes.

Treatment. Static sprain of this type will not respond well to treatment indicated for acute sprains but should receive the treatment given for flatfoot, namely, support of the arch, improvement of the posture of the foot and reconstructive exercises (Fig. 610) to improve the muscle tone of the foot. The muscles of the foot are very similar to those of the hand, and therefore the importance of proper specific exercises for the so-called weak foot or chronic sprain should be recognized. Participation in sports cannot be permitted without either adequate arch supports or adequate strapping, since every recurrence of symptoms simply makes it more difficult to effect a complete recovery. This type of condition is not at all limited to "flatfoot." In fact, some of the most painful arches are the very high ones, which cause most of the body weight to be carried on the metatarsal heads and on the heel. This subjects the plantar ligament and other inferior ligaments of the foot to considerable stress on weight-bearing. A carefully outlined program, meticulously followed by the patient, will give gratifying results. It should be emphasized again that during the violent exercise of athletics the arch should be protected by flexible cork and leather arch supports once it has been subject to chronic sprain.

Chronic sprain of the intermetatarsal ligaments is evidenced by pain in the area of the metatarsal heads. This may be a sequela of acute sprain or may be due to static stretching of the ligaments. It must be treated by circumferential strapping, metatarsal pad and anterior heel, but here again the treatment will be incompatible with athletic activity. Chronic sprain may be accompanied by or confused with plantar neuroma.

PLANTAR NEUROMA (MORTON'S TOE)

Plantar neuroma is a static condition of the foot that occurs relatively frequently in athletes (Fig. 611). The player usually complains of a "sprain" of the anterior arch. The symptom

Figure 610. Reconstructive exercises for the foot. Position: The patient sits with the feet on a smooth, flat surface. These exercises should be done slowly and forcibly with maximum effort maintained for three seconds, 1–2–3. *A*, Actively lift the toes, keeping the ball of the foot on the floor. This should be done 30 times. *B*, Slide the foot forward so that the toes protrude beyond an edge. Flex toes downward 30 times. *C*, Spread the toes widely 30 times. At first it may be necessary to assist this movement with the hands. *D*, Raise the inner margin of the foot with the weight thrown on the outer margin. Curl the toes downward and backward in an attempt to "make a fist." *E*, Holding one foot firmly on the floor, place the other foot forward until it rests on the heel. In this position, rotate the anterior part of the foot from the outside inward so that the tip of the right big toe makes a complete circle in a clockwise direction. Definite effort must be made to force this motion to the extreme. The left should turn counterclockwise.

These exercises must be done slowly to the count of 1–2–3 seconds, with a similar period between each movement. Distinct effort must be made to get the most possible motion, and if this is done a definite strain will be felt upon the involved muscles. Exercises should be begun at about ten times apiece, gradually increasing the numbers to 30 times apiece. The series should be done twice daily.

You must not hurry through these exercises.

that distinguishes it from sprain is intermittent, excruciating pain in the lateral part of the forefoot, usually running into the adjacent sides of the third and fourth toes and occasionally up the dorsum of the foot toward the ankle. There is often a feeling of an electric shock running out into one or both of the toes. Numbness of the adjacent sides of these two toes frequently may be present, but it is not as common as the tingling sensation or shock feeling which runs down into the toes. The condition is not ordinarily brought on by any specific motion or any specific sprain. It comes on spontaneously when least expected. The patient usually feels much more comfortable barefooted, whereas in sprain of the arch, the patient is not comfortable without the support of shoes. On examination, tenderness will be found between the third and fourth metatarsal heads, and it will be exquisite upon localized pressure in the plantar surface of the web between the third and fourth toes when pressure is directed back toward the third and fourth heads. This finding is best elicited by exerting pressure with the rubber end of a pencil. Compression of the metatarsal heads,

particularly by rolling the heads across each other by lateral pressure, will often elicit a definite click accompanied by pain that is usually referred to the third and fourth toes. An almost diagnostic description by the patient is

Figure 611. Plantar neuroma. Plantar aspect. In this approach the nerve is subcutaneous and readily treated. The more commonly used incision is dorsal, as described in the text.

that while he is walking, dancing or running, he may suddenly get a severe pain in the forefoot; he snatches off his shoe and massages his foot with almost immediate relief.

The cause of this condition is a thickening of the plantar nerve at the point where the medial and lateral branches join and then separate to pass to the adjacent sides of the third and fourth toes. The thickened area where the "x" is formed is subject to trauma when caught between the metatarsal heads. A predisposing factor is relaxation of the inter-metatarsal ligaments, which permits splaying of the forefoot. As a result of this irritative pressure, an extremely large mass of nerve and fibrous tissue may gradually be formed. The larger the mass, the more frequently it is caught between the metatarsal heads, resulting in more severe symptoms.

Treatment. Nonsurgical measures for treatment of plantar neuroma may occasionally be successful and should always be tried. Perhaps the most effective treatment of this kind is a longitudinal arch support fitted with a meta-tarsal pad just behind the metatarsal heads. This tends to permit the heads to spread out over the pad, thus separating them a little and relieving the pressure between them. An anterior heel or so-called metatarsal bar put on the shoe may be effective. This is made by filling in the area at the very back of the sole at the point where the weight-bearing stops. Thus the sole is about ⅛ in. thicker here than elsewhere, so that the initial weight-bearing thrust comes on the bar before it comes over into the sole of the shoe. Since the pinching is usually quite transient, measures such as heat, massage and elevation usually are not effective. *Surgical treatment* usually is extremely effective if properly carried out. It is extremely important to resect the mass completely. While this may be done through the sole of the foot, the general aversion to leaving an open sore on the plantar surface of the foot has made the dorsal incision much more popular, although it is considerably more complicated.

It should be recalled that the medial plantar nerve ordinarily supplies three and a half toes and the lateral plantar nerve supplies one and a half. As a rule, the lateral plantar nerve sends a communicating branch over to the most lateral component of the medial plantar nerve and they join just proximal to the heads of the third and fourth metatarsals. As they pass distally, they divide to form the lateral digital nerve to the third toe and the medial digital nerve to the fourth toe. The resulting thickening makes the nerve particularly sus-

ceptible to pressure between the adjacent metatarsal heads. The nerve courses in the plantar surface of the foot beneath the intermetatarsal ligaments but superior to the plantar aponeurosis, lying in the interval between the long flexor tendons.

The surgical approach is as follows: A linear incision is made, beginning at the web between the third and fourth toes and extending parallel to these two metatarsals and between their extensor tendons. The skin is divided and the extensor tendons are retracted, exposing the dorsal interossei tendons adjacent to each metatarsal. These are retracted, exposing the ligament extending between the two metatarsal heads. This is divided transversely, and the two metatarsal heads are retracted, permitting access to the space just superficial to the plantar subcutaneous tissue. The digital nerves should be defined and cut distally. They are then reflected back, freeing the tumor mass, which can be pushed up by pressure applied under the sole of the foot. The mass is carefully elevated out of the intermetatarsal space, and dissection is carried proximally until the normal nerve trunk is identified. Ordinarily there will be a medial and a lateral trunk.

Dissection of the nerves should continue as far as the middle of the metatarsal shaft before they are divided. This should prevent recurrence of pain from constriction of the nerve in the scar. Usually there will be a discrete mass of fatty, fibrous and nerve tissues with two digital nerves and two proximal nerves that appear relatively normal. We recently have reoperated on a patient who had intractable pain following excision of a plantar neuroma. We found an extremely large edematous nerve extending right into the masses of scar and very adherent to it. It did not have a neuroma on the end but its adherence to the scar between the two metatarsal heads caused the pain, which was promptly relieved by resection of the nerve back up under the metatarsals. In the repair, care should be taken to approximate the divided intermetatarsal ligament, and in the aftercare, the metatarsal heads must be supported by a snug bandage in order to prevent further separation between them.

TENOSYNOVITIS

The foot is quite subject to tenosynovitis because its tendons are charged with the responsibility both of motion and of supporting considerable weight. The cause of tenosynovitis here is the same as in other locations, namely, a direct blow or chronic overuse. The latter is a more important factor in the athlete. Frequently tenosynovitis is combined with other conditions, such as strain of the tendon attachment. The resultant irritation causes friction between the tendon and its surrounding sheath with edema, inflammation and adhesions, all of which cause pain on active function. Characteristic findings are pain on passive stretching of the involved tendon, pain on active motion of the involved tendon and tenderness over the tendon at the point of the irritation. Careful palpation over the tendon during active motion will often elicit "snowball" crepitation, which is diagnostic of tenosynovitis. The tendon sheath usually does not distend with excess fluid as does the joint with synovitis. Tenosynovitis is particularly prone to occur in the early phases of training, especially in track men when they are training on the boards.

Treatment. Tenosynovitis is another of those conditions which can be treated well only by elimination of the stress involved. This of necessity means elimination of competitive athletics. Other measures of importance in expediting the cure are local injection into the sheath, not the tendon, local physical therapy and protection of the tendon. In the foot it is difficult to prevent stress on the tendon without giving support to the arch. These cases frequently should be treated by a splint to prevent motion altogether, followed later by adequate strapping and wrapping to prevent excess motion. At the same time the splint and the strapping should support the arch of the foot. Caution should be used in applying the strapping so that it does not compress the tendon between the strapping and the underlying bone; this may increase the irritation rather than diminish it.

Tenosynovitis involving the dorsiflexors, namely, the anterior tibial, peroneus tertius and toe extensors, should be treated by strapping the foot to prevent plantar flexion (see Fig. 14). In tenosynovitis of the posterior structures, such as the calf, peroneals and posterior tibial, the foot should be strapped so that it will not dorsiflex beyond neutral and also to provide lateral support (see Fig. 559). All too often, however, the irritating factor is function of the muscle rather than of passive stretching of the tendon, and continued forcible motion is incompatible with prompt recovery. Once recovery is complete, strapping is of great importance in preventing recurrence. If strapping does not give complete relief, the patient should spend about 10 to 14 days in a walking cast before the strapping. This will expedite recovery.

BURSITIS

Bursitis is not a common problem in injury to the foot, although it is well to bear in mind that it may occur. A particularly distressing type of bursitis is that of the bursa between the calcaneus and skin on the plantar surface of the heel. This can be readily mistaken for strain of the attachment of the plantar ligament, particularly if spurs happen to be demonstrable at this attachment. The bursitis can usually be distinguished by the fact that tenderness is considerably further posterior on the heel than is usually the case in involvement of the plantar ligament. *Treatment* is by local injection, local application of heat, wearing of protective sponge rubber in the shoes and, in severe cases, excision of the bursa. There may be a bursitis of the bunion joint but this does not occur frequently in athletes and requires no discussion here.

Another bursa frequently involved in the foot is that between the tendo Achilles and the back of the calcaneus. The symptoms here may be readily confused with those of strain of the attachment of the tendo Achilles. However, active contraction of the calf should not cause increase of symptoms in bursitis, although local pressure does. Careful examination will usually distinguish the condition, the pain being just proximal to the attachment of the tendon to the calcaneus and anterior to the tendon. Tenderness may also be elicited by applying pressure in the space anterior to the tendo Achilles. Rarely does the bursa enlarge enough to permit the fluid to be palpated or aspirated. *Treatment* consists of local injection and protection of the space against pressure. In the acute phase, dorsiflexion of the foot should be prevented by strapping. This bursitis is not usually as resistant as apophysitis and not as recurrent as strain of the tendo Achilles attachment.

Another common bursitis which particularly frustrates the athlete, especially a track person, involves the bursa lying under the first metatarsal head between the skin and the medial sesamoid. A callus often develops in this area and the skin becomes quite firm and hard. This is apposed to the tendon aponeurosis containing the medial and lateral sesamoids, and the increased weight-bearing on these two hard surfaces encourages the development of the bursa between them. While this bursa may be protective, permitting the surfaces to slide more freely over each other, it often becomes inflamed and causes severe pain on weight-bearing, particularly on running. This requires the treatment given for all bursitis conditions, that is, protection against irritation, aspiration and injection if indicated. The condition may be extremely distressing to the athlete, since any attempt to resume his athletic endeavors before the bursa is entirely healed will simply result in aggravation of the bursitis. This should not be confused with involvement of the articular cartilage on the sesamoid itself, although the subjective symptoms may be quite similar. If the inflammation of the bursa becomes chronic, with thickened walls, it may be necessary to excise it surgically.

SYNOVIAL HERNIA (GANGLION)

Although synovial hernia is not particularly common in the ankle, it frequently occurs in the foot. This is explained by the multiplicity of joints and tendons in the foot, making legion the areas where chronic sprain followed by weakness of the capsule and herniation of the synovium may occur. It is not necessary to discuss these in detail in their various locations, but one or two deserve special mention here.

One frequent area is near the peroneal tendon distal to the lateral malleolus. In this instance the herniation may be of extremely large size, as in a patient recently operated upon in whom the mass was about the size and shape of the third finger but came down to a single defect in the tendon sheath no larger than the point of a lead pencil (Fig. 612). Another frequent area of involvement is the dorsum of the foot in the long extensor tendons, where the hernia may come off the tendon sheath or occurs in the tarsal joints.

The *treatment* is the same as treatment of synovial hernia elsewhere (page 69). It cannot be overemphasized that if surgical treatment is undertaken, it should be done as a major procedure under general anesthesia so that the sac can be meticulously dissected out. If at all possible the defect in the sheath or capsule should be repaired. Chopping off the top of the mass through a ½ in. "medical" incision only results in scarring, which makes a later surgical procedure extremely difficult. Surgical excision should be followed by complete immobilization for at least the three weeks needed for the ligament or capsule to begin to heal. Resulting stiffness is not as common in the foot as it is in the wrist. No particular rehabilitation is necessary other than for the muscles which have been immobilized.

Figure 612. Lateral side injury of the peroneal tendons, with resulting painful tumor alongside peroneal tendons. Section proved it to be a synovial hernia off the tendon sheath. A, The exposed mass. B, The dissection. C, Down to match-stem pedicle. D, The intact mass removed.

The treatment of these lesions by violent direct trauma, such as a sharp blow, should be abandoned. Aspiration of the mass followed by application of a pressure dressing can be readily done in the foot and is an acceptable measure. Some have reported unbelievably good results from injection of steroids, but in my experience this has rarely had any more effect than simple aspiration of the lesion. Repeated aspiration, particularly in the foot, entails the hazard of ultimate infection and is probably not justified by the results. In several cases in which surgery has followed corticoid injections, we have seen plaques of calcium-like material within the sac or in the adjacent tissues. These have been ascribed to irritation from the injection, but the matter requires further investigation.

A synovial hernia of moderate size is not incompatible with athletic activity. There is really no objection to permitting athletic competition and postponing removal of the hernia to a later time, provided adequate strapping is utilized and symptoms are not severe enough to prohibit active use of the foot.

DISLOCATION

Dislocation of the foot is not a frequent injury in athletics. It is much more infrequent than ankle dislocation, for obvious reasons. The foot is protected by the shoe and frequently by wrapping and is not subject to the violent disruptive stresses that may dislocate the ankle or knee. When a severe injury to the foot occurs, the x-rays should be carefully studied and compared with films of the opposite foot. Particularly to be looked for is a possible separation of the tarsal joints. A common type of dislocation is one extending along the foot between the first and second metatarsal bases, between the internal and middle cuneiforms, and across the foot laterally at the level of the metatarsal cuboid joints (Figs. 613 and 614). This may be suspected from a tendency of the foot to be broader in this area with characteristic widening of the joint space, the wider space angulating across the foot. The base of the fifth metatarsal is more prominent than it normally is and pressure here is quite painful. The tip of the base of the metatarsal may be broken off so that the shaft is actually lateral to the proximal tip. This represents a serious disruption of the ligaments of the foot and should be treated by complete reduction and internal fixation. If it is not treated or is treated overcasually, the result is broadening of the forefoot, chronic strain of the tarsal joints and marked incapacity, which are extremely difficult to treat at a later stage (Fig. 615). In such obviously severe injuries of the forefoot, a particular effort must be made to be sure that the swelling, pain and disability are not actually due to a persistent displacement or to a spontaneously reduced dislocation.

Other examples of dislocation are illustrated in Figures 616 to 618.

Figure 613. *A*, Dislocation between the first and second metatarsals, the inner and middle cuneiforms, the middle cuneiform and navicular, and the navicular and cuboid. Note definite increase in space between middle and medial cuneiform and the medial cuneiform and distal side of the navicular. *B*, Early, very firm fixation with three screws was done. Immobilization in a walking cast for four weeks was followed by weight-bearing in a stout boot for four weeks. *C*, Twelve weeks postoperative: The screws were removed and arch support was recommended for one year, with no athletic activity permitted. Good recovery.

Figure 614. Overlooked dislocation. It was necessary to fuse the two middle and medial cuneiforms. There was some resultant disability. This dislocation is between the first and second metatarsals, medial and middle cuneiforms. The joint between the proximal end of the medial cuneiform and the navicular was not seriously damaged.

Figure 615. Result of unreduced dislocation similar to that in Figure 613 with gross disability. Note the displacement between the first and the second metatarsals extending along the metatarsal cuneiform and cuboid joints with lateral displacement. Note base of M-5 displaced proximally and laterally. *Right,* The normal foot for comparison.

Figure 616. Fracture-dislocation of the foot. Note fracture extending across the base of metatarsals 2–3–4 with lateral dislocation of the base of M-5. The whole unit is displaced laterally. This is a disabling type injury if not reduced by approximating the shaft of M-2 to M-1. This is similar to the injury in Figure 613.

Figure 617. Unusual case of compound dislocation of ankle and foot. Note that the talus is tipped out of the ankle mortice but the deltoid ligament is apparently intact. Talus is also dislocated on the tarsus.

Figure 618. *A,* Fracture-dislocation in tarsal-metatarsal region. This injury is similar to that of Figure 613, except that the defect continued back through the navicular by breaking its middle third. *B,* The follow-up shows good healing of the navicular but widening of the space between the first and the second rays. This probably could have been prevented by early open reduction and internal fixation.

Dislocations of the toes are not frequent but should be promptly recognized and completely reduced. Adequate support is usually provided by strapping the injured toe to the adjacent toes, which are used as splints. If the athlete wears well-fitted shoes and firm soles, continued activity is permissible. The habit of playing competitive sports without shoes is to be deplored, since the shoe is an excellent protection for the foot.

FRACTURE

The anatomical division of the foot into posterior, middle and anterior portions has definite clinical value in the consideration of fractures.

Fracture of the Posterior Portion of the Foot

This section of the foot, including as it does the talus and calcaneus, is rarely fractured in athletics if sprain-fractures are excluded. The ordinary fracture here is direct compression, as occurs in a fall from a height or from driving the foot into the floor board of a car (Figs.

619 to 621). Fortunately, direct compression injuries are not common in athletics. Certain fractures do occur in special situations such as have been described in the section on the ankle. Abnormal forceful motion may cause avulsion (Figs. 622 to 624) or snubbing fractures of the talus (Fig. 625), and the sustentaculum tali may be broken by forceful eversion of the foot (see Fig. 619). It is extremely important to restore the contour of the calcaneus and particularly the integrity of the talo-calcaneal joint. Adduction or abduction of the foot may cause a snubbing or avulsion fracture of the superior portion of the calcaneus at the calcaneocuboid joint. If the fragment is large and displaced, it should be replaced surgically if necessary. The smaller fragment may be treated as a sprain and recovery will be good (Fig. 626).

Fracture of the Central Portion of the Foot

This portion of the foot includes the navicular, cuboid, and first, second and third cuneiforms. This section is extremely well bound together by the various ligaments and moves almost as a unit. Compression fractures may

Figure 619. Compression fracture of the calcaneus as this pole vaulter landed on the edge of the pit. *A*, Showing medial and lateral expansion of the calcaneus, with fracture through the sustentaculum tali. This could easily be overlooked. *B*, Lateral view is not definitive.

Figure 620. Professional football player sustained injury to foot with immediate swelling. Stayed off it for four weeks then continued playing, but with increased trouble. *A*, X-ray six months post-injury revealed fracture of anterior process of the calcaneus. At removal, the fragment was found to be one in. long, extending right into the talocalcaneal joint. *B*, There was a normal anterior process on the opposite foot. *C*, One month postoperative. *D*, Two months postoperative.

Figure 621. Persistently painful heel after sharply striking the ground. *A*, The negative lateral film. *B*, Two weeks later condensation shown at the ball of the calcaneus, indicating a compression fracture.

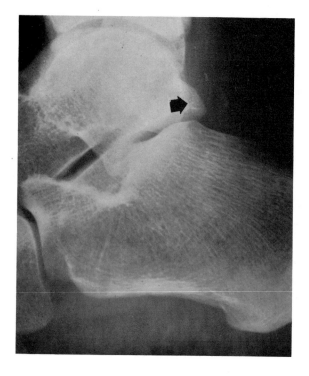

Figure 622. Avulsion of the posterior portion of the talus three weeks old. Note the shape of the avulsed fragment which would fit right on the posterior end of the talus. This is not an os trigonum. This is the result of a dorsiflexion injury, the same forces that cause tibiofibular separation.

Figure 623. *A*, A forcible dorsiflexion injury. Note the separate fragment at the back of the talus. This is an actual fracture of the posterior process of the talus, not os trigonum. Note normal foot *(B)* showing unusually long posterior process. The mechanism here is probably snapping off of this posterior process as the back of the talus comes forcibly against the top of the calcaneus. This patient had been treated for a "minor strain" and was still very symptomatic three months later. Removal of the fragment relieved the symptoms.

Figure 624. Avulsion of the superior margin of the head of the talus. Detachment of the anterior capsule. This should be treated by excision of the fragment and repair of the capsule.

Figure 625. *A,* Fracture through anterior portion of the body of the talus, result of forcible plantar flexion injury. *B,* Result nine months after open reduction and internal fixation.

occur in these bones but they are usually not recognized as such unless there has been a major injury to the foot. A much more common fracture in athletics is avulsion of an adjacent fragment of bone by the ligament at the time of dislocation or subluxation of the joint. This may be between the cuneiforms or between the cuneiforms and the cuboid or navicular. In the dislocation between the first and second metatarsals, then between the first and second cuneiforms and then across between the navicular and cuboid, there may be one or more areas of fracture (see Fig. 618). That is, the injury may split the middle cuneiform rather than cause dislocation between the first and second; the posterior portion of the cuboid may fracture rather than dislocate between the cuboid and navicular. These are modifications of the same injury and require the same treatment, namely, firm fixation in perfect position until union occurs. Surgery may be necessary to accomplish this end. Bony fusion of the joint is considerably more functional than hypermobility or painful motion and results in little handicap. Several weeks will be needed for union to take place, and during this period the foot should be carefully immobilized in a cast that molds the arch into perfect position. A walking cast is not advisable. When the cast is removed and tape applied, protection should be supplied by a molded arch support for many months, since

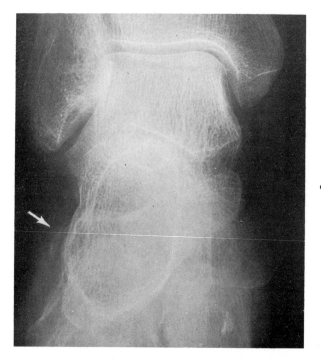

Figure 626. Sprain-fracture of lateral margin of calcaneus, an inversion injury.

Figure 627. Typical avulsion fracture at the base of the fifth metatarsal.

chronic disability of the foot is frequent following fractures in this area.

Fracture of the Anterior Portion of the Foot

By far the most common area for fracture is the anterior portion of the foot, which consists of the long bones of the metatarsals and phalanges.

Fracture of the Metatarsals

The five metatarsals are long bones that are firmly bound together by overlapping layers of ligament at their bases, held together in the midshaft by the interosseous membrane and at the distal ends by the plantar and dorsal divisions of the distal intermetatarsal ligament.

Fracture of the Base of the Metatarsal. The most frequently occurring fracture is at the base of the fifth metatarsal (Fig. 627). This conical base, with its tip posterior, is considerably weaker than the quadrilateral bases of the other metatarsals (Fig. 628). The strong attachment of the peroneus brevis plus the massive lateral ligament attachments tends to fix the base of this metatarsal as the forefoot is sharply inverted and adducted, and a greater or lesser fragment of the base of this bone may be pulled away. This is essentially a sprain-fracture and may be treated as such. Nonunion of the fragment is not unusual, and while not necessarily disabling, it may be quite painful. Immobilization in plaster splints followed by wearing of a walking cast for a total of four weeks will usually give firm enough fixation so

that taping and a good stout shoe may be used afterward for support. If painful nonunion persists, the fragment, if small, may be removed and the attachments replaced to the metatarsal. If the fragment is large, internal fixation may be necessary.

On the medial side of the foot the base of

Figure 628. Fracture of the bases of the second, third and fourth metatarsals caused by a sharp hyperflexion injury as the player was hit on the leg from behind. This is one of the hazards of "clipping."

the first metatarsal is not often the site of fracture owing not only to its sturdy structure but also to the fact that the stresses applied to this side are not as great as those on the lateral side.

The metatarsal bases may be involved in a fracture-dislocation in which a portion of the base is snubbed off as the shaft is forced away from its normal position (see Fig. 616). These fractures are usually caused by sharp dorsiflexion or forcible plantar flexion of the foot. The result may be extremely distressing, particularly if the lesion is not recognized. Careful x-ray study will usually reveal the fracture, particularly when one's attention is called to it by sharply localized tenderness. It is important that the integrity of the joint surfaces be restored as fully as possible, particularly if there is a tendency for a portion of the bone to subluxate. In these cases, reduction should be followed by fixation with a transfixion Kirschner wire, the wire being passed across the bases of the intact bones and through the involved bone after complete reduction.

Fracture of the Shaft of the Metatarsal. Metatarsal shaft fractures are similar to those of long bones elsewhere. The presence of five bones in the same plane allows each one to protect the other to some extent. The cause may be a crushing force applied over the dorsum of the foot as it is resting on the ground or forcible torsion of the forefoot on the tarsus. Examination reveals tenderness over the involved area with swelling and hematoma formation. Diagnosis can be confirmed by x-ray study. If there is gross displacement, the fracture should be reduced and held in good position. This may require open reduction. Frequently if only one shaft is involved, it may hold well without internal fixation (Figs. 629 and 630). In a comminuted, oblique or spiral fracture of several shafts, skeletal traction may be needed through the toes to secure proper alignment of the bones (Figs. 631 and 632). Particular attention should be paid to the space between the metatarsals, best judged by comparison with the opposite foot. If the bases of these bones tend to separate, they can frequently be held in a firm position by threaded Kirschner wires transfixed through several metatarsals after the bones have been placed in a normal position. Fracture of the metatarsals is an extremely disabling injury to an athlete, and complete healing must be secured before competition is permitted. An arch support should be worn, particularly in athletic shoes.

Isolated fatigue fracture of the metatarsal

Figure 629. This 15 year old male fumbled a hand-off, and he and another player jumped on the ball. He had pain in his foot and pain on walking. Examination revealed very marked tenderness over the shaft of the second metatarsal. A, This fracture through the middle of the shaft with intact bones on either side will heal without any significant displacement, as shown in B.

Fracture of the Head and Neck of the Metatarsals. Fracture through this area in the foot is not nearly so frequent as in the hand. Ordinarily there is little displacement, and simple fixation and protection from weight-bearing will suffice (Fig. 633). However, if the fracture is unrecognized and malunion or non-union occurs, the metatarsal head may be removed, but this may be quite disabling. This is not to be recommended for an acute injury, since union can usually be obtained without it if good fixation is secured. It may be necessary to pass a Kirschner wire through the head of the metatarsal and down into the shaft in order to hold the head in proper position.

Fracture of the articular cartilage of the metatarsal head is infrequent in athletics and does not constitute a serious hazard. If a portion of the head is broken off in any way and heals in an irregular manner, that head may be removed. It is not advisable to remove more than one head or to remove the first or fifth in an athlete.

Fracture of the Toes

Fractures of the toes do not present as serious a problem as fractures of the fingers, in spite of the fact that similar anatomical structures are involved. While fracture of the toe seems to arouse a sardonic amusement in the minds of everyone else, to the athlete the fractured toe may be extremely disturbing, and may cause him to miss an entire season's play. While it is usually not necessary to carry out

Figure 630. Fracture of the proximal end of the shaft of the fifth metatarsal. Note bipartite medial sesamoid to first toe. This may be mistaken for a fracture.

shaft may occur from strain (pages 69 and 667). Indeed, excessive strain may cause complete fracture with displacement as the leverage is applied to the metatarsal heads with the foot in equinus.

Figure 631. *A*, Metatarsal fracture resulting from a fall from a horse when the foot was caught between the horse and the road. *B*, Skeletal traction was ineffectual. *C*, Open reduction with transfixion pin and threaded wire resulted in a normal foot. There is no epiphyseal disturbance of the metatarsals.

Figure 632. *A*, Fracture of shaft of first metatarsal, treated by skeletal traction. *B*, Six months postreduction.

the methods for fixation in the toes that are used in the fingers, one should at least take sufficient pains in the treatment of these conditions to be sure that the end result will be compatible with normal and not unduly delayed function. Many of these accidents occur in the dressing room rather than on the playing field, by slipping on a wet floor or stubbing the toes against articles of furniture. The tendency among team players for a certain amount of horseplay to work off excess exuberance makes these accidents more probable. While the ordinary person may get by pretty well by simply wearing a heavy shoe, the athlete, who needs to wear extremely flexible shoes and constantly must forcibly flex and

Figure 633. Typical fracture of the neck of the fourth metatarsal. This view shows a little plantar rotation of the head of the metatarsal, and clinically the head was quite prominent in the sole of the foot. This deformity should be corrected to prevent painful metatarsal head. There is an incomplete fracture of M-3.

extend the toes, presents a wholly different problem.

Fracture of the First Toe. The first toe should be considered separately, since it is much more vital in the mechanics of the foot than the smaller toes. In normal stride, considerable stress is applied to the first toe, and after the strike phase, when the first toe reaches the ground, it is forcibly flexed to assist in the walkover from heel to toe. As the opposite leg is moved forward, the big toe of the hind foot is kept on the ground in a marked degree of dorsiflexion; and as the toe leaves the ground to swing the leg forward again, sharp flexion of the toe aids in propulsion. A stiff or painful metatarsophalangeal or interphalangeal joint in the first toe that is disabling for ordinary walking is usually remedied by a stiff sole or an anterior heel, but this is not compatible with athletics.

The first toe may be injured by direct force, such as when a locker room bench falls on it. This results in a more severe contusion with or without comminuted fracture of the distal or proximal phalanx. This is a painful injury, with extravasation of blood into the tissues, swelling, throbbing and severe discomfort. Careful x-ray study is required to determine whether there is fracture involving the joint, since this has much more serious implications than fracture of the tuft or shaft (Fig. 634). If the x-ray findings are negative, careful study of the toe itself will reveal the extent of the hematoma. Any blood under the nail should be drained, preferably by drilling through the nail rather than by lifting the nail further away from the nail bed, unless avulsion has already taken place. The foot should be elevated and packed in ice and walking forbidden. Concentrated treatment during the first few hours or days may well prevent a long period of disability.

Fracture of the Distal Phalanx. This fracture probably will not require manipulation or even rigid immobilization. If it is at the base of the distal phalanx (Fig. 635), particularly if it extends into the joint, careful reduction should be carried out and a toe spica cast applied. If the fracture is of the articular surface, the fragment may require pinning in place with a small wire. The same rules for treatment of fractures of weight-bearing joints apply to fractures above the joint of the first toe.

Fracture of the Proximal Phalanx. This fracture is much more serious than fracture of the distal phalanx. The fracture may be of the head, the neck (Fig. 636), the shaft or the base. Any deformity should be corrected and

Figure 634. Tuft fracture of distal phalanx of first toe. Note also avulsion fracture of lateral margin of the articular surface of the distal phalanx.

may be held with intramedullary fixation by a Kirschner wire. This is a satisfactory method and obviates the need for long periods of immobilization with a plaster cast. Athletic competition cannot be permitted with these injuries as long as there is a danger of stress causing recurrence of the deformity.

An extremely painful fracture of the first toe comes as the result of a forceful kick that drives the base of either the distal (Fig. 637) or proximal phalanx into the opposing head. This results in osteochondral damage and occasionally in comminution of the base of the bone. In some cases the displacement from a comminuted fracture of the proximal phalanx will be enough to require traction with a wire through the distal phalanx and on an outrigger.

Should a painful traumatic arthritis of the interphalangeal joint occur, it can best be treated by removal of the articular surface and fusion of the joint in the straight position. This results in little disability.

Involvement of the *metatarsophalangeal joint* is much more serious, since fusion of this joint is not compatible with the best function of the foot. In this joint one is justified in attempting to remove the irregularity rather than fusing the joint. An irregularity occasionally forms around the bases of the bones from

Figure 635. Avulsion fracture of the lateral margin of the proximal end of the distal phalanx of the first toe caused by forcing the distal phalanx inward.

sprain or sprain-fracture. Spurs may arise which seriously interfere with dorsiflexion (Fig. 638). Good function may be expected following resection of these spurs provided they are not manifestations of chronic degenerative arthritis involving the articular cartilage.

With the advent of artificial turf, there seems to be a sharp increase in snubbing-type injuries to the first toe. As the shoe holds in the turf, the foot slides forward within the shoe and forces the distal phalanx into the end of the shoe. The result may be injury to the nail with avulsion. It may be to the interphalanageal joint or to the metatarsophalangeal joint. These injuries may be quite disabling and require careful consideration as to protection of the toe.

Fractures of the Smaller Toes. While fractures of the smaller toes are much less disabling than those of the first toe, they can be extremely exasperating. The most common is fracture of the proximal phalanx of the fifth toe, often occurring as the result of a nighttime attempt to move furniture with the toe (Fig. 639). This causes sharp abduction of the toe, resulting in a spiral, oblique fracture. In the second, third and fourth toes the fracture is usually from overflexion or overextension and is often a transverse fracture, generally near the joint (Fig. 640). Avulsion of a portion of

Figure 636. Fracture of neck of proximal phalanx of first toe, treated by plaster cast and later by shoe with a metal plate. The stability of the fracture permitted it to be held without internal fixation.

Figure 637. Osteochondral damage of the base of the distal phalanx of the first toe from soccer kicking. This injury may occur from forcing the toe into the end of the shoe as the shoe sticks to the turf.

Figure 638. Spur over the dorsum of the distal end of the first metatarsal, apparently the result of kicking. The opposite foot and the rest of the joints are normal. Complete relief followed excision. The same injury may occur from forcing the toe into the end of the shoe.

Figure 639. Spiral fracture of shaft of little toe involving the interphalangeal joint. In this toe this fracture can be treated by simple coaptation dressing.

Figure 640. Spiral fracture of proximal phalanx of third toe. Treated by strapping of the second, third and fourth toes together. The forefoot should also be strapped and a shoe with a hard sole worn.

the articular surface frequently occurs. These fractures have a tendency to heal with the toe in flexion so that a painful hammer toe may result, which requires definitive treatment. X-ray study will reveal the fracture.

An effort should be made to realign the toe. In the fifth toe, abduction deformity usually persists. This can be corrected without anesthesia by inserting a pencil or pen shaft between the fourth and fifth toes at the base and exerting quick, firm pressure outward on the pencil and inward on the head of the first phalanx. Perfect position, while not necessary, is desirable. Following reduction, the toe should be strapped to its fellow if it is the fifth toe or to the toe on either side if it is one of the others. Because of swelling extending back into the forefoot and difficulty in gait, it is also advisable to extend the strapping backward and circumferentially to include the forefoot (Fig. 641). This will result in less disability in the toe and a great deal more discomfort on weight-bearing. The patient should be able to walk in a shoe that has been cut out to relieve the pressure at the tender area. The decision as to participation in athletic competition may be a difficult one, since the player may feel very good when he walks or even runs. To his dismay, however, he may find that as he goes full speed or cuts sharply, throwing the foot into varus or valgus, he will experience sharp pain which may cause him to fall or lose stride and so cost him a great deal of his effectiveness. A period of rest is probably very worthwhile. In such an injury, packing the toe in ice overnight may mean the difference between

rapid, uneventful healing and tedious convalescence since, once the toe becomes badly swollen and edematous, the restoration of pain-free function becomes increasingly difficult.

Avulsion fractures of the toes (Fig. 635) are, strictly speaking, muscle tendon or ligament injuries, and here again there is a tendency for hammer toe deformity to occur. A common avulsion is that of the extensor aponeurosis by sharp plantar flexion. The toe is flexed and painful. At the time of the initial injury, the toe should be strapped straight if the condition is recognized. Usually the patient is not seen by the physician until persistence of pain brings him in weeks later. At this time fusion of the involved joint is the best treatment.

Figure 641. Strapping for fractured third toe. Note that the adjacent toes are strapped to the broken one. The whole is strapped to the forefoot.

Figure 642. This female developed gradual soreness in forefoot, noticed when running up and down stairs. *A*, Negative film, diagnosed a stress fracture. *B*, One month later. Note light abundant callus. *C*, Two months later. Note indefinite, healing fracture line.

Stress Fracture (Fatigue Fracture)

The fatigue fracture was first described in the foot. This so-called "march" fracture was reported following mobilization for World War II, when many young males who were unaccustomed to being on their feet were equipped with a pack and required to walk long distances in heavy shoes. The resulting stresses on bones not used to this degree of activity caused a great deal of strain, particularly in the area of the metatarsal necks. The patient develops symptoms similar to those of an arch strain, with pain along the forepart of the arch, increased on weight-bearing or other activity and relieved by rest. Examination reveals local tenderness over the metatarsals with pain on stretching of the plantar arch but usually none on other motions of the foot. X-ray examination made in an early stage usually shows no abnormality. The patient is treated for arch sprain with pads and heat, but the condition persists, with local tenderness and increasing disability. Subsequent x-rays made after a few weeks will show callus formation around the metatarsal shaft (Figs. 642 to 644). This is sometimes accompanied by evidence of a crack across the shaft, but there may be absolutely

Figure 643. "March" fracture. A sketch showing a classic "march" fracture through the neck of the second metatarsal. This fracture usually occurs through the metatarsal shaft, the callus appearing before the fracture itself is evident.

Figure 644. Typical "march" fracture in a young athlete. Note complete absence of any fracture line as such. Uneventful healing.

no indication of a break in the continuity of the bone. This condition has frequently been confused with bone tumor, and instances have been reported in which amputation had been recommended under the diagnosis of osteogenic sarcoma with periosteal reaction. A little patience will usually answer the question, since in march fracture callus rapidly consolidates, becomes harder and smaller and ultimately disappears.

This condition is incompatible with active competitive sports during the acute stage, and competition should be permitted only after consolidation of the callus mass is complete. If the lesion is recognized early, the best treatment is wearing of a plaster boot for two to three weeks followed by adequate strapping for a week or ten days, and then the use of an arch support and a firm shoe. This type of condition graphically illustrates the value of re-examination by x-ray. If findings on the initial x-rays have been negative but the symptoms persist, careful follow-up films will often reveal the pathologic changes. It should be emphasized again that x-ray is simply an adjunct to the diagnosis, and a normal x-ray by no means rules out a bone lesion.

OTHER CONDITIONS OF THE FOOT

Hammer Toe

It is not necessary to detail the treatment of hammer toe. This condition results from a combination of contracture of the flexor and extensor tendons so that one or more joints are in flexion and another in extension (Fig. 645). A frequent combination is for the interphalangeal joints to be in flexion and the metatarsophalangeal joint in extension. This causes pressure on the tip of the distal phalanx and on the dorsum of the proximal interphalangeal joint. Painful corns may result. Hammer toes may result from unrecognized poliomyelitis, from a high-arched, cavus-type foot, as a result of short shoes or socks, or from previous injury. Proper care of the primary condition should minimize the deformity. Hammer toe can be successfully treated and athletics can be resumed. In the meantime, a properly fitted shoe with the leather split at the pressure point or the application of suitable pads may add materially to the patient's comfort. A very frequent instance of disabling hammer toe involves the fifth toe. In fact, this toe is very frequently in the hammer toe position, which presents the knuckle of the proximal interphalangeal joint dorsally and the tip of the toe on the plantar surface, each of which may develop a very painful corn. A simple method for treatment of this condition may save many months and even years of discomfort. The head of the proximal phalanx should be resected and tenotomy of the extensor tendon performed. This does not leave any residual deformity; in fact, the toe looks more normal than it did in its previous hammer toe condition. It almost always relieves the corn on the dorsum on the inner side of the head of this proximal phalanx and on the tip of the distal phalanx.

Subungual Exostosis

This is a painful condition of the distal phalanx, usually of the first toe, which is not uncommon in athletes (Fig. 646). The pathology is the development of an exostosis on top of the distal phalanx extending up under the nail bed. Trauma may be a definite etiological factor. The condition may develop in a basketball player as a result of having his toe repeatedly trampled. Once the exostosis develops it is extremely sensitive to pressure or trauma. The patient presents with a very painful, swollen, edematous toe. In many instances the nail has been cut away to permit the tumor mass to push up without the pressure of the nail over it. While these lesions look vicious clinically, they are always benign and may be cured by removal of the exostosis. If it is extensive and the nail bed has been destroyed, removal of the distal one half of the distal phalanx, with plastic closure of the toe after removal of the entire nail and nail bed, may be the best solution. This condition is often confused with ingrown toenail or simple contusion and hematoma. The frightening appearance may suggest a malignant tumor.

Ingrown Toenail

Ingrown toenail may occur on any toe but is most severe on the first. Basically, the cause is a rolling of the toenail in a scroll-like fashion so that the two lateral margins tend to roll under the central portion to make a tube rather than a flat plane. This is a natural tendency of the nail, as evidenced in some species of mammals in which a conical claw is formed by a

Figure 645. Hammer toes, corrected by fusion of the proximal interphalangeal joints. The severe hallux valgus has been corrected. The wires may be removed once fusion is solid.

complete circling of the toenail. The resulting convexity causes the edge of the nail to dig into the side of the toe. The paronychial fold bulges to the outside and extends out over the dorsum of the nail.

Treatment. In the early stages ingrown toenail can usually be managed conservatively. Prophylaxis is of prime importance; well-fitting shoes and socks, careful hygiene to avoid inflammation, and proper trimming of the nail will prevent serious deformity. The nail should be trimmed straight across without rounding off the pointing. If the nail tends to be heavy, the center portion may be thinned by an emery board or suitable nail file so that, in the middle of the nail extending from the root to the tip, the substance is quite thin. This permits the lateral margins to roll upward by breaking the arc of the nail. A similar but incorrect thing has been done by others, who have split the nail down its center, but this often results in serious complications. The flattening may be

Figure 646. Subungual exostosis. Note the sharp spurring upward of the distal end of the distal phalanx. This was treated by resection of the tuft of the distal phalanx. It should be emphasized that the entire tip of the distal phalanx should be removed. To simply remove the spur invites recurrence.

aided by placing very small pledgets of cotton under the nail corners, once the tendency for ingrowing is noted. This must be carefully done or the pledgets may break off the corner of the nail and do more harm than good. They should not be made large enough to lift the nail away from the nail bed lest the problem be further complicated. If infection occurs, it should be adequately treated by drainage, application of hot packs and administration of suitable antibiotics, both local and general. The patient should be barred from the general dressing room while his toe is acutely infected. Surgery of the toenail can usually be avoided by adequate attention in the early stages.

If the deformity persists and defies conservative treatment, surgery will usually give very satisfactory results. I cannot condemn too strongly the prevalent practice of simply removing the nail. In the first place, this is not simple, and in the second place, when the nail regenerates it is even more curled than before so that the problem is increased. A suitable procedure is illustrated in Figure 647, great care being taken to eliminate all of the nail root and nail bed so that a recurrence or spur formation does not result that will require further treatment.

Active athletic competition with a serious ingrown toenail is scarcely permissible, since excruciating pain may result if the foot is trod upon. Active forcible flexion and extension may cause pain and increased inflammation.

An ingrown toenail involving the smaller toes is much less serious but should receive essentially the same treatment. This, however, is more difficult to carry out in the small toes. Surgical removal of all or part of the nail bed is not a mutilating operation and is far more acceptable in the small toes than a similar procedure on the first toe.

Corns

The best way to prevent disability from a corn in an athlete is to prevent the corn. The shoe must be carefully fitted and no pressure points permitted to develop. The most common locus is the toes, where definite pressure occurs between the toe and the shoe. The little toe, particularly, is an offender, since it will frequently tend to curl up in the hammer toe position. Many athletes have a very high arch with some degree of hammer toe in all the small toes. These tend to get corns along the dorsum of the proximal interphalangeal joints. It does little good to remove a corn and not eliminate the condition that caused it. The area should be padded to protect it from pressure. The corn should be softened with lanolin. If necessary, judicious trimming may be done. Careless application of medicated corn plasters has often resulted in painful ulcers. Careful fitting of the shoe and sock and avoidance of wrinkles are important.

Calluses

Calluses of the foot are the result of friction and pressure. They tend to be extremely dis-

Figure 647. Surgical treatment of ingrown toenail. Care is taken to eliminate all the nail root and nail bed to prevent recurrence of spur formation. This may be done on each side of the nail if indicated. There should be no permanent disability if properly done.

abling, since the piling up of keratin, presumably as a protective measure, results in interposition of a very hard mass between the bone and the shoe. Painful bruising of the underlying tissues or periosteum may result. The obvious measure is to prevent the imbalance of the foot and get a more even distribution of weight by building up or padding the shoe in such a manner as to relieve the weight on the involved area. The most frequent pressure on the foot is under the metatarsal heads. Painful callus under the first head may be relieved by shifting the weight to the lateral side of the foot. An anterior heel or metatarsal bar may protect against direct weight-bearing. In running on the toes, however, the metatarsal bar which ordinarily protects a person by taking the weight off the metatarsal head is, of course, not functioning. Careful attention to the callus by buffing it down with an emory board, softening it with lanolin, and so forth, will pay dividends.

Athlete's Foot

Fungal infections of the foot are endemic in almost the entire population. They are particularly prevalent in the locker room, where too often little attention is paid to ordinary precautionary measures. For details of prevention and treatment, see page 50. Enteric medication seems to offer definite promise in resistant cases.

Verrucae

The verruca, or wart, must be distinguished from the callus. The callus arises as a direct result of too much pressure on a certain area. Multiple verrucae, on the other hand, is a skin disease probably caused by a virus which may spread over the entire sole of the foot and be extremely disabling. Confusion may arise when a verruca is at a weight-bearing point and is surrounded by a callus. Treatment should be carried out by one who is especially proficient in the treatment of conditions of the foot. Radiation should be used only under the careful guidance of an expert and probably not more than one series should be given to any one area.

Freiberg's Disease

Freiberg's disease is necrosis of the metatarsal head, usually before the closing of the epiphysis, similar to Perthes' disease at the hip (Fig. 648). Early Freiberg's disease should be treated by prevention of weight-bearing, but this condition is frequently not recognized until it is well advanced. If the bone is seriously deformed, the painful metatarsal head should be removed. If the lesion heals without deformity, it is of no consequence.

Congenital Deformities of the Foot

There are many other deformities of the foot that are simply developmental and of little significance. They may at times be the precursors of later disability due to static imbalance, but they should not bar participation in athletics. The congenital hallux valgus (Fig. 649) or bunion is amenable to surgical treatment if

Figure 648. Freiberg's disease. *A,* The unaffected foot. Note extra long second metatarsal shaft with large head, which bears undue proportion of the weight. This contributes to the osteochondritis. *B,* The healed osteochondritis of the metatarsal head (Freiberg's disease) with joint irregularity and pain. *C,* Removal of the second metatarsal head resulted in considerable improvement.

Figure 649. Congenital hallux valgus, right. Note bifid epiphysis on the proximal phalanx of first toe, left. This is not pathological but may require treatment. The primary pathological change here is the adduction of the first metatarsal, which is trying to act like a thumb. Correction of the "bunion joint" will fail unless the metatarsal adduction is corrected by osteotomy.

necessary (Fig. 650). In the male it usually can be handled without surgery. Congenital short first metatarsal (Fig. 651) may be helped by suitable padding of the shoe. Pronation or supination similarly can be improved by improving the weight-bearing stance. The accessory navicular (Figs. 652 to 654) or prehallux may become symptomatic during pronation of the foot and may be completely relieved by application of a suitable arch support. Athletic shoes with little or no arch, often with no heel, may often give inadequate support to the pronated or flat foot and need to be supplemented by a molded flexible arch support.

Fracture of a Sesamoid

Various sesamoid bones in the foot are subject to injury.

Accessory Navicular. The most common sesamoid injury occurs in the prehallux or accessory navicular. In an eversion injury with a tight posterior tibial tendon, an avulsion force is applied to the accessory bone and is pulled away from its attachment to the navicular or, in the occasional case, pulled in two. This is similar to avulsion of the tendon attachment to the navicular. It may be misleading because the accessory navicular may be recognized as an extra bone and the injury may be overlooked. A history of forceful eversion of the foot or of active contraction of the posterior tibial is characteristic. On examination, tenderness will be sharply localized to the accessory bone and to the navicular. Forced passive eversion or strong active inversion against resistance is painful. X-ray studies may be confirmatory.

Treatment for this condition may be nonsurgical. The patient is placed in a cast with the foot inverted for about three weeks, followed by inversion-type strapping for another three weeks. However, if there is separation of the fragment or if the navicular is large, it is advisable to remove the accessory navicular and complete the sling operation by positioning the posterior tibial tendon under the navicular. This type of operation is particularly gratifying because the arch is usually good and correction of the pronation will give markedly improved function of the foot.

While this condition may be overlooked, the opposite situation also must be guarded against. One must not interpret an accessory navicular as being a fracture of the tubercle of the navicular. Careful comparison with the opposite foot and careful analysis of the clinical findings will usually distinguish between the two conditions. As indicated previously, the two may coincide and require sharp diagnostic acumen. In case the accessory bone remains persistently painful, it should be removed in any event.

Figure 650. *A*, Film 13 years before shows very marked hallux valgus on both sides with formation of exostosis on the metatarsal head and widening of the space between the first and second metatarsals. Note the longer length of the second metatarsal. This should be classified as congenital adductus primus varus. *B*, Film 13 years later; note the marked advancement of the changes. No intervening treatment. Note the deformity of the proximal phalanx of the second toe on the left with considerable hammer toe and overlapping of the first and second toes. There is marked migration of the lateral sesamoid with extensive increase in the size of the exostosis and bursa. The prognosis would have been very much more favorable if surgery had been carried out when the patient was first seen.

Figure 651. Congenital short first metatarsal with separation of the first and second heads. This throws unusual weight on the second head and is likely to cause a painful foot. The first metatarsal not only is short but is adducted. Correcting the deformity by open wedge osteotomy will give additional length to the first metatarsal.

Figure 652. Note accessory navicular at the medial border of right foot. This should not be interpreted as an injury. Note the much smaller one of the left side. Although the accessory navicular is not primarily traumatic, it is quite subject to injury either by a single episode with avulsion of the accessory bone or by repetitive strain. If symptomatic, the bone may be removed and the posterior tibial tendon placed under the navicular, the "sling operation."

Figure 653. Patient has long-standing pronated feet with recent development of severe symptoms on the right over the medial portion of the navicular. No known history of injury, although one might suspect there had been an avulsion of this bone with subsequent nonunion. Note the accessory bone is very much larger on the right. This should be treated by resection of the accessory bone and some of the protruding medial border of the navicular, transferring the posterior tibial tendon to a new course under the navicular.

Sesamoid in the Flexor Tendon to the Big Toe. The medial sesamoid under the first metatarsophalangeal joint is subject to trauma when the toe is in forced dorsal flexion and a blow is applied to the ball of the foot. The mechanics of this injury resembles that of patellar fracture in which the combination of tension on the patella plus a localized blow fractures the bone. This injury can be extremely distressing, since it prevents the athlete from running on his toes. He may have very persistent pain and the true pathology may be overlooked. This history of sudden, severe pain under the ball of the foot with tenderness and inability to "drive" is significant. Examination will reveal sharply localized tenderness with localized swelling, pain on dorsiflexion of the toe and pain on active plantar flexion of the toe. X-rays are confirmatory.

Treatment consists of immobilization of the foot for several weeks. Usually the acute condition is not recognized and it is seen as a chronic condition, at which time the best treatment will be excision of the sesamoid (Fig. 655). In case nonsurgical treatment has been elected and has failed, or in certain instances when surgical treatment has been chosen as the primary treatment, the injury often occurs in a person with a high arch and a tight plantar ligament. In such a case, one should consider the advisability of carrying out a plantar fasciotomy at the time of the surgery for the sesamoid in order to relieve the tension of the plantar fascia. This would not unduly prolong the patient's morbidity, since the plantar fasciotomy could be done at the same time the sesamoid is removed and the recovery period would be parallel. There can be no question

Figure 654. Acute injury simulating accessory navicular. *A*, This is actually a fracture of the medial tubercle of the navicular. *B*, Normal foot. This fracture may heal if properly protected. A painful fibrous union can be treated by resection of the fragment and repositioning the posterior tibial tendon.

Figure 655. Unrecognized fracture of sesamoid. Note the difference from bipartite sesamoid. Here there is an irregular fracture line and calcification around the area. This sesamoid was removed. Note the high arched foot, which probably contributed to the injury. A plantar fasciotomy was done at the time of the removal of the irregular sesamoid in order to reduce some of the stress caused by the high arch.

that the cavus-type foot with a high arch and tight plantar fascia contributes to pressure on the metatarsal head. This should be considered in the management.

Bipartite Sesamoid of the First Toe

This is a congenital condition in which the medial and occasionally the lateral sesamoid will show transverse separation of the two segments at the midline (see Fig. 630). This must not be confused with fracture, which is much less frequent. Since many fractures are not recognized until late, on x-ray they may,

indeed, resemble the rounded-off margins of the partite bone. The history will be quite different as a rule, however, in that discomfort in the case of the bipartite sesamoid will be gradual in onset and mild in character. The symptoms are ordinarily those of accompanying metatarsal arch strain, and the bipartite sesamoid is found coincidentally and usually is of no significance whatever. Careful analysis of the case and comparison with the opposite foot will give a lead as to the true nature of the condition. Chronic symptoms definitely localized in the sesamoid merit its surgical removal. Disappointment will follow removal if these clear indications are not present.

22

Rehabilitation Following Athletic Injuries

FRED L. ALLMAN, JR.

INTRODUCTION

Rehabilitation of the athlete following injury or surgery is perhaps the most important aspect of treatment, for often the degree of rehabilitation determines the ability of the athlete to safely and effectively return to competition. Kraus (1959) stated, "Injuries which are sustained during athletic participation are usually produced by circumstances inherent in respective athletic performance, and they are, therefore, characterized by exposure to recurrent identical trauma, making reinjury likely."

It is very unlikely that an athlete will be restored to a safe performance level unless specific measures are taken for a return to normal function. Rarely is an injury so mild that some form of rehabilitation is not necessary, and as a rule, the more serious the injury, the more prolonged and necessary is the rehabilitation.

Yet, in spite of the importance of adequate rehabilitation, many athletes either are never rehabilitated or are inadequately rehabilitated. Numerous studies have indicated that this inadequacy of rehabilitation is most certain to result in a very high incidence of re-injury and an unnecessary restriction of future participation in sports by the athlete. In order to insure that rehabilitation is effective, each individual responsible for determining whether a previously injured athlete should play must develop and fully understand certain basic guidelines to be followed during the rehabilitative process. It is hoped that this chapter on rehabilitation will help those involved with the treatment of athletes to be more specific and more knowledgeable in this regard.

Athletic injuries tend to occur in rather definite patterns and to some parts of the body more than others. Certain principles of rehabilitation may be applied generally; however, there are certain parts of the body in which injury is particularly prevalent and in which rehabilitation is extremely important. These are grouped together as thigh and knee, calf and foot, shoulder and arm, forearm and wrist, and head and spine. Included throughout the text have been recommendations concerning rehabilitation related to the specific area of the body being discussed, with suitable reference to this special chapter on rehabilitation.

Goal of Rehabilitation

The goal of rehabilitation is restoration of function to the greatest possible degree and in the shortest possible time. In order to reach this goal and achieve a safe performance level, the best protection is balanced bilateral muscular strength as well as antagonistic muscle balance.

Rehabilitation following injury is better when an exercise can be applied selectively and when resistance can be used where it is most needed and avoided where it is not needed or wanted.

Rehabilitation must be individualized, and the missing quality of muscle function must be identified and restored. Properly performed exercises to build strength not only will improve strength but also will improve speed, flexibility and functional ability. Neuromuscular re-education is also an essential objective of training.

Progressive Resistive Exercise

In 1945, scientific experimentation and clinical application by DeLorme proved that the best way to build muscular strength and endurance was a program of progressive resistive exercise. This has since been confirmed many times.

More recently, Jones has shown that properly performed progressive resistive exercise increases range of motion and improves flexibility. This is beneficial because injury is far less likely to occur when flexibility has improved as much as possible in association with good strength.

The SAID Principle

In reconditioning for vigorous sports activity following injury, it is necessary to understand the SAID principle (Wallis and Logan, 1964). The letters SAID stand for Specific Adaptation to Imposed Demands. Simply stated, this means that the training program must attempt to adapt the individual to the demands that may be made upon him during athletic performance. Adaptation is specific and refers to the alteration of the structure or function of an organ or part as a result of an altered environment. Function increases with use, and that which we do not use, we lose. The intensity, duration and frequency of activity are all related to the functional capacity that is developed.

Rehabilitation of the athlete deals primarily with the restoration of muscle function—that is, the missing quality of muscle function must be identified and restored (muscle strength, endurance and flexibility). Strength is general, but the application of strength is selective. The proper use of strength in any activity comes only from the practice of the particular activity.

In formulating the exercise prescription, exercise should be applied selectively, depending upon the sport in which an athlete is involved.

Types of Rehabilitative Exercises

Rehabilitative exercises are prescribed body movements that help to restore or favorably alter specific functions in an individual following an injury. Active exercise is purposeful voluntary motion that is performed by the injured individual himself, with or without resistance and with or without the aid of gravity. Active exercise may be static, kinetic or isokinetic. Static exercise is that which is performed without producing joint motion. In an isometric contraction, the muscle being utilized maintains a fixed length. Kinetic exercise is that which is performed to produce joint movement. The contracting muscle shortens, producing the movement which is isotonic. Isokinetic exercises are those in which joint motion occurs at a controlled rate. Concentric (positive) contraction occurs when a muscle is contracted from the extended to the shortened position. Eccentric (negative) contraction occurs when the tensed muscle lengthens.

In a positive contraction, tension develops in the muscle, a resistance is overcome and the length of the muscle decreases. In isometric contraction, muscle length remains constant as muscle tension is developed. In negative contraction, the muscle develops tension, and the muscle increases in length. Generally speaking, when a weight is lifted, "positive" work is performed. When a weight is lowered, "negative" work is involved.

It requires at least twice as much oxygen to do positive work as negative work. Therefore, negative work has little or no training effect on the cardiovascular system.

Muscular soreness and discomfort usually accompany an intense bout of negative work. However, this soreness has proved to be more bearable if a break-in period of several days precedes the actual training or if the actual training is continued for at least three consecutive days. Never should the trainee discontinue exercising and just rest. He will become even sorer in this case.

Strength increases are produced by exercises in proportion to the intensity of work, and "negative only" exercise provides an intensity of work that cannot be achieved in any other manner.

The superiority of negative exercise for strength building can be seen in the studies of Doss and Karpovich, Olson's group, and Komi and Buskirk. Some attempts were made on the part of these researchers to equate the training routines of the positive and negative groups, and the quality of negative work was clearly demonstrated.

High intensity of muscular contraction is undoubtedly the single most important factor in exercises performed for the purpose of increasing muscular strength.

Muscle Tension

Baer and associates concluded from a study they conducted that neither total work done nor power in the physical sense is a major factor in determining the improvement of muscular strength. They contended that the common denominator which accounts for strength improvement is the *tension developed* by the muscle during exercise. Earlier studies by others demonstrated that the tension which a muscle produces during contraction decreases as the speed of shortening increases. Thus, in isotonic exercise, greatest tension is developed at a slower rather than a faster rate of contraction, thereby establishing a condition which is conducive to greater improvement in muscular strength.

Maximum Intensity of Contraction

Maximum intensity of contraction is produced when the highest possible percentage of the muscular mass is involved at a given moment, and certain factors are required to produce this situation.

Good form, or the style of performance, is very important if maximum benefit is to be obtained with progressive resistive exercise. Proper form includes the speed of movement, the range of movement and beginning the movement from a prestretched position. Also, the resistance should be moved in a smooth fashion and briefly stopped in the position of full muscular contraction. *Jerking movements should be avoided.*

1. The speed of movement must not be too fast or too slow. If it takes 2 to 3 seconds to raise a weight, then it should take 4 to 5 seconds to lower that same weight.

2. The range of movement must be as great as possible. Prevention of injury is most likely when the muscles have been strengthened in every position and over a full range of possible movement.

3. The movement must start from a prestretched position. Prestretching is involved when a relaxed muscle is pulled into a position of increased tension prior to the start of contraction. Prestretching properly applied enables one to handle heavier weights and thus bring into action a greater percentage of the muscle mass during each repetition. For example, the weight should be lowered from the contracted position in a controlled manner until the bar (or resistance arm) is about 1 in. from the position of full extension. At that point, there should be a very quick "twitch" or "thrust." Immediately following the quick "twitch," the movement should be slowed in a controlled manner. The only rapid move-

ment of the bar or resistance arm should be during the first portion of the raising (positive) part of the repetition. The remaining portion of each repetition should always be smoothly performed.

4. The load must be heavy enough to require a maximum intensity of contraction. High-intensity exercise requires the repetitive performance of a resistance movement that is carried to the point of momentary muscular failure. When performing high-intensity exercise, at least 8 repetitions should be performed and usually not more than 12 to 15. If 8 repetitions cannot be completed, then the resistance is too high, and if one can perform more than 12 to 15, it is too light. Consider a set completed when it is momentarily impossible to perform another full repetition in good form.

High-intensity contraction must be practiced on an infrequent basis, with adequate allowance for total recovery between training sessions; that is, the work should not be done too long or too often. Total recovery from a high-intensity training session requires at least 48 hours. *During the early stages of rehabilitation, the intensity of the work is so low that training is possible on a daily basis.* Later, as the intensity increases, the workouts are reduced to three times per week and, during in-season training, to only twice per week.

The Sequence of Exercises

The sequence in which the various muscle groups are to be worked should be such that the largest muscle group is worked first, proceeding down to the smallest group. Working the largest muscles first causes the greatest growth stimulus. Also, it is sometimes impossible to reach the required condition of momentary muscular exhaustion while working a large muscle group if the system has been previously exhausted by exercises for other smaller muscles.

Neuromuscular Re-education

Neuromuscular re-education primarily involves development of a proprioceptive awareness. Normal function will in most cases return more quickly to the athlete who is allowed to continue with activities that permit near normal function but do not interfere with the normal healing process.

Evaluation for Return to Sports Activity

Prior to being given permission to return to full activity, the athlete must be evaluated from the standpoint of strength, range of movement and girth, and finally there should be some form of functional evaluation of the involved body area (Figs. 656 to 658).

It should be remembered that although normal strength may have been restored by a properly conducted therapeutic exercise program, skill is required for the proper use of strength, and skill is produced in only one way—by the practice of a particular activity. Therefore, in order to fully determine whether the injured athlete has returned to normal high-level performance, he must be evaluated while participating in athletic activity.

Even after the athlete has achieved a safe performance level and is allowed to return to full participation, he should be recalled for periodic re-evaluation at appropriate times. It is only through periodic re-evaluation that an athlete can maintain a safe performance level. Although many will be able to maintain such a performance level with relative ease, others will have to continue with some form of rehabilitation to maintain such a high level, even after their return to activity.

Further, it should be remembered that rehabilitation must deal with the total organism, not just with the involved injured part. Therefore, although most of the initial effort will be directed toward the injured area, attention must also be given to maintaining overall fitness as much as possible for the duration of rehabilitation. Measures that will enable uninvolved parts of the body to remain active should be encouraged, and as soon as possible, the overall program should include activities that will aid in cardiovascular-pulmonary reconditioning.

Stationary cycling and swimming are often possible long before the injured athlete is ready to return to full participation in his specific sports activity. Other similar activities can often be initiated at an early stage in the rehabilitation program.

The ability of the athlete to continue to use the uninvolved parts of his body to the fullest extent possible will surely shorten the recovery period and allow safe return to full sports participation at the earliest possible time.

REHABILITATION PROCEDURES FOR SPECIFIC AREAS

As indicated in the preceding discussion, it is of utmost importance that the entire musculoskeletal system be maintained at the optimal level. Interest in the injured area should not preclude general conditioning. However,

Date _____

Name _____

Record Number_____

	Right	Left
Girth		
Quadriceps		
at cc above patella.....................	___	___
midpatella	___	___
Calf	___	___
Strength		
Quadriceps.............................	___	___
Hamstrings	___	___
Gastroc soleus.........................	___	___
Hip flexor	___	___
Hip abductor...........................	___	___
Hip extensor	___	___
Hip adductor...........................	___	___
Goniometric		
Extension	___	___
Flexion.............................+......	___	___

Comments

Figure 656. Knee evaluation form.

Date _____
Name _____
Record Number _____

	Right	Left
Girth		
Arm...		
Forearm		
Strength		
Hand		
Shoulder		
Internal Rotation.......................		
External Rotation.......................		
Flexion......................................		
Extension		
Abduction..................................		
Goniometric		
Abduction..................................		
Flexion......................................		
Internal Rotation.......................		
External Rotation.......................		
Extension		

Comments

Figure 657. Shoulder evaluation form.

Date _____
Name _____
Record Number _____

	Right	Left
Girth		
Foot		
Ankle..		
Strength		
Plantar flexion		
Dorsiflexion		
Internal Rotation.......................		
External Rotation.......................		
Goniometric		
Plantar flexion		
Dorsiflexion		
Inversion		
Eversion....................................		

Comments

Figure 658. Ankle evaluation form.

it is obvious that the rehabilitation should be concentrated on the injured area. Specific measures are necessary for each different location.

These areas have been grouped in certain combinations which in general require similar measures. A detailed discussion of each of these areas follows and should be quite useful as rehabilitation proceeds.

Head and Spinal Injuries

Head and spinal injuries are the number one cause of deaths directly related to athletic participation. Although proper technique is very important, it is also mandatory that all athletes participating in contact sports provide themselves with the greatest possible degree of protection by maintaining good strong musculature with a full range of painless, unrestricted motion. Maximum strength and flexibility in the spinal muscles can be obtained with proper progressive resistive exercises.

Many less serious conditions involving the spine and low back respond very well to conservative measures when the appropriate exercise routine is utilized. The following exercises are examples of the type used at the Sports Medicine Clinic.

Neck Exercises

Phase 1. (Do these exercises as long as pain exists at the site of injury. Do not progress to more strenuous exercises.) These exercises consist of moving the neck and head through the entire range of motion and *then* continuing to contract the neck muscles at the completion of the movement for an additional 5 seconds. Repeat each movement 10 times. The movements are as follows:

1. Head rotation—to right; to left (Fig. 659*A*).

2. Side tilt—ear toward right shoulder with head held erect; ear toward left shoulder with head held erect (see Fig. 659*B*).

3. Forward thrust—chin forward and down, touching low on chest (see Fig. 659*C*).

4. Head backward—Note: *Do not* move head backward past the neutral or "natural" position. That movement will aggravate most neck problems.

Phase 2. (Start these exercises only when pain and stiffness are no longer a problem.) This phase includes all the preceding exercises with resistance added by means of the following:

1. Partner resisting movement in all directions with his hands.

2. Self-applied resistance with a towel or your hands.

3. Spring-loaded or weight-loaded head strap.

William's Flexion Exercises (Low Back)

Abdominal Curl. Regular sit-ups can aggravate back injuries. *Do not do them!* The following exercise should permanently replace regular sit-ups in your training. If it is necessary, show these instructions to your coaches.

Assume the starting position shown in Figure 660*A*: knees bent, arms folded on the chest, back flat on floor or mat. Now, roll your body up as one rolls a rug; start by pulling the neck forward so that your chin is on your chest. Now roll your shoulders forward (see 660*B*) and then attempt to push your head as far forward between your legs as possible. You will not go far, but if you try as hard as possible for 5 seconds, your abdominal muscles will get very good exercise. Relax; repeat as many times as desired. Athletes should do 25 to 40 repetitions. Others may perform at least 10 at a time and gradually build to 25.

Knees to Chest Stretching. Perhaps the worst exercise one can do, in terms of aggra-

Figure 659. Neck exercises.

Figure 660. See text for details.

vating back problems, is the double leg raise, done lying on one's back. *Do not, under any circumstance, do this exercise.* Rather, perform the following:

Assume the same starting position as in Exercise A. Pull the knees as far into your chest as possible while forcing your head toward your stomach (see Fig. 660*C* and *D*). Hold this position for 10 to 30 seconds. Repeat as many times as it takes to feel a relaxing stretch to the back.

Back Stretch on Chair. Sit on the edge of a chair that is supported against the wall. Drop your head and shoulders between your knees while attempting to touch your elbows to the floor (see Fig. 660*E* and *F*). Relax and stay in this position for 10 to 30 seconds. If your back is quite painful, do more of *C* and *D*, and do not do this exercise until you have less pain.

Posture. Proper posture can be explained in terms of the relationship between the knees and the spine. When a person stands or walks continually with the knees held very straight (even locked-out), as in Figure 660*G*, his spine will exhibit an excess curve. This will cause

pain and weakness in the small of the back. If the individual maintains a slight bend at the knees (10 to 15 degrees) as in Figure 660*H*, then back alignment is normal and stresses are reduced. Assume this posture and practice maintaining it.

Shoulder and Arm

The shoulder and arm play a critical role in all major sports, but most especially in the throwing sports. The action of throwing is an extremely complex activity, with a sequential pattern of movements in which each part of the body must perform a number of carefully timed and executed acts. Synergistic fluid agonist-antagonist function for each associated movement in the shoulder and arm is extremely important, but just as important are the coordinated footwork, leg action, hip motion and trunk rotation, plus some action of the other arm.

Fast body movements require the greatest muscle forces, and therefore throwing produces the highest forces at the greatest number of joints. It therefore becomes obvious that the entire body must be carefully and properly conditioned or reconditioned—not just the involved throwing arm.

Rehabilitation Following Shoulder Injuries in Athletes

The following program is that used at the Sports Medicine Clinic in Atlanta, Georgia, by William Andrews, R.P.T.

Rotator Cuff Injuries

Early Rehabilitation. At this stage the rotator cuff is compromised by its subacute or postsurgical status. The shortness of the cuff muscles and the disproportionate strength of the other musculature of the pectoral girdle make conventional full-range exercise inappropriate, even if active range of motion is possible. The following exercises are indicated.

Gripping Exercises. Grip a hand dynamometer or tennis ball at several points along the arc from full (pain-free) abduction-flexion–external rotation to full adduction-extension–internal rotation. This brings the rotator cuff into synergistic (fixative) contraction, as well as conditions forearm muscles, which have probably atrophied if inactivity has been of long duration.

Codman (Pendulum) Exercises. This exercise increases the range of motion while stimulating contraction of the rotator cuff owing to the gentle traction applied to the muscle systems (see Fig. 163A).

Bench Press Supports. Lie supine on the bench, holding the barbell in a "locked-out"

position. A freely held barbell or dumbbells are preferable to a statically held weight machine, since four-way control is stimulated by the free barbell and not by the weight machine. The weight should be only heavy enough to stimulate fixation of the cuff gently. Progression is accomplished by widening the grip gradually from about 20 to 30 in. (to pain tolerance). This increases the external rotation gradually. The weight is also increased gradually.

Deadlift Supports. Hold the barbell or corresponding lever of the multistation weight-training apparatus with an overhand grip at the front of the thighs. The shoulders are held in a shrug position. Single efforts of 10 seconds are performed. Progression is obtained by widening the grip and increasing the weight.

Hanging from Chinning Bar. A bench or chair is used to elevate the body so that the bar can be grasped regardless of a deficient range of motion. The bar is gripped but no effort is made to support full or partial weight until the arms can be painlessly held over the head. The patient merely grips the bar and isometrically sets the latissimus muscle group in a comfortable range. Once full weight-bearing is possible, progression is obtained by widening the grip.

Intermediate Rehabilitation. At this stage the rotator cuff should be able to contract fully without pain, but full range is not present and strength is not yet fully developed. The cuff is, however, adequate for performance of conventional shoulder conditioning exercises that will develop strength and further increase the range of motion. The following exercises are carried out.

Light Dumbbell Circles. This is an extension of the pendulum exercises. Done while standing upright, the dumbbell is directed upward and outward in a rotary manner and then upward and inward in the opposite direction. These circles progress by widening the excursion of the circle and increasing the weight.

Bench Presses. Progressing from supports, the patient gradually adds bending to the movement until a full range bench press is possible. More weight is added. Once again, because of the need to support the weight in all directions, freely held weights are preferable to weight machines. Although dumbbell bench exercises, or "flyes," may present a safety problem, they offer a wider range of motion.

Upright Rowing. This is a progression of the deadlift supports, using the same grip, in which the weight is raised to a position high on the chest. Varying the width of the hand grips is desirable.

"Lat" Machine Pull-Downs to the Rear of Neck. A shoulder-width grip is used at first, with later progression to a wider grip. Weight is added until the patient is able to progress to behind the neck pull-ups (only if a minimum of six can be performed).

Advanced Rehabilitation. The progression through the intermediate stage has probably left the athlete at near normal development. To develop extra strength of the structures in question, along with increased flexibility, the following program of exercise might be utilized:

1. Alternate dumbbell presses or presses behind the neck.

2. Dumbbell bench presses, incline presses, "flyes" or parallel bar dips.

3. Bent-arm pull-overs.

4. High pulls with a snatch grip, or repetition "cleans."

All of the preceding are done for strength at the level of weight, repetitions and number of sets that will assure maximum development in accordance with the individual's potential. The exercises are done to the extremes of motion so that flexibility is improved. If properly done in this manner, no specific flexibility exercise is needed. To supplement any deficiency, however, the following exercises can be performed:

5. Straight arm pull-overs across the width of a bench, using a progressively wider grip. The weight is kept at a permanently light setting (30 lb.)

6. Light dumbbell "flyes," with a medicine ball between the shoulder blades, or elastic cable stretching at pulley weights. In the latter, the cable is held in back of the shoulders, with the palms facing forward at shoulder height; the cable is worked forward and backward, stretching the pectoral girdle and rib cage.

Glenohumeral Dislocations and Subluxations

All stages of rehabilitation for glenohumeral dislocations and subluxations are similar to those for the rotator cuff, with the following exceptions.

1. If surgical intervention has not been instituted to correct the dislocation, no exercise should be done which places the shoulder in a compromised position (abducted and externally rotated). Thus, grips should never be wide, bench work should only be done in the top one third of the movement and presses are best performed in only the lower half of the range. To accomplish this, the use of a "power rack" is beneficial. If unavailable, the barbell, with the assistance of two spotters, is used.

2. When the extent of damage to the cuff and surrounding structures is extensive, progress will be slower, and there will be greater atrophy and limitation of range.

3. Special emphasis is given to strengthening the internal rotator muscles (subscapularis muscle).

Acromioclavicular Injuries

Early Rehabilitation. At the subacute or postoperative stage, pain is often a limiting factor, with associated tightening of all the shoulder musculature (trapezius, pectoral, deltoid, latissimus, etc.) as well as the possibility of tightness and weakness in the adjacent arm muscles. For this reason, the following exercises are used:

1. Light, active range of motion for shoulder flexion and abduction and internal and external rotation for flexion and extension of the elbow and for supination and pronation of the forearm.

2. Light resistive exercise for the trapezius (shrug).

3. Light resistive exercise for the anterior deltoid (upright row).

4. Resistive exercise, to tolerance, for the forearm, biceps and triceps muscles. All should be done so that little or no downward pull is effected at the shoulder (lying or seated rather than standing).

5. Codman (pendulum) exercises are done to increase the tolerance of the shoulder to weight-support with a limited range of motion (see Fig. 163A).

Intermediate Rehabilitation. At this stage pain should be absent and the range of motion should be nearly full. The main goal is strengthening the muscular attachments of the trapezius and deltoids in the area of the clavicle and acromion near the acromioclavicular joint. This is done by strengthening the entire deltoid-trapezius group. The following exercises should be done:

1. Dumbbell presses done alternately (emphasis on the anterior deltoid).

2. Wide grip press behind the neck (emphasis on the lateral deltoid and trapezius).

3. Shoulder shrug (emphasis on the trapezius).

4. Upright row (emphasis on the anterior deltoid and trapezius).

Advanced Rehabilitation. Increasing the general muscle bulk in the anterior shoulder area should have a strengthening effect on the acromioclavicular joint. All of the preceding exercises are appropriate when done intensively with a heavy progression of weight. Also beneficial are all incline presses, all "cleans," snatches and deadlifts, bench presses and pullovers.

Injuries Related to the Throwing Sports

It is easier to prevent than to correct injuries related to the throwing sports. Essential aspects for prevention include the following: assuring general fitness of the musculature through adequate strength training, the establishment of fluid agonist-antagonist function for each associated movement at the shoulder and elbow and, most important, the development of appropriate flexibility and coordination of movement, as well as of a proper kinesthetic sense by the athlete. To achieve these goals, the following program is recommended.

1. Full range strength training, mostly with dumbbells. Done to extremes of stretch and with "ballistic" movement to assure the maintenance of quick, fluid reaction in the muscles.

Figure 661. Stretching for shoulders and upper back. See text for explanation.

2. Additional stretching movements for the entire shoulder-elbow area.

3. Maintenance of flexibility and fluid motion in the thoracic and lumbar spines. This can have a beneficial effect on the general state of flexibility in the extremities.

4. Thoughtful practice of the throwing skill to establish the most fluid and efficient pattern possible.

5. Proper warm-up, taking care not to abuse the endurance and recovery capabilities of the structures involved (not throwing too often or too much at one time or too soon after a lay-off).

Stretching for Shoulders and Upper Back

Dead Hang. Grip overhead bar and hang (till grip fails) (Fig. 661*A*).

Variations:

1. Pull knees to chest while hanging (see Fig. 661*B*).

2. Perform partial (not full) pull-ups while hanging (see Fig. 661*C*).

3. Swing side to side while hanging (see Fig. 661*D*).

4. Do "frog kick" while hanging (see Fig. 661*E*).

Bar Dips. Use 24 inch width parallel bars or chair backs (chairs must be sturdy!). Lower body into the stretched, fully lowered position (see Fig. 661*F*). Remain in this position 15 seconds. Repeat 5 to 10 times.

Variations:

1. Use weight strapped about waist for added resistance.

2. Do "push-up" dips between chair seats (see Fig. 661*F*).

Upper Back Extension. Lie face down across an exercise bench or use the "hyperextension" unit on the Universal Gym. The bench provides support at the level of the rib cage (Fig. 662). Do the exercise as follows:

1. Fold hands behind neck and point elbows outward (see Fig. 662*A*).

2. Lift body to fully extended (up) position.

3. Hold 2 seconds.

4. Lower body and repeat 10 times.

Variations:

1. Maintain extended position while raising dumbbells to side; 10 repetitions (see Fig. 662*B*).

2. Maintain extended position while raising dumbbells forward (see Fig. 662*C*).

3. Maintain extended position while "rowing" barbell to chest (see Fig. 662*D*).

Figure 662. Upper back extension. See text for details.

Wrist-Elbow Exercises

Wrist Flexion. Place the wrist in a palms-up position, supported at the edge of a table or on the knee so that only the hand will be allowed to move. Grasp the weighted dumbbell (_____ pounds)* or weighted bag. Perform the exercise as follows:

1. Flex (bend upward) the wrist as far as possible (Fig. 663*A*).

2. Hold 2 to 3 seconds.

3. Lower fully; repeat up to 15 times.

_____

*The initial starting weight must be determined. It will vary according to the patient's sex, size and disability and other factors. It is determined by trial and error.

Figure 663. Wrist-elbow exercises. See text for details.

4. Increase weight if 15 proper repetitions can be performed with no pain at the site of injury.

Wrist Extension. Performed in similar fashion to wrist flexion except that palm faces down. Start with _____ pounds.*

Gripping Exercise. Use a tennis ball or other gripping-type device. Start with moderate-intensity gripping, which is held 2 to 3 seconds and repeated 15 times. Increase intensity of grip to correspond to increased intensity in wrist flexion and wrist extension exercises.

Thumbs-Up Elbow Flexion. Hold a dumbbell or weighted bag (_____ pounds)* at your side so that your thumb points straight forward. Perform the exercise as follows:

1. Slowly bend elbow to 90 degrees only. Allow no upper arm movement (see Fig. 663B).

2. Hold in this position 2 to 3 seconds.
3. Lower slowly; repeat up to 12 repetitions.
4. Increase weight if 15 repetitions can be achieved without pain at the site of the injury or a break in strictness of form.

Lever-Bar Rotation (In). Use a dumbbell bar arranged as shown in Figure 663C.

Place the wrist at the edge of the table, as in wrist flexion exercise. Grip the bar at the non-weighted end, with the weight (_____ pounds)* outboard. Perform as follows:

1. Rotate hand inward as far as possible (see Fig. 663D).
2. Hold momentarily.
3. Allow weight to return to starting posi-

—————————

*The initial starting weight must be determined. It will vary according to the patient's sex, size and disability and other factors. It is determined by trial and error.

tion *slowly* (2 to 3 seconds). Repeat up to 15 times.

4. Effective weight can be increased by using a fixed weight and increasing distance A–B as strength increases.

Lever-Bar Rotation (Out). Place the wrist at edge of the table as in the wrist extension exercise. Use _____ pounds* to start, gripping the nonweighted end of the bar with the weights inboard. Perform as in previous exercise, except that the wrist should be rotated out rather than in during Step 1 (see Fig. 663*E*).

KNEE AND THIGH

Injury to the knee constitutes the most frequent disabling injury in sports. The frequency of knee injuries in recent years is related to the increase in the number of participants in competitive sports, the increased tempo of most sports activities and failure of adaptation to imposed demands. Many factors are related to the incidence and severity of knee injuries. However, no other factor is more important than adequate musculature to provide maximum protection.

No other areas of the body are as prone to atrophy following injury as are the knee and thigh. The muscular atrophy that usually follows injury or surgery is a neurological phenomenon. It causes a very rapid loss of strength and muscle bulk in the supporting musculature of the knee.

It is possible, however, to prevent a significant amount of this muscle atrophy through the use of preoperative and postoperative exercises. These exercises should be instituted as soon as possible, and in order to achieve the desired result in the shortest possible time, a definite plan with pre-established goals must be formulated.

Muscle action stabilizes the knee joint and helps to defend the ligaments against abnormal stress. The stretch effect of the normal ligament to which stress is applied is a proprioceptive stimulation to the surrounding musculature, causing these muscles to support the stressed joint. The knee with ligamentous laxity and muscular weakness is much more injury prone than the knee without such laxity and weakness. It should also be remembered that although the response is much less visible or

measurable, ligaments respond to a training program as do muscles and over a period of time become stronger and thus more resistant to injury.

In rehabilitating the knee and the lower extremities, it is very important to seek equal bilateral strength as well as antagonistic muscle balance. Numerous studies have indicated that a disparity of 10 per cent or greater in the lower extremity makes injury or reinjury much more likely. Testing is therefore essential to determine the strength level of the various muscle groups about the knee, hip and leg.

Rehabilitation Following Knee Injuries in Athletes

The following program outlined is that used at the Sports Medicine Clinic in Atlanta, Georgia, by William Andrews, R.P.T.

Injury Classification

It is important to classify injuries by type and extent, since the course of rehabilitation will differ from one type to another. The injury classification and specified therapy routines should not be considered to be inflexible or to limit further elaboration or specialization. Types of injury include the following:

1. Single ligament or uncomplicated meniscus injury.
2. Multiple ligament injury or complicated single ligament or meniscus injury.
3. Multiple ligament injury associated with other complicating factors, such as a fracture.
4. Chondromalacia of the patella or femoral condyle erosion, either alone or in combination with any of the preceding types.

Stages of Rehabilitation

Rehabilitation following knee injury or surgery can be divided into five stages: presurgical, immediate postoperative, early intermediate, late intermediate and advanced.

Presurgical Stage. The presurgical stage is usually significant only when elective surgery is to be performed. If a specific diagnosis has not been made, therapeutic exercise may be instituted to aid in diagnosis as well as to provide functional benefits. Therapeutic exercise at this stage is designed to build or maintain strength without aggravating the existing injury. Thus, the exercise must be, for the most part, not through a full range of motion. Isokinetic exercise is especially desirable dur-

---

*The initial starting weight must be determined. It will vary according to patient's sex, size, and disability and other factors. It is determined by trial and error.

ing this stage because of its readily controlled, noncompelling nature. The following exercises should be carried out.

1. Quadriceps setting: 10 second contractions for 5 minutes each hour while awake. See Figure 664D.

2. Straight leg raising: 15 nonstop repetitions with the maximum possible resistance each hour while awake. See Figure 664A.

If, owing to pain and subsequent reflex inhibition of the quadriceps femoris muscle, the athlete is unable to initiate quadriceps setting or straight leg raising, then the special "negative" resistance exercises described in the following section should be utilized. In negative resistance exercises, the patient raises the leg with assistance, then actively lowers it without assistance.

3. Isometric knee extension (at or near full extension): 15 repetitions each hour while awake.

4. Isometric or isokinetic knee flexion: 15 repetitions (optional).

5. Hip extension (wall pulley): 20 to 25 repetitions (optional).

6. Hip flexion (wall pulley): 20 to 25 repetitions (optional).

7. Hip abduction (wall pulley): 20 to 25 repetitions (optional).

8. Hip adduction (wall pulley): 20 to 25 repetitions (optional).

The above routine should be performed daily for 10 to 14 days prior to surgery. In so doing, the preservation of muscle tone and the improved kinesthetic sense will help in preparation for the practice of similar exercises immediately postoperative. Instruction in three-point gait training should also be given during this stage. Touch weight-bearing on the injured extremity is allowed; however, while the involved extremity is in the weight-bearing phase of gait, the knee is fully extended and the quadriceps muscle is "set." Complicated or more serious injuries are usually treated by elective surgery and therefore are not included in this stage of therapy, since surgery is most often indicated immediately.

Immediate Postoperative or Postinjury Stage. The optimal time for commencement of therapeutic exercise is approximately 24 hours following surgery or injury. An earlier beginning is often met by an unreceptive and confused patient. Any beginning later than 24 hours must be considered a loss of valuable time. As soon as normal function ceases, atrophy and other debilitating mechanisms begin to occur and serve to delay further return of normal function. Exercises in this stage are similar to those in the presurgical stage, except for those movements that are precluded by the presence of a cast, dressing, or associated immobilization. The following exercises should be carried out.

1. Quadriceps setting: 10 second contractions for 5 minutes each hour while awake.

2. Straight leg raising: 10 repetitions each hour while awake, with maximum possible resistance.

If, owing to pain and subsequent reflex inhibition of the quadriceps femoris muscle, the athlete is unable to initiate quadriceps setting or straight leg raising, then the following routine should be used.

a. Manually, by using appropriate slings and pulleys or by using the opposite leg for assistance, passively elevate the involved extremity to a position of 90 degrees of hip flexion (or as much hip flexion as the patient will comfortably tolerate.)

b. Have athlete "hold" the involved limb in this position by active contraction of the involved muscles. Slowly remove the passive support and have the patient lower the limb to the starting position.

c. Repeat Step a, but this time elevate the limb only two thirds the height obtained in Step a. Then slowly lower it, as described in Step b.

d. Repeat Step a, but this time elevate the involved limb only one third the height obtained in Step a. Then slowly lower it, as described in Step b.

e. If the athlete is able to actively hold the involved limb at 30 degrees, then he probably will be able to initiate elevation on his own without manual support or slings and pulley assistance.

f. If the athlete is unable to initiate elevation of the limb from the starting position, then have him "hold" at the lowest possible position that he can maintain actively and then raise the extremity as high as possible. Several such repetitions should enable the athlete to initiate quadriceps setting and straight leg raising with no assistance.

3. Isometric hip extension: 10 second "presses" onto the bed for 10 repetitions each hour while awake.

4. Abduction and adduction of the hip: 10 second presses against resistance for 10 repetitions each hour while awake.

5. Ankle plantar flexion: 10 second presses against resistance for 10 repetitions each hour while awake.

6. Ambulation. As soon as the patient is able voluntarily to elevate the involved extremity from the bed, he is allowed to ambulate on crutches, using a three-point gait, with touch weight-bearing on the involved extremity. The touch weight-bearing stimulates proprioceptive receptors that provide the central nervous system with an awareness of body segments (in the involved extremity). Proprioceptive awareness has been shown to be of primary importance in neuromuscular re-education.

The goal during this stage of rehabilitation is maintenance of muscle mass, strength and function during the period of time that immobilization is indicated. These exercises should be progressive and continuous during the entire immobilization period. It is important that exercises be prescribed for the entire extremity as well as for other major body segments, since bed rest and immobilization deprive all these segments of normal activity.

The preceding exercises are recommended for uncomplicated single ligament and meniscectomy cases. More complicated injuries are characterized by increased instability, increased pain, increased potential for hemorrhage and the need for more extensive tissue repair; these conditions are indications for the most judicious choice of activity and dosage. In most patients, however, given time and proper supervision, the level of activity can approach that of patients with less complicated injuries. Careful control of the rate of exercise progression is the key to success, with the obvious presence of pain and edema serving as primary guidelines. Thus, the following immediate postsurgery, or postinjury, routine is usually possible, even with very complicated cases:

7. Quadriceps setting: 10 second sets, for 5 minutes each hour while awake.

8. Straight leg raising: to tolerance for 30 seconds each hour while awake.

9. Hip extension (isometric): to tolerance for 30 seconds each hour while awake.

Early Intermediate Rehabilitation. At the end of the immobilization period, the patient proceeds immediately into the early intermediate stage of rehabilitation. This stage is a continuation of the postsurgical stage and the exercises are similar, but with added emphasis on progression. Exercises are also included to increase the active range of motion (ROM). Passive stretching is seldom used, as active ROM exercises usually provide full ROM within a reasonable period of time. In cases in which terminal extension is a problem, the patient is instructed in passive-active exercise

to correct this deficit. The following exercises should be carried out:

1. Straight leg raising: using maximum resistance.

2. Pulley exercises:
   Hip extension—progressive to 15 to 20 repetitions
   Hip flexion—progressive to 15 to 20 repetitions
   Hip abduction—progressive to 15 to 20 repetitions
   Hip adduction—progressive to 15 to 20 repetitions

3. Knee extension-flexion utilizing isokinetic exercises, beginning with a relatively low speed and gradually increasing the speed.

Or, if using another type of weight-loading apparatus, lift the weight or perform the exercise effort by using both legs in a steady lift fashion—taking two full seconds to lift the weight. In the "lifted" position, hold for 1 to 2 seconds. Then, lower the weight with injured leg only, taking four full seconds: 2 Up—Hold 2—Lower 4.

4. Ankle plantar flexion: progressive to 15 to 20 repetitions.

5. Terminal extension exercise (hurdler's exercise): with the addition of a towel looped over the forefoot for additional stretching of the popliteal area (see Fig. 666A, for details of exercise).

One set of the preceding exercises are done during the first session, two sets at the next, three sets at the next and never more than three sets subsequently. Progression is consistent and judicious. As soon as a pain-free ROM in excess of 90 degrees is present at the knee, with no apparent swelling and no significant pain, the following changes are made:

6. Leg raises are eliminated.

7. Isotonic leg extension is added: one leg at a time, alternating legs. Resistance is added progressively, 15 to 20 repetitions.

8. Isotonic knee flexion: resistance is added progressively, 15 to 20 repetitions.

9. Terminal extension is continued if necessary.

10. Active stretching of the rectus femoris muscle, the hamstring muscles and the Achilles tendon is initiated at the same time that isotonic exercises are introduced.

11. Stationary bicycling is added to tolerance, usually 2 to 4 miles at one sitting, with a resistance based upon the capability of the individual.

12. At this stage the leg press is added to tolerance. Resistance is progressive, 20 to 30 repetitions.

Each of these exercises is performed 2 to 3 times daily. The rationale at this stage is no longer maintenance of function but building (rebuilding) muscle mass and function. Still, aggressiveness should not gain the upper hand over judicious choice of exercise dosage. Of primary importance at this stage are mobilization and achievement of pain-free flexion and full extension. Secondarily, proper form in the performance of the exercise is indicated. Of third importance is the actual amount of resistance used in the exercise, although once motion and proper form have been achieved, the resistance load becomes all-important. More complicated or extensive injury may call for a slower beginning at this stage. However, if the physician observes closely for signs of pain and swelling and follows basic precautions concerning the rate of progression, most of these patients can eventually progress to the same level of performance as those with less complicated injuries, although at a slower rate. *In many cases of extensive erosion of the joint surfaces on either the patella or the femoral condyle, resistive ROM exercise may be permanently contraindicated.* In these cases, isokinetic types of exercise are usually helpful.

Late Intermediate Rehabilitation. The criteria for advancement to this stage are pain-free full range of motion of the involved joint and a strength deficit in the quadriceps group of no more than 25 per cent. The following exercises should be carried out:

1. Leg extension: both legs simultaneously, 15 to 20 repetitions.

2. Leg flexion: both legs simultaneously, 15 to 20 repetitions.

3. Leg press: 15 to 20 repetitions.

Accentuate the "negative." Take 2 full seconds to lift weight. With weight in this position, hold for 1 to 2 seconds. Then lower it, taking 4 seconds.

4. Stationary bicycle: emphasize high speed and high resistance. Progress with distance up to 5 miles.

5. Running: preferably uphill or, if on the treadmill, with a grade of 5 to 10 per cent. Gradually increase distance and speed.

At this stage of rehabilitation the emphasis is more on sports conditioning and less on therapy. Sports conditioning focuses on development of "functional power." Considerations must include resistance, speed of movement, range of movement and repetitions. By this stage it has been determined whether or not intensive exercise is indicated. If not, then exercise is limited to nonresistive exercise of the isokinetic type and to non-ROM exercises,

such as straight leg raises, isometrics at various angles and full ROM hip and ankle movements.

Advanced Rehabilitation. The criteria for entry into this phase of rehabilitation are that the athlete is deemed able to participate in competitive sports and has no more than 5 to 10 per cent strength deficit in the quadriceps mechanisms. The following exercises are to be carried out:

1. Warm-up using a stationary bicycle or jump rope: maximum performance, 3 to 5 minutes' duration.

2. Leg press: to exhaustion, 15 to 20 repetitions.

Accentuate the "negative" by taking twice as long to lower the weight than was required to raise it.

3. Leg extension: to exhaustion, 15 to 20 repetitions.

4. Three-quarter knee bends: to exhaustion, 15 to 20 repetitions.

5. Leg curl: to exhaustion, 15 to 20 repetitions.

6. Toe raise: to exhaustion, 15 to 20 repetitions.

7. Stationary bicycle: taper off. Moderate resistance for 3 to 5 minutes' duration.

The preceding exercises should be performed, with absolutely no rest between them, in approximately 5 minutes, excluding the time necessary to perform the jump rope and bicycle exercises. The central focus of advanced rehabilitation is exactly the same as advanced sports conditioning. Done properly, sports conditioning should simultaneously provide maximum benefit in developing power, endurance and flexibility.

Special Circumstances That Require Alteration of Rehabilitation Procedures

Cruciate Ligament Instability

Following injuries to the anterior cruciate or capsular ligament, varying degrees of anterior and rotary instability may be present. If so, maximum loading or fast, jerky extension of the knee may cause anterior subluxation of the tibia on the femur. It is therefore very important, following such injuries and following surgery for anterior cruciate ligament repair or reconstruction, that precautions be taken and the rehabilitation procedure be so modified that maximum loading and fast, jerky movement be avoided when performing knee extension exercises. This phenomenon is progressively less likely to occur as the range of motion approaches full extension.

Terminal Extension Exercises

Occasionally following surgery or injury, the patient has difficulty in obtaining full extension of the knee. This lack of complete extension is most often due to weakness in the extensor mechanism during the last 10 to 15 degrees of extension. If allowed to persist for a long period of time, in addition to a subjective feeling of weakness or "instability," the loss of complete extension tends to produce a "flexion contracture" resulting from shortening of the hamstring muscles. The injured knee with a weak quadriceps will require a special precaution. *In doing active extension exercises, one must be sure that the knee reaches complete extension at each level of weight.* If the exercises do not bring the knee to complete extension, a distressing extensor lag may develop, with a devastating effect on the athlete. He must be able to lock the knee in complete extension in order to participate in athletic activity. Extensor lag means that the player can passively extend to zero degrees but can actively extend to only 15 or 20 degrees. The knee is completely unstable between zero and 15 or 20 degrees and so will tend to give way with every stride. This is a much more important handicap than a flexion contracture of the same degree. The latter can be controlled by the quadriceps, whereas the extensor lag cannot. Also, if the athlete is allowed to participate in too much activity prior to regaining full extension, chronic synovitis is likely to occur. The existence of flexion contracture, quadriceps weakness and swelling usually results in pain, and in turn the pain is likely to cause continuation of the aforementioned conditions.

It is therefore very important to obtain full knee extension as soon as possible following surgery or injury.

The following exercises are recommended:

1. Sit on the floor with the involved knee extended as much as possible, a bath towel around the forefoot, with foot dorsiflexed; while pulling the ends of the towel toward the body, set the quadriceps muscle and simultaneously exert downward pressure on the knee—stretching the posterior structures of the knee.

2. Place a small rolled pad beneath the involved knee. "Set" the quadriceps muscle and elevate the heel and leg while exerting downward pressure on the knee.

Chondromalacia Patella

Rehabilitation of athletes with this condition necessitates alteration of the usual progressive resistive exercise program. If the condition is mild and there is no similar involvement of the underlying femur, then a continuation of straight leg raising exercises beyond the usual period of time is usually all that is necessary for rehabilitation. However, in more severe cases or in those complicated by femoral involvement, the following exercises should be performed.

1. Straight leg raising, as described earlier.
2. Isokinetic exercise using a "self-adjusting resistance" so that undue pressure will not be placed on the patella during maximum patella-femoral contact.
3. Isometric exercises performed at varying degrees of knee extension against a fixed object or the uninvolved limb.
4. Negative resistance exercise performed by lifting the weight with the uninvolved extremity and lowering the weight with the involved extremity, as described earlier under Intermediate Stage, Knee Rehabilitation.
5. "Bench technique" modified so that the starting position of the exercise permits only 10 to 15 degrees of knee flexion. As the legs are straightened, the major action of the patella is upward in line with the quadriceps mechanism, and little pressure is placed on the patella against the femur in this terminal phase.

The Single Boot Progressive Exercise Program*

1. After a mild warm-up, determine the single maximum lift as follows. Ascertain the load which the muscle can lift to full extension and return to position, but which the muscle cannot lift a second time to full extension. If a second lift is accomplished with the initial load, allow a short rest and add weight to the boot; the amount of weight added depends on the ease of the second lift. Repeat the process again and readjust the weight if necessary. The establishment of this single maximum lift is the most difficult part of the program. Accuracy

---

*Klein, K. and Allman, F.: The Knee in Sports. Texas, Pemberton Press, 1969.

A Straight leg raise

Gym bag for weights

B Standing front leg raise

C Side leg raise

D "Quad-setting" exercise

E Seated leg extension

F Standing knee flexion

Figure 664. Home knee exercises. See text for details.

here is necessary in the development of the total program. In the rebuilding of strength and bulk, it would be better to slightly underload the boot rather than to overload it.

2. Once this single lift factor has been determined, the exercise pattern may be developed as follows. Subtract five pounds from the single maximum lift (quadriceps) to establish the loading for ten repetitions of the exercise for the first set, for the quadriceps. This load should include the boot weight. If the muscle ' is only strong enough to lift the "boot" (5 lb. more or less), then it is obvious that the muscle is very weak indeed. Removal of all the weight would leave only the weight of the leg, and possibly that would be enough weight during the initial workout period. In the first ten days to two weeks, moderate resistance exercise would be best, that is, the lifting of the weight that is comfortable to the individual without undue stress.

3. The hamstring loading is determined by taking a percentage of the initial quadriceps loading (i.e., 50 to 55 per cent for upper high school and beginning college age level and 60 per cent for college varsity football age level). For quadriceps, for example, 10 repetitions of motion load equals 30 pounds times 55 per cent, or 16.50 pounds for the initial hamstring load. This would include the weight of the boot and clamp attachments. If the wall-pulley system is used, then the total 16.50 pounds would be placed on the pulley rack. If adjustments in the weight loading have to be made, an accurate initial loading program should be established during the first day or two. From this point, the loading program follows an established weekly increase pattern. Occasionally, small adjustments will have to be made in the third to eighth week.

4. Each exercise week consists of three to four exercise periods, in which both muscle groups are exercised according to the individual's program.

5. At the beginning of each new week, a 10 pound increase in weight loading is added for both muscle groups. This addition is a constant factor and continues throughout the entire length of the program or as long as the person is able to do the work. In the latter few weeks it might be necessary to reduce each increment slightly, which would be indicative that the muscle groups are reaching their maximal strength. If the person is unable to complete the three sets of exercises at the beginning of the week, he should be able to do so by the latter part of the week. As strength and endurance are gradually increased, the program

should be completed daily. This is a progressive challenge to the muscles, which will be in effect throughout the program.

6. In quadriceps exercise, the most important factor is full extension of the knee for maximal effect on the vastus medialis muscle. If the person is unable to fully extend the knee in all exercise sets, then the following adjustments should be made: (1) the total loading should be slightly reduced, or (2) specific terminal exercises should be added to the program.

Home Knee Exercises

1. Lie on your back. Keep the knee absolutely straight as you lift it to 45 degrees. Lower it slowly. Do not relax the leg, but repeat 15 times. As you get stronger, add weights by means of putting weight in a gym bag or "flight bag" and draping the handles over the ankles (see Fig. 664A).

2. Standing front leg raise is done exactly as the preceding exercise, only you stand to do the lift. Perform 15 repetitions. Add weight when you are able (see Fig. 664B).

Standing side raise is done exactly as the preceding exercise, only the weight is lifted to the side. Do 15 repetitions (see Fig. 664C).

3. This "quad-setting" exercise is performed seated on the floor. Place a couple of rolled-up towels under the knee. While pushing the back of the knee down into the towel as hard as possible, attempt to keep the entire surface of your leg in contact with the floor. Hold 5 seconds. Repeat 10 times (see Fig. 664D).

4. Sit on a high table, with the back of the knee just at the edge of the table. You may wish to use towels to pad the back of the knee. From the fully bent position, straighten the knee as much as possible and hold for 3 seconds. Repeat 15 times. As you get stronger, add weight by means of a weighted bag. Continue using this exercise only as long as there is no increased pain or swelling as a result of the exercise (see Fig. 664E).

5. Stand erect and balance by holding onto a stable piece of furniture. Bend the exercising knee backwards. Use the weighted bag, as in the preceding exercises. Do 15 repetitions (see Fig. 664F).

Knee Exercises (Fig. 665)

Note: Because you will not be using your leg normally for some time, you will lose

Figure 665. Early knee exercises. See text for details.

muscle size and strength. This loss must be regained by physical therapy after you are out of the cast or bandage. Much of the possible loss can be prevented by starting exercise *now*. You can speed your recovery and insure a more successful recovery by doing your best *now*.

Leg Push-Down. Push down as hard as you can with the entire leg; hold 5 seconds. Perform 10 times at once and repeat 10 times per day. Once home, this exercise should be done through the full range of motion (from overhead to floor) against a helper's resistance; i.e., you push down as helper pushes up (see Fig. 665A).

Straighten Knee. If in an elastic bandage, straighten your knee as hard *and as far* as you can; hold 5 seconds. Perform 10 times; repeat 10 times per day. If in cast, do same effort and imagine you are "breaking" the cast (see Fig. 665B).

Leg Lift. *Lying flat,* lift the leg overhead as far as possible; hold 3 seconds and then lower slowly. Perform 5 to 10 times and repeat up to 200 total lifts per day. This can be done against a helper's resistance, as in the leg push-down exercise (see Fig. 665C).

Myositis Ossificans Traumatica Rehabilitation

During Stage I, or the inflammatory phase of myositis ossificans traumatica, the involved extremity should be protected from further injury. Immobilization is usually helpful, and limitation of motion at adjacent joints is usually beneficial. No active exercise should be given to the involved area during this stage. Use of ice and compression to aid in limiting the extent of the hematoma is indicated.

During Stage II, or the proliferative stage, it is usually helpful to begin quadriceps setting exercises for the thigh; or, in case of myositis ossificans traumatica involving the arm, hand grip and upper extremity, "setting" exercises are helpful. Active range of motion exercises are allowed as pain and soreness subside, but no attempt is made to forcibly increase motion.

During Stage III, or the repair stage, it is usually possible to begin light resistive exercises through the available range of motion. Joint motion should be monitored daily, and if there is a decrease in motion or return of symptoms, the exercises must be reduced or completely omitted. If the response to light resistive exercise is favorable, then gradually progress to the normal progressive resistive exercise routine, as outlined for rehabilitation elsewhere. In patients with myositis ossificans, these exercises must be carefully controlled. Pain in the involved muscle indicates overload. The exercises should be pain-free.

Stretching Exercises for Hips and Legs (Fig. 666)

Note: Before you do the following exercises, which are meant to be done intensely, you

Hamstring stretch

A

Thigh stretch

B

Groin stretch (side lunge)

C

Figure 666. Stretching exercises for hips and legs. See text for details.

must warm up. This may include any light exercise or jogging, which does not cause pain. Allow ten minutes for warm-ups.

Ice Massage. You may wish to precede your stretching with ice massage if you are in real pain or if your muscles are in spasm. If you do the massage, omit the warm-ups mentioned previously.

Use a large piece of ice frozen in a 10 or 12 oz. paper cup. Massage the injured muscle, using firm, overlapping circular movements. Attempt to massage an area no greater than a softball, with the center being the point of most pain. Allow 15 minutes, then proceed directly to the stretching exercises that follow:

Hurdler's Stretch. Assume a seated position on the ground with one leg stretched straight in front of you and the other bent under itself in back of you (see Fig. 666A).

Note: In any stretching exercise, it is more beneficial to stretch slowly and steadily until the stretch is complete, usually in 15 seconds (it will be quite painful); release slowly. Never jerk or fall into a stretched position.

This exercise is done in two parts. First is the hamstring stretch. While keeping the knee straight, attempt to bring the chin as close to the knee as possible. If necessary, loop a belt over the foot and pull. Do one hamstring stretch and then one thigh stretch, described in the following paragraph.

Second is the thigh stretch. While keeping the point of the knee on the floor and the ankle directly under your hips, bend your entire body backwards until you are as far as you can get; full range should be with your elbows resting on the floor in back of you (see Fig. 666B).

Now reverse your entire position and perform both exercises in the new position. Avoid overflexing the injured knee, e.g., deep knee bends.

Groin Stretch. Assume a stance with feet planted about double shoulder width and feet pointing forward and flat on the floor (keep them this way throughout the exercise). Now, lower your body to one side so that your fingertips support your balance by being placed on either side of your supporting leg. The opposite leg will experience a stretch from the inside of the knee clear into the groin area (see Fig. 666C). Release and stretch the other leg.

CALF AND FOOT

The susceptibility of the ankle to ligamentous injury in athletics necessitates complete rehabilitation following injury. Instability of the ankle joint cannot be tolerated in the athlete, and inadequately treated or poorly rehabilitated ankle injures often result in instability. Also, regardless of the excellence of repair or the completeness of healing, any period of inactivity causes a progressive decline in the strength and flexibility of the involved part.

Ankle and Lower Leg Exercises

Toe Raises. These can be done on the floor if the ankle is stiff or painful (Fig. 667A). When it becomes more flexible, stand on the edge of a step or other elevated structure, so that your heel stretches below the level of your toes (see Fig. 667B).

Start doing this exercise using your body weight only and standing on both feet; do 20 to 25 repetitions. When able, switch to standing on one foot only, using the elevation as

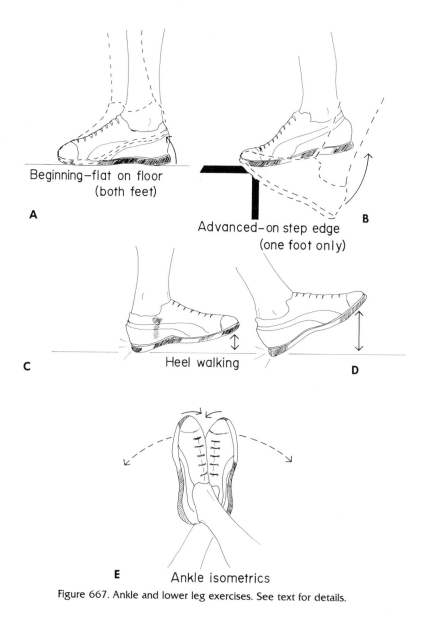

Figure 667. Ankle and lower leg exercises. See text for details.

mentioned earlier. When able to perform 20 to 25 repetitions while standing on one foot only, progress to holding a weighted object in one hand.

Heel Walking. Walk, keeping your toes as far off the ground as possible. Take short "choppy" steps; use shoes with good solid heels; walk on a firm surface (see Fig. 667C).

When able to walk in such a manner for two full minutes, or approximately 100 feet, progress to carrying weighted objects or walking in the same manner up a hill or incline (see Fig. 667D).

Isometric Ankle "Wrestling." Sit and place one ankle over the other (halfway through, switch ankles). Exert an outward force with both ankles so that your feet are firmly pressing against each other. Hold for 10 seconds, release, and repeat 10 times (see Fig. 667E).

As your ankles become stronger and less painful or stiff, allow them to move in and out against each other as you exert the outward force. Make each full movement last 10 full seconds. Repeat 10 times.

REFERENCES

DeLorme, T. L.: Restoration of muscle power by heavy-resistance exercises. J. Bone Joint Surg. 27:645–667, 1945.

Doss, W. S., and Karpovich, P. V.: A comparison of concentric, eccentric, and isometric strength of elbow flexors. J. Appl. Physiol. 20:351–353, 1965.

Jones, A.: Metabolic cost of negative work. Ath. J. 56:40–41, 80, 1976.

Komi, P. V., and Buskirk, E. R.: Effect of eccentric and concentric muscle conditioning on tension and electrical activity of human muscle. Ergonomics, 15:417–434, 1972.

Kraus, H.: Evaluation and treatment of muscle function in athletic injury. Am. J. Surg. 98:353–362, 1959.

Olson, V. L., Smidt, G. L., and Johnston, R. C.: The maximum torque generated by the eccentric, isometric, and concentric contractions of the hip abductor muscles. J. Am. Phys. Ther. Assoc. 52:149–157, 1972.

Wallis, E. L., and Logan, G. A.: Figure Improvement and Body Conditioning through Exercise. Englewood Cliffs, Prentice-Hall, 1964.

INDEX

Page numbers in **boldface** indicate illustrations. Page numbers followed by t indicate tables.